Optometry

Optometry

Edited by

Keith Edwards, BSc, FBCO, DCLP

Coordinator of Examinations,
The British College of Optometrists;
Ophthalmic Adviser, The Association of Optometrists;
former Secretary, The London Refraction Hospital

Richard Llewellyn, BSc, FBCO, DOrth

Practising Optometrist,
50 St Mary Street, Bridgwater, Somerset;
former Secretary, The London Refraction Hospital

Butterworths

London   Boston   Singapore   Sydney   Toronto   Wellington

First published, 1988

© Butterworth & Co. (Publishers) Ltd, 1988

British Library Cataloguing in Publication Data

Optometry.
  1. Optometry.
  I. Edwards, Keith H.   II. Llewellyn,
Richard D.
  617.7′5

  ISBN 0–407–00309–6

Library of Congress Cataloging in Publication Data

Optometry.
  Includes bibliographies and index.
  I. Optometry. I. Edwards, Keith H.   II. Llewellyn,
Richard D.   [DNLM: 1. Optometry.   WW 704 062]
RE951.068   1988   617.7′5   88–4278
ISBN 0–407–00309–6

Typeset by TecSet Ltd, Wallington, Surrey
Printed in Great Britain at the University Press, Cambridge

Foreword

It was a great pleasure and an honour to have been asked to write the foreword to *Optometry*.

The last textbook on the optometric visual examination published in the UK was written by George Giles in 1960 and has been out of print for a long time. Since then, the discipline of optometry has become an established university field in the same vein as physics, chemistry or medicine. It has extended its sphere of activity to include new tests, together with some old established tests which have since received scientific confirmation or been altered.

New materials have emerged and sophisticated electronic instruments controlled by microcomputers are being relentlessly introduced into the modern visual eye examination.

Such new challenges required more profound knowledge of the fundamental sciences of optometry and the introduction of other basic sciences (e.g. biochemistry) into the training of the optometric practitioner. The limited sight test of yesterday is finally being replaced by a full eye examination, and the modern optometric practitioner is the best trained person to carry it out. This person devotes more time to consultation, diagnoses ocular and even some systemic diseases, manages some ocular conditions, provides visual training, corrects subnormal vision, chooses the most appropriate material to correct vision for the working distance or distances which will sustain comfortable vision for long periods of time, advises on illumination and ocular hygiene etc.

To achieve this goal, an up-to-date text was vital. This book edited by Keith Edwards and Richard Llewellyn thoroughly fulfills this need. It is a gigantic text written by some 31 authors and comprising 38 chapters with the wide breadth of topics that modern optometry demands. Each author is an expert in his or her own field. The chapters are well written, clear and up to date. There are some variations of style which is to be expected with so many authors. It is to the credit of the editors that the overall presentation and the flow of the text have attained such good uniformity. I believe that this book has reached the object envisaged and that it will become the indispensable textbook of the discipline of optometry for many years to come.

Michel Millodot
Professor and Head,
Department of Optometry, University of Wales
Institute of Science and Technology, Cardiff

Preface

Over a number of years, both of us have been involved with undergraduate and postgraduate teaching, and have perceived a need for a textbook covering the broad range of subjects with which an optometrist is required to be familiar. All the subjects involved are specialities in their own right, the number of textbooks devoted to single topics, such as contact lenses, pharmacology, anatomy and physiology etc., bearing witness to this fact.

However, no existing single volume fulfilled the perceived need or covered the theoretical background to the visual and perceptive processes together with the techniques for the practical investigation and subsequent management of the normal and abnormal. It is beyond our abilities to write authoritatively on the range of subjects to be covered, so using contacts gained while serving at the London Refraction Hospital, we invited authors with special knowledge, skills and experience to contribute to this text. Each writer has brought a unique insight to their contribution.

No apology is made for the 'balance' of this book. Internationally, optometrists have an increasing role to play in many aspects of a patient's visual and general welfare. An understanding of the processes which lead to visual and binocular perception is vital, as is an awareness of the circumstances which can delay, impede or inhibit such development. Refractive techniques are constantly being refined and communicative skills can always be improved. Within the practice environment, photography and electrophysiological techniques offer recording and investigative possibilities that are little exploited at present. Gonioscopes and blood pressure measuring devices are beginning to be used by more and more practitioners and instrumentation is becoming increasingly sophisticated with the use of microprocessors.

The newly qualified graduate is up-to-date but inexperienced. The experienced practitioner is mature but may well be out-of-date. This text has been designed to appeal to both. It is hoped that the former will find it useful in coalescing information from various disciplines and that the latter will find the up-to-date coverage useful as a source of new material and as a refresher and revision aid.

In most cases the authors have included comprehensive references and some have added further reading lists to facilitate additional study of topics of special interest.

We wish to express our thanks to all of the contributing authors. Sadly, Deryck Humphriss died soon after finishing his chapters. It is hoped that their inclusion within this text will serve as a small memorial to his great contribution to optometry.

This book was conceived about eight years ago and active production started three years later. During this time it has lived jointly with us and our families, the latter having to suffer its intrusion into what might otherwise have been leisure time. To our respective wives and children, we both wish to express our thanks for the tolerance and patience that we have been shown and look forward to being able to devote a little more time to domestic matters.

Keith Edwards
Richard Llewellyn

Contributors

Geoffrey Ball, RD, MSc
Professor Emeritus, The University of Aston and
Former Head, Department of Ophthalmic Optics,
The University of Aston, Birmingham, UK

Simon Barnard, FBCO, FAAO, DCLP
Lecturer in Clinical Optometry, Department of
Optometry and Visual Science, The City
University, London, UK

Jennifer Birch, MPhil, FBCO, SMSA
Lecturer in Clinical Optometry, Department of
Optometry and Visual Science,
The City University, London, UK

Alan Bird, MD, FRCS
Professor of Clinical Ophthalmology,
Institute of Ophthalmology, London;
Consultant Ophthalmologist, Moorfields Eye
Hospital, City Road, London, UK

Richard Earlam, FBCO, FADO
Department of Optometry, University of Wales
Institute of Science and Technology,
Cardiff, UK

Keith Edwards, BSc, FBCO, DCLP
Coordinator of Examinations,
The British College of Optometrists;
Ophthalmic Advisor,
Association of Optometrists, London, UK

Colin Fowler, PhD, FBCO
Lecturer, Department of Vision Sciences,
University of Aston, Birmingham, UK

Jim Gilchrist, MPhil, FBCO
Lecturer, Department of Optometry,
University of Bradford, Bradford, UK

John Grundy, BSc, FBCO
Independent Optometrist, Co. Durham, UK

Graham Harding, PhD, FBPsS
Professor of Clinical Neurophysiology
and Head of Department,
Department of Vision Sciences, University of
Aston, Birmingham, UK

Kenneth Harwood, FBCO, DOrth, DCLP
Former Senior Staff Refractionist,
London Refraction Hospital,
London, UK

Colin Hood, AIMBI, MIST, ABIPP
Head, Department of Medical Illustrations,
Moorfields Eye Hospital,
London, UK

The late **Deryck Humphriss**
Research Associate, National Institute of
Personnel Research,
Johannesburg, South Africa

Sarah Janikoun, MB BS, DO
Clinical Assistant, Guy's Hospital and Croydon
Eye Unit, London, UK

Richard Llewellyn, BSc, FBCO, DOrth
Practising Optometrist,
50 St Mary St, Bridgwater,
Somerset, UK

Elizabeth McClure, FBCO
Principal Optometrist, Tennent Institute of
Ophthalmology, Western Infirmary, Glasgow, UK

Ronald Mallett, FBCO, FAAO, DOrth
Senior Lecturer, The London Refraction Hospital,
London, UK

Jerry Nelson, PhD
Working Group in Biophysics, Department of
Physics, Philipps University,
West Germany

Rachel North, PhD, FBCO
Department of Optometry,
University of Wales Institute of Science and
Technology, Cardiff, UK

Henri Obstfeld, MPhil, FBCO, FBOA, HD, DCLP
Lecturer, Department of Optometry and Visual
Science, The City University, London, UK

Daniel O'Leary, PhD, FBOA
Lecturer, Department of Optometry, University of
New South Wales, Kensington, Australia.

Rogers Reading, MOpt, PhD
Professor, School of Optometry,
Indiana University,
Bloomington, USA

Gordon Ruskell, MSc, PhD, DSc, FBCO
Professor of Ocular Anatomy, Department of
Optometry and Visual Science,
The City University, London, UK

Janet Silver, MPhil, FBCO, FBIM
Principal Optometrist, Moorfields Eye Hospital,
London, UK

Harry Stockwell
Former Director of Research and Development,
Clement Clarke International, London, UK

Janet Stone, FBCO, FBOA HD, DCLP
Optometrist and Contact Lens Practitioner,
Shrewsbury, UK

John Storey, MSc, PhD, FBCO, DCLP
Principal Ophthalmic Optician,
Manchester Royal Eye Hospital,
Manchester, UK

Stephen Taylor, PhD, FBCO, FAAO
Director of Professional Services,
Melson Wingate Ltd and
Visiting Lecturer, Department of Optometry,
University of Wales Institute of Science and
Technology, Cardiff, UK

Janet Vale, MSc, MPS
Lecturer in Ocular Pharmacology,
Department of Physiological Sciences,
University of Manchester,
Manchester, UK

Michael Wolffe, JP, PhD, FBCO
Director of Training, Dolland & Aitchinson
Group plc,
Yardley, Birmingham, UK

Ivan Wood, PhD, FBCO
Lecturer in Ophthalmic Optics,
Department of Optometry,
University of Manchester Institute of Science and
Technology, Manchester, UK

Geoffrey Woodward, PhD, FBCO, DCLP
Head of Department and Professor of Optometry
and Visual Science,
Department of Optometry and Visual Science,
The City University,
London, UK

Contents

Part 1

Visual perception

1

Neurology of visual perception

Gordon Ruskell

Any practitioner involved with vision and the vision sciences must, as a basis for his work, have a knowledge of the fundamental neurology of vision and visual perception.

The structures involved in the neurology of visual perception, which form the subject of this chapter, commence with the retina, progress through the neural pathways conducting visual information to the brain, and terminate in the striate cortex (*Figure 1.1*). Extrageniculate pathways, prestriate cortex and the basis of central integration are also mentioned briefly.

Retina

The retina, which is thin, delicate and mostly transparent, is interposed between choroid and vitreous and forms the innermost of the three coats of the eye. The outer layer of the retina, the pigment epithelium, is firmly attached to the choroid, but the inner or neural retina has a weak and vulnerable attachment to the pigment epithelium. Anteriorly, the retina is continuous with the ciliary epithelium at the ora serrata and posteriorly with the optic nerve and, in these positions, the neural retina is firmly attached. It is thinnest at the foveola, a small area providing the greatest visual resolution at the centre of the retina, and close to the ora serrata (0.1 mm), and thickest at the parafovea (0.23 mm) and at the optic disc margin where retinal nerve fibres emerge from the eye to form the optic nerve.

Yellow pigment is present in the central part of the retina at the macula lutea, and varies in density and area between individuals. The pigment is least dense at the foveola at the centre of the macula and most dense in the slopes of the foveal pit, diminishing gradually to a background level at about 1.0 mm or 4° eccentricity (Stabell and Stabell, 1980;

Snodderley *et al.*, 1984a, b). The pigment, which is discussed later in the chapter, may be lutein, a derivative of xanthophyll (Bone and Landrum, 1984).

The visual process is initiated in the retina which houses the light receptive cells of the eye, the rods and cones and, unlike other end-organs, much of the interneuronal processing occurs within the retina

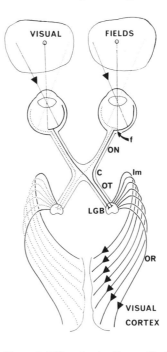

Figure 1.1 The visual pathway. Excitation of the visual pathway by objects in the left half of each visual field is conducted to the right lateral geniculate body (LGB) and visual cortex. f, fovea; lm, loop of Meyer; C, chiasma; ON, optic nerve; OR, optic radiations; OT, optic tract

3

before transmission of impulses to the brain. Accordingly, much of the structure of the retina compares with that of the central nervous system.

Histology

The most striking feature of the stained retina in cross-section is the sharply defined layers in which are located receptors and nerve cells in the regular, sequential order of the visual pathway. The layers and membranes are numbered conventionally from the outermost layer as follows: (1) retinal pigment epithelium, (2) rod and cone layer, (3) outer limiting 'membrane', (4) outer nuclear layer, (5) outer plexiform layer, (6) inner nuclear layer, (7) inner plexiform layer, (8) ganglion cell layer, (9) nerve fibre layer and (10) inner limiting membrane. The layers and their neurones are summarized in *Figure 1.2*.

Pigment epithelium

The pigment epithelium (layer 1) (*Figure 1.2*) is the versatile servant of the neuroretina, and it is composed of a single layer of pigment epithelial cells packed tightly together in a polygonal, mainly hexagonal, array. The principal functions of the pigment epithelium are:

(1) Transport of metabolites for the receptors from the choroidal blood circulation, including vitamin A or retinol, which are vital for the visual process (Heller, 1976), and facilitated by the large surface area provided by the infoldings and processes of the outer and inner surfaces.
(2) Absorption by the melanosomes of transretinal light that has failed to bleach receptors, thus preventing back scattering and degradation of the retinal image.
(3) Provision of attachment sites for rods and cones, without which metabolite transfer cannot occur and receptors become unreceptive to light.
(4) Phagocytosis of outer segment discs shed from receptor tips.

Regarding the third of these functions, receptor and apical process membranes are apposed, but structural modifications indicative of junctional complexes are not present. A viscous ground substance containing two glycoaminoglycans, shown in a coagulated form in *Figure 1.3*, probably provides a bond between the two (Berman and Bach, 1968). The bond is broken in the clinical condition of retinal detachment.

Rod and cone cells

Rod and cone cells make up the rod and cone layer (layer 2) of the retina; their inner processes traverse

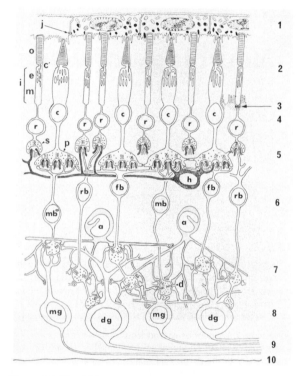

Figure 1.2 The 10 layers and the neurones of the retina (the names of the layers numbered on the right are given in the text). Junctional complexes (j) near the apices of pigment epithelial cell interfaces include zonula occludens (tight junction), zonula adherens (intermediate junction) that completely girdle each cell, and a large macular gap junction that is probably responsible for electrical coupling of the cells. Rod tips are buried in the pigment epithelium whereas processes extend from the epithelium to enclose cone tips. The outer limiting 'membrane' (layer 3) consists of intermediate junctions between receptors and Müller cells in perfect register at the bases of myoids. Horizontal (h) and amacrine (a) cells conduct across the retina and are shown heavily and lightly shaded. Bipolar and ganglion cells conduct through the retina and are shown unshaded. Intracellular lines drawn at synapses represent synaptic ribbons. c, cone nucleus; c' connecting stalk containing cilium; d, dyad synapse; dg, diffuse ganglion or alpha cell; e, ellipsoid; fb, flat bipolar; i, inner segment; mb, invaginating midget bipolar; mb°, flat midget bipolar; mg, midget ganglion or beta cell; p, cone pedicle; r, rod nucleus; rb, rod bipolar; s, rod spherule. (Largely derived from the work of Polyak (1957), Missotten (1965), Dowling and Boycott (1966), Boycott and Dowling (1969) and Kolb, Boycott and Dowling (1969))

the outer limiting membrane, then the other nuclear layer where their nuclei are located, and finally terminate in the outer plexiform layer (layer 5). The highly distinctive compartments of these cells are indicated diagrammatically in *Figure 1.2*.

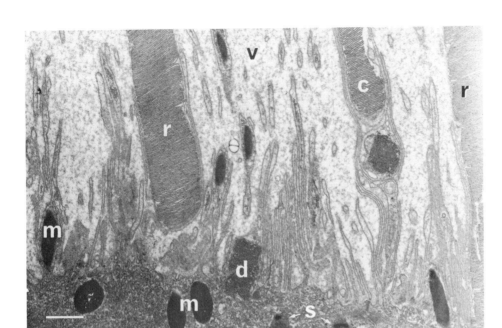

Figure 1.3 Processes extend from the apical surfaces of retinal pigment epithelial cells to enclose the tip of a cone (c) in the parafoveal region of a rhesus monkey retina. A group of about 25 outer segment discs is broken away from one of the cone tips prior to delivery by the processes to the epithelium where the disc cluster becomes an engulfed phagosome. A larger cone cluster (d) half enclosed by epithelium is also shown. The rod outer segments (r) contact the body of the pigment epithelium and the one on the right edge of the figure is embedded. m, melanosomes; s, secondary lysosomes or lipofuscin granules; v, viscous ground substance in interreceptor space. Marker = 1μm

Shape, dimensions and distribution of rods and cones

The rod inner segment is cylindrical maintaining the same width throughout its length from the external limiting membrane to the connecting stalk. The outer segment is also cylindrical, about 1.4 μm wide (Marshall *et al.*, 1979), and just noticeably thinner than the inner segment. The cone inner segment departs slightly from the shape of a cylinder as the width increases from the outer limiting membrane to a maximum of 5 or 6 μm near its centre and then tapers as it approaches the connecting stalk. At the stalk the inner and outer segments have the same width but the outer segment continues to taper to give the cone its characteristic shape. Cones, unlike rods, display some variation in shape. At the fovea, where only cones are present, they have a maximum width of about 2.5 μm in man and rather less in rhesus monkeys and they lack the usual taper, assuming the appearance of rods (*Figure 1.4*); their staining characteristics confirm their identity as cones (Wolff, 1948).

The inner and outer segments of cones together are approximately 65 μm long at the fovea reducing to about 40 μm at the parafovea and beyond. Rods are slightly longer than cones of the same region.

According to Østerberg (1935) there are between 110 and 125 million rods and between 6 and 8 million cones in the human retina; their distribution along the horizontal meridian is shown in *Figure 1.5*. Visual acuity reduces across the retina from 6/6 or better at the fovea to 6/30 or worse at 10° (Ludvigh, 1941; Mandelbaum and Sloane, 1947), then gradually worsens. The foveal lattice of photoreceptors, revealed in tangential section at the external limiting membrane (*Figure 1.6*), is a highly regular hexagonal structure probably providing the metrics with which the visual system determines spatial separation even for tasks involving hyperacuity (Hirsch and Hylton, 1984).

Receptor outer segments

Receptor outer segments consist of a dense stack of between 700 and 1200 disc-shaped double membranes enclosed by the cell membrane. Discs are unattached to each other or to the cell membrane in rods, except at the base where they consist of invaginations and, as Sjøstrand (1961) first suggested, the discs are formed from the cell membrane in this manner. The cone discs differ from those of the rods in that they maintain their connection with the cell membrane and are connected to each other,

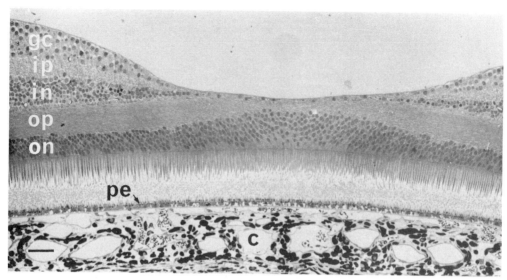

Figure 1.4 The fovea of a rhesus monkey. The fovea is reduced to a thickened outer nuclear layer (on), part of the outer plexiform layer (op) and the internal limiting membrane at the centre of the foveal pit (in man the outer nuclear layer may be reduced to a few cells). The inner nuclear layer (in) consists of a few nuclei close to the centre, thickening rapidly at the edges of the figure where the inner plexiform (ip) and ganglion cell (gc) layers appear. The fibres of rod and cone cells radiate from the centre of the fovea to reach their synapses with bipolar cells (Henle's fibre layer). Receptor outer segments have turned and present as dots; the inner segments are all slender at the centre, thickening slightly towards the edges of the figure where faintly stained rods first appear. c, choroid; pe, pigment epithelium. Marker = 10 μm

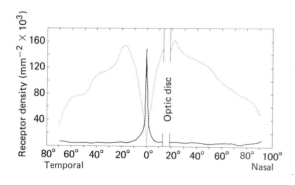

Figure 1.5 Rod and cone density along the horizontal meridian of a human retina. Cone density (solid line) is far greater at the fovea (0°) than elsewhere and drops rapidly with distance from the fovea. Rods (dotted line) are absent from the fovea and reach a peak density at 20°. No receptors are present at the optic disc. (After Oesterberg, 1935)

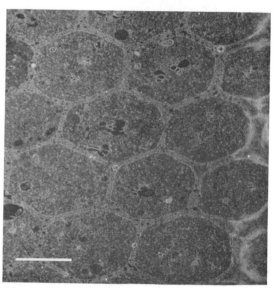

Figure 1.6 Foveal mosaic of a rhesus monkey retina. The section is cut almost exactly tangentially, close to the outer limiting membrane. The mainly six-sided receptor myoids contain neurofilaments, microtubules and agranular endoplasmic reticulum organized into Golgi membranes in some instances. Small rounded profiles interposed between receptors are the basket fibres of Müller neuroglial cells. The dense thickened cell membranes to the right are the outer limiting membrane; it appears unusually broad due to the orientation of the section. Marker = 2 μm

but from the evidence of electron micrographs it appears that this arrangement occurs only at irregular intervals and that intervening discs may have no attachment (*Figure 1.7*).

The neural process of vision begins with the bleaching of receptor photopigments by light. One of these, rhodopsin, is incorporated in and contributes a substantial part of the proteinaceous structure of the rod disc membranes (Blaurock and Wilkins, 1972; Basinger, Bok and Hall, 1976). The highly specialized structure of the outer segment provides an efficient photon-catching device because the regular disposition of photopigment molecules on each disc reduces the chance of photons traversing the receptor unabsorbed.

Mammalian cone photopigments have not been isolated (Crescitelli, 1972), but it is known that there are three of them which differ according to their light-absorbing qualities (Rushton, 1957; Weale, 1959; Brown and Wald, 1964; Marks, Dobelle and MacNichol, 1964; Dartnall, Bowmaker and Mollon,

1983), and that individual cones contain one of the three pigments. Thus, one may refer to red, green and blue cones according to the wavelength maximally absorbed and, in the baboon, 33% of cones are red cones, 54% green cones and 13% blue cones, with the proportion of blue cones reducing to 3% in the central retina (Marc and Sperling, 1977). A similar distribution in man would partly account for the well-known 'blue blindness' or tritanopia of the foveal region.

Receptor inner segments

A narrow eccentrically placed connecting stalk containing a cilium joins inner and outer segments (*see Figure 1.7*). Inner segments are composed of two easily distinguishable zones within a single compartment: the outer zone or ellipsoid which is packed with mitochondria and the inner zone or myoid which contains free ribosomes, granular and agranular endoplasmic reticulum, Golgi membranes, vesicles and neurotubules. The importance of the myoid lies in its major responsibility for the manufacture of practically all of the principal classes of molecules involved in the production and repair of outer segment discs. Protein molecules are synthesized in the myoid in association with ribosomes and a few enter the nucleus, others passing the nucleus into the fibre to reach the terminals; some are transported to the mitochondria of the ellipsoid but the bulk, probably mainly opsin (the protein of visual pigment), passes through the connecting stalk to the stacks of discs in the outer segment.

Receptor nuclei and fibres

A slender outer fibre connects the rod cell body to the inner segment and an inner fibre terminates at the synaptic seam of the outer plexiform layer (*see Figure 1.2*). The cell body is little more than the nucleus because the perikaryon is extremely thin. All cone cell bodies are adjacent to their inner segments, except at the fovea, and have an inner fibre only, which is relatively long and thick. The fibres contain neurotubules and, in general, they have the appearance of axons. Receptor fibres are directed centripetally in most of the retina, but centrally they radiate from the fovea and lie in the plane of the retina, with successive fibres gradually changing orientation with distance from the fovea. The membranes of the radiating fibres (of Henle) probably contain the bulk of the yellow macula pigment (Bone and Landrum, 1984). The linear arrangement of pigment molecules, so produced, is responsible for the pigment's dichroic nature and the consequent polarization of incident light. The entoptic phenomenon of Haidinger's brushes is an expression of macular pigment dichroism and has proved clinically useful (Stanworth and Naylor, 1955).

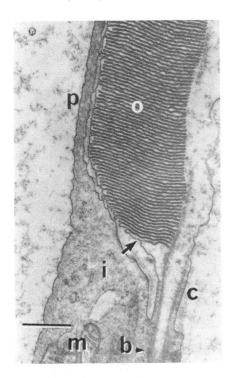

Figure 1.7 Connecting stalk (c) joining inner (i) to outer (o) segment of a rhesus monkey foveal cone. Two of the nine doublets (sectioned longitudinally) of the cilium lie within the connecting stalk and terminate in the dense basal body (b). The inner segment forms a shallow socket or calyx for the outer segment, deepened by means of 15 finger-like extensions or calyceal processes one of which (p) is seen in the figure. New outer segment discs are formed by invagination of the cell membrane on one side of the connecting stalk (arrow). m, mitochondria of ellipsoid. Marker = 0.5 μm

Receptor terminals

The wide cone pedicles and rod spherules, and the terminals of bipolar neurones and horizontal cells with which they synapse, are shown in *Figure 1.2*. Their morphology indicates that they are chemical synapses, but the neurotransmitter involved is uncertain although there is tentative evidence that receptor cells release acetylcholine (Schwartz and Bok, 1979). In addition, there is good structural and functional evidence of electrical synapses between the terminals of cones and between those of rods and cones (Cohen, 1965; Uga *et al.*, 1970; Lasansky, 1972) by means of gap junctions (Raviola and Gilula, 1973; Raviola, 1976; Reale, Luciano and Spitznas, 1978). Evidence for electrical coupling between cones in the turtle retina (Baylor, Fuortes and O'Bryan, 1971) revealed the interesting property of selective linkage between cones of similar spectral responses (Detwiler and Hodgkin, 1979). Whether or not smaller contacts between receptors at the level of the outer limiting membrane (Raviola, 1976) represent further sites for electrical coupling is debatable, but appears unlikely in man (Reale, Luciano and Spitznas, 1978).

Receptor orientation

Traditionally, receptor axes were considered to lie perpendicular to the surface of the retina, yet such an arrangement is inefficient for they would be directed towards the centre of the eye and not to the incoming light (posterior receptors excepted). Receptors are known to display a marked directional sensitivity (Stiles–Crawford effect 1), only axial or nearly axial rays being accepted and funnelled to the outer segments (Enoch, 1963). Consequently, Laties, Liebman and Campbell (1968) reassessed receptor alignment and observed an increasing inclination from the normal to the retinal surface with distance from the fovea in monkeys, so that all receptors were directed towards the front of the eye in the vicinity of the exit pupil (Laties and Enoch, 1971); man appears to have a similar arrangement. Disordered receptor orientation is spontaneously corrected during recovery from certain pathological disturbances of the retina suggesting the presence of an orientation mechanism (Enoch, van Loo and Okun, 1973). Abnormal orientation, as determined by measuring the centration of the Stiles–Crawford effect sometimes may be a factor in the pathology of amblyopia (Enoch, 1959; Bedell, 1980).

Protein metabolism of receptors

Amino acids, when injected into a laboratory animal, are predominantly utilized by cells that reproduce or renew their organelles most rapidly. The progress of incorporation of amino acids into structural protein may be monitored autoradiographically and, using this method, Droz (1963) and Young (1967) noted that receptor cells of the retina renewed their protein at a far faster rate than any other part of the retina. Most of the protein is used in the renewal and repair of outer segment discs.

Protein is utilized in rods by the continuous formation of new discs at the base and by molecular renewal in existing discs (Young, 1974), i.e. discs are both renewed and repaired. The new discs move through the outer segment and break off in groups of 30 or 40 at the tips and become engulfed by the pigment epithelium to form phagosomes. A disc takes 6–8 weeks to move through the outer segment from formation to destruction in frogs, about 8 days in mice and 9–13 days in monkeys (Young, 1967, 1971).

The renewal of cone outer segment protein appears to proceed in a different manner from that of rods when studied by autoradiography. Aggregations of new protein in growing membranes at the base of the outer segment, and the subsequent displacement of the labelled membranes, have not been observed in mammalian cones; instead the molecules are dispersed throughout the outer segment suggesting a mechanism of disc repair rather than replacement. However, phagosomes are present in the pigment epithelium opposite the all-cone fovea and in the processes of epithelial cells extending to peripheral cones in man (Hogan, Wood and Steinberg, 1974) and monkeys (*see Figure 1.3*), and in the all-cone retina of squirrels (Anderson and Fisher, 1976). So disc shedding is also a feature of the cone renewal process, but perhaps, in contrast to rods, the emphasis is on disc repair. If one makes the reasonable assumption that availability of protein for repair reduces with distance from the cilium, the gradual reduction in disc diameter and tapering of cones is readily understood.

Rod disc shedding is cyclic in monkeys peaking 1 hour after the onset of light (La Vail, 1976; Young, 1978; Fisher, Pfeffer and Anderson, 1983), when rod contribution to vision is, at least, diminished. The raised threshold of the rod electroretinogram observed shortly after light onset in man (Birch, Berson and Sandberg, 1984) may result from a similar cycle.

The vigorous visual cell renewal system which, of course, includes lipid and carbohydrate in addition to protein utility, is potentially vulnerable and, in those diseases, especially metabolic and inherited ones that selectively affect rods and cones, the renewal system is probably disrupted (Young, 1976; Szamier *et al.*, 1979). The assembly of new outer segment discs practically stops in experimental retinal detachment (Kroll and Machemer, 1969; Anderson *et al.*, 1983).

Receptor membrane potential and sensitivity

Intracellular recordings from mudpuppy visual receptors revealed a resting membrane potential of approximately 30 mV negative internally, increasing maximally in a graded fashion by only 5 mV upon exposure to light (Werblin and Dowling, 1969). Thus the response to light was hyperpolarization rather than depolarization and an action potential was not generated. The response characteristics are slightly different for rods and cones as demonstrated in turtles (Schwartz, 1973); cones require approximately four times the light energy required by rods to achieve an equivalent response. Hence the difference in sensitivity is negligible and fails to account for the several orders of difference in sensitivity separating scotopic and photopic vision.

The sensitivity difference is attributable to the summation permitted by the substantial convergence of rods to bipolar and ganglion cells which constitutes a wide quantum-catching system. In contrast, cones, at least central cones, display minimal summation because they lack neural convergence and are thus at a disadvantage when the quantity of impinging light quanta is low. In order to reach visual threshold with a small stimulus field, the intensity required is similar for the fovea and the periphery. As an expression of the power of summation, if the size of the stimulus field is now substantially increased, peripheral threshold intensity is reduced to perhaps a thousandth of the original value, whereas lowering of the threshold at the fovea is moderate (Weale, 1958) and at least in part due to the introduction of rod stimulation with the larger field.

Rod and cone synapses in the outer plexiform layer

Practically all the synapses of this layer lie at a single locus, the synaptic seam, near the inner nuclear layer (*see Figure 1.2*). Cones synapse with midget, flat midget and flat bipolar cells. Midget bipolar cells possess a tight cluster of dendrites in contact with a single cone (Polyak, 1941, 1957; Dowling and Boycott, 1966), each dendrite invaginating the flat cone pedicle as the centre piece of one of its numerous triads (*see Figure 1.2*). Flat midget bipolar dendrites do not invaginate the pedicle, but contact the cone base, one on each side of the invaginations. This one-to-one relationship of cones and bipolars is not maintained away from the fovea in man. In contrast, the broader group of dendrites of flat bipolar cells contact about six cones without invaginating the base of the pedicle (Missotten, 1965). Rod bipolar cells constitute a single class and they have the broadest spread of up to 45 dendrites which invaginate a similar number of rod spherules (Boycott and Dowling, 1969). So at the first

synapse, convergence of rod input is evident whereas convergence is lacking in the cone/midget bipolar pathway.

Horizontal cells also synapse in the outer plexiform layer with their dendrites invaginating cones (from 6 to 12 cones centrally and from 30 to 50 cones peripherally) as the two lateral elements of the triad (Kolb, 1970; Boycott and Kolb, 1973). Horizontal cell axons are extremely fine (0.2–0.4 μm) and are up to 1 mm long, ending in a rich arborization extending over a much larger area than the dendrites and they contact from 80 to 150 rods (Kolb, 1974; Gallego and Sobrino, 1975). Applying conventional notions of nerve conduction, one would suppose that this arrangement indicates that horizontal cells are excited by cone activity and transmit to rod spherules. However, this is doubtful because, lacking the capacity to produce an impulse, conduction is by electrotonic spread which is limited by the resistance of the fine axon (Gallego and Sobrino, 1975). Hence the cell would provide local interaction between cones and between rods but not between rods and cones.

Synapses of the inner plexiform layer

Bipolar, ganglion and amacrine cells synapse in a complex manner and at several levels within the inner plexiform layer (Dowling and Boycott, 1966; Foos and Miyamasu, 1973). Examples of their relationships are given in *Figure 1.2*, but the two amacrines are representative without expressing the multitude of forms and transmitters employed by these cells (Ehinger, 1983). Mention must be made of several varieties of interplexiform cells (Gallego, 1971) which form a distinct subgroup of amacrines. They have dendritic communications with other amacrines, but are unique in possessing an axon which passes back to the outer plexiform layer where they synapse with bipolar dendrites and horizontal cells (Dowling, Ehinger and Floren, 1980).

Ganglion cells

The term 'retinal ganglion cell' refers to all neurones having a cell body in the retina and an axon that joins the optic nerve. The ganglion cell layer is made up of their cell bodies with a small number of displaced amacrines. Oppel (1967) estimated that 1.2 million ganglion cells are present in the human retina with the greatest density at the macula where they lie eight deep, reducing rapidly in density up to 10° from the fovea and then gradually to the periphery, interrupted only by a modest peak at about 20° opposite the region of peak rod density. The layer may reduce to a single cell thickness at the periphery.

Numerous varieties of ganglion cells have been described but here the familiar Polyak (1941) classi-

Table 1.1 Ganglion cell types and their properties in cats

Anatomical classification	Cell type		
	Alpha	Beta	Gamma
Cell diameter (μm)	24–28	12–25*	5–15
Dendritic spread (μm)	300–600	25–250*	Wide
Proportions (%)	4	55	41
Projections	LGN, SC	LGN	LGN, SC
Physiological classification	Y	X	W or Q
Response characteristics	Brisk Transient	Brisk Sustained	Sluggish Sustained
Receptive field size	Large	Small	Large
On-centre, off-centre	Both	Both	Both
Spatial summation	Non-linear	Linear	Linear
Conduction velocity	Relatively fast	Slower	Slowest
Possible function	Movement detection	Visual resolution	Uncertain

*Diameter and dendritic spread increase with eccentricity.
Derived from the data of Enroth-Cugell and Robson (1966, 1984), Stone and Hoffman (1972), Boycott and Wässle (1974), Cleland and Levick (1974a, b), Rowe and Stone (1976) and Wässle, Boycott and Illing, 1981.
LGN = lateral geniculate nucleus; SC = superior colliculus.

fication and that of Boycott and Dowling (1969) will be passed over in favour of the simpler alpha, beta, gamma classification Boycott and Wässle (1974) derived for cats but which is partly applicable to primates. Apart from its simplicity, it has the added virtue that some physiological correlates are known (Illing and Wässle, 1981; Wässle, Boycott and Illing, 1981;) (*Table 1.1*).

In primates, small ganglion cells are far more common than large ones and few or no large cells are present in the central retina (Webb and Kaas, 1976; Perry and Cowey, 1981). The central small or *beta* cells are the midget ganglion cells of Polyak's (1941) terminology (Leventhal, Rodleck and Dreher, 1981; Perry and Cowey, 1981) and they have small dendritic fields (6–16 μm). With increasing retinal eccentricity, the dendritic field increases (up to 60 μm) but the cells are arguably still of the same beta class, even though Polyak would not have called them midget cells. Large or *alpha* cells have large dendritic fields increasing very substantially with eccentricity from about 35 μm at 3° to 170 μm at 18°. Some anatomical details and physiological properties of alpha and beta cells in cats are presented in *Table 1.1* including the well-known X, Y (Enroth-Cugell and Robson, 1966, 1984) and W (Stone and Hoffman, 1972) physiological types.

X-like properties are discernible in primate cells with colour-opponent properties (De Monasterio, 1978) and they are probably morphologically equivalent to beta cells (Perry and Cowey, 1981). Y-like properties are associated with cells responding to broad spectral bands which correspond to the alpha cells. A third class of ganglion cell, the gamma cell, which has less discrete properties than alpha or beta cells, is found in the cat retina (*Table 1.1*); other morphological types of cell are also present in primates (Leventhal, Rodieck and Dreher, 1981), but none can be equated with gamma (W) cells. A comparison of morphological cell types in the human retina is hindered by the observation that cell size range is unimodal at any point in the retina (Hebel and Holländer, 1983), and by the lack of reliable data on dendritic field size. Central cells are uniformly small, the mean diameter increasing up to 30–40° and then decreasing in the periphery.

Spectral transmission through the retina

Modification of colour signals, with progress from the three varieties of cones to the ganglion cells, has been recorded electrophysiologically in several animals as noted above, but, with the exception of cyprinid fish (Scholes, 1975), virtually no progress has been made in understanding their anatomical substrates (Mariani, 1984). Consequently, endeavours to explain the connectivity of wavelength-specific cells found here or in the lateral geniculate nucleus and visual cortex must be speculative.

Rod and cone pathways through the retina

There are probably no exclusive rod pathways through the retina, and the direct cone pathway through midget bipolars and midget ganglion cells is arguably subject to the influence of rod activity, perhaps even at the fovea. Where do the rod and cone pathways converge? There is broad agreement that mainline conduction from rods and cones to the inner plexiform layer is separate at bipolar cell level, hence the appelations of rod and cone bipolar cells, but already the inter-receptor gap junctions provide an opportunity for interaction. Although horizontal cells join cones with rods, the argument that functional links occur only between groups of cones or groups of rods is popular.

There is no doubt that mixed inputs occur at inner plexiform level and first one must ask if rod and cone bipolars synapse directly with the same ganglion cell. The answer to this question is unclear in primates, but flat cone bipolars and rod bipolars may do so (*see Figure 1.2*). In cats, which have been most fully studied, it appears not to be the case (Kolb, 1979). Cone bipolars synapse directly but rods use the amacrine cell as an intermediary before converging on the same ganglion cell. Cone pathway dyads usually include an amacrine element so any cone pathway has the potential to contribute to rod pathways through the amacrine cell (*see Figure 1.2*). Single amacrines also have conventional presynaptic contacts with both rod and cone bipolars permitting interaction either way. Inner plexiform amacrine cells may also introduce cross-connections, and finally a so-called ganglion cell connecting other ganglion cells and not contributing an axon to the optic nerve has been described in man and dogs (Gallego and Cruz, 1965).

On the basis of neuroanatomical studies, ganglion cells cannot be designated as rod or cone types in cats (Kolb, 1979) and Rodieck and Rushton's (1976) microelectrode recordings from a sample of ganglion cells revealed a mixed rod and cone input when an appropriate manipulation of stimuli was used. Perhaps a different result might be expected from primate midget ganglion cells at the fovea where the possibility of rod input is least likely.

Nerve fibre layer

Axons of ganglion cells turn into the plane of the retina and are partitioned into bundles by sheet-like Müller cell processes augmented by another glial cell — the astrocyte. The axons of fibres pass to-

wards the optic disc to form the optic nerve and those from areas nasal to the disc take the shortest, radial course, but the remainder form a discrete and largely predictable pattern (*Figure 1.8*) dictated by the need to avoid crossing the foveal pit (Vrabec, 1966). Important points to note are:

(1) No fibre crosses the horizontal meridian, hence a fibre originating in the upper retina enters the upper half of the optic disc.
(2) As a consequence temporal fibres form a horizontal raphe, often regarded as a horizontal locus extending to the periphery from which fibres are angled away.

Figure 1.8 shows that this is true for a short distance only (approximately 4 mm or 15°), and more peripherally fibres run parallel to the horizontal locus before arcing around the fovea.

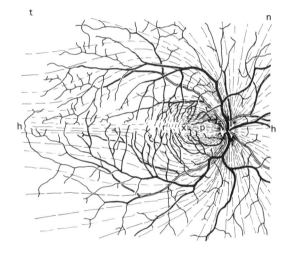

Figure 1.8 Blood vessel arborization and nerve fibre direction in the retina. Venules (solid) are shown crossing in front of arterioles (clear) to assist recognition; the direction of bundles in the nerve fibre layer is indicated by fine interrupted lines. All vessel trunks issue from the clear, elliptical optic disc or papilla on the right of the figure and the larger branches avoid the fovea (x) and central region (the fovea is free of vessels). Nerve fibres pass radially to the nasal (n) side of the optic disc whereas fibres on the temporal (t) side are diverted to avoid crossing the fovea. Some of the nerve fibres from the fovea and central region pass straight to the optic disc and others arc above and below the fovea: together these form the papillomacula bundle (p). A raphe (r) is formed by the central fibres temporal to the fovea. No nerve fibres and few vessels cross the horizontal meridian (hh). After Polyak's (1941) representation of the blood vessels and nerves of a rhesus monkey retina and slightly modified according to Vrabec's (1966) illustration of the nerve fibre layer of the human retina. Only part of the nasal retina is shown

The thickness of the fibre layer is minimal peripherally and thickest at the disc (up to 30 μm), especially on the temporal side, where the greatest number of macula fibres enter the optic nerve head. It seems likely that, in man, the longer fibres (of peripheral origin) lie on the vitreal side of the layer at the disc as in rhesus monkeys (Minckler, 1980). If this is so, then peripheral fibre vulnerability in glaucoma is probably a consequence of ischaemia rather than of pressure against the hard scleral angle at the disc margin.

Optic nerve

The optic nerve conducts nerve fibres from the retina to the chiasma. The full length of the nerve averages nearly 50 mm made up of intraocular (nearly 1 mm), intraorbital (20–30 mm), intracanicular (about 6 mm) and intracranial (3–16 mm) portions. Within the cranium the nerve is slightly flattened, measuring about 5 mm horizontally and 3 mm vertically. Within the optic canal and the orbit the nerve is cylindrical measuring between 3 and 4 mm. In the scleral canal of the eye, where nerve fibres lose their myelin sheaths, the diameter reduces sharply to approximately 1.5 mm.

The intraorbital course of the nerve roughly corresponds to the long axis of the orbit but it is not straight. The nerve curves laterally nearer the orbital apex and bends downwards closer to the eye which it enters 3 mm medial and just above the posterior pole. The slack of 5 or 6 mm provided by the gentle bending allows for ocular movement and presumably, in extreme rotations, the optic nerve straightens.

Although the optic nerve is traditionally regarded as a peripheral nerve, its structure compares with a fibre tract of the central nervous system connecting two parts of the brain. Like the brain itself, the optic nerve is invested with meningeal sheaths. A thin pia mater is tightly adherent to the full length of the optic nerve up to the scleral canal, and connective tissue septa extend from the pia to divide the nerve into several hundred fascicles. The septa are often incomplete and fasciculation is less marked intracranially. Pial vessels follow the septa into the nerve and the central retinal artery and vein penetrate the nerve inferiorly between 5 and 17 mm behind the eye (Steele and Blunt, 1956), then pass obliquely to a central position and enter the eye near the centre of the optic disc (*Figure 1.9*). The vein usually lies lateral to the artery. Arachnoid mater covers the nerve intracranially shortly before it enters the optic canal and extends forward up to the scleral canal. Dura mater lining the cranium continues into the optic canal forming the outermost sheath of the optic nerve and, at the orbital exit from the canal, the outer lamina of the dura is continuous with the

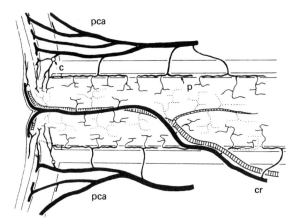

Figure 1.9 Blood vessels of the intraorbital optic nerve. Arteries are in solid black, veins are hatched or dotted. The central retinal artery has few branches within the optic nerve and none in the region of the scleral canal until it reaches the prelaminar level. A cilioretinal artery (not shown in the figure) passes directly from a posterior ciliary artery and turns into the retina at the rim of the optic disc in one or both eyes of 15–20% of individuals (Hayreh, 1963). c, arterial circle of Zinn; cr, central retinal vessels; p, pial artery; pca, posterior ciliary arteries

periosteum of the orbit. The three meningeal sheaths fuse and attach part of the circumference of the optic nerve firmly to the bone of the canal so that the nerve has no capacity to move within it, yet adequate space remains for circulation of cerebrospinal fluid to and from the subarachnoid and subdural spaces of the optic nerve. At the eye the dura fuses with the sclera (*Figures 1.10 and 1.11*).

Histology of the optic nerve

Nerve fibres of the optic nerve vary in diameter from 0.25 to 2.5 μm with a maximum frequency at 0.5 μm (Potts *et al.*, 1972a,b). Axon diameters range between 0.2 and 2.0 μm with a peak at 0.4 μm. Although the distribution of fibre sizes is strongly skewed to the smaller diameters, it is unimodal and they total from 1 to 1.2×10^6 (Potts *et al.*, 1972a) or even more (Hughes and Wässle, 1976). All fibres possess a myelin sheath that is thin compared with those of peripheral somatic nerves but some variation is found, the smaller axons tending to possess the thinnest sheaths (Anderson and Hoyt, 1969).

Since the optic nerve is a central nervous system tract rather than a true peripheral nerve, the fibres lack a Schwann cell investment and oligodendroglia are the cells responsible for fibre myelination. Each oligodendrocyte provides a myelin investment for 12–40 axons for a length of about 30 μm only. The oligodendrocytes display evidence of oxidative

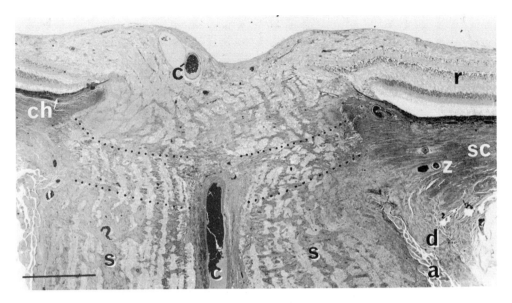

Figure 1.10 Section through a human optic nerve head. Nerve fibres are lightly stained compared with the adjacent connective tissue septa, cribriform plate and astrocytic sleeves. The limits of the lamina cribrosa (not clearly shown in the figure) are indicated by dotted lines. Detachment of part of the retina on the right is an artefact of preparation. a, arachnoid mater; c, central retinal artery; c′, blood-filled branch of central retinal artery and adjacent branch of the central retinal vein; ch, choroid; d, dur mater; r, retina; s, septa of postlaminar optic nerve; sc, sclera; z, circle of Zinn. Stained with toluidine blue; marker = 0.5 mm

enzyme activity whereas the axons do not, suggesting that they act as energy donors to the axons (Blunt *et al.*, 1967). A second glial cell, the astrocyte, is also present within and at the perimeter of fascicles (*Figure 1.11*).

Centrifugal (efferent) nerve fibres are known to occur in most of the major sensory pathways, but whether or not they are present in the visual pathway below the level of the lateral geniculate nucleus is uncertain. Reports supporting the presence of centrifugal fibres in the optic nerve and retina are numerous (Brook, Downer and Powell, 1965; Noback and Mettler, 1973; Wolter, 1974; Repérant and Gallego, 1976), yet some experienced observers appear unconvinced (Polyak, 1957; Dowling and Boycott, 1966).

The retinotopic projections of nerve fibres through the optic nerve and the remainder of the visual pathway are shown in *Figure 1.12*.

Optic nerve head

Considerable modification of the optic nerve occurs as it penetrates the sclera (*see Figures 1.10* and *1.11*). The nerve is no longer ensheathed by meninges and it is penetrated by collagenous trabeculae extending from the inner third of the sclera and bridging the scleral canal. This region of the optic nerve is the lamina cribrosa and its trabeculae give strength to the optic nerve head, which would otherwise be subject to backward displacement by the high intraocular pressure.

Upon entering the scleral canal, the nerve fibres lose their myelin sheaths almost in perfect register and the rows of oligodendrocytes terminate. Only astrocytes (and possibly microglia) are present in the laminar and prelaminar regions. The association of oligodendrocytes with myelination is emphasized by their presence in the rabbit retinal nerve fibre layer, only in the regions exhibiting the characteristic myelinated nerve fibres of this species (Steele and Blunt, 1956). Myelinated nerve fibres sometimes continue into the retina for a short distance in man, particularly from the upper and lower temporal regions of the disc (Straatsma *et al.*, 1981).

The prelaminar nerve fibres may hump forward slightly forming an optic papilla as they change direction to enter the retina and they leave a central pit (the physiological cup) which varies in depth, width and position between individuals. The cup is often asymmetrical with a steeper wall most commonly on the nasal side of the optic disc, but the less steep temporal side of the cup extends closer to the disc margin. The central retinal vessels appear at the disc from the deepest region of the cup. In glaucoma, the tissues of the optic nerve head are pushed backwards by the raised intraocular pressure and the cup extends to the margin of the disc in the late stages of the disease.

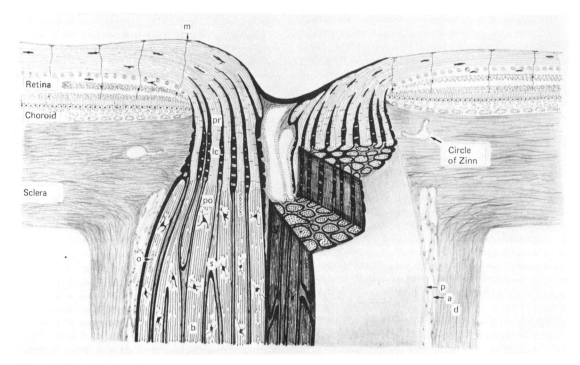

Labels on figure: m, Retina, Choroid, pr, lc, Circle of Zinn, Sclera, po, o, s, p, a, d, b

Figure 1.11 Section through the optic nerve head (partly represented in three dimensions). Unmyelinated nerve fibres of the retina turn through the scleral canal to form the optic nerve. Trabeculae pass from the sclera into the scleral canal anteriorly forming the cribriform plate and the retinal fibres leave the eye through the spaces of the plate. The scleral trabeculae and the fibres together form the lamina cribrosa (lc) permitting the designations *prelaminar* (pr) and *postlaminar* (po) to the optic nerve on the ocular and orbital sides of it. All items of the optic nerve drawn in solid black are composed of astrocytes which provide a thin, complete sheath for the cylindrical bundles (b) of myelinated fibres of the postlaminar optic nerve and thus separate nerve fibres from the connective tissue septa (s). At the level of the lamina cribrosa, astrocytes continue to line the bundles, separating fibres from the connective tissue (largely collagenous) trabeculae and thickening between the separate layers of laminar meshes and at the border of the scleral canal. Astrocytes become the sole component of the meshes in the prelaminar optic nerve, gradually thinning as the bundles turn into the retina, where only scattered astrocytes are present. The layer of astrocytes separating the optic nerve head from the vitreous often thickens at the base of the cup formed near the centre of the optic nerve head or disc where the central retinal vessels are first exposed. At the border of the disc the astrocyte layer terminates and Müller cell (m) footplates provide a cellular interface between retina and vitreous. Astrocytes form a peripheral collar for the intraocular part of the optic nerve, separating the nerve from sclera, choroid and outer retina in turn. Dendritic astrocytes are present within nerve fibre bundles, but in the laminar and prelaminar regions they are few and astrocytes are represented within bundles mainly by the processes of those lining the bundles.

Oligodendrocytes (o) provide the myelin for optic nerve fibres and consequently they are present only in the postlaminar region. The posterior part of the sclera is continuous with the dura mater (d) cover of the optic nerve and is separated from the nerve proper by the arachnoid mater (a) and pia mater (p). Spaces formed between the three meningeal sheaths are filled with cerebrospinal fluid and end blind at the optic nerve head. Meningocytes line all the spaces. The pia mater is tightly applied to the optic nerve surface and connective tissue septa (s) extend from the pia and separate the nerve into several hundred bundles. Of the rich vascular supply to the optic nerve head only the central retinal vessels and the arterial circle of Zinn are represented. (Partly based on the studies of Anderson and Hoyt (1969) and Anderson (1969))

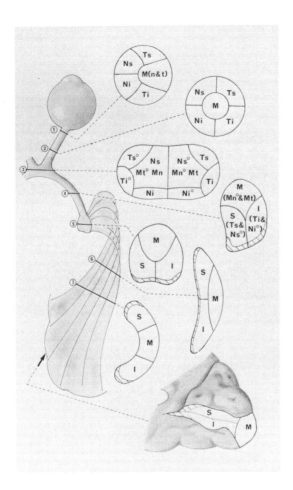

Figure 1.12 Retinotopic projections through the visual pathway. Immediately behind the eye at (1), the macular fibres (M) separate the superior (Ts) and inferior (Ti) temporal fibres but, further back at (2), they are centrally placed with approximate symmetry of the surrounding nasal (N) and temporal fibres. All temporal fibres including temporal macular fibres (Mt) are uncrossed at the chiasma (3), but all nasal fibres cross to the opposite side. Equivalent fibres from the left eye are indicated by the superscript o. Inferior nasal fibres occupy an inferior position in the chiasma whereas superior nasal and macular fibres are intermingled centrally in the upper part of the chiasma. In the optic tract (4) onwards, inferior (I), superior (S) and macular (M) fibres consist of ipsilateral temporal and contralateral nasal fibres and the inferior fibres are disposed laterally. This arrangement is maintained at the lateral geniculate body (5), then twisting and elongating in the early optic radiations (6) so that the superior fibres are uppermost but in contact with inferior fibres centrally. Further on at (7), the macular separate superior and inferior fibres. At the striate cortex macular fibres occupy the inferior and lateral aspects of the occipital pole cortex with a limited medial representation as shown. Much of the remainder of the striate cortex lies buried in the calcarine sulcus with the horizontal meridian located approximately at the base of the sulcus. The projections shown are somewhat arbitrary, e.g. in the optic nerve towards the chiasma some observers claim that the quadrant fibres rotate clockwise 45°. Macular fibres have a broader spread than shown, at least in the infrageniculate pathway, and M represents only the greatest concentration. Extreme peripheral fibres occupy the perimeter of the optic nerve and they are indicated by a separate cross-hatched zone elsewhere. (Based on the experimental and clinical studies of Spalding (1952), Polyak (1957), Teuber, Battersby and Berde (1960) and Hoyt and Luis (1962))

Vessels of the optic nerve head (*see Figure 1.9*)

Short posterior ciliary arteries penetrate the sclera close to the scleral canal and give off branches contributing to a partial or complete arterial circle, the circle of Zinn, which passes circumferentially about the optic nerve within the sclera. Arterioles pass centripetally from the circle or directly from the ciliary arteries and either continue into the nerve centripetally or provide precapillaries that turn circumferentially or radially at the sclera/nerve interface for a short distance before turning again to enter the nerve. Vessels enter the optic nerve at laminar and prelaminar levels and form a rich capillary network. Venules drain the capillary network and join the central retinal vein.

Once it has moved to the centre of the nerve, the central retinal artery contributes little to optic nerve nourishment; its branches are infrequent and none occur at laminar and immediate postlaminar levels. However, small arterioles issue from the central retinal artery or its branches before they leave the optic disc and distribute to the prelaminar optic nerve and are, therefore, partly responsible for the remarkably dense capillary network of this region. Some branches of the prelaminar region pass beyond the boundaries of the disc to form a radial peripapillary network (Henkind, 1967).

Passage of arteriolar branches from the choroid to the optic nerve head has been noted by numerous workers (*see* Anderson and Braverman, 1976) and small venules may pass from the disc to the choroid. All capillaries of the intraocular portion of the optic nerve are unfenestrated.

A variety of anastomoses between the small vessels of the optic nerve head have been proposed and challenged, especially in recent years. One of these, between the scleral arterial circle and the central retinal artery, appears unlikely except at capillary level. A capillary connection would account for the limited focal leak of fluorescein into the central retinal artery using a fluorescence angiography technique after blocking the central retinal artery behind the eye (Hayreh, 1972). A link between capillary branches of pial arterioles and laminar vessels and between their venous counterparts does occur.

Obliteration of prelaminar disc vessels caused by raised intraocular pressure in glaucoma leads to atrophic changes in the nervous tissue (Hayreh, 1970).

Chiasma

Position and relations

The chiasma (chiasm) is a midline structure of the hypothalamus of the brain and is formed by the junction of the two optic nerves. It is flattened vertically with a height of 3–5 mm and an average width of 13 mm and lies slightly above or may rest upon a thick endothelial-lined sheet of tissue, the diaphragma sella, which is continuous with the dural lining of the cranial cavity forming the roof of the hypophyseal fossa. The diaphragm separates the chiasma from the hypophysis which may be immediately below, slightly forward or behind the chiasma. On each side of the chiasma lie the two internal carotid arteries on the point of contributing to the arterial circle of Willis.

Disorders of the adjacent structures may lead to stretching or pressure on the chiasma with impairment of its function (O'Connell, 1973). For example, arterial aneurysms and meningeal or hypophyseal tumours may produce loss of visual field relating to the retinotopic projections exposed to the space-occupying lesions. Pressure on the chiasma from below, as a consequence of a hypophyseal tumour expanding upward through the diaphragm, selectively damages inferior retinotopic projection fibres with the resultant superior field loss.

Decussation

Nerve fibres from the temporal hemiretinas occupy lateral positions within the chiasma and continue into the optic tracts on the same side. Nasal fibres, which make up about 53% of the total in monkeys (Kupfer, Chumbley and Downes, 1967), cross to the other side (*see Figure 1.12*). Compliance with the rule of sensory transfer from one side of the body to the opposite hemisphere of the brain is achieved for vision by means of this semi-decussation (*see Figure 1.1*). Inferior nasal fibres, having crossed in the anterior chiasma, are often depicted advancing for a short distance in the opposite optic nerve before passing back in the contralateral optic tract, and superior nasal fibres are shown looping into the ipsilateral tract before crossing in the posterior chiasma and progressing to the contralateral tract. Accounts of these fibre excursions are probably exaggerated (Strachan and Cleary, 1972) and the paths taken by fibres in crossing are likely to be confined within the chiasma. Well-controlled studies of macular fibre projections in monkeys show that they are dispersed throughout most of the chiasma (but substantially located as shown in *Figure 1.12*), bordered inferiorly and mixed superiorly with the peripheral fibres (Hoyt and Luis, 1962).

Optic tract

An overwhelming majority of nerve fibres of the chiasma continue into the optic tracts (*see Figure 1.1*), but a few leave it dorsally as the retinohypothalamic pathways to enter the bilateral suprachiasmatic nuclei (Moore, 1973; Sadun, Schaechter and Smith, 1984). The nucleus is an important pacemaker for the generation of circadian rhythms. It is partly, but not exclusively, responsible for the light–dark entrainment of the 24-hour cycle of the rhythms (Albers *et al.*, 1984). The tracts pass laterally and posteriorly, skirting the body of the hypothalamus and terminate in the lateral geniculate bodies, which lie half buried in the substance of the brain.

The bulk of the nerve fibres in each tract enter and terminate in the lateral geniculate nucleus but an important fraction of fibres, probably all branches of retinogeniculate neurones (Cajal, 1893; Bunt *et al.*, 1975), leave the tract in the superior brachium, which lies immediately anterior to the lateral geniculate body. Beta (X) cell fibres are unlikely to enter the brachium (Leventhal, Rodieck and Dreher, 1981). Brachial fibres are distributed to a variety of nuclei including:

(1) The pregeniculate (ventral lateral geniculate) nucleus (Tigges, Bos and Tigges, 1977), possibly providing a photic input utilized in the reflex regulation of eye movements.
(2) The pretectal nuclei (Lowenstein, Murphy and Loewenfeld, 1953; Dineen and Hendrickson, 1983) mediating the pupillary light reflex.
(3) The superior colliculus (Hubel, Levay and Wiesel, 1975; Wurtz and Albano, 1980) contributing to the government of eye movements.
(4) The pulvinar (Chalupa, Coyle and Lindsley, 1976; Wong-Riley, 1977; Bender, 1981; Mizuno *et al.*, 1982; Itaya and van Hoesen, 1983), again possibly involved in eye movement control.
(5) The accessory optic nuclei (Pasik, Pasik and Hamori, 1973; Westheimer and Blair, 1974; Grasse and Cynader, 1984) which may provide information on the direction and velocity of whole-field motion to the central nervous system.

Destruction of the occipital cortex eliminates geniculostriate visual pathway function and inevitably produces total blindness. This conventional and currently actively supported view has been challenged by a substantial body of experienced workers who claim that at least an awareness of visual space may remain intact, attributable to the fibres leaving the retinogeniculate pathway in the superior brachium (Trevarthen, 1968; Campion, Latto and Smith, 1983). The pulvinar and accessory optic nuclei are most favoured as the mediators of any residual vision or 'blindsight'.

The pulvinar projects to the prestriate cortex and receives projections from striate and prestriate neurones, but the suggestion that it may represent a second visual pathway running parallel to the geniculostriate radiations is questionable (Bender, 1983).

An optic tract carries visual information from the contralateral half-field of each eye with the retinotopic projections from the two retinas superimposed or homonymous, but in the lateral geniculate nucleus the terminations of the two sets of neurones are segregated.

Lateral geniculate body

The lateral geniculate body houses a nucleus consisting of six roughly dome-shaped layers of neurones stacked one above another concentrically around the hilum (*Figure 1.13*). Two magnocellular layers lie closest to the hilum and four parvocellular (small cell) layers farthest from it. Numbered from the hilum, crossed retinogeniculate fibres terminate in layers 1, 4 and 6 and uncrossed fibres in layers 2, 3 and 5 (Kupfer, 1965). The morphological and physiological characteristics of retinal neurones are duplicated in the lateral geniculate nucleus with alpha or Y neurones confined to the magnocelluiar and beta or X neurones to the parvocellular layers (Bunt *et al.*, 1975; Leventhal, Rodieck and Dreher, 1981). Measurement of the spatial resolution of cells in cats led Ikeda and Wright (1976) to attribute amblyopia associated with squint to selective malfunctioning of beta cells.

Approximate retinotopic fibre projections in the nucleus are shown in *Figure 1.12*, and these should be distinguished from the loci of fibre terminations. Macular fibre terminations occupy the full width of all six layers posteriorly and terminals representing the central 20° of visual field fills the posterior half (Kaas, Guillery and Allman, 1972; Malpeli and Baker, 1975).

The precise functions of the nucleus remain obscure but it is clearly not a simple relay station. A clue for substantial integrative activity is provided by the presence of small interneurones in each layer (Wong-Riley, 1972; Szentágothai, 1973). The activity of interneurones is confined within their layer. Inputs from occipital cortex (Lund *et al.*, 1979), brainstem reticular formation (Leger *et al.*, 1975) and other brain loci indicate that retinal visual

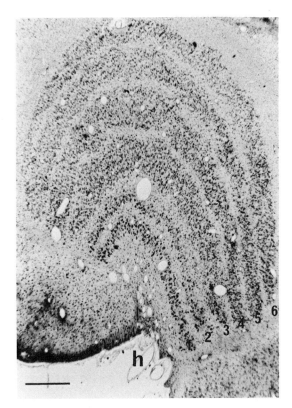

Figure 1.13 Frontal section through the lateral geniculate nucleus of a rhesus monkey. The greater size of cells of laminae 1 and 2 is evident. The hilum (h) is a shallow, sagittal sulcus at the base of the lateral geniculate body. Vascular infiltration, unrivalled in any other structure of the brain, is indicated by the numerous clear spaces. Marker = 0.5 mm

information is subject to a variety of influences preceding conduction to the optic radiations and striate cortex.

Optic radiations

The optic radiations issue from the lateral geniculate nucleus dorsolaterally as the optic peduncle and soon fan out into a thin, vertically orientated band lying close to the wall of the posterior horn of the lateral ventricle and directed towards the occipital lobe. However, the band is twisted as it expands from the peduncle with inferior fibres directed forwards into the lateral lobe of the brain, skirting the inferior horn of the lateral ventricle, before turning back sharply (*see Figure 1.1*). Evidence for the initial forward looping (loop of Meyer) of the inferior fibres comes from the incidental observation of upper contralateral field loss in both eyes associated with temporal lobectomy treatment for severe epilepsy (Marino and Rasmussen, 1968; Bender and Bodis-Wollner, 1978). Radiations buckle and fold within the occipital lobe shortly before terminating in the involuted and complexly shaped striate cortex.

Do radiation fibres terminate exclusively in the striate cortex? In the knowledge that extrastriate terminations are present in cats, endeavours were made to seek them in primates with consistent failure until recently. It now appears incontrovertible that some geniculate fibres in monkeys terminate in prestriate cortex equivalent to areas 18 and 19 in man (Yukie and Iwai, 1981; Bullier and Kennedy, 1983) providing a firm foundation for supposing that they also occur in man.

Macular sparing is a phenomenon associated with contralateral half-field loss as a consequence of radiation lesions; current anatomical knowledge is inadequate to account for it (Koerner and Teuber, 1973).

Striate cortex

The striate cortex (Brodmann's area 17, primary visual cortex) is distinguished from all other cortical areas in possessing a thin band of medullated nerve fibres (the white line of Gennari) running parallel to the cortical surface approximately centrally. It lies in the occipital lobe mainly on the medial aspect of each hemisphere (*Figures 1.14* and *1.15*) with some individual variation (Brindley, 1972). Representation of the visual field and retina is disproportionate, with a much greater area in receipt of central retinal projections. Linear cortical representation is almost 35 times greater for the central field than at 40–50° eccentricity in monkeys (Daniel and Whitteridge,

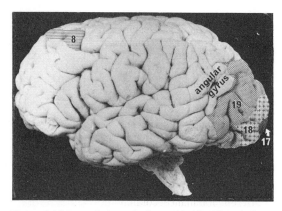

Figure 1.15 Lateral view of a human brain. The whole occipital lobe is shaded to distinguish areas 17, 18, 19 and area 8, which is the frontal eye field governing voluntary eye movements, is also indicated

1961; Hubel and Wiesel, 1974; Dow *et al.*, 1981), and man displays a similar order of magnification (Drasdo, 1977; Rovamo and Virsu, 1979). Thus, the extra demands of central vision are met by a greater cortical area for unit angle of field, reducing gradually with eccentricity, rather than by greater cell density; one part of the striate cortex is cytologically indistinguishable from another.

The six cortical layers numbered from the brain surface have different mixtures of nerve fibres and cell types (Lund, 1973; Billings-Gagliardi, Chan-Palay and Palay, 1974). The greatly expanded layer 4 of the striate cortex receives the terminating fibres of the optic radiations which retain their myelin thus producing the white line of Gennari. A few radiation fibres terminate in layer 1 (Blasdel and Lund, 1983). With the introduction of new axon marking techniques, knowledge of the intrinsic relations of striate cortical cells and their projections to adjoining and contralateral areas and subcortical structures has advanced rapidly (Lund *et al.*, 1975; Macko *et al.*, 1982; Fries and Distel, 1983; Swadlow, 1983).

Animal experimentation reveals that striate cortex has a discrete physiological organization for cells with differing binocular responses. Initial reception of visual information in layer 4 remains monocular in the cortex (Hubel and Wiesel, 1977) but degrees of binocularity are found in most cells of the other layers, i.e. cells that respond to a light stimulus presented to the right or left eye. All cells along a locus perpendicular to the cortical surface display ocular dominance of varying degree from total dominance by one eye (monocular), partial dominance, to none (equal binocular). Cells with these characteristics occupy a column about 0.4 mm in width, neighboured on each side by dominance columns for the opposite eye and of the same width. In fact the columns, so defined, extend through the

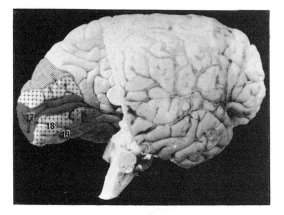

Figure 1.14 Lateral view of a human brain with the posterior part of the right hemisphere removed exposing the medial aspect of the left hemisphere. The whole occipital lobe is shaded differently to indicate its three regions—Brodmann's areas 17, 18 and 19. The calcarine sulcus divides the striate cortex (area 17) into upper and lower halves

cortex for considerable distances constituting slabs rather than columns. Despite this, the word *column* is retained in order to be consistent with nomenclature used for other sensory cortex. A topographical map of alternate right and left eye dominance columns for the central field is shown in *Figure 1.16* — the dark stripes represent all the columns or slabs of underlying cells preferring the same eye. An anatomical correlate of the pattern is discernible at layer 4 level where fine, poorly stained lines of reduced fibre connections are observed, in perfect register with the borders of physiological columns, when a silver technique is used. The lines express the sparsity of tangential spread of cell processes between dominance columns at this level. At all other levels, the linear pattern cannot be seen and the regular density of stain is uninterrupted at the column edges where, presumably, the abundant cell processes permit lateral interaction thereby explain-

ing the degrees of binocularity introduced into columns away from layer 4. A similar anatomical pattern observed in man (Hitchcock and Hickey, 1980) is the strongest evidence that a similar functional organization obtains in human striate cortex.

Cells of the striate cortex also display a preference for orientation of the visual stimulus and again, cells with the same preference are organized into columns apparently independent of the dominance columns (Hubel and Wiesel, 1977; Hubel, Wiesel and Stryker, 1978).

Prestriate cortex

Brodmann's areas 18 (parastriate) and 19 (peristriate) complete the cortex of the occipital lobe of the brain in man (*see Figures 1.14* and *1.15*) and the old argument persists that they are visuopsychic areas where perceptual analysis occurs, as distinct from the visual *imprint* of area 17 (Campbell, 1905; Whitnall, 1932), based partly on clinical evidence of perceptual deficits associated with lesions of these areas. Such a distribution of function now appears most unlikely (Phillips, Zeki and Barlow, 1984) and experiments on monkeys show that the occipital cortex consists of visual areas dealing with separate features of the visual input. Thus, the occipital cortex consists of visual areas of which five have been identified so far in the macaque (*see Figure 1.16*). The visual areas of cortex each receive the full or central part of the visual half-field in a retinotopic manner (with the exception of V4; Zeki, 1980) and respond exclusively to visual stimuli. However, V4 and V5 are complexes containing more than one representation of the visual half-field, but only one in each has been examined in detail. Perhaps the firmest examples of functional allocation are motion analysis in V5 and colour analysis in V4 (Zeki, 1978a). The prestriate areas receive their inputs directly or indirectly from V1, but the recent discovery of a direct geniculate projection to the prestriate cortex dismisses the notion that the V1 source is exclusive.

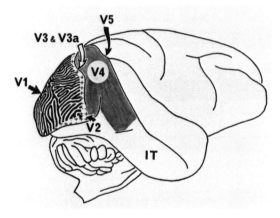

Figure 1.16 Lateral view of the right side of a rhesus monkey brain with the visual areas indicated. The position of dominance colums at the brain surface is marked on the striate cortex or area Vl (the columns are transposed approximately from the data of Hubel and Freeman (1977)). The dark stripes correspond to the dominance columns of one eye and the light stripes to those of the other; right and left eye columns are of equal thickness as are the columns relating to all parts of the retinal projection (the apparent diminution towards the brain profile is intended to represent attenuation due to the third dimension). The exposed striate cortex of the figure corresponds to a fraction more than the central 4° of visual field with representation of the fovea indicated by the arrow head and of the vertical meridian by the border with area V2 (marked by crosses). Much of area V2, the whole of areas V3 and V3a and part of the V4 complex (shaded) lie in the cortex lining the lunate sulcus, indicated by the unfilled arrow, and thus obscured from view. The anterior border of V4 is uncertain and that shown is speculative. The V5 complex lies deep within the superior temporal sulcus. Most of the inferior temporal cortex (IT) is probably also concerned exclusively with vision (Desimone and Gross, 1979). Areas V2 to V5 are referred to collectively as prestriate visual cortex. (Mainly after Zeki, 1978a,b, 1983)

The boundaries distinguishing cortical areas by their structure (Brodmann's areas) translate imperfectly for the cortical mapping efforts of the physiologist and, consequently, designations such as VI (vision 1) and A1 (audition 1) are widely used. Relationships between the systems are usually disregarded, but if one is to accept data obtained from monkeys as a guide to functional organization in the human brain for which only structural maps are available, it is helpful to know that the striate cortex is precisely V1 and area 17 in the monkey, V2 and V4 probably lie in area 18 and V5 in area 19 (Zeki, 1978b). Clinically, the prestriate areas and the angular gyrus (*see Figure 1.15*) are of interest because lesions here give rise to those agnosias and aphasias associated with visual disconnection (Damasio and Damasio, 1983).

References

ALBERS, H.E., LYDIC, R., GANDER, P.H. and MOORE-EDE, M.C. (1984) Role of the suprachiasmatic nuclei in the circadian timing system of the squirrel monkey. II. Light-dark cycle entrainment. *Brain Res.*, **300**, 285–294

ANDERSON, D.H. and FISHER, S.K. (1976) The photoreceptors of diurnal squirrels: outer segment structure, disc shedding and protein renewal. *J. Ultrastruc. Res.*, **55**, 119–141

ANDERSON, D.H. STERN, W.H. FISHER, S.K. ERICKSON, P.A. and BORGULA, G.A. (1983) Retinal detachment in the cat — the pigment epithelial–photoreceptor interface. *Invest. Ophthalmol. Vis. Sci.*, **24**, 906–926

ANDERSON, D.R. (1969) Ultrastructure of human and monkey lamina cribosa and optic nerve head. *Arch. Ophthalmol.*, **82**, 800–814

ANDERSON, D.R. and BRAVERMAN, S. (1976) Reevaluation of the optic disc vasculature. *Am. J. Ophthalmol.*, **82**, 165–174

ANDERSON, D.R. and HOYT, W.F. (1969) Ultrastructure of intraorbital portion of human and monkey optic nerve. *Arch. Ophthalmol.*, **82**, 506–530

BASINGER, S., BOK, D. and HALL, M. (1976) Rhodopsin in the rod outer segment plasma membrane. *J. Cell Biol.*, **69**, 29–42

BAYLOR, D.A., FUORTES, M.G.F. and O'BRYAN, P.M. (1971) Receptive fields of cones in the retina of the turtle. *J. Physiol.*, **214**, 265–294

BEDELL, H.E. (1980) Central and peripheral retinal photoreceptor orientation in amblyopic eyes as assessed by the psychophysical Stiles–Crawford function. *Invest. Ophthalmol. Vis. Sci.*, **19**, 49–59

BENDER, D.B. (1981) Retinotopic organization of macaque pulvinar. *J. Neurophysiol.*, **46**, 672–693

BENDER, D.B. (1983) Visual activation of neurons in the primate pulvinar depends on cortex but not colliculus. *Brain Res.*, **279**, 258–261

BENDER, M.B. and BODIS-WOLLNER, I. (1978) Visual dysfunctions in optic tract lesions. *Ann. Neurol.*, **3**, 187–193

BERMAN, E.R. and BACH, J. (1968) The acid mucopolysaccharides of cattle retina. *Biochem. J.*, **108**, 75–88

BILLINGS-GAGLIARDI, S., CHAN-PALAY, V. and PALAY, S.L. (1974) A review of lamination in area 17 of the visual cortex of macaca mulatta. *J. Neurocytol.*, **3**, 619–629

BIRCH, D.G. BERSON, E.L. and SANDBERG, M.A. (1984) Diurnal rhythm in the human rod ERG. *Invest. Ophthalmol. Vis. Sci.*, **25**, 236–238

BLASDEL, G.G. and LUND, J.S. (1983) Termination of afferent axons in macaque striate cortex. *J. Neurosci.*, **3**, 1389–1413

BLAUROCK, A.E. and WILKINS, M.H.F. (1972) Structure of retinal photoreceptor membranes. *Nature*, **236**, 313–314

BLUNT, M.J., WENDELL-SMITH, C.P., PAISLEY, P.B. and BALDWIN, F. (1967) Oxidative enzyme activity in macroglia and axons of cat optic nerve. *J. Anat.*, **101**, 13–26

BONE, R.A. and LANDRUM, J.T. (1984) Macular pigment in Henle fiber membranes: a model for Haidinger's brushes. *Vision Res.*, **24**, 103–108

BOYCOTT, B.B. and DOWLING, J.E. (1969) Organization of the primate retina: light microscopy. *Philos. Trans. R. Soc. Lond. Ser. B Biol. Sci.*, **255**, 109–176

BOYCOTT, B.B. and KOLB, H. (1973) The horizontal cells of the rhesus monkey retina. *J. Comp. Neurol.*, **148**, 115–139

BOYCOTT, B.B. and WÄSSLE, H. (1974) The morphological types of ganglion cells of the domestic cat's retina. *J. Physiol.*, **240**, 397–419

BRINDLEY, G.S. (1972) The variability of the human striate cortex. *J. Physiol.*, **225**, P1–P3

BROOKE, R.N.L., DOWNER, J. DE C. and POWELL, T.P.S. (1965) Centrifugal fibres to the retina in the monkey and cat. *Nature*, **207**, 1365–1367

BROWN, P.K. and WALD, G. (1964) Visual pigments in single rods and cones of the human retina. *Science*, **144**, 145–151

BULLIER, J. and KENNEDY, H. (1983) Projection of the lateral geniculate nucleus onto cortical area V2 in the macaque monkey. *Exp. Brain Res.*, **53**, 168–172

BUNT, A.H., HENDRICKSON, A.E., LUND, J.S, LUND, R.D. and FUCHS, A.F. (1975) Monkey retinal ganglion cells: morphometric analysis and tracing of axonal projections, with a consideration of the peroxidase technique. *J. Comp. Neurol.*, **164**, 265–286

CAJAL, S.R. (1893) *La Retine des Vertebrés*. English version translated by D. Maguire and R.W. Rodieck in *The Vertebrate Retina* by R.W. Rodieck, San Francisco, Freeman, 1973

CAMPBELL, A.W. (1905) *Histological Studies on the Localisation of Cerebral Function*. London: Cambridge University Press. Cited by Whitnall (1932)

CAMPION, J., LATTO, R. and SMITH, Y.M. (1983) Is blindsight an effect of scattered light, spared cortex, and near-threshold vision? *Behav. Brain Sci.*, **6**, 423–486

CHALUPA, L.M., COYLE, R.S. and LINDSLEY, D.B. (1976) Effect of pulvinar lesions on visual pattern discrimination in monkeys. *J. Neurophysiol.*, **39**, 354–369

CLELAND, B.G. and LEVICK, W.R. (1974a) Brisk and sluggish concentrically organized ganglion cells in the cat's retina. *J. Physiol.*, **240**, 421–456

CLELAND, B.G. and LEVICK, W.R. (1974b) Properties of rarely encountered types of ganglion cells in the cat's retina and an overall classification. *J. Physiol.*, **240**, 457–492

COHEN, A.I. (1965) Some electron microscopic observations on interreceptor contacts in the human and macaque retinae. *J. Anat.*, **99**, 595–610

CRESCITELLI, F. (1972) The visual cells and visual pigments of the vertebrate eye. In *Photochemistry of Vision*, edited by H.J.A. Dartnall, *Handbook of Sensory Physiology Volume VII/I*, pp. 245–363. Berlin: Springer Verlag

DAMASIO, A.R. and DAMASIO, M. (1983) The anatomic basis of pure alexia. *Neurology*, **33**, 1573–1583

DANIEL, P.M. and WHITTERIDGE, D. (1961) The representation of the visual field on the cerebral cortex in monkeys. *J. Physiol.*, **159**, 203–221

DARTNALL, H.J.A., BOWMAKER, J.K. and MOLLON, J.D. (1983) Human visual pigments: microspectrophotometric results from the eyes of seven persons. *Proc. R. Soc. Lond. B. Biol.Sci.*, **220**, 115–130

DE MONASTERIO, F.M. (1978) Properties of concentrically organized X- and Y-ganglion cells of macaque retina. *J. Neurophysiol.*, **41**, 1394–1417

DESIMONE, R. and GROSS, C.G. (1979) Visual areas in the temporal cortex of the macaque. *Brain Res.*, **178**, 363–380

DETWILER, P.B. and HODGKIN, A.L. (1979) Electrical coupling between cones in turtle retina. *J. Physiol.*, **291**, 75–100

DINEEN, J.T. and HENDRICKSON, A. (1983) Overlap of retinal and prestriate cortical pathways in the primate pretectum. *Brain Res.*, **278**, 250–254

DOW, B.M., SNYDER, Z.A., VAUTIN, R.G. and BAUER, R. (1981) Magnification factor and receptive field size in foveal striate cortex of the monkey. *Exp. Brain Res.*, **44**, 213–228

DOWLING, J.E. and BOYCOTT, B.B. (1966) Organization of the primate retina: electron microscopy. *Proc. R. Soc. Lond B Biol.Sci.* **166**, 80–111

DOWLING, J.E., EHINGER, B. and FLOREN, I. (1980) Fluorescence and electron microscopical observations on the amine-accumulating neurons of the cebus monkey retina. *J. Comp. Neurol.*, **192**, 665–686

DRASDO, N. (1977) The neural representation of visual space. *Nature*, **266**, 554–556

DROZ, B. (1963) Dynamic conditions of proteins in the visual cells of rats and mice as shown by autoradiography with labeled amino acids. *Anat. Rec.*, **145**, 157–167

EHINGER, B. (1983) Connexions between retinal neurons with identified neurotransmitters. *Vision Res.*, **23**, 1281–1291

ENOCH, J.M. (1959) Receptor amblyopia. *Am. J. Ophthalmol.*, **48**, 262–273

ENOCH, J.M. (1963) Optical properties of retinal receptors. *J. Opt. Soc. Am.*, **53**, 71–85

ENOCH, J.M., VAN LOO, J.A. and OKUN, E. (1973) Realignment of visual photoreceptors disturbed in orientation secondary to retinal detachment. *Invest. Ophthalmol.*, **12**, 849–853

ENROTH-CUGELL, C. and ROBSON, J.G. (1966) The contrast sensitivity of retinal ganglion cells of the cat. *J. Physiol.*, **187**, 517–552

ENROTH-CUGELL, C. and ROBSON, J.G. (1984) Functional characteristics and diversity of cat retinal ganglion cells. Basic characteristics and quantitative description. *Invest. Ophthalmol. Vis. Sci.*, **25**, 250–267

FISHER, S.K., PFEFFER, B.A. and ANDERSON, D.H. (1983) Both rod and cone disc shedding are related to light onset in the cat. *Invest. Ophthalmol. Vis. Sci.*, **24**, 844–856

FOOS, R.Y. and MIYAMASU, W. (1973) Synaptic analysis of inner plexiform layer in human retina. *J. Comp. Neurol.*, **147**, 447–454

FRIES, W. and DISTEL, H. (1983) Large layer VI neurons of monkey striate cortex (Meynert cells) project to the superior colliculus. *Proc. R. Soc. Lond. B Biol. Sci.*, **219**, 53–59

GALLEGO, A. (1971) Horizontal and amacrine cells in the mammal's retina. *Vision Res.* **11** (Suppl.), 33–50

GALLEGO, A. and CRUZ, J. (1965) Mammalian retina: Association nerve cells in ganglion cell layer. *Science*, **150**, 1313–1314

GALLEGO, A. and SOBRINO, J.A. (1975) Short-axon horizontal cells of the monkey's retina. *Vision Res.*, **15**, 747–748

GRASSE, K.L. and CYNADER, M.S. (1984) Electrophysiology of lateral and dorsal terminal nuclei of the cat accessory optic system. *J. Neurophysiol.*, **51**, 276–293

HAYREH, S.S. (1963) Arteries of the orbit in the human being. *Br. J. Surg.*, **50**, 938–953

HAYREH, S.S. (1970) Pathogenesis of visual field defects. Role of the ciliary circulation. *Br. J. Ophthalmol.*, **54**, 289–311

HAYREH, S.S. (1972) Optic disc changes in glaucoma. *Br. J. Ophthalmol.*, **56**, 175–185

HEBEL, R. and HOLLÄNDER, H. (1983) Size and distribution of ganglion cells in the human retina. *Anat. Embryol.*, **168**, 125–136

HELLER, J.A. (1976) A specific receptor for retinal binding protein as detected by the binding of human and bovine retinal binding protein to pigment epithelial cells. *Am. J. Ophthalmol.*, **81**, 93–97

HENKIND, P. (1967) Radial peripapillary capillaries of the retina. 1. Anatomy: human and comparative. *Br. J. Ophthalmol.*, **51**, 115–123

HIRSCH, J. and HYLTON, R. (1984) Quality of the primate photoreceptor lattice and limits of spatial vision. *Vision Res.*, **24**, 347–356

HITCHCOCK, P.F. and HICKEY, T.L. (1980) Ocular dominance columns: evidence for their presence in humans. *Brain Res.*, **182**, 176–179

HOGAN, M.J., WOOD, I. and STEINBERG, R.M. (1974) Phagocytosis by pigment epithelium of human retinal cones. *Nature*, **252**, 305–307

HOYT, W.F. and LUÍS, O. (1962) Visual fiber anatomy in the infrageniculate pathway of the primate. Uncrossed and crossed retinal quadrant fiber projections studied with Nauta silver stain. *Arch. Ophthalmol.*, **68**, 94–106

HUBEL, D.H. and FREEMAN, D.C. (1977) Projection into the visual field of ocular dominance columns in macaque monkey. *Brain Res.*, **122**, 336–343

HUBEL, D.H., LeVAY, S. and WIESEL, T.N. (1975) Mode of termination of retinotectal fibers in macaque monkey: an autoradiographic study. *Brain Res.*, **96**, 25–40

HUBEL, D.H. and WIESEL, T.N. (1974) Uniformity of monkey striate cortex: a parallel relationship between field size, scatter and magnification factor. *J. Comp. Neurol.*, **158**, 295–306

HUBEL, D.H. and WIESEL, T.N. (1977) Ferrier lecture. Functional architecture of macaque monkey visual cortex. *Proc. R. Soc. Lond. B Biol. Sci.*, **198**, 1–59

HUBEL, D.H., WIESEL, T.N. and STRYKER, M.P. (1978) Anatomical demonstration of orientation columns in macaque monkey. *J. Comp. Neurol.*, **177**, 361–380

HUGHES, A. and WÄSSLE, H. (1976) The cat optic nerve: fiber total count and diameter spectrum. *J. Comp. Neurol.*, **169**, 171–184

IKEDA, H. and WRIGHT, M.J. (1976) Properties of LGN cells in kittens reared with convergent squint: a neurophysiological demonstration of amblyopia. *Exp. Brain Res.*, **25**, 63–78

ILLING, R.B. and WÄSSLE, H. (1981) The retinal projection to the thalamus in the cat: a quantitative investigation and a comparison with the retinotectal pathway. *J. Comp. Neurol.*, **202**, 265–286

ITAYA, S.K. and VAN HOESEN, G.W. (1983) Retinal projections to the inferior and medial pulvinar nuclei in the old-world monkey. *Brain Res.*, **269**, 223–230

KAAS, J.H., GUILLERY, R.W., and ALLMAN, J.M. (1972) Some principles of organization in the dorsal lateral geniculate nucleus. *Brain Behav. Evol.*, **6**, 253–299

KOERNER, F. and TEUBER, H.L. (1973) Visual field defects after missile injuries to the geniculo-striate pathway in man. *Exp. Brain Res.*, **18**, 88–113

KOLB, H. (1970) Organization of the outer plexiform layer of the primate retina: electron microscopy of Golgi-impregnated cells. *Philos. Trans. R. Soc. Lond. Ser. B Biol. Sci.*, **258**, 263–283

KOLB, H. (1974) The connections between horizontal cells and photoreceptors in the retina of the cat: electron microscopy of Golgi preparations. *J. Comp. Neurol.*, **155**, 1–14

KOLB, H. (1979) Inner plexiform layer in the retina of the cat — electron microscopic observations. *J. Neurocytol.*, **8**, 295–330

KOLB, H., BOYCOTT, B.B. and DOWLING, J.E. (1969) A second type of midget bipolar cell in the primate retina. *Philos. Trans. R. Soc. Lond. Ser. B Biol. Sci.*, **255**, 177–184

KROLL, A.J. and MACHEMER, R. (1969) Experimental retinal detachment in the owl monkey. *Am. J. Ophthalmol.*, **67**, 117–130

KUPFER, C. (1965) The distribution of cell size in the lateral geniculate nucleus of man following transneuronal cell atrophy. *J. Neuropathol. Exp. Neurol.*, **24**, 653–661

KUPFER, C., CHUMBLEY, L. and DOWNER, J. DE C. (1967) Quantitative histology of optic nerve, optic tract and lateral geniculate nucleus of man. *J. Anat.*, **101**, 393–401

LASANSKY, A. (1972) Cell junctions at the outer synaptic layer of the retina. *Invest. Ophthalmol.*, **11**, 265–275

LATIES, A.M. and ENOCH, J.M. (1971) An analysis of retinal orientation: Angular relationship of neighbouring photoreceptors. *Invest. Ophthalmol.*, **10**, 69–77

LATIES, A.M., LIEBMAN, P.A. and CAMPBELL, C.E.M. (1968) Photoreceptor orientation in the primate eye. *Nature*, **218**, 172–173

LA VAIL, M.M. (1976) Rod outer segment disc shedding in relation to cyclic lighting. *Exp. Eye Res.*, **23**, 277–280

LEGER, L., SAKAI, K., SALVERT, D., TOURET, M. and JOUVET, M. (1975) Delineation of dorsal lateral geniculate afferents from the cat brain stem as visualized by the horseradish peroxidase technique. *Brain Res.*, **93**, 490–496

LEVENTHAL, A.G., RODIECK, R.W. and DREHER, B. (1981) Retinal ganglion cell classes in the Old World monkey: morphology and central projections. *Science*, **213**, 1139–1142

LOWENSTEIN, O., MURPHY, S.B. and LOEWENFELD, I.E. (1953) Functional evaluation of the pupillary light reflex pathways. *Arch. Ophthalmol.*, **49**, 656–670

LUDVIGH, E. (1941) Extrafoveal visual acuity as measured with Snellen test-letters. *Am. J. Ophthalmol.*, **24**, 303–310

LUND, J.S. (1973) Organization of neurons in the visual cortex area 17 of the monkey (*Macaca mulatta*). *J. Comp. Neurol.*, **147**, 455–496

LUND, J.S., HENRY, G.H., MACQUEEN, C.L. and HARVEY, A.R. (1979) Anatomical organization of the primary visual cortex (area 17) of the cat. A comparison with area 17 of the macaque monkey. *J. Comp. Neurol.*, **184**, 599–618

LUND, J.S., LUND, R.D., HENDRICKSON, A.E., BUNT, A.H. and FUCHS, A.F. (1975) The origin of efferent pathways from the primary visual cortex, Area 17, of the macaque monkey as shown by retrograde transport of horseradish peroxidase. *J. Comp. Neurol.*, **164**, 287–304

MACKO, K.A., JARVIS, C.D., KENNEDY, C., MIYAOKA, M., SHINOHARA, M., SOKOLOFF, L. and MISHKIN, M. (1982) Mapping the primate visual system with $(2-^{14}C)$-deoxyglucose. *Science*, **218**, 394–397

MALPELI, J.G. and BAKER, F.H. (1975) The representation of the visual field in the lateral geniculate nucleus of *Macaca mulatta*. *J. Comp. Neurol.*, **161**, 569–594

MANDELBAUM, J. and SLOAN, L.L. (1947) Peripheral visual acuity. *Am. J. Ophthalmol.*, **30**, 581–588

MARC, R. and SPERLING, H.G. (1977) Chromatic organization of primate cones. *Science*, **196**, 454–456

MARIANI, A.P. (1984) Bipolar cells in monkey retina selective for the cones likely to be blue-sensitive. *Nature*, **308**, 184–186

MARINO, R. and RASMUSSEN, T. (1968) Visual field changes after temporal lobectomy in man. *Neurology*, **18**, 825–835

MARKS, W.B., DOBELLE, W.H. and MacNICHOL, E.F., Jr (1964) Visual pigments of single primate cones. *Science*, **143**, 1181–1182

MARSHALL, J., GRINDLE, J., ANSELL, P.L. and BORWEIN, B. (1979) Convolution in human rods: an ageing process. *Br. J. Ophthalmol.* **63**, 181–187

MINCKLER, D.S. (1980) The organization of nerve fiber bundles in the primate optic nerve head. *Arch. Ophthalmol.*, **98**, 1630–1636

MISSOTTEN, M.L. (1965) The synapses in the human retina. In *The Structure of the Eye II. Symposium*, edited by J. W. Rohen, pp. 17–28. Stuttgart: Schattauer

MIZUNO, N., ITOH, K., UCHIDA, K., UEMURA-SUMI, M. and MATSUSHIMA, R. (1982) A retino-pulvinar projection in the macaque monkey as visualized by the use of anterograde transport of horseradish peroxidase. *Neurosci. Lett.*, **30**, 199–204

MOORE, R.Y. (1973) Retinohypothalamic projection in mammals: a comparative study. *Brain Res.*, **49**, 403–409

NOBACK, C.R. and METTLER, F. (1973) Centrifugal fibers to the retina in the rhesus monkey. *Brain Behav. Evol.*, **7**, 382–399

O'CONNELL, J.E.A. (1973) The anatomy of the optic chiasma and heteronymous hemianopia. *J. Neurol. Neurosurg. Psychiat.*, **36**, 710–723

OPPEL, O. (1967) Untersuchungen über die Verteilung und Zahl der retinalen Ganglienzellen beim Menschen. *Graefe's Arch. Clin. Exp. Ophthalmol.*, **172**, 1–22

ØSTERBERG, G.A. (1935) Topography of the layer of rods and cones in the human retina. *Acta Ophthalmol. [Suppl.]*, **6**

PASIK, T., PASIK, P. and HAMORI, J. (1973) Nucleus of the

accessory optic tract. Light and electron microscopic study in normal monkeys and after eye enucleation. *Exp. Neurol.*, **41**, 612–627

PERRY, V.H. and COWEY, A. (1981) The morphological correlates of X- and Y-like retinal ganglion cells in the retina of monkeys. *Exp. Brain Res.*, **43**, 226–228

PHILLIPS, C.G., ZEKI, S. and BARLOW, H.B. (1984) Localization of function in the cerebral cortex: past, present and future. *Brain*, **107**, 327–361

POLYAK, S. (1941) *The Retina*. Chicago: University of Chicago Press

POLYAK, S. (1957) *The Vertebrate Visual System*. Chicago: University of Chicago Press

POTTS, A.M., HODGES, D., SHELMAN, C.B., FRITZ, K.J., LEVY, N.S. and MANGNALL, Y. (1972a) Morphology of the primate optic nerve. I. Method and total fiber count. *Invest Ophthalmol.*, **11**, 980–988

POTTS, A.M., HODGES, D., SHELMAN, C.B., FRITZ, K.J., LEVY, N.S. and MANGNALL, Y. (1972b) Morphology of the primate optic nerve. II. Total fiber size distribution and fiber density distribution. *Invest. Ophthalmol.*, **11**, 989–1003

RAVIOLA, E. (1976) Intercellular junctions in outer plexiform layer of retina. *Invest. Ophthalmol.*, **15**, 881–894

RAVIOLA, E. and GILULA, N.B. (1973) Gap junctions between photoreceptor cells in the vertebrate retina. *Proc. Natl Acad. Sci. USA*, **70**, 1677–1681

REALE, E., LUCIANO, L. and SPITZNAS, M. (1978) Communicating junctions of the human sensory retina. A freeze-fracture study. *Graefe's Arch. Clin. Exp. Ophthalmol.*, **208**, 77–92

REPÉRANT, J. and GALLEGO, A. (1976) Fibres centrifuges dans la rétine humaine. *Arch. Anat. Microsc. Morphol Exp.*, **65**, 103–120

RODIECK, R.W. and RUSHTON, W.A.H. (1976) Cancellation of rod signals by cones, and cone signals by rods in the cat retina. *J. Physiol.*, **254**, 775–785

ROVAMO, J. and VIRSU, V. (1979) An estimation and application of the human cortical magnification factor. *Exp. Brain Res.*, **37**, 495–510

ROWE, M.H. and STONE, J. (1976) Properties of ganglion cells in the visual streak of the cat's retina. *J. Comp. Neurol.*, **169**, 99–126

RUSHTON, W.A.H. (1957) Physical measurement of cone pigment in the living human eye. *Nature*, **179**, 571–573

SADUN, A.A., SCHAECHTER, J.D. and SMITH, L.E.H. (1984) A retinohypothalamic pathway in man: light mediation of circadian rhythms. *Brain Res.*, **302**, 371–378

SCHOLES, J.H. (1975) Colour receptors, and their synaptic connexions, in the retina of a cyprinid fish. *Philos. Trans. R. Soc. Lond. Ser. B Biol. Sci.*, **270**, 61–118

SCHWARTZ, E.A. (1973) Responses of single rods in the retina of the turtle. *J. Physiol.*, **232**, 503–514

SNODDERLEY, D.M., BROWN, P.K., DELORI, F.C. and AURAN, J.D. (1984a) The macula pigment. I. Absorbance spectra, localization and discrimination from other yellow pigments in primate retinas. *Invest. Ophthalmol. Vis. Sci.*, **25**, 660–673

SNODDERLEY, D.M., BROWN, P.K., DELORI, F.C. and AURAN, J.D. (1984b) The macula pigment. II. Spatial distribution in

primate retina. *Invest. Ophthalmol. Vis. Sci.*, **25**, 674–685

SJØSTRAND, F.S. (1961) Electron microscopy of the retina. In *The Structures of the Eye*, edited by G.K. Smelser, pp. 1–28. New York: Academic Press

SPALDING, J.M.K. (1952) Wounds of the visual pathway: I. The visual radiation. *J. Neurol. Neurosurg. Psychiatr.*, **15**, 99–109

STABELL, V. and STABELL, B. (1980) Variation in density of macular pigmentation and in short-wave cone sensitivity with eccentricity. *J. Opt. Soc. Am.*, **70**, 706–711

STANWORTH, A.J. and NAYLOR, E.J. (1955) The measurement and clinical significance of the Haidinger effect. *Trans. Ophthalmol. Soc. UK*, **75**, 67–78

STEELE, E.J. and BLUNT, M.J. (1956) The blood supply of the optic nerve and chiasma in man. *J. Anat.*, **90**, 486–493

STONE, J. and HOFFMAN, K.P. (1972) Very slow-conducting ganglion cells in the cat's retina: a major, new functional type? *Brain Res.*, **43**, 610–616

STRAATSMA, B.R., FOOS, R.Y., HECKENLIVELY, J.R. and TAYLOR, G.N. (1981) Myelinated retinal nerve fibres. *Am. J. Ophthalmol.*, **91**, 25–38

STRACHAN, I.M. and CLEARY, P.E. (1972) The study of the human optic nerve with elliptically polarised light. In *The Optic Nerve*, edited by J.S. Cant, pp. 292–297. London: Henry Kimpton

SWADLOW, H.A. (1983) Efferent systems of primary visual cortex: a review of structure and function. *Brain Res. Rev.*, **6**, 1–24

SZAMIER, R.B., BERSON, E.L., KLEIN, R. and MEYERS, S. (1979) Sex-linked retinitis pigmentosa — ultrastructure of photoreceptors and pigment epithelium. *Invest. Ophthalmol.*, **18**, 145–160

SZENTÁGOTHAI, J. (1973) Neuronal and synaptic architecture of the lateral geniculate nucleus. In *Handbook of Sensory Physiology VII/3*, edited by R. Jung, pp. 141–176. Berlin: Springer Verlag

TEUBER, H-L., BATTERSBY, W.S. and BENDER, M. (1960) *Visual Field Defects after Penetrating Missile Wounds of the Brain*. Cambridge: Harvard University Press

TIGGES, J., BOS, J. and TIGGES, M. (1977) An autoradiographic investigation of the subcortical visual system in chimpanzee. *J. Comp. Neurol.*, **172**, 367–380

TREVARTHEN, C.B. (1968) Two mechanisms of vision in primates. *Psychol. Forsch.*, **31**, 299–327

UGA, S., NAKAO, F., MIMURA, M. and IKUI, H. (1970) Some new findings on the fine structure of the human photoreceptor cells. *J. Electron Microsc.*, **19**, 71–84

VRABEC, FR. (1966) The temporal raphe of the human retina *Am. J. Ophthalmol.*, **62**, 926–938

WÄSSLE, H., BOYCOTT, B.B. and ILLING, R.B. (1981) Morphology and mosaic of on-and-off-beta cells in the cat retina and some functional considerations. *Proc. R. Soc. Lond. B Biol. Sci.*, **212**, 177–195

WEALE, R.A.(1958) Retinal summation and human visual threshold. *Nature*, **181**, 154–156

WEALE, R.A. (1959) Photo-sensitive reactions in fovea of normal and cone-monochromatic observers. *Opt. Acta*, **6**, 158–174

cating junctions of the human sensory retina. A freeze-fracture study. *Graefe's Arch. Clin. Exp. Ophthalmol.*, **208**, 77–92

WEBB, S.V. and KAAS, J.H. (1976) The sizes and distribution of ganglion cells in the retina of the owl monkey *Aotus trivirgatus*. *Vision Res.*, **16**, 1247–1254

WERBLIN, F.S. and DOWLING, J.E. (1969) Organization of the retina of the mudpuppy, *Necturus maculosus*. II. Intracellular recording. *J. Neurophysiol.*, **32**, 339–355

WESTHEIMER, G. and BLAIR, S.M. (1974) Unit activity in accessory optic system in alert monkeys. *Invest. Ophthalmol.*, **13**, 533–534

WHITNALL, S.E. (1932) *The Anatomy of the Human Orbit and Accessory Organs of Vision*. Oxford: Oxford University Press

WOLFF, E. (1948) *The Anatomy of the Eye and Orbit*. London: H.K. Lewis

WOLTER, J.R. (1974) Electron microscopic demonstration of centrifugal nerve fibers in the human optic nerve. *Graefe's Arch. Clin. Exp. Ophthalmol.*, **210**, 31–42

WONG-RILEY, M.T.T. (1972) Neuronal and synaptic organization of the normal dorsal lateral geniculate nucleus of the squirrel monkey, *Saimiri sciureus*. *J. Comp. Neurol.*, **144**, 25–60

WONG-RILEY, M.T.T. (1977) Connections between the pulvinar nucleus and the prestriate cortex in the squirrel monkey as revealed by peroxidase histochemistry and autoradiography. *Brain Res.*, **134**, 249–268

WURTZ, R.H. and ALBANO, J.E. (1980) Visual-motor function of the superior colliculus. *Annu. Rev. Neurosci.*, **3**, 189–226

YOUNG, R. (1967) The renewal of photoreceptor cell outer segments. *J. Cell Biol.*, **33**, 61–72

YOUNG, R. (1971) The renewal of rod and cone outer segments in the rhesus monkey. *J. Cell. Biol.*, **49**, 303–318

YOUNG, R.W. (1974) Biogenesis and renewal of visual cell outer segment membranes. *Exp. Eye Res.*, **18**, 215–223

YOUNG, R.W. (1976) Visual cells and the concept of renewal. *Invest. Ophthalmol.*, **15**, 700–725

YOUNG, R.W. (1978) Daily rhythm of shedding and degradation of rod and cone outer segment membrane in chick retina. *Invest. Ophthalmol.*, **17**, 105–116

YUKIE, M. and IWAI, E. (1981) Direct projection from the dorsal lateral geniculate nucleus to the prestriate cortex in macaque monkeys. *J. Comp. Neurol.*, **201**, 81–97

ZEKI, S.M. (1978a) Functional specialization in the visual cortex of the rhesus monkey. *Nature*, **274**, 423–428

ZEKI, S.M. (1978b) Uniformity and diversity of structure and function in rhesus monkey prestriate visual cortex. *J. Physiol.*, **277**, 273–290

ZEKI, S.M. (1980) The representation of colours in the cerebral cortex. *Nature*, **284**, 412–417

ZEKI, S.M. (1983) The distribution of wavelength and orientation selective cells in different areas of monkey visual cortex. *Proc. R. Soc. Lond. B Biol. Sci.*, **217**, 449–470

2

The psychology of vision

Jim Gilchrist

Understanding visual perception

The study of visual perception is a multidisciplinary adventure. Vision begins with the information in the retinal image, which may be studied through physics, and is ultimately mediated through the responses and connection of visual neurones, which may be studied through physiology. The perceptual interpretation of the image which gives the actual experience of seeing may be studied through psychophysics, the technique of measuring subjective visual responses developed by Gustav Fechner (1860). The psychology of vision is really a bridge spanning all three of these disciplines, though its development probably owes most to psychophysics.

In recent years, visual psychology has advanced considerably through the study of vision as information processing. During the 1960s, psychophysical studies by Fergus Campbell and others at Cambridge showed that many of the information processing principles used in optical physics could also be applied to vision. This insight inspired much further psychophysical research which, alongside important physiological studies, particularly those of David Hubel and Torsten Wiesel at Harvard, led to many significant developments in understanding vision. (*See* Hubel (1982) and Wiesel (1982) for fascinating accounts of their work, and Frisby (1979, Chap. 3) for an excellent introduction to visual neurophysiology.)

The information processing approach forces the distinction between processes and mechanisms in perception. As an example, consider the problem of trying to understand how a computer plays chess. Probes could be placed inside the machine to measure the voltages on individual pins of integrated circuits, rather like putting electrodes into brain cells and measuring their responses. Although the responses of the computer may be interesting, we have virtually no chance of inferring from these responses how the computer plays chess. It is necessary to distinguish between what the computer hardware does and what the program software does, and understanding one does not necessarily help in understanding the other. Similarly, to understand vision the processes of perception must be distinguished from the mechanisms of brain physiology. This sort of analogy has recently encouraged an approach to vision research known as computational theory, closely associated with the work of David Marr at the Massachusetts Institute of Technology (MIT). Marr pointed out that complex processes must be explained at a number of levels, and argued that, in vision research, a start should be made by asking what the visual system is trying to achieve. If the goals of visual processing can be accurately identified, possible ways can be devised of achieving them and we may then work towards understanding the mechanisms by which the brain actually does achieve them. In the period since the mid-1970s, this approach has produced a good deal of new theory about visual processing which has been tested using psychophysical techniques. Marr's work is summarized in one volume (Marr, 1982), which makes essential reading.

The aim of this chapter is to provide an introduction to the psychology of vision. A number of aspects of visual perception and current explanations of how they work will be reviewed. Many interesting and important topics cannot be covered in a chapter of this size, e.g. after-effects, illusions and perceptual constancies. In particular, the study of colour vision has been omitted because, in spite of its perceptual significance, it has been much less central to the recent development of perceptual theory than, for example, luminance, stereo and movement processing. Also, early visual perception is primarily dependent on luminance information rather than on colour.

Levels of visual processing

Perceptual interpretation of visual information involves building mental images or representations of the scene (Shepard, 1978). Marr (1980) suggests that visual representations are developed through a hierarchy of processing stages, and he identifies three principal levels. First, a primal sketch is created by locating the edges of objects in the scene and constructing their outline shapes. This is followed by a two-and-a-half dimensional ($2\frac{1}{2}$ D) sketch in which surface characteristics such as curvature, texture and colour are determined. Perception at this stage is considered to depend upon the position from which the scene is viewed, and is called viewer-centred. Finally, a three-dimensional (3 D) model representation is developed through which the complete structure of objects can be appreciated. This full representation is considered to be object-centred, so the observer may judge what an object would look like from any viewpoint even though it may only be seen from one viewpoint. This is the stage of 'turning' something over in the mind' (Shepard and Metzler, 1971; Cooper and Shepard, 1984). (*See* Oatley (1978) for a readable introduction to perceptual representation and processing.)

Our study in this chapter is limited to the 'early' visual processes of edge detection and some aspects of surface perception. These form the basis of, and are more clearly understood than, higher-level 'cognitive' processing (*see* Spoehr and Lehmkuhle (1982) for a text dealing with aspects of higher-level processing and Pinker (1984) for a review of recent cognition research). I will begin by considering what information is available for edge detection and how it can be specified.

Specifying visual information

The image received on the retina is just a pattern of different light intensities and wavelengths which may change from moment to moment. These spatial and temporal variations in the image provide the only information available for visual processing. Objects can be seen only if their luminance and/or colour distribution differs from that of their background. Pictures can be created with the same luminance at every point, so that objects are distinguished from backgrounds only by colour differences, but subjects have difficulty in focusing on such isoluminant stimuli (Wolfe, 1983). This indicates that luminance differences are essential for accurate edge perception.

The spatial information in a scene can be determined by moving a small photocell across it and measuring the luminance of every point. The average of these measurements is the mean luminance of the scene and determines the state of adaptation of

the eye. The luminance of any individual point will be the product of the amount of light falling on it (*illuminance*) and the amount it reflects (*reflectance*), assuming the surface on which the point lies is not a light source. Spatial luminance variations are usually, therefore, caused by illuminance changes, e.g. shadows, reflectance changes, e.g. patterned wallpaper, or both. In some cases, luminance variations occur, even when illuminance and surface reflectance are uniform, due to irregularities in surface curvature or texture, e.g. wood-chip wallpaper. Knowing whether a luminance change results from illuminance or reflectance differences is important for accurate perception of the lightness and colour of surfaces (Land and McCann, 1971; Land, 1977; Gilchrist, 1979). In early processing, however, the priority is edge detection; classification of edges comes later (Gilchrist, Delman and Jacobsen, 1983). Edges are generally defined by the following characteristics (*Figure 2.1*):

1. Contrast — the magnitude of a luminance change between two image points. The contrast indicates the 'strength' of an edge and determines how easily it can be seen.
2. Spatial frequency — the 'scale' at which luminance changes occur in the image. High spatial frequencies correspond to many luminance changes between two points and are, therefore, associated with fine detail or texture. Low spatial frequencies correspond to changes which extend over larger areas in the image such as those produced by large objects or shadows on a surface.

A careful study of the gratings in *Figure 2.1* reveals that changing the contrast or spatial frequency of a sine-wave also changes the luminance gradient of the edge. The luminance gradient is the rate of luminance change across the image. Steep luminance gradients give sharp edges and shallow gradients give smooth (or blurred) ones (*Figure 2.2a, b*).

Although this figure shows a change of edge gradient with fixed contrast and spatial frequency, the effect can, in fact, be explained by considering each edge as consisting of a number of components of different contrast and spatial frequency. This is the principle of frequency analysis, a general technique which may be used for analysing luminance variations in an image, developed by the eighteenth century mathematician Joseph Fourier. The principle of Fourier synthesis (*Figure 2.2c*) is simply that any waveform, however complicated, can be built up from a number of sine-waves of different frequencies and amplitudes. The same principle is used in music synthesizers which can build up sounds of any complexity from sine-wave sound profiles. Fourier analysis (*Figure 2.2d*) is just the

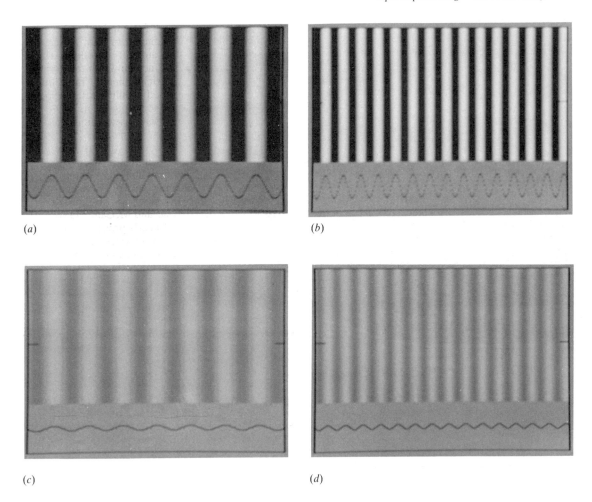

(a)

(b)

(c)

(d)

Figure 2.1 Contrast and spatial frequency. Pairs (a)+(c), (b)+(d): sine-wave gratings with different contrasts but the same spatial frequency. Contrast is calculated by measuring the peak and trough luminances and dividing their difference by their sum. Pairs (a)+(b), (c)+(d): different spatial frequencies but the same level of contrast. Spatial frequency is calculated by measuring the number of cycles of the waveform per degree of visual angle (1 cycle = 2 bars)

reverse process of taking a waveform and working out the set of sinusoidal frequencies it contains. Frequency analysis of visual stimuli has been widely employed since the 1960s but was, in fact, proposed in 1866 by the physicist and philosopher Ernst Mach (*see* Ratliff, 1965).

Temporal information may be determined by measuring the luminance of each image point over a period of time. The luminance profiles produced can be defined in the same terms, and analysed in the same way as those representing spatial information except that they are referred to as temporal frequency rather than spatial frequency, and are measured in cycles/s or hertz (Hz).

Optical processing — the retinal image

When an image is formed by an optical system, aberrations cause the amplitude (*contrast*) of all spatial frequencies to be reduced, and frequencies are lost if their contrast falls to zero. Knowing the amount of contrast loss for every spatial frequency gives a complete description of system quality. The relationship between contrast loss and spatial frequency is called the *modulation transfer function* (MTF) of the system. (*See* Cornsweet (1970, Chap. 12) for an introduction to frequency analysis and MTFs.)

The spatial performance of the visual system can be described by an MTF (Selwyn, 1948; Schade, 1956). The complete visual MTF is determined partly by the optical system of the eye and partly by the neural processing of the image. Since retinal image quality depends on the optical performance of the eye, it can be distinguished by referring only to the *optical transfer function* (OTF). The precise form of the ocular OTF depends critically on the pupil size, which determines the contribution of ocular aberrations, but generally shows progressive contrast reduction as spatial frequency increases with a loss of high spatial frequencies (*Figure 2.3a*). The distinction between the 'sharp' edges of a square-wave grating and the 'blurred' edges of a sine-wave is, as mentioned previously, the presence of

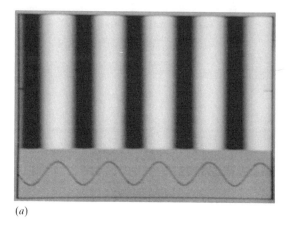

(a)

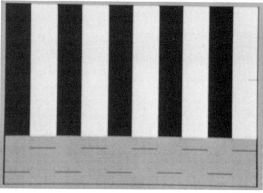

(b)

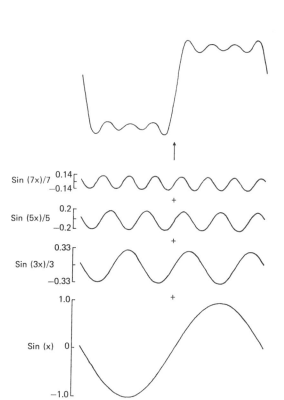

(c)

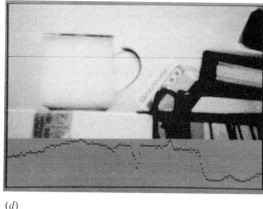

(d)

Figure 2.2 Luminance gradient and spatial frequency analysis. (*a, b*) Sine-wave and square-wave gratings with the same contrast and spatial frequency, but significantly different luminance gradients at the light/dark edge. (*c*) Fourier synthesis: square waves (or other complex waveforms) may be produced by combining a number of sine-waves of different contrast and spatial frequency. (*d*) Each line of an image has a luminance profile which can be treated as a complex waveform. Fourier analysis can be used to determine its sine-wave components

high frequency components in the former, so that high frequency loss is equivalent to blurring the image. The consequence of the ocular OTF, therefore, is a retinal image which has lower contrast and is slightly more blurred than its corresponding object (Campbell and Gubish, 1966).

The blurring out of high spatial frequencies by the eye has an advantage for visual processing. Earlier it was described how the luminance distribution in an image can be measured by taking a photometric reading at each point. The retina is organized as a large number of very small photocells, the rods and cones, which sample the image at many different points simultaneously. The spacing of the receptors determines how frequently the image is sampled. If the image contains spatial frequencies which are close to the sampling frequency and, if the sampling points are very regular, a form of image distortion called aliasing can occur (*Figure 2.3b*). Sampling frequency is highest at the fovea to increase resolution, and foveal regularity is essential for positional accuracy (*see* later), and to reduce sensitivity to noise

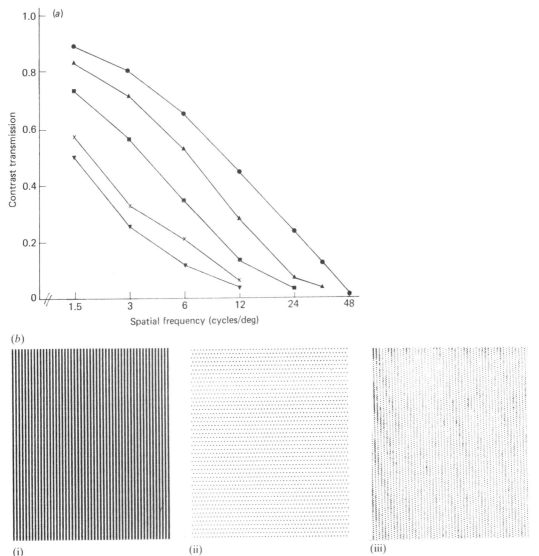

Figure 2.3 Optical performance of the eye. (*a*) The optical transfer function (OTF) with different pupil sizes shows how higher spatial frequencies are progressively filtered out. Pupil size: ●, 2 mm; ▲, 3 mm; ■, 4 mm; ×, 5 mm; ▼, 6 mm. (After Campbell and Gubisch, 1966.)

(*b*) The effect of aliasing, which would occur if very high frequencies were received at the retina. A high frequency grating (i) is sampled by an array of receptors of similar frequency (ii) and the result is a distorted moiré pattern (iii)

(Bossomaier, Snyder and Hughes, 1985). Optical aberrations effectively eliminate all spatial frequencies which may be high enough to give rise to foveal aliasing (Williams, 1985). In the peripheral retina, where the sampling frequency is lower, aliasing may be avoided by irregularity of the receptors (Yellott, 1982).

The OTF of the eye can also be used to describe the effect of defocusing the retinal image (Green and Campbell, 1965; Charman, 1979). Not only do people with refractive errors suffer a blurred image, i.e. loss of high spatial frequencies, but they also suffer reduced contrast of remaining spatial frequencies. The contrast loss at any spatial frequency increases with the amount of defocus and the ophthalmic implications of this are discussed in detail by Smith (1982). Comprehensive discussions of the eye as an optical system may be found in Charman (1983) and Fry (1984).

Neural processing — receptive fields and edge detection

The neurophysiological studies of Barlow (1953), Kuffler (1953) and Hartline and Ratliff (1957) gave the first clear indication that interpretation of the visual image begins in the retina and not in the visual cortex, and it is now known that the retina is responsible for the early processing stage of edge detection. The theoretical aspects of edge detection have been discussed by Marr and Hildreth (1980) who point out two requirements of any edge detection scheme. The first is to detect spatial luminance changes across the image. The second is to distinguish between large and small scale variations, such as shadows and texture, which may coexist in the same image area. In other words, the system must be able to measure luminance gradients at different spatial frequencies. The human visual system meets these requirements through the structure of the retinal receptive fields.

Receptive fields measure luminance gradients

Each retinal ganglion cell will only respond to a stimulus if it falls within a circular group of rods and cones known as the *receptive field* (RF) of the ganglion. Ganglion cell RFs comprise two concentric zones which produce opposite responses to spots of light falling on them (*Figure 2.4*).

The spatially opponent organization of retinal RFs means that maximum excitation of an on-centre ganglion occurs when a spot of light fills the RF centre. A larger spot which also covers part of the surround will give a lower response due to lateral inhibition, and filling the RF with light will produce

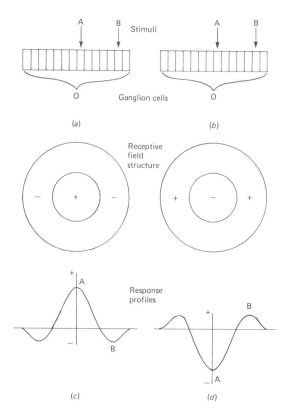

Figure 2.4 Spatially opponent receptive fields. (*a*) A spot of light falling in the central area of an 'on-centre' receptive field excites a response from the ganglion cell, while another spot falling simultaneously on the surround inhibits this response. (*b*) The situation is reversed for an 'off-centre' ganglion cell. (*c, d*) Response profiles from on and off-centre RFs show how the amount of excitation or inhibition depends on where the stimulus falls in the receptive field

minimum response. The effect of this is to make ganglion cells more sensitive to contrast than to uniform luminance in their RFs. On-centre ganglion cells respond best to light spots on a dark background and off-centre cells to dark spots on a light background.

The way that this arrangement measures the luminance gradient can be more precisely understood as follows. The two-dimensional response profile of an off-centre RF contains a strong inhibitory (negative) centre flanked by two weaker excitatory (positive) portions of the surround. The 'weighting function' of the entire RF profile can, therefore, be approximated as $+1/-2/+1$ which can further be thought of as a combination of two weighting functions of $+1/-1$. The significance of this idea becomes apparent if an edge being examined at every point by such an RF is considered (*Figure 2.5*).

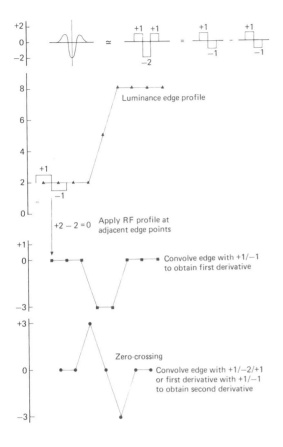

Figure 2.5 Convolution and zero-crossings. The shape of an off-centre RF response profile can be approximated by $+1/-2/+1$. If such an RF looks at every point on an edge profile, the 'convolution' of edge and RF profiles produces a result known as a 'zero-crossing' (zc). This is mathematically equivalent to taking the second derivative of the edge profile, i.e. measuring the luminance gradient

Applying the weighting function $+1/-1$ at each point on the edge profile has the effect of calculating the difference between every adjacent pair of luminance values, i.e. differentiating. Since our full RF profile represents two such profiles together, applying the $+1/-2/+1$ RF directly at each point has the effect of differentiating twice. Thus, retinal RFs actually measure the gradient of a luminance profile by computing its second derivative. The process of applying the same RF profile to every point on the edge profile is called convolution and the retina achieves this by having an array of RFs looking at every part of the edge simultaneously. Differentiating edge profiles in this way gives a result known as a zero-crossing because of the characteristic shape of the function obtained. It may then be said that the retina detects edges by locating zero-crossings in the image.

The idea that the visual system differentiates the image was also proposed by Mach in 1865 to explain the phenomenon of 'spatial induction' or 'simultaneous contrast'. This can best be seen in luminance staircase patterns, where darker bands appear on the dark side of each edge and lighter bands appear on the light side, even though the luminance across each bar of the pattern is uniform (*see* Cornsweet, 1970, p.276). Note that the same result can be obtained from *Figure 2.5* if the second derivative 'zero-crossing' profile is subtracted from the original edge profile. These contrast enhancement effects are now called Mach bands and they are important because they illustrate that the retina, not only detects edges, but also uses the results of the process to amplify them. Introductions to this form of processing may be found in Ratliff (1972) and Lindsay and Norman (1977), and a comprehensive study of lateral inhibition in the retina with details of Mach's work in Ratliff (1965). An excellent introduction to edge detection and classification, with examples of Mach bands and related illusions, may be found in Frisby (1979, Chap. 6).

Receptive fields act as spatial frequency filters

In addition to measuring luminance gradients, the RF also fulfils Marr and Hildreth's requirement for a spatial frequency filter. There are two aspects to this, related to the size and shape of the RF profile.

The convolution scheme outlined above uses an RF profile of fixed size. It can readily be seen that an RF looking at an area of the edge will be sensitive only to luminance gradients within that area. Detecting luminance gradients at different scales (spatial frequencies) therefore requires different sized RFs. It has long been established that retinal ganglion cells have different sized RFs. Small RFs are traditionally associated with high resolution foveal vision and larger ones with summation of responses from many receptors for increased sensitivity in the peripheral retina (Robson, 1975). The function of RFs as spatial frequency filters, however, alters our concept of how the retina is organized. Since foveal vision is capable of detecting low spatial frequencies as well as high ones, there must be RFs of different sizes at the fovea and, indeed, in other retinal areas too. This suggests a model of retinal organization in which small RFs are embedded within larger ones in a given retinal region, so that an area of the image falling on that region can be simultaneously analysed at a number of scales (Koenderink, 1977). This makes sense because high frequency details of a scene are always embedded within lower frequency outlines. It also enables sharp edges to be distinguished from blurred ones, because the former will have frequency components detectable at the same spatial location by a number of RF sizes. Filtering of the image at different scales is also helped by the shape of the RF. Unlike the approximate weighting function used above to illustrate differentiation, the actual retinal RF profile has a smooth shape. Indeed, the excitatory and inhibitory parts of this profile each take the form of the normal, or Gaussian, distribution which is common in statistics, and the RF profile is often described as a *difference-*

of-Gaussians (DOG) function. Convolution of an image with a Gaussian function smooths or blurs any information that does not correspond to the scale of the Gaussian. Convolution with a DOG-shaped receptive field profile has the effect of detecting only those edges (zero-crossings) that correspond to the size of the receptive field (*Figure 2.6*).

It must be remembered that each retinal RF can

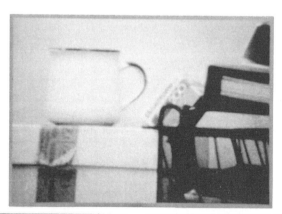

(*a*)

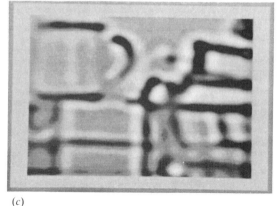

(*b*)   (*c*)

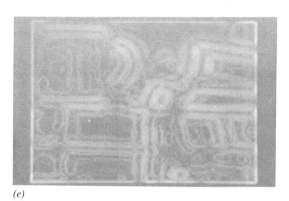

(*d*)   (*e*)

Figure 2.6 Convolution with different sized receptive fields. An original image (*a*) after convolution with a small (*b*) and a large (*c*) 'difference-of-Gaussians' receptive field profile. Note that images (*b*) and (*c*) are blurred according to the scale of the RF and edges which occur at the appropriate scale are revealed. Images (*d*) and (*e*) show the edges in (*b*) and (*c*), respectively

detect only small 'local' elements of object edges. Also, because it is circular, the RF is not sensitive to the orientation of the edge-elements it detects. At a later stage in processing, therefore, these local edge-elements must be combined into edge-segments of different orientations which, in turn, must be combined into complete 'global' outlines of the objects they represent. The simple cells of the visual cortex have RFs which are not circular and so will respond best to edges in particular orientations. This would seem to make them suitable for combining groups of edge-elements into orientated edge-segments. Marr and Hildreth (1980) propose that this could be achieved by simple cells having RFs composed of a suitable arrangement of on-centre (X+) and off-centre (X−) retinal ganglion cells.

At this stage an appreciation of a very simplified scheme for the perception of object shape can begin. Edge-elements are detected in every part of the image simultaneously by retinal RFs. At a higher level of processing, cortical neurones combine the edge-elements to extract object outlines and this process also acts on every part of the image simultaneously. This method of handling information across the whole image at the same time is called parallel processing.

The terms X+ and X− have been used in reference to spatially opponent ganglion cells. These were called X cells to distinguish them from other ganglions (Y cells) which have larger RFs and are fewer in number (Enroth-Cugell and Robson, 1966). The Y cells respond best to rapidly moving or flickering stimuli, indicating that the retina contains a system for detecting temporal as well as spatial luminance changes. Neurophysiological studies suggest that Y cells detect flicker by measuring temporal luminance gradients (Rodieck and Stone, 1965), and psychophysical evidence supports this (Wilson, 1979). Parallel processing in the visual system, therefore, incorporates both spatial and temporal pathways for edge detection. Detailed reviews of parallel X and Y pathways may be found in Lennie (1980a, b).

The concept of lateral inhibition in the receptive fields of retinal ganglion cells provides a model of early visual processing which has strong theoretical and physiological support. Recently, however, an alternative model has been proposed which operates at the level of the retinal receptors. This has been called the *intensity-dependent spatial summation* (IDS) model, the principles of which are as follows:

1. Each individual retinal receptor has a Gaussian-shaped response profile.
2. The height (magnitude) of a receptor's response is proportional to the intensity of the point of light which falls on that receptor.
3. The area under the response profile remains constant, so that bright points of light give rise to

tall narrow responses, while dim points give rise to short broad responses.

According to this scheme, the interactions that occur between the responses from a large array of retinal receptors will predict centre-surround antagonism, spatial frequency filtering, Mach bands and many other manifestations of low-level visual processing. An introductory discussion of this simple but powerful model may be found in Cornsweet (1985), and a more theoretical account is given by Cornsweet and Yellott (1985).

Spatial visual performance
Contrast sensitivity and spatial frequency channels

Since the basic requirement for edge detection is contrast and since any edge can be analysed into component sine-waves, a measurement of how much contrast is needed to detect sine-waves of different spatial frequencies provides a useful way of determining the spatial performance of the visual system. The amount of contrast needed for a grating to be just detectable is called the contrast threshold and its reciprocal is the contrast sensitivity. A graph showing the amount of contrast required to detect gratings of different spatial frequencies is known as the threshold spatial *contrast sensitivity function* (CSF) (*Figure 2.7a*; Campbell and Green, 1965a; *see* Campbell and Maffei, 1974 for an introduction).

The CSF is a form of MTF of the visual system which incorporates both the optical performance of the eye and the neural performance of the visual pathway. The threshold CSF indicates a number of interesting things about everyday vision:

1. More contrast is needed to detect fine details than large objects because sensitivity is good for lower frequencies and gets much worse as frequency increases. For example, when driving in fog, a situation where contrast is very low, the outline of another vehicle is more easily detected than the detail of characters on a number plate.
2. Since sharp edges always contain high frequencies, more contrast is needed to recognize whether an edge is sharp than to simply detect that it is present.
3. Detection of all frequencies is easier if the mean luminance is high (van Meeteran and Vos, 1972). This emphasizes the importance of good illumination for good visibility (Sheedy, Bailey and Raasch, 1984).
4. *Visual acuity* (VA) can be predicted from contrast sensitivity but not vice versa. Acuity tests measure the smallest size of detail (highest spatial frequency) which can be resolved using high

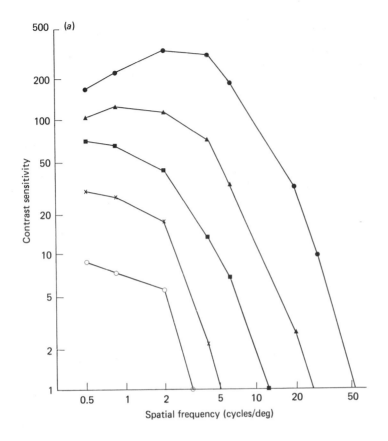

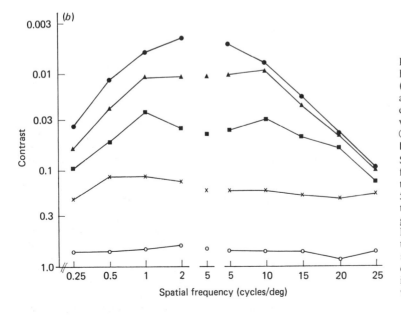

Figure 2.7 Threshold and suprathreshold contrast sensitivity functions. (*a*) Threshold contrast sensitivity against spatial frequency to different mean luminance levels (after van Meeteran and Vos, 1972). $\bigcirc$, 10^{-4}cd/m^2; $\times$, 10^{-3} cd/m^2; $\blacksquare$, 10^{-2} cd/m^2; $\blacktriangle$, 10^{-1} cd/m^2; $\bullet$, 10 cd/m^2 Suprathreshold contrast sensitivity functions obtained by fixing the contrast of a grating of spatial frequency 5 cycles/deg, and matching the contrast of higher and lower frequency gratings to that of the fixed one. Note that the upper curve represents the threshold CSF and that the sensitivities at different spatial frequencies become more equal as contrast increases (after Georgeson and Sullivan, 1975)

contrast targets. VA can therefore be found by taking the point on the threshold CSF where the graph cuts the spatial frequency axis. This shows that VA measurement indicates very little about the visual system because it represents only the upper limit of spatial performance. It is exactly like measuring hearing by finding the highest frequency tone that can be heard. In both cases vital information about other frequencies is being overlooked. It is fundamental to an understanding of vision that performance at different spatial frequencies is measured.

5. Contrast sensitivity is usually measured with vertical sine-wave gratings. Sensitivity to oblique gratings is lower than that to horizontal or vertical ones (Watanabe *et al.*, 1968).

In addition to the threshold CSF for detection of gratings, the CSF can also be plotted at levels of contrast above threshold. One way of doing this is to measure how much difference in contrast can be detected between two gratings of the same frequency. These measurements may, of course, be taken at a number of contrast levels, so it is possible to obtain a number of suprathreshold CSFs (Watanabe *et al.*, 1968; Georgeson and Sullivan, 1975). It should be noted that, as the contrast level increases, the CSF becomes flatter (*Figure 2.7b*). This indicates that, in good contrast, edges of any spatial frequency can be detected more or less equally.

Contrast sensitivity measures using compound gratings provide evidence that the edges detected by different RFs are processed in separate *spatial frequency channels*. Compound gratings are those consisting of more than one sinusoidal frequency component. If all frequencies were processed within a single visual channel, then summation of responses to each component should make a compound grating more visible than a simple one. Campbell and Robson (1968) showed that the visibility of compound gratings was not significantly higher than that of their most visible component alone — psychophysical evidence for mutiple channels. The notion of separate channels for different spatial frequencies explains why a stimulus can be made less visible (masked) if combined with another stimulus of similar spatial frequency, but masking does not occur if the frequencies are very different (Stromeyer and Julesz, 1972). It also indicates why adaptation to stimuli of one spatial frequency or orientation will reduce sensitivity to similar frequencies or orientations but not to different ones (Blakemore and Campbell, 1969). In fact, these principles of masking and adaptation have been used experimentally to determine the likely number of channels and their bandwidth, i.e. the range of spatial frequencies that each channel carries. Mathematical modelling based on psychophysical data indicates that at least four channels are necessary (and six channels are enough)

to account for spatial visual performance (Wilson and Bergen, 1979; Wilson, 1983). Detailed reviews of the subject of spatial frequency channels can be found in Braddick, Campbell and Atkinson (1978), Robson (1980) and Graham (1981).

Contrast sensitivity measurement has proved to be clinically valuable in detecting a range of pathological conditions (*see* Arden, 1978; Ginsburg, 1984; Hess, 1984; Woodhouse, 1987), and the principle can readily be adapted for routine use simply by using low contrast letter charts (Regan and Neima, 1983). It is interesting to note that the shape of the Mach band luminance profile discussed earlier is a mathematical transform of the CSF. This means that psychophysical measurement of the extent of Mach bands can be used as an alternative way of assessing spatial visual performance, and may provide more sensitive measures in some clinical situations, e.g. measurement of corneal oedema (Remole, 1979, 1980) and even fixation disparity measurement (Remole, 1983, 1984).

Hyperacuity

The limit of grating acuity predictable from the threshold CSF is about 50–60 cycles/deg, equivalent to a bar width of about 30″ arc. This limit is set by the spacing of the foveal cones which is about 25″ arc. In some types of visual task, however, spatial judgements can be made which are much finer than the normal acuity limit. The classic example is vernier judgement in which differences as small as 5″ can be noticed in the positions of two lines placed end to end. Another example is stereopsis which may provide depth judgements of 5″ or less. Generally, these fine spatial judgements are called hyperacuities (Westheimer, 1975). Hyperacuity can be measured using many different stimulus configurations (Westheimer and McKee, 1977). In addition to displaced vernier lines, we may judge the displacement of one dot in a regular array or from the centre of a circle, the curvature of an arc or an angular deflection of one part of a line etc. In all these examples, the critical judgement does not depend on resolving spatial separation between parts of the stimulus, but on the precision with which one part can be located relative to another. The nature of hyperacuity processing is not yet clear, though it must involve a system by which position signals from a number of cones can be averaged. Averaging, or interpolation, is likely because the mean of a set of measurements will give a more accurate estimate of position than any one measurement. It also follows that a high degree of regularity in the arrangement of foveal receptors would aid position judgements.

Although hyperacuity is usually considered in vernier terms, it is important to note that judgements of spatial displacement when a target moves from one location to another also reveal hyperacuity. This indicates that the higher level interpolation process draws on spatial and temporal information and is a significant factor in motion detection. A review of the subject is given by Westheimer (1981). Since hyperacuity processing must occur at a level of the visual pathway beyond the retina, hyperacuity performance may also be used clinically to evaluate central visual function (Enoch and Williams, 1983; Whitaker and Buckingham, 1987).

Stereopsis

Having two eyes is a major advantage in vision. First of all, edge detection is improved since binocular contrast sensitivity is some 40% higher than monocular (Campbell and Green, 1965b; *see* Blake and Fox (1973) and Blake, Sloane and Fox (1981) for comprehensive reviews of this binocular summation). In addition, stereopsis provides a way of seeing a structure in a scene. Structure-from-stereo can provide information about two-dimensional contours and three-dimensional surface shape. This is possible even when such structure is not visible monocularly, as in *random-dot stereograms* (RDS) (*Figure 2.8*), indicating the value of the process for 'camouflage breaking'. Stereopsis works by interpreting geometrical disparities between the images of each eye (*see* Moses, 1975; Frisby, 1979, Chap. 7).

When a pencil is held up vertically at eye level and then each eye closed in turn, the position of the pencil appears to change with respect to the background because each eye views it from a different location. When the monocular views are fused, the amount of horizontal disparity between the two positions of the pencil can be used to calculate its distance from the background. The smallest disparity that can be detected is a measure of stereoacuity, and may be as little as a 5″ arc. The largest disparity that can be fused without diplopia is called 'Panum's fusional limit'.

Stereo processing can be considered in two stages, the first of which involves matching the two monocular images so that fusion is possible (the correspondence stage). Gregory (1979) has shown that stereopsis is not possible in isoluminant stimuli, so it may be concluded that detection of luminance edges by each eye independently is a prerequisite for achieving correspondence. The threshold CSF indicates how much contrast is necessary for monocular edge detection, but stereoscopic CSF measurements show that higher contrast is needed to perceive depth (Frisby and Mayhew, 1978).

Random-dot stereograms were popularized by Julesz (1971) and highlight the problems of the correspondence stage. How do we determine which point in one stereo-half should correspond to a given point in the other? The probability of matching points incorrectly is so high that some strategy must be used to limit the number of possible matches. The visual system solves this by matching the edges detected in each spatial frequency channel separately (Julesz and Miller, 1975). The actual matching process used by the visual system is complex and not fully understood, but possible schemes are discussed by Nelson (1975), Marr and Poggio (1979) and Mayhew and Frisby (1980).

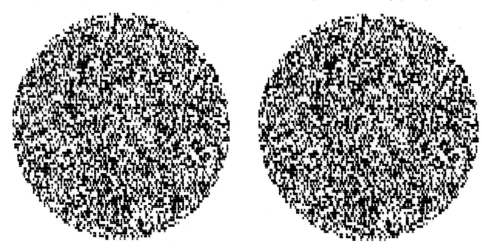

Figure 2.8 Random-dot stereogram. Random-dot stereograms (RDS) comprise two monocular halves consisting of identical arrangements of dots, except that a central portion (in this case a square) is displaced laterally in one half relative to the other. When the stereo-halves are fused, the central disparate portion is clearly seen standing out from the background, even though it cannot be detected monocularly. The RDS can be viewed by converging the eyes to a point in front of the page and relaxing accommodation until the fused image is in focus

The second stage of stereopsis (the interpretation stage) involves analysis of the fused image to reveal depth information. Solving the correspondence problem gives a set of matched points. All this means is that some point in the left image is correctly associated with some point in the right, not that they coincide in space. It is essential for stereopsis that some matched points do not coincide spatially since these provide the disparity on which the interpretation of surface shape depends.

The stereogram of *Figure 2.8* shows a square standing out from its background. The depth (disparity) between every point on the square and its background is constant. If the square were slanted relative to the background, however, the disparity would vary. To interpret the orientation of surfaces, therefore, changes in disparity across the image must be analysed, as well as the disparity at each point. This situation is essentially the same as in edge detection where changes of luminance across the image had to be measured. This was achieved by having RFs (spatial frequency channels) measuring luminance gradients, and stereopsis appears to work by having RFs designed to measure disparity gradients. This has been established psychophysically using disparity gratings (Tyler, 1974), which are sine-wave gratings in depth, produced by modulating disparity in an RDS. When fused, the grating appears like a sheet of corrugated metal. As in conventional luminance gratings, spatial frequency and amplitude (of disparity in this case) can be varied independently. This enables measurement to be made of the disparity necessary to perceive depth at different spatial frequencies, giving a disparity sensitivity function similar in shape to the CSF. This function can be regarded as the combined response of a number of channels, each of which responds to a range of disparity gradients. To distinguish them from the spatial frequency channels which measure luminance gradients, these have been called hypercyclopean channels (Tyler, 1975; Schumer and Ganz, 1979). The realization that stereopsis measures disparity gradients changes the concept of the fusional limit. The maximum disparity between two points that can be fused depends on their spatial separation, i.e. on their disparity gradient (Burt and Julesz, 1980).

The lateral separation of the eyes determines that horizontal disparities are the most important for depth perception, but vertical disparities may also occur if an object is imaged eccentrically (i.e. not on the fovea), or if the eyes fix asymmetrically (i.e. not straight ahead). Vertical disparities, when present, are much smaller than horizontal ones. Magnifying one image vertically to cause such disparity produces an unexpected change in depth perception, as though the image of the other eye had been magnified horizontally. This has been called the induced effect (Ogle, 1972). The role of vertical disparities in stereopsis has only recently been understood. Mayhew (1982) proposes that they are used to calculate two important viewing parameters: the angle of gaze and the viewing distance. This explains the induced effect, since artificially creating vertical disparity causes the visual system to compute an incorrect gaze angle, resulting in a misinterpretation of any horizontal disparity (*see also* Gillam and Lawergren, 1983; Frisby, 1984).

A comprehensive review of binocular disparity processing is given by Tyler (1983). For general reviews of spatial vision *see* DeValois and DeValois (1980) and Westheimer (1984).

Spatiotemporal visual performance

Perceiving flicker — the temporal modulation transfer function

Most visual scenes present temporal as well as spatial information. Temporal changes alone can be important in edge detection as in the case of stationary flickering lights, and temporal information processing also starts in the retina. The electrical activity of the receptors following one brief flash of light continues for much longer than the flash itself, indicating a period of temporal summation which increases the chance of detecting the flash. Receptors with long summation periods (rods) have greater sensitivity, while those with short summation periods (cones) provide good temporal resolution, i.e. they can detect rapid changes in the stimulus. This is analogous to having large RFs to increase spatial sensitivity and small ones for spatial resolution. When a number of brief light flashes occur successively, the visual system responds to their average luminance. This is called temporal integration and is thought to occur at some processing stage after the retinal receptors. It is analogous to spatial integration which determines that the eye adapts to the mean luminance in a scene (Haber and Hershenson, 1980).

The temporal performance of the visual system can be assessed by measuring the contrast needed to detect a light flickering at different frequencies. The luminance of the flickering light is varied sinusoidally. These measurements give a temporal contrast sensitivity function (*Figure 2.9*), often called the 'deLange curve' or temporal MTF (deLange, 1952; Kelly, 1961).

The shape of the temporal and spatial MTFs, and their implications, are very similar:

1. More contrast is needed to detect rapidly flickering lights and the greatest sensitivity to flicker is at about 10–20 Hz.
2. Flicker is more easily detected at high luminance.

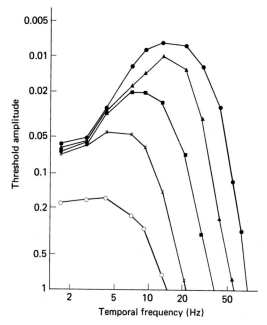

Figure 2.9 The temporal MTF at different luminance levels (after Kelly, 1961). The amplitude at which flickering lights of different luminances are just detectable is plotted against the flicker frequency, o, 0.06 troland; ×, 0.65 troland; ■, 7.1 trolands; ▲, 77 trolands; ●, 850 trolands

3. The highest detectable flicker frequency at maximum contrast is about 60 Hz. This is the *critical fusion frequency* (CFF) above which flicker is no longer visible. Note that the CFF, which has often been used as a measure of visual performance, represents only the high frequency limit of the temporal MTF, analogous to the relationship between VA and the spatial CSF.

It has been shown that the spatial CSF can be considered as the combined responses of a number of spatial frequency channels. It is interesting to consider whether there are also channels in temporal vision, each sensitive to its own range of flicker frequencies. Evidence for this is less convincing than for spatial vision, but it is generally agreed that low and high temporal frequencies appear to be processed separately in 'sustained' and 'transient' channels, respectively (Watson and Robson, 1981).

Measurement of temporal MTFs has also been adopted clinically (*see* Manny and Levi, 1982; Kayazawa *et al*, 1984; Wright, Drasdo and Harding, 1984).

Sustained and transient channels

The concept of separate channels for low and high temporal frequencies requires consideration of inter-

actions between spatial and temporal processing, because object detection at very low flicker frequencies must depend primarily on spatial information. Spatiotemporal interactions have been explored by measuring contrast sensitivity for spatial gratings which are also temporally modulated. This is achieved either by having the grating drift across a screen at various speeds, or by flickering a stationary grating at various temporal frequencies.

Spatial contrast sensitivity for drifting gratings was measured by van Nes (1968) and Kelly (1979) who found a loss of sensitivity at high spatial frequencies and an increase at low. This means that visual acuity is reduced if an image is moving, but the detectability of larger objects, e.g. vehicles, is improved. Contrast sensitivity for stationary flickering gratings was measured by Kulikowski and Tolhurst (1973) who found two distinct thresholds. At one contrast level, the flicker became noticeable while at another the spatial pattern appeared. These two thresholds vary independently with changes of spatial or temporal frequency, suggesting that each is the response of a separate processing channel. The flicker sensitive channel responds best to rapid temporal changes, so it has been called a 'transient channel' or 'movement detector'. The other responds best to stationary or slowly changing stimuli and has been called a 'sustained channel' or 'pattern detector' (*see Table 2.1*). The characteristics of sustained and transient channels have been identified with those of X and Y ganglion cells, respectively (*see* Breitmeyer (1984) for a review of sustained and transient visual channels).

The terms 'pattern detector' and 'movement detector' have the unfortunate implication that pattern and movement are independent aspects of visual stimuli. A static pattern may contain only spatial information, but all temporally varying stimuli also have a spatial component. In the case of a flickering target, the spatial content of the scene is fixed while the temporal varies. In the case of a moving target, both spatial and temporal changes occur in the image. Pattern and movement processing cannot, therefore, be independent.

Motion

As has been shown, motion is a consequence of spatiotemporal change. However, all spatiotemporal changes are not perceived as motion. For example, we are normally not aware of the movement of a clock hand but, rather, conclude that it has moved from a change in its position over a period of time. The significance of this distinction can be seen in experiments measuring motion thresholds, the smallest amount of target movement that can be detected. When positional cues are present in a stimulus the threshold depends on the amount of target displacement and this is essentially a hyper-

Table 2.1 Characteristics of sustained and transient channels

Property	Sustained	Transient
Response latency	Long	Short
Temporal conditions for maximum response	Static targets/low frequency flicker	Moving targets/high frequency flicker
Spatial conditions for maximum response	High SFs	Low SFs
RF size	Small	Large
Retinal location	Central (especially fovea)	Peripheral
Sensitive to blur	Yes	No

Adapted from Haber and Hershenson (1980).

acuity judgement as mentioned earlier. However, if positional information is removed, the threshold depends on the velocity of target movement (Nakayama and Tyler, 1981). Since velocity is a vector, this means that perception of motion depends on simultaneous perception of both the magnitude and direction of spatiotemporal change.

Direction sensitivity (DS) in vision has long been suspected because of motion after-effects. If adaptation to a target which moves in one direction occurs, a stationary target will then appear to move in the opposite direction. Barlow, Hill and Levick (1964) found DS ganglion cells in the rabbit which responded to stimulus movement in one direction, but not in the opposite direction. Psychophysical evidence for DS mechanisms in humans was reported by Levinson and Sekuler (1975) who concluded that direction sensitivity was a property of the transient channels (*see* Sekuler and Levinson (1977) for an introduction).

The visual processing of motion is not yet clearly understood. The finding that isoluminant stimuli are ineffective for motion perception (Ramachandran and Gregory, 1978), again indicates that luminance edge detection is an essential first stage. Following edge detection, information must be analysed by a set of DS units. Marr and Ullman (1981) suggest that this could be achieved by having cells whose RFs consist of three components: a sustained on-centre cell $(X+)$ and a sustained off-centre cell $(X-)$ together locate an edge, and these are combined with a transient Y cell which signals temporal changes. The sign of the Y cell's response indicates the direction of motion.

It is naturally assumed that the purpose of motion perception is the detection of moving objects. In fact it gives much more information than this and, in particular, it can be used like stereopsis to determine the structure in a scene. Stereo vision operates on spatial disparities between two simultaneous views of an image. Motion may provide spatial disparities between successive views of an image. Just as object

outlines and three-dimensional shape not previously apparent can be seen stereoscopically in RDS, so such structure may be perceived in certain stimuli when they move, but not when they are stationary.

A classic example of our ability to perceive structure-from-motion is described by Johansson (1975). This is a film of two people dancing in the dark! Each dancer is made visible only by spots of light on the shoulders, elbows, wrists, hips, knees and ankles so that individual frames of the film show just a collection of bright dots. When the film is run two moving figures can easily be seen. Braddick (1974, 1980) using similar displays, called *random-dot kinematograms* (RDKs), showed that a central square of dots which were disparate between two successive views could only be seen if all the dots moved in the same direction. Direction sensitivity is, therefore, also important in processing structure-from-motion. The distinction between perceiving motion and perceiving structure-from-motion is highlighted in the work of Rogers and Graham (1982) who produced perceptions of corrugated surfaces (like stereo disparity gratings) from RDKs. In these cases, the structure which emerges is stationary, even though motion processing is responsible. (For a comprehensive text on depth perception through motion, *see* Braunstein (1976).)

The similarity between RDS and RDK displays suggests that the perception of structure from stereo and motion may involve similar processing principles. Ullman (1979) has taken this approach, proposing the same two stages of achieving correspondence between edges in successive views of the image, and then interpreting disparities in the set of matched points obtained. His mathematical analysis indicates that unambiguous structure can be perceived from three successive views of just four points in the image, explaining why Johansson's demonstration works so effectively. Evidence that the visual system may actually use the same physiological mechanisms for both stereopsis and the perception of structure-from-motion is reported by Richards and Lieberman

(1985). (A comprehensive, though advanced, review of motion processing is given by Nakayama (1985).)

Marr and Ullman's (1981) theory of movement detection makes some unexpected predictions about movement perception. Perhaps the most striking of these are that:

(1) The detection of movement can be affected by changing the luminance of an edge at the moment of its displacement.
(2) An edge which is physically stationary may appear to move if its onset is associated with a simultaneous change in luminance.

These and other predictions of the Marr–Ullman model have recently been tested psychophysically by Moulden and Begg (1986). Their results confirm all the predictions of the model and lead to a number of suggestions of how it may be tested further. This is a good example of the power which computational theory has brought to the psychology of vision. If possible, it is generally better to have a theory of how something works that can be tested in practice, rather than hoping for a theory to emerge from a lot of diverse practical observations.

Finally, Moulden and Begg (1986, p.154) make a point which may help keep the study of visual perception in perspective:

'It is not possible to prove the correctness of a model. The best that one can do is to expose it rigorously to the possibility of disproof.'

Our whole understanding of vision depends on a model, or theoretical framework, which helps us to make sense of perception. We cannot ultimately prove the truth of this framework. The best we can do is work to expose its weaknesses and be prepared to accept the new theories and practices that will follow.

Acknowledgement

The author would like to thank a number of colleagues who read earlier drafts and contributed to the preparation of this chapter: David Pickwell, Maurice Yap, Usha Dhanesha, Shahina Pardhan, Caroline Perrins who provided the stereogram, and Tony Shakespeare who assisted in the preparation of photographs.

References

ARDEN, G.B. (1978) The importance of measuring contrast sensitivity in cases of visual disturbance. *Br. J. Ophthalmol.*, **62**, 198–209

BARLOW, H.B. (1953) Summation and inhibition in the frogs retina. *J. Physiol.*, **119**, 69–88

BARLOW, H.B., HILL, R.M... and LEVICK, W.R. (1964) Retinal ganglion cells responding selectively to direction and speed of image motion in the rabbit. *J. Physiol.*, **173**, 377–407

BLAKE, R. and FOX, R. (1973) The psychophysical inquiry into binocular summation. *Percept. Psychophys.*, **14**, 161–185

BLAKE, R., SLOANE, M. and FOX, R. (1981) Further developments in binocular summation. *Percept. Psychophys.*, **30**, 266–276

BLAKEMORE, C. and CAMPBELL, F.W. (1969) On the existence of neurons in the human visual system selectively sensitive to the orientation and size of retinal images. *J. Physiol.*, **203**, 237–260

BOSSOMAIER, T.R.J., SNYDER, A.W. and HUGHES, A. (1985) Irregularity and aliasing: Solution? *Vision Res.*, **25**, 145–147

BRADDICK, O.J. (1974) A short range process in apparent motion. *Vision Res.*, **14**, 519–527

BRADDICK, O.J. (1980) Low-level and high-level processes in apparent motion. *Philos. Trans. R. Soc. Lond. Ser. B Biol. Sci.*, **290**, 137–151

BRADDICK, O.J., CAMPBELL, F.W. and ATKINSON, J. (1978) Channels in vision: basic aspects. In *Handbook of Sensory Physiology*, edited by R. Held *et al.*, Vol. VIII, *Perception*, pp. 3–38. New York: Springer Verlag

BRAUNSTEIN, M.L. (1976) *Depth Perception through Motion*. New York: Academic Press

BREITMEYER, B.G. (1984) Sustained and transient neural channels. *Visual Masking*, Chap 6. New York: Oxford University Press

BURT, P. and JULESZ, B. (1980) Modifications of the classical notion of Panum's fusional area. *Perception*, **9**, 671–682

CAMPBELL, F.W. and GREEN, D.G. (1965a) Optical and retinal factors affecting visual resolution. *J. Physiol.*, **181**, 576–593

CAMPBELL, F.W. and GREEN, D.G. (1965b) Monocular versus binocular visual acuity. *Nature*, **208**, 191–192

CAMPBELL, F.W. and GUBISCH, R.W. (1966) Optical quality of the human eye. *J. Physiol.*, **186**, 558–578

CAMPBELL, F.W. and MAFFEI, L. (1974) Contrast and spatial frequency. *Sci. Am.*, **231**, 106–114

CAMPBELL, F.W. and ROBSON, J.G. (1968) Application of Fourier analysis to the visibility of gratings. *J. Physiol.*, **197**, 551–566

CHARMAN, W.N. (1979) Effect of refractive error in visual tests with sinusoidal gratings. *Br. J. Physiol. Opt.*, **33**, 10–20

CHARMAN, W.N. (1983) The retinal image in the human eye. In *Progress in Retinal Research*, edited by N. Osborne and G. Chader, Vol. 2, pp. 1–50. New York: Pergamon Press

COOPER, L.A. and SHEPARD, R.N. (1984) Turning something over in the mind. *Sci. Am.*, **251**, 114–121

CORNSWEET, T.N. (1970) *Visual Perception*. New York: Academic Press Inc.

CORNSWEET, T.N. (1985) A simple retinal mechanism that has complex and profound effects on perception. *Am. J. Optom. Physiol. Opt.*, **62** (7), 427–438

CORNSWEET, T.N. and YELLOTT, J.I. (1985) Intensity-dependent spatial summation. *J. Opt. Soc. Am. (A)*, **2**, 1769–1786

DELANGE, H. (1952) Experiments on flicker and some calculation on an experimental analogue of the foveal systems. *Physica*, **18**, 935–950

DEVALOIS, R.L. and DEVALOIS, K.K. (1980) Spatial vision. *Annu. Rev. Psychol.*, **31**, 309–341

ENOCH, J.M. and WILLIAMS, R.A. (1983) Development of clinical tests of vision: initial data on two hyperacuity paradigms. *Percept. Psychophys.*, **33**, 314–322

ENROTH-CUGELL, C. and ROBSON, J.G. (1966) Contrast sensitivity of retinal ganglion cells of the cat. *J. Physiol.*, **187**, 517–522

FECHNER, G.T. (1860) *Elements of Psychophysics*, translated by H.E. Adler, edited by D.M. Howes and E.G. Boring. 1966. New York: Holt

FRISBY, J.P. (1979) *Seeing: Illusion, Brain and Mind*. Oxford: Oxford University Press

FRISBY, J.P. (1984) An old illusion and a new theory of stereoscopic depth perception. *Nature* **307**, 592–593

FRISBY, J.P. and MAYHEW, J.E.W. (1978) Contrast sensitivity function for stereopsis. *Perception*, **7**, 423–429

FRY, G.A. (1984) The eye as an optical system. In *Optical Radiation Measurements*, edited by C.J. Bartleson and F. Grum, Vol. 5. New York: Academic Press

GEORGESON, M.A. and SULLIVAN, G.D. (1975) Contrast constancy: deblurring in human vision by spatial frequency channels. *J. Physiol.*, **252**, 627–656

GILCHRIST, A.L. (1979) The perception of surface blacks and whites. *Sci. Am.*, **240**, 88–97

GILCHRIST, A.L., DELMAN, S. and JACOBSEN, A. (1983) The classification and integration of edges as critical to the perception of reflectance and illumination. *Percept. Psychophys.*, **33**, 425–436

GILLAM, B. and LAWERGREN, B. (1983) The induced effect, vertical disparity and stereoscopic theory. *Percept. Psychophys.*, **34**, 121–130

GINSBURG, A.P. (1984) A new Contrast Sensitivity Vision Test Chart. *Am. J. Optom. Physiol. Opt.*, **61**, 403–407

GRAHAM, N. (1981) Psychophysics of spatial frequency channels. In *Perceptual Organisation*, edited by M. Kubovy and J. Pomerantz, pp. 1–25. New Jersey: Erlbaum

GREEN, D.G. and CAMPBELL, F.W. (1965) Effect of focus on the visual response to a sinusoidally modulated spatial stimulus. *J. Opt. Soc. Am.*, **55**, 1154–1157

GREGORY, R.L. (1979) Stereo vision and isoluminance. *Proc. R. Soc. Lond B Biol. Sci.*, **204**, 467–476

HABER, R.N. and HERSHENSON, M. (1980) *The Psychology of Visual Perception* New York: Holt, Rinehart and Winston

HARTLINE, H.K. and RATLIFF, F. (1957) Inhibitory interaction of receptor units in the eye of Limulus. *J. Gen. Physiol.*, **40**, 357–376

HESS, R.F. (1984) On the assessment of contrast threshold functions for anomalous vision. *Br. J. Orthop.*, **41**, 1–14

HUBEL, D.H. (1982) Exploration of the primary visual cortex, 1955–78. *Nature*, **299**, 515–524

JOHANSSON, G. (1975) Visual motion perception. *Sci. Am.*, **232** (6), 76–88

JULESZ, B. (1971) *Foundations of Cyclopean Perception*. Chicago: University of Chicago Press

JULESZ, B. and MILLER, J.E. (1975) Independent spatial frequency tuned channels in binocular fusion and rivalry. *Perception*, **4**, 125–143

KAYAZAWA, F., SONODA, K., NISHIMURA, K., NAKAMURA, T., YAMAMOTO, T and ITOI, M. (1984) Clinical application of temporal modulation transfer function. *Jap. J. Ophthalmol.*, **28**, 9–19

KELLY, D.H. (1961) Visual response to time-dependent stimuli (i): Amplitude sensitivity measurements. *J. Opt. Soc. Am.*, **51**, 422–429

KELLY, D.H. (1979) Motion and vision II: stabilised spatio-temporal threshold surface. *J. Opt. Soc. Am.*, **69**, 1340–1349

KOENDERINK, J.J. (1977) Current models of contrast processing. In *Spatial Contrast*, edited by H. Spekreijse and L.H. van der Tweel. Amsterdam: North Holland Pub. Co.

KUFFLER, S.W. (1953) Discharge patterns and functional organisation of mammalian retina. *J. Neurophysiol.*, **16**, 37–68

KULIKOWSKI, J.J. and TOLHURST, D.J. (1973) Psychophysical evidence for sustained and transient detectors in human vision. *J. Physiol.*, **232**, 149–162

LAND, E.H. (1977) The retinex theory of color vision. *Sci. Am.*, **237**, 108–128

LAND, E.H. and McCANN, J.J. (1971) Lightness and retinex theory. *J. Opt. Soc. Am.*, **61**, 1–11

LENNIE, P. (1980a) Parallel visual pathways: a review. *Vision Res.*, **20**, 561–594

LENNIE, P. (1980b) Perceptual signs of parallel pathways. *Philos. Trans. R. Soc. Lond. Ser. B Biol. Sci.*, **290**, 23–37

LEVINSON, E. and SEKULER, R. (1975) The independence of channels in human vision selective for direction of movement. *J. Physiol.*, **250**, 347–366

LINDSAY, P.H. and NORMAN, D.A. (1977). *Human Information Processing*, 2nd edn, p.192. New York: Academic Press

MANNY, R.E. and LEVI, D.M. (1982) Psychophysical investigations of the temporal modulation sensitivity function in amblyopia: uniform field flicker. *Invest. Ophthalmol. Vis. Sci.*, **22**, 515–524

MARR, D. (1980) Visual information processing: the structure and creation of visual representations. *Philos. Trans. R. Soc. Lond. Ser. B Biol. Sci.*, **290**, 199–218

MARR, D. (1982) *Vision*. San Francisco: W.H. Freeman and Co.

MARR, D. and HILDRETH, E. (1980) Theory of edge detection. *Proc. R. Soc. Lond. B Biol. Sci.*, **207**, 187–217

MARR, D. and POGGIO, T. (1979) A computational theory of human stereo vision. *Proc. R. Soc. Lond. B Biol. Sci.*, **204**, 301–328

MARR, D. and ULLMAN, S. (1981) Directional selectivity and its use in early visual processing. *Proc. R. Soc. Lond. B Biol. Sci.*, **211**, 151–181

MAYHEW, J.E.W. (1982) The interpretation of stereo-disparity information: the computation of surface orientation and depth. *Perception*, **11**, 387–403

MAYHEW, J.E.W. and FRISBY, J.P. (1980) Spatial frequency tuned channels: implications for structure and function from psychophysical and computational studies of stereopsis. *Philos. Trans. R. Soc. Lond. Ser. B Biol. Sci.*, **290**, 95–116

MOSES, R.A. (1975) *Adler's Physiology of the Eye — Clinical Application*. St Louis: C.V. Mosby

MOULDEN, B. and BEGG, H. (1986) Some tests of the Marr–Ullman model of movement detection. *Perception*, **15**, 139–155

NAKAYAMA, K. (1985) Biological image motion processing: A review. *Vision Res.*, **25**, 625–660

NAKAYAMA, K. and TYLER, C.W. (1981) Psychophysical isolation of movement sensitivity by removal of familiar position cues. *Vision Res.*, **21**, 427–433

OATLEY, K. (1978) *Perceptions and Representations*. London: Methuen and Co. Ltd.

OGLE, K.N. (1972) *Researches in Binocular Vision*. New York: Hafner Publ. Co.

PINKER, S. (1984) Visual cognition: an introduction. *Cognition*, **18**, 1–63

RAMACHANDRAN, V.S. and GREGORY, R.L. (1978) Does colour provide an input to human motion perception? *Nature*, **275**, 55–56

RATCLIFF, F. (1965) *Mach Bands: Quantitative Studies on Neural Networks in the Retina*. San Francisco: Holden-Day Inc.

RATLIFF, F. (1972) Contour and contrast. *Sci. Am.*, **226** (6), 90–101

REGAN, D. and NEIMA, D. (1983) Low contrast letter charts as tests of visual function. *Ophthalmology*, **90**, 1192–1200

REMOLE, A. (1979) Contrast thresholds versus border enhancement: sensitivity to retinal defocus. *Am. J. Optom. Physiol. Opt.*, **56**, 153–162

REMOLE, A. (1980) Contrast thresholds versus border enhancement: effect of scattered light. *Am. J. Optom. Physiol. Opt.*, **57**, 85–94

REMOLE, A. (1983) Border enhancement as a function of binocular fixation performance. *Am. J. Optom. Physiol. Opt.*, **60**, 567–577

REMOLE, A. (1984) Binocular fixation misalignment measured by border enhancement: a simplified technique. *Am. J. Optom. Physiol. Opt.*, **61**, 118–124

RICHARDS, W. and LIEBERMAN, H.R. (1985) Correlation between stereo ability and recovery of structure-from-motion. *Am. J. Optom. Physiol. Opt.*, **62**, 111–118

ROBSON, J.G. (1975) Receptive fields: neural representation of the spatial and intensive attributes of the visual image. In *Handbook of Perception*, edited by E.C. Carterette and M.P. Friedman, Vol 5. New York: Academic Press

ROBSON, J.G. (1980) Neural images: the physiological basis of spatial vision. In *Visual Coding and Adaptability*, edited by C.S. Harris, pp. 177–214. New Jersey: Lawrence Erlbaum Ass.

RODIECK, R.W. and STONE, J. (1965) Analysis of receptive fields of cat retinal ganglion cells. *J. Neurophysiol.*, **28**, 833–849

ROGERS, B.J. and GRAHAM, M. (1982) Similarities between motion parallax and stereopsis in human depth perception. *Vision Res.*, **22**, 261–270

SCHADE, O.H. (1956) Optical and photoelectric analog of the eye. *J. Opt. Soc. Am.*, **49**, 425–428

SCHUMER, R. and GANZ, L. (1979) Independent stereoscopic channels for different extents of spatial pooling. *Vision Res.*, **19**, 1303–1314

SEKULER, R. and LEVINSON, E. (1977) The perception of moving targets. *Sci. Am.*, **236** (1), 60–73

SELWYN, E.W.H. (1948) The photographic and visual resolving power of lenses: Part 1 — visual resolving power. *Photogr. J.*, **88B**, 6–12

SHEEDY, J.E., BAILEY, I.L. and RAASCH, T.W. (1984) Visual acuity and chart luminance. *Am. J. Optom. Physiol. Opt.*, **61**, 595–600

SHEPARD, R.N. (1978) The mental image. *Am. Psychol.*, **33**, 125–137

SHEPARD, R.N. and METZLER, J. (1971) Mental rotation of three dimensional objects. *Science*, **171**, 701–703

SMITH, G. (1982) Ocular defocus, spurious resolution and contrast reversal. *Ophthal. Physiol. Optics*, **2**, 5–23

SPOEHR, K.T. and LEHMKUHLE, S.W. (1982) *Visual Information Processing*. San Francisco: W.H. Freeman and Co.

STROMEYER, C.F. and JULESZ, B. (1972) Spatial frequency masking in vision: critical bands and spread of masking. *J. Opt. Soc. Am.*, **62**, 1221–1232

TYLER, C.W. (1974) Depth perception in disparity gratings. *Nature*, **251**, 140–142

TYLER, C.W. (1975) Stereoscopic tilt and size after-effects. *Perception*, **4**, 187–192

TYLER, C.W. (1983) Sensory processing of binocular disparity. In *Vergence Eye Movements: Basic and Clinical Aspects*, edited by C.M. Schor and K.J. Ciuffreda. New York: Academic Press.

ULLMAN, S. (1979) *The Interpretation of Visual Motion*. Cambridge, Mass: MIT Press

VAN MEETERAN, A. and VOS, J.J. (1972) Resolution and contrast sensitivity at low luminances. *Vision Res.*, **12**, 825–833

VAN NES, F.L. (1968) Enhanced visibility by regular motion of retinal images. *Am. J. Psychol.*, **81**, 366–374

WATANABE, A., MORI, T., NAGATA, S. and HIWATASHI, K. (1968) Spatial sine wave responses of the human visual system. *Vision Res.*, **8**, 1245–1263

WATSON, A.B. and ROBSON, J.G. (1981) Discrimination at threshold; labelled detectors in human vision. *Vision Res.*, **21**, 1115–1122

WESTHEIMER, G. (1975) Visual acuity and hyperacuity. *Invest. Ophthalmol.*, **14**, 570–572

WESTHEIMER, G. (1981) Visual hyperacuity. *Prog. Sens. Physiol.*, **1**, 1–30

WESTHEIMER, G. (1984) Spatial vision. *Annu. Rev. Psychol.*, **35**, 201–226

WESTHEIMER, G. and McKEE, S.P. (1977) Spatial configurations for visual hyperacuity. *Vision Res.*, **17**, 941–947

WHITAKER, D. and BUCKINGHAM, T. (1987) The resistance of displacement thresholds for oscillatory movement to optical image degradation. *Ophthal. Physiol. Opt.* (in press)

WIESEL, T.N. (1982) Postnatal development of the visual cortex and the influence of environment. *Nature*, **229**, 583–591

WILLIAMS, D.R. (1985) Aliasing in human foveal vision. *Vision Res.*, **25**, 195–205

WILSON, H.R. (1979) Spatiotemporal characterisation of a transient mechanism in the human visual system. Unpublished manuscript cited by Marr (1982), p. 170

WILSON, H.R. (1983) Psychophysical evidence for spatial channels. In *Physical and Biological Processing of Images*, edited by O.J. Braddick and A. Sleigh. Berlin: Springer-Verlag

WILSON, H.R. and BERGEN, J.R. (1979) A four mechanism model for spatial vision. *Vision Res.*, **19**, 19–32

WOLFE, J.M. (1983) Hidden visual processes. *Sci. Am.*, **248** (2), 72–85

WOODHOUSE, J.M. (1987) Contrast sensitivity measurement. *Optician*, **193**, 19–27

WRIGHT, C.E., DRASDO, N. and HARDING, C.F.A. (1984) Electrophysiological and psychophysical studies on suspected unilateral retrobulbar neuritis. *Trans. Int. Cong. Br. Coll. Ophthal. Opt.*, **1**, 69–93

YELLOT, J.I. JR (1982) Spectral analysis of spatial sampling by photoreceptors: topological disorder prevents aliasing. *Vision Res.*, **22**, 1205–1210

3

Neurophysiology of vision and its clinical application

Graham Harding

Neurophysiology is the scientific study of the functioning of the nervous system. In the case of vision the neurophysiology begins after the initial transduction which allows the visual environment to be represented as electrochemical events in the receptors of the eye. This change in potential is transmitted via the bipolar cells to the ganglion cells. Both the bipolar and ganglion cells perform a type of spatial averaging and inhibition by receiving additional inputs from the horizontal and amacrine cells, respectively.

The optic nerve in man contains approximately 1×10^6 fibres, unevenly distributed in terms of retinal distribution and providing an exaggerated representation of the macula in proportion to peripheral retina. At the optic chiasma, approximately 55% of fibres cross to the opposite hemisphere of the brain. Fibres originating in the temporal retina in general remain ipsilateral, whereas those from the nasal retina cross over. The division between nasal and temporal retina is probably not sharp and represents, at best, a statistical probability rather than a clear division. Beyond the optic chiasma most fibres proceed to a synapse in the lateral geniculate bodies, although a small proportion of fibres decussate to tectal terminations. The lateral geniculate bodies, although representing both the temporal retina of the ipsilateral eye and the nasal retina of the cross lateral eye, still generally keep the synaptic connections of the two eyes separate in a series of layers.

From the lateral geniculate bodies, new fibres proceed to area 17 of the visual cortex where they terminate in layer 4C. The neural representation of the visual field present in each optic nerve is still maintained at this point.

All these stages of visual transmission are probably reflected as electrophysiological events. Some of these events, such as the *electroretinogram* (ERG)

and *visual evoked cortical potential* (VECP), are easily recorded simply because it is easy to place non-invasive electrodes close to the site. Other signals, such as those from lateral geniculate or tectal sites, are much more difficult to record, probably due to their inconvenient anatomical placement, although recently success has been achieved using far-field recording techniques (Harding and Rubinstein, 1980). Within the space of this chapter only a resumé of each electrophysiological system can be presented, but further reading is given at the end of the chapter.

Recording techniques

The problem of electrode design and application has always been critical to electrophysiology. The initial connection to the subject or patient limits the efficiency of the whole system. It is imposed on a biological system which it must faithfully record without itself affecting the operation of the system. Modern electrophysiological recorders provide no 'load' on the biological system, i.e. very little current is taken from the tissue and the recording itself does not affect the electrophysiological behaviour of the biological system. Electrophysiological techniques are concerned with amplifying the potential difference between two electrodes or their 'leads', and care must be taken to reduce potentials occurring external to the biological system under study. The mode of application of the electrode to the living tissue is governed by the need to produce low resistance between the electrode and the tissue. As a general rule, the resistance between a pair of electrodes should be reduced to approximately 5 kΩ. If the potential difference generated by the source is to be applied efficiently to the input of the amplifier, the skin resistance should be as small as practicable.

Electrodes

For most electrophysiological recording, the most commonly used electrode is the silver–silver chloride 'stick-on' electrode. This consists of a small dished silver cup, with a narrow flange and the lead soldered to a tag on one side. This connection is enclosed in epoxy resin. The complete electrode is about 1 cm in diameter. The electrode is chlorided in its entirety and is applied using a special glue. A small amount of this non-toxic glue (*collodion*) is distributed around the edge of the electrode flange and then dried by a stream of air. When the electrode is in position, it is filled with electrode jelly using a hypodermic syringe with a blunt-ended needle. The needle is inserted through the hole in the back of the electrode, pressed gently onto the scalp and rotated to penetrate the superfluous 'dead' layer. The electrode is then filled with jelly, the notched flat-ended needle allowing the electrolyte to fill the electrode cavity. The electrode jelly penetrates the skin ensuring low electrode–skin resistance.

Electrodes for electroretinography are naturally a special consideration. The 'standard' corneal electrode is now the Henkes type. This consists of a fairly large plastic lens which is placed in direct contact with the cornea and which, due to its bulk, keeps the eyelids open. Within this is the actual electrode, usually consisting of silver wires wrapped around a black artificial pupil within the 'cup' of the lens and kept away from contact with the cornea. Although there have been many variations on this electrode involving more refined contact lens types of electrodes, all interfere with vision to some extent. They are also not easily tolerated by young children and this creates severe clinical problems. With the advent of 'averaging' computers, it became possible to enhance the signal relative to background noise, and electrodes more distant from the source of the signal became tolerable. A variety of electrodes were used, either standard silver–silver chloride electrodes placed on the lower lid or more specialized electrodes in contact with the eye itself. Two types of electrodes of this latter type have been developed. The first consists of a nylon gold-coated fibre which is cut into small strips (Arden *et al.*, 1979). Each small strip is soldered to a lead and then bent over at its tip so it will hook into the fornix of the eye. The electrode has only a limited number of re-use applications. The second electrode is a gold–cotton spun wire, the use of which was pioneered by Dawson, Trick and Maida (1981). The electrode is laid along the tarsal surface where capillary action keeps it in contact with the eye.

The problems of electrode placement are obviously unique to the type of signal to be recorded, i.e. ERG, electro-oculogram (EOG), or visual evoked potential (VEP). Related to this topographical distribution is the problem of electrode linkage, but a few general principles can be stated.

Amplifiers and recorders

All amplifiers require two inputs. Conventionally, one input is known as the black lead and the other as the white lead. The amplifier records the difference in potential between the two leads. Visual evoked potentials usually follow the rule that, if the black lead is negative with respect to the white, there is an upward deflection of the trace. This convention is the opposite of that for electroretinograms.

In reference recording, such as the ERG, it is always easy to 'reverse' the signal. If the black lead is connected to the active electrode, i.e. the electrode close to the signal source, when the signal is positive, there will be a downward deflection of the trace. If the white lead is connected to the active electrode, positive will be indicated by an upward deflection, and this is the technique used in ERGs.

VEP studies frequently use either convention, i.e. 'negative up' or 'positive up' depending on the training and experience of the investigators, and how the signal is to be related to other parameters. It is, therefore, essential that the convention used should be stated in diagrams and text. In this chapter, all figures will show the convention used but both types of conventions will be used as appropriate.

In reference recording, one electrode is considered the 'active' electrode, i.e. it is placed over the source of the signal, and the other lead placed as 'reference' over some inactive site. In actual practice, the definition of the reference is impossible to fulfil. The 'reference' site has been a continuing source of controversy as an inactive site does not exist, and the best compromise that can be obtained is to use a site which is relatively inactive in terms of the signal being investigated and, in addition, is not particularly susceptible to other electrophysiological artefacts. Thus, with visual evoked potentials (VEPs) the further forward the reference point on the head the less it is affected by the VEP but the more the electrode is affected by eye-movement potentials and the ERG. A good compromise is either a midfrontal site or linked rolandic electrodes. For ERGs a reference distal to the outer canthus, i.e. a frontotemporal site, is used.

Once two or more recording channels are used, this problem may be overcome by using the same electrode as the reference for all channels. This form of recording is known as 'common reference'.

Obviously, in this situation the relative amplitude of different active sites may be compared in relation to the same reference electrode. Equally, any signal arising from the reference electrode will appear in the same phase and be of the same amplitude in all channels, i.e. it will be a common signal. This common reference system of recording has recently dominated VEP recordings, and its use certainly allows easy comparability between different centres in the world, because, since the interelectrode distances are large, minimal changes in active electrode location will have little effect. In addition, the use of common reference recording allows computer synthesis of other forms of record including 'bipolar' recording between pairs of active electrodes.

In one sense, all recordings are bipolar in that they record potential differences between pairs of electrodes. However, the term 'bipolar recording' is usually used to describe the situation in which both leads of a channel (and their associated electrodes) are considered to be active. However, because the channel will record the potential difference between the two electrodes, this does mean that changes of opposite polarity and equal amplitude at the two sites will produce the same signal. Thus, if the black lead becomes 100 μV negative in relation to the white, then in the bioelectrical convention the trace will deflect upwards by 100 units. In the same way, if the white lead becomes 100 μV positive in relation to the black, the same deflection will be produced. Of course, if both leads become equally negative (or positive), no signal will be recorded. It is this technique that is used for recording the electro-oculograms. Since the front of the eye is positive and the rear negative as the eye moves to one side, one electrode becomes more positive (on the side to which the eyes deflect) and the other more negative.

Signal enhancement systems

Techniques of signal enhancement which have contributed to electrophysiology are many and varied. This chapter will only be concerned with techniques which are commonly used in visual electrodiagnosis and which are commercially available. In general, therefore, this means restricting the chapter to a special case of cross-correlation, i.e. signal averaging.

It was Dawson (1951) who first utilized this technique to define the signal and those 'components which are time-locked to the stimulus' and utilized a superimposition technique to enhance this signal. The amplified signal is monitored and is taken to the analog–digital converter of an averaging computer where the signal is converted into digital quantities and stored in the computer's memory. The computer provides a trigger for the stimulus and then stores the activity for a short period following the stimulus. At the end of each storage sweep, the computer, after a brief delay, retriggers the stimulus and repeats the operation. Obviously, with this procedure any event that is time-locked to the stimulus will increase in amplitude relative to the decay of background noise which is random.

The electroretinogram

The electroretinogram is a recording of the retinal action potential, triggered by changes in illumination. The potential itself is a complex one affected by many variables and represents an algebraic summation of all the potentials developed in a variety of retinal layers and cells. By modifying stimulus parameters, it is of course possible to reduce the response from some receptors while still stimulating others. Thus, a blue background can be used to attenuate the activity of rods (and relatively few cones) while intermittent bright red light elicits a 'pure' cone response. The ERG consists of three main waves known as a, b and c (*Figure 3.1*). Granit (1933) proposed that the ERG was composed of the output of three separate subsystems: PI, PII and PIII; PIII was a negative potential the leading edge

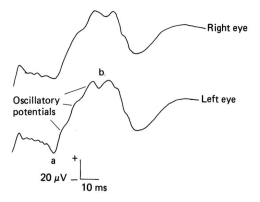

Figure 3.1 The electroretinogram as recorded under scotopic conditions. Both a- and b-waves are shown with, in addition, three oscillatory potentials superimposed on the rising edge of the b-wave. These responses are entirely normal from both eyes and are recorded with the ERG convention of positive up

of which formed the a-wave of the ERG. It is produced by the cell body of photoreceptors and this has two components from cone (a1) and rod (a2). PII is a positive potential probably produced by bipolar cells or Müller cells and contains two components. The first is a positive peak forming the b-wave of the ERG and underlying this is a slow positive DC shift. PI appears to constitute the c-wave of the ERG and, because it appears to be generated by pigment epithelium, it is also reflected in the standing potential of the EOG. In addition to these relatively slow potentials, there are the oscillatory waves which appear on the positive moving b-wave of the ERG. They were first described in man by Cobb and Morton (1954). Their origin is unknown although they may arise in amacrine cells.

In its simplest relationship, the ERG represents the sum of potentials developed by the whole of the retina. Because of this, it obviously relates to the *amounts* of active retina, assuming that the entire retinal area is stimulated. Thus, it is possible, by studying the amplitude of the components of the ERG, to deduce the area of retinal stimulation. There is no simple relationship to which particular area has been activated — only one to the amount of area. This simple relationship coupled to the concept of differential stimulation forms the basis for the clinical use of ERG.

As a basic clinical technique, ERGs can be used to provide an overall estimate of the amount of active retina remaining (Crews, Thompson and Harding, 1978). Thus, if 50% of the retina is detached or damaged, the photopic ERG would be reduced by 50% compared to the fellow eye. Obviously there is a normal variation in amplitude of the signal but this is usually small (Crews, Thompson and Harding, 1978). The amplitude is usually conventionally measured as the peak-to-peak amplitude of the a- and b-waves. Such techniques are simplistic and crude but have been shown to be of great use in a variety of conditions in which retinal damage has occurred. Obviously the signal is affected by the relative brightness of stimulus and this must be considered in uniocular clinical conditions. It has been shown that bright direct light produces faster, higher amplitude ERGs than those produced by less bright stray light. Thus the intensity, diffusion, distance and location relative to the point of fixation of the stimulation are critical. To standardize these factors there has been a recent revival of the ganzfeld stimulator. Using this technique, both background illumination and stimulation parameters can be fully controlled and even illumination of the retina produced. The full field bowl stimulator consists of a plastic sphere with an inner matt white surface. A central LED (light emitting diode) provides a fixation point. The bowl is illuminated by either an incandescent lamp or a flash tube (Chatrain *et al.,* 1980). Interposed coloured or neutral density filters allow independent changes in both background and stimulation illumination. Using these techniques a 'rod ERG' is elicited by dim blue flashes with an absence of background illumination and dark adaptation or a 'cone ERG' by rapid (30 Hz) white flashes against a blue background illumination designed to saturate rod receptors. The various combinations of stimulation and background can of course be computer controlled.

Similar techniques are used in non-ganzfeld situations in the clinic. A few dim blue stimuli are applied to the dark adapted eye to produce a rod response. A flickering (30 Hz) light with or without steady background illumination is used to produce a cone response. It was thought that rods cannot follow rapid flicker, but it has been shown that these follow up to 28 Hz.

Although control of stimulus, colour, duration and intensity obviously makes a major contribution to standardization of the technique, other subjective factors also influence the signal. These are: the level of dark adaptation, pupil size, age, sex and refraction. Of these factors the first two are the most important.

The normal ERG shows both photopic and scotopic features. Indeed the b-wave has early and late features, the early features predominating under light-adapted conditions and later features under dark adaptation. The a-wave has similar features (Armington, Johnson and Riggs, 1952), but these are less clear and not usually seen in clinical investigations. In general, the b-wave should increase in amplitude during dark adaptation with the development of a more rounded shape.

The amplitude and latency of the b-wave is obviously affected by stimulus intensity as is the amplitude and latency of the a-wave. As the intensity of stimulation is increased, there is an increase in amplitude of the b-wave with a shortening in latency. With continued increase in intensity, the b-wave amplitude stabilizes at about the time the a-wave increases in amplitude and reduces its latency. With further increase in intensity, small oscillatory potentials are seen on the ascending (positive) portion of the b-wave. Although the oscillatory potentials increase in amplitude with intensity, their latency appears to remain fixed. There are usually 4–6 wavelets and they are differentially affected by disease states when compared to the a- and b-waves. If the effect of pupil size is now considered, then obviously the maximum amplitude of the a- and b-wave will be reached at a higher intensity for normal pupils than if the eye is artificially dilated. For this reason, in many clinics pupils are dilated as part of the test. The inconvenience for the patient is, however, greater and, certainly for scotopic ERG where the undilated pupil cannot react to a 12-μs flash before the electrical response of the ERG occurs, the effect is negligible. Other variations in the ERG are produced by artefacts such as blinking, eye movements etc. and patient cooperation should always be obtained.

Mention should be made of the *early retinal potential* (ERP) although this does not really form part of neurophysiology since it is thought to be an electrical manifestation of the bleaching of retinal photopigment. It is only elicited by very bright stimuli and consists of a tiny triphasic wave with a latency of 60 μs occurring shortly before the a-wave.

A recent development has been the technique of 'pattern' ERG. Under this condition, the overall level of illumination remains a constant but local changes in luminance occur. A pattern consisting either of alternate black and white bars or checks is moved back and forth or optically reversed so that small local areas of retina change from light to dark and vice versa. Since accurate focusing of the pattern is obviously essential, electrodes which interfere with vision cannot be used. The gold foil or the Dawson electrode are entirely satisfactory.

Pattern ERGs are maximally obtained when the parafoveal area is stimulated. Obviously stimuli containing checks or bars as small as 7.5' of visual angle can be visualized and produce clear responses. For stimulating large retinal areas, checks of 30' of arc or bars of 2 cycles/deg are used. Since the response is a local luminance response, the contrast of the black and white stimuli also affect the amplitude of response. Care must be taken to ensure that the bright white areas of the stimulus are not inducing stray light to other retinal areas.

The electro-oculogram

Electro-oculography entails recording the standing corneoretinal potential, usually during eye movements. Skin electrodes are placed on the temporal area lateral to the outer canthi and on the nose close to the medial canthi. The patient is asked to look at the two fixation lights, 30° apart which are successively illuminated at 1/s for 10 s/min. Eye movements are recorded on an oscillograph with slow paper speed and a relatively short time constant of 0.2 s. This will not allow the oscillograph to follow eye position but will show clearly the eye movements. The patient is placed in complete darkness for 20 min and the eye movements are carried out for 12 min in the dark and then for a further 10 min while exposed to bright background illumination. The amplitude of the pen excursions following the eye movements is measured in both dark and light conditions (*Figure 3.2*) and a ratio calculated. This light:dark ratio is usually expressed as a percentage and is commonly known as the Arden Index (Arden, Barrada and Kelsey, 1962). In general the normal index should exceed 185%. The index varies randomly over time by up to a third within any individual. Indeed the standard deviation on a mean index of 215% is 25% (Van Lith and Balik, 1970).

Visual evoked potentials

The visual evoked potential is usually taken to indicate the cortical potential, although the very earliest components may be subcortical in origin (Harding and Rubinstein, 1980). The VEP is elicited by either a diffuse flash stimulus, an alternating pattern of white and black checks which reverse at fixed intervals of time (*pattern-reversal*) or a pattern or stimulus which appears from a grey background with no overall change in luminance (*pattern-appearance*). It is essential that the two pattern stimuli are *not* considered together as the responses

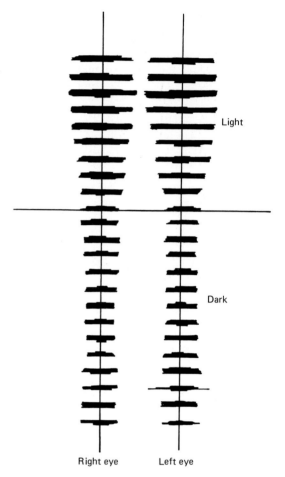

Figure 3.2 A normal electro-oculogram. The increase in amplitude of the eye movement potential is seen to change from dark conditions to light conditions. In this case the dark/light ratio equals 200% from the right eye and 208% from the left eye

that they elicit are entirely different. The response is recorded by electrodes placed close to the occipital poles and referred to a relatively inactive site such as the frontal or rolandic regions. Although some techniques of electrode placement specify the location of the electrodes in terms of fixed distances from bony landmarks (commonly the inion), the preferred system uses measurements as a percentage of head size and are thus equally applicable to babies and adults (10–20 system, *see Figure 3.3*).

The normal VEP to flash stimulation consists of a complex series of waves beginning around 20 ms. Under normal conditions of stimulation recording and averaging, a bright flash of around 1300 cd/m^2 per s is repeated about 32 times at a rate of 2/s and the responses averaged as described earlier. The typical response is shown in *Figure 3.4*. The nomenclature

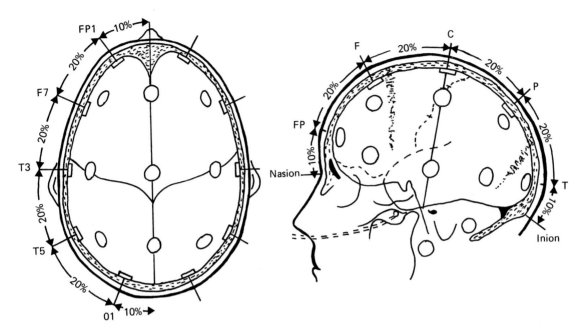

Figure 3.3 The plan and side view of the head with the standard 10/20 system electrode position marked in. It is known as the 10/20 system because all interelectrode distances are 10% or 20% of the measurement between the bony landmarks. In the plan view, the electrodes can be seen to be placed 10% or 20% of the distance between the nasion (bridge of the nose) and the midline at the back of the head. In the side view, the distance is taken between the nasion and the inion and the distance is then divided into 10% and 20% derivatives for each electrode position. It should be noted that the system is therefore proportional to head size and may be used on very tiny babies or adults

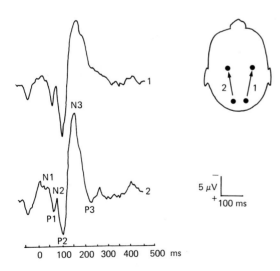

Figure 3.4 The normal flash-evoked visual potential. The components are labelled according to the method of Harding (1974). The major positive component (P_2) occurs shortly after 100 ms and is the component most used in both clinical and normal studies. The recording is shown from both the right and left occiputs when referred to ipsilateral central electrodes

used for this response is that of Harding (1974). There is little doubt that the flash response is more variable than the pattern response and the normal interocular variation may reach 25% in terms of amplitude. The latency is however relatively stable. The early components up to and including P_2 are thought to be most affected by physiological variables, psychological variables only affecting later components. The amplitude of the response increases and the latency shortens with intensity but only up to a relatively low saturation threshold. Above this threshold, intensity has little effect and therefore patient variation, such as pupil size and refractive error, has little effect. This is in contrast to the effect of refractive error on both pattern-reversal and appearance (*Figure 3.5*) (Wright, 1983). This insensitivity of the flash response provides a degree of clinical robustness in conditions where patients cannot or will not fixate a pattern and where refractive errors are unknown. Because the light is bright and diffuse, accurate fixation is not necessary as entoptic stray light appears to fairly evenly illuminate the entire retina. For this reason, half-field stimulation is impossible to accurately produce and only patients with hemianopia accurately reflect this situation (Harding, Smith and Smith, 1980). Under these conditions, however, the distribution of a flash

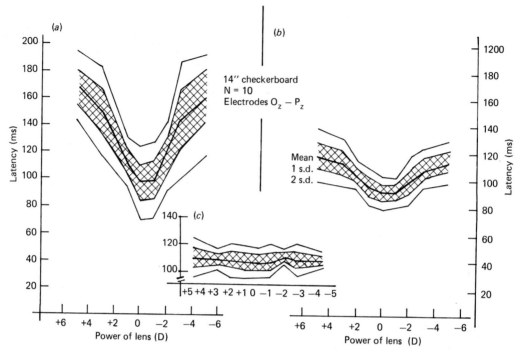

Figure 3.5 The effect on the visual evoked response of increasing and decreasing the power of the lens from the subject's correct refraction. As can be seen, the most marked effect on the latency of the VER is on the CII component of pattern appearance (*a*). A similar, although less marked, effect is seen on the pattern reversal P_{100} component (*b*). The P_2 component of flash (N = 6)(*c*) is completely unaffected by ±5 increases or reduction in the power of the lens. Thus, for pattern responses, patients must be correctly refracted, but for flash response this is not significant. (From Wright, 1983)

response on the scalp is seen to be clearly contralateral (i.e. it is recorded over the visual cortex contralateral to the stimulated half-field), as is the appearance response; both of these contrast with the pattern-reversal response which is clearly ipsilateral (i.e. anatomically 'wrong') to a 16° radius half-field pattern reversal checkerboard using large checks (Harding, Smith and Smith, 1980).

The age of the patient alters the latency of the flash-evoked VEP much more than the latency of the pattern reversal VEP (Wright, 1983). Norms for latency of flash and pattern VEPs are given in *Table 3.1*.

Since the VEP lasts for more than 250 ms, it is important that the stimulus rate is slow. Many authors have shown that at greater than 4 stimuli/second each response affects the subsequent one either positively or negatively. To avoid this complication, transient responses should not be recorded at stimuli rates exceeding 2/second. The only exception to this statement is in 'steady-state' recording in which the cortex is deliberately 'driven' at higher rates, usually around 8–10/second, by a sinusoidally modulated light. This technique has not been shown to have any significant advantages and will not be

further considered. Pattern-reversal VEPs are an exceptionally popular clinical tool. They have the advantage that the waveform is simpler than that of the flash-evoked potential, and has less variability (Halliday and Mushin, 1980). In addition, pattern-reversal VEPs are more sensitive to ocular factors and even fairly accurate refraction to within a range of 1 D can be performed (*see* Figure 3.5).

Stimulus parameters also greatly influence the pattern-reversal VEP, particularly when it is recorded over a variety of scalp sites. The luminance, contrast levels, check size, field size and sharpness of contour all alter the latency and amplitude of the VEP. Check size and field size interrelate logically with small checks producing the largest earliest response from macular stimulation, and large checks producing them from peripheral stimulation. To control for luminance and contrast, relatively bright stimuli (100 cd/m²) are used with a contrast level between black and white squares of between 80 and 100%.

The ability to provide discrete stimuli at specific locations in the visual field is one of the great advantages of pattern stimuli. Providing stimuli to particular parts of the visual field allows accurate location of the signal over the scalp. There is now no

Table 3.1 Norms for latency of flash and pattern VEPs

Age group (years)	Flash P₂ component	Pattern reversal P₁₀₀ (56' check)	Pattern-onset CI (56' check)	Pattern-onset CII (56' check)
10–19	114.5 ± 9.84	108.56 ±10.9	*	*
20–29	120.75 ±10.99	101.78 ±7.64	71.7 ±9.3	98.0 ±14.0
30–39	121.7 ±7.8	106.78 ±4.91	71.1 ±7.5	99.0 ±4.6
40–49	126.8 ±11.26	104.6 ±5.15	71.65 ±9.8	102.9 ±9.95
50–59	122.5 ±15.45	102.89 ±6.75	71.0 ±5.6	105.6 ±13.1
60–69	127.28 ±11.28	109.22 ±10.45	74.2 ±5.7	110.5 ±9.8
70–79	134.25 ±12.72	111.00 ±8.7	73.0 ±5.0	116.4 ±9.2

*Pattern-onset data not available due to ambiguity of waveforms.

doubt that half-field stimulation using large checks in a large half-field produces a maximal response apparently ipsilateral to the field stimulated. There is no doubt that the signal is actually originating over the correct contralateral hemisphere, but the position of active and reference electrodes used by many workers produce this pseudo-ipsilaterality (Kriss and Halliday, 1980). As checks become smaller (less than 15′ of visual angle) and targets smaller (less than 10° visual angle), the maximal response swings over to the correct contralateral side (Harding, Smith and Smith, 1980). The elegant simplicity and lower variability of the pattern reversal VEP (*Figure 3.6*) allow a simple form of nomenclature using polarity (as in flash) with a subscript of latency. The main part is the P₁₀₀ component occurring at around 100 ms. This is seen ipsilateral to the field stimulated and appears to be maximally generated by the macula. It is this wave that closely approximates the P₂ wave of the flash response and may well be contained in that more complex and rounded component.

The pattern-appearance response, or more correctly the pattern onset–offset response, appears markedly different to the pattern-reversal response (*Figure 3.7*). Unlike pattern-reversal and flash response, it is usually shown positive up. The components which are present are usually referred to as CI (positive at 72 ms), CII (negative at 105 ms) and CIII (positive at 155 ms) (Jeffries, 1977). These components are often differently affected by different stimuli and subjective parameters. The CII component appears markedly affected by the contour or sharpness of the pattern and is easily the most sensitive to defocusing of any technique. Other

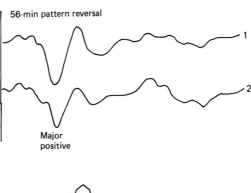

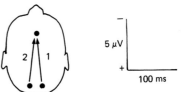

Figure 3.6 The visual evoked response to pattern reversal is shown recorded from a normal subject. The responses in this case are shown recorded from each occiput and referred to the midfrontal electrode F_z. The response is of much simpler waveform than the flash VEP and to a large extent consists of a high amplitude positive component around 100 ms usually known as the P₁₀₀ component

components are affected by contrast (CI) and by meaning of significance (CIII). These components follow the flash response in being recorded maximally over the hemisphere contralateral to the half-

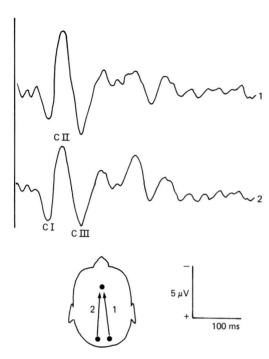

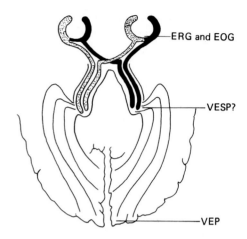

Figure 3.8 The visual system in relation to the location of the various electrophysiological signals. It is apparent that occular lesions will affect the ERG or the EOG, that optic nerve lesions will affect VESPs and VEPs bilaterally, but only on stimulation of the affected eye, whereas postchiasmal lesions will affect the VESP and VEP from one hemisphere, whichever eye is stimulated

Figure 3.7 The VEP elicited by pattern-onset/offset with a 56′ checkboard. The onset components of CI, CII and CIII are clearly apparent, as is the off response which tends to be a smaller mirror image of the onset component. It should be noted that pattern-onset/offset recordings are quite often made with the opposite convention, i.e. positive up and negative down

field stimulated (Shagass, Amadeo and Roemer, 1976).

However, in spite of this elegant sensitivity, or indeed because of it, the pattern appearance response has been less clinically useful. The sensitivity of this and other techniques to ocular factors, means that subjective cooperation of the patient is almost always essential. Accurate refraction should be carried out prior to testing with pattern stimuli and great care should be taken to make sure that the stimulus itself is not blurred.

Clinical electrodiagnosis

In this section, the previous emphasis on individual techniques will be ignored and complementary results from all applicable techniques will be considered in relation to specific clinical conditions. Only a thumbnail sketch of the most common referrals for electrodiagnosis can be given and, for a wider review, the reader is referred to the further reading at the end of this chapter.

One of the essential features of electrodiagnosis is its ability to localize the lesion (*Figure 3.8*). Even neglecting the visual evoked subcortical potential (VESP), by providing monocular stimulation and recording the ERG and EOG from each eye and the VEP from both visual cortices, it is possible to localize lesions to the globe, the optic nerve, the optic chiasma and the tracts and visual cortices. The other eye, if unaffected, can act as the normal control for the affected eye and equally the signals arising from the two visual cortices can act as controls for each other.

It should, of course, be remembered that signals such as the visual evoked potential may be affected by any lesion affecting the pathway at any prior level. Thus, lesions affecting the retina, the optic nerve, the optic chiasma and the optic tracts can all affect the visual evoked potential.

The eye

The three most common electrodiagnostic referrals for conditions affecting the eye itself are opacities of the media, retinitis pigmentosa and retinal detachment. Disturbances of the vascular system of the retina constitute a fourth but less common group.

Cataract

Investigation of opacities of the media has in general concentrated on cataracts. If the amplitude of the ERG is maintained then, of patients with normal pre-operative ERGs, 92% achieve a post-operative visual acuity of 6/6. Patients with a reduced b-wave amplitude, however, usually do not achieve such good vision, only 22% of this group having a visual acuity of 6/6. It should be remembered that, in some patients, the b-wave amplitude is greater in the eye with the cataract than in either the normal eye or aphakic eyes, and it has been suggested by Burian and Burns (1966) that the lens with a cataract is acting as a diffuser.

There is at present no evidence to suggest that lens opacities affect the pre- and post-operative electro-oculogram, but the flash VEP is clearly affected. In the series of patients studied, Thomson and Harding (1978) found that the amplitude of the flash VEP was a good predictor of the visual outcome in patients with cataracts. The amplitude of the P_2 wave of the flash VEP from the affected eye was compared to the amplitude from the unaffected eye and, if the reduction in amplitude was greater than that found as a normal intraocular variation, the visual outcome was poor, the vision achieved being 6/24 or worse. If, however, the amplitude was not reduced, then the visual outcome was good, the patients achieving 6/12 or better post-operatively (*Figure 3.9*).

Vitreous haemorrhages obscure the fundus and retina and often one of the few accurate means of assessment of damage and prognosis that can be made is by electrodiagnosis. If the vitreous haemorrhage is associated with retinal detachment, the electroretinogram is reduced according to the amount of retina involved. The relationship appears to be simple and purely related to areal scores of retinal involvement since the ERG is not reflective of foveal magnification. The VEP under these conditions usually does not provide a great deal of assistance, only correlating with the length of time since the detachment took place. If the vitreous haemorrhage follows a central retinal vein thrombosis, most components of the ERG are reduced, but the oscillatory potentials are absent (*Figure 3.10*). In most other vitreous haemorrhages, including that associated with diabetic retinopathy, the oscillatory potential is partly reduced.

With the recent development of techniques of vitrectomy, the prediction of retinal and visual function through opaque media has become more important. It is essential under these conditions to use a very bright stimulus (intensity 16 on a Grass stroboscope, i.e. 9661 cd/m² or 483 nit seconds). The electroretinogram has been claimed to be superior to other tests of retinal function under these conditions (Fuller, Knighton and Machemer, 1975). Experience at Aston has shown that the VEP is also of use with a very bright flash stimulus using the same simple relationship of amplitude of the P_2 component as was discussed with cataracts.

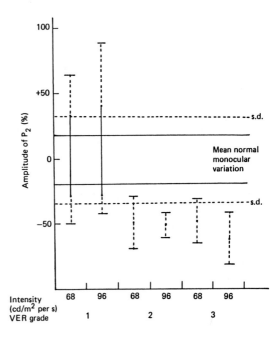

Figure 3.9 The mean monocular variation from a normal sample between fellow eyes. To this is added one standard deviation in each direction providing a normal limit of around 35% difference between eyes. The patients with cataracts fall into three grades: grade 1 has no difference between the cataract eye and the normal eye; grade 2 shows a reduction of less than 50% and grade 3 a reduction of more than 50% when the differences between the eyes actually increase as the intensity of the stimulus is increased

Retinal damage

Traumatic damage to the eye obviously affects all electrodiagnostic tests. Usually the EOG is more markedly affected than the ERG. Even with blunt injury, the EOG is depressed for a few days whereas the a- and b-waves of the ERG are really only affected by severe injuries. The use of both the ERG and the VEP to give a combined score produces the best prognostic indication in eyes with severe penetrating wounds. The method of scoring both the ERG and the VEP is simple. For the ERG the only score is that of amplitude; if the amplitude of the ERG is reduced by less than 25% it is considered as grade I, between 25% and 50% as grade II, and more than 50% as grade III; if the ERG is absent it is considered as grade IV. Almost identical ratings are used for the VEP, except that, if the VEP is markedly delayed, then the score is increased by one grade. Under these conditions, a lid ERG which is reduced less than 50% and the VEP which is either reduced less than 50% or not

Binocular

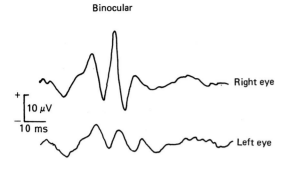

Right eye

10 μV
10 ms

Left eye

Binocular

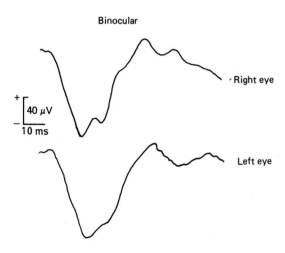

Right eye

40 μV
10 ms

Left eye

Figure 3.10 The results from a patient with a central retinal vein occlusion of the left eye. The top two traces show the oscillatory potentials recorded using a short-time constant to remove the a- and b-waves of the electroretinogram. It can be seen that all the oscillatory potentials are markedly reduced from the left eye. The lower two traces show the ERG under photopic conditions recorded with a longer time constant. The a- and b-waves can be seen and superimposed on the b-wave from the right eye are the oscillatory potentials. These are markedly reduced or missing from the left eye

delayed, invariably predict a good visual outcome. It should be remembered that the two techniques are measuring different levels of the pathway and are therefore complementary. The ERG is measuring the area of retina that has been damaged, whereas the VEP is reflecting foveal magnification and the normal functioning of the optic nerve and visual cortices. Many severe eye injuries may be associated with other head trauma and it is essential that the entire visual system is considered. Obviously indirect or direct optic nerve trauma could cause an

extinguished VEP in the presence of a completely normal ERG. By combining these two techniques, electrodiagnostic tests produce a better prognostic indication than any other technique of assessing damage.

Inherited retinal degenerations

Inherited retinal degenerations form an important area of electrodiagnostic investigations. The move towards early diagnosis and recognition of genetic counselling has increased the demand for electro-diagnostic assistance. Much of the clinical work is directed to the problems of retinitis pigmentosa. Both the ERG and the EOG are markedly affected and most observers believe that the ERG is affected slightly earlier in the course of the disease. The ERG is often affected at a very early stage when fundus changes are minimal or absent. The response is usually extinguished in the recessive form of the disorder in which marked changes of retinal function occur at an early stage and on which the prognosis for vision is poor. In the autosomal dominant type, the ERG is relatively well preserved, being only slightly reduced in amplitude at the time when there is only a mild effect on vision (*Figure 3.11*). Since, in the recessive condition, the ERG appears to be extinguished early, there is no simple relationship with the severity of the disease. Indeed, it has been suggested that the electroretinogram may be extinguished from birth (Franceschetti, Francoise and Babel, 1963). However, other workers suggest that when there is a history of late onset and mild form of the disease, the ERG is relatively well preserved and correlates with the functioning area of the retina (Armington *et al.*, 1961).

The EOG usually shows an absent response to light at an early stage of the disease. The absence of an increased light/dark ratio is very marked being abnormal in 96% of eyes (Babel *et al.*, 1977). The VEP in retinitis pigmentosa is quite often well preserved, being recordable when the ERG cannot be detected. This is not surprising because the ERG reflects only the amount of retina involved, whereas the VEP is dependent on macular function as represented by cortical magnification and, of course, it is the macular function which is relatively spared in retinitis pigmentosa.

Optic nerve

Conditions affecting the optic nerve can similarly be divided into acquired or inherited types. Among the most common referrals for acquired conditions are acute optic neuritis, direct and indirect optic nerve trauma, various toxic conditions and atrophies.

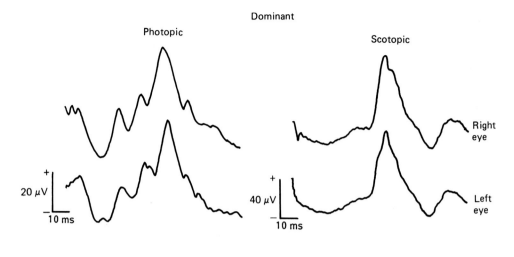

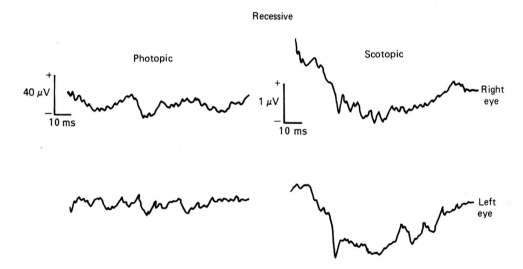

Figure 3.11 Recordings taken under photopic conditions from two separate patients with retinitis pigmentosa. The upper trace shows a patient with autosmal dominant type of retinitis pigmentosa with a well preserved ERG. The lower trace shows a severe reduction in a patient with a recessive form of retinitis pigmentosa. The responses in this case were all recorded using corneal electrodes.

Optic neuritis

Acute optic neuritis must provide by far the most common referral for VEPs. As would be expected from a condition affecting the optic nerve, the ERG and EOG are unaffected, but the VEP is markedly delayed. The delay is seen in the flash, pattern-reversal and pattern-appearance VEPs, but by far the greatest delay is shown in the two responses to change in pattern (*Figure 3.12*). The amplitude of the VEP is reduced in the acute condition when visual acuity is severely impaired and, indeed,

the response to pattern stimuli may be completely abolished. Under these conditions, the flash evoked potential comes into its own as a response which can still be elicited and which is often delayed. Although the visual evoked response correlates to some extent with the visual acuity in terms of amplitude, the latency is completely dissociated with the delay which has occurred, persisting even after the visual acuity has apparently returned to normal. This finding is of great assistance in the diagnosis of multiple sclerosis since clinically silent lesions can be recognized even when the patient does not report

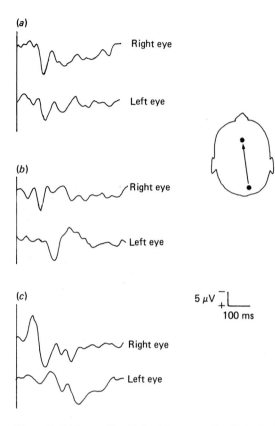

Figure 3.12 The results obtained in a case of unilateral acute optic neuritis affecting the left eye. The flash response (*a*) only shows a mild reduction in amplitude and only a slight delay of the P_2 component. Pattern reversal, however, shows a marked shift of the P_{100} and pattern-onset—offset shows a similar delay to the entire complex. (*a*) Flash; (*b*) 56′ pattern-reversal; (*c*) 56′ pattern-onset–offset

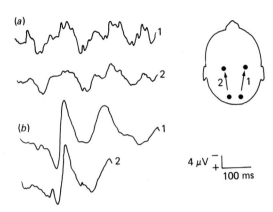

Figure 3.13 A case of direct optic nerve trauma. The patient had a gunshot wound in which the bullet entered the left temple, traversed the left orbit, hit the floor of the right orbit and richocheted out through the right temple. The visual evoked response from the left eye (*b*) is well maintained with a clear P_2 component affected by flash stimulation. The response from the right eye (*a*) is absent with only background EEG activity being present. The bullet has therefore spared the left optic nerve but completely ablated the right optic nerve

the occurrence of any visual symptoms. Obviously, since multiple sclerosis should represent a disseminating lesion, it is important that other pathways are investigated using evoked responses. In cases where delays have occurred, it is of course possible to state whether the apparently normal optic nerve has also been affected and whether any lesions have also occurred postchiasmally since, under these conditions, the response over the visual cortices will be asynchronous, occurring earlier on one hemisphere of the brain than on the other.

Trauma

Direct optic nerve trauma is quite frequently associated with injuries to the globe although, on some occasions, the injury may avoid the globe but penetrate the optic nerve (*Figure 3.13*). However, cases of indirect optic nerve trauma do occur, usually as a result of a fall in which the head is severely struck.

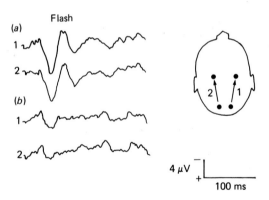

Figure 3.14 A case of indirect optic nerve trauma. This young boy, while climbing over the railway lines, was electrocuted and fell onto the lines below. Although he survived the electrocution, the head injury caused an indirect optic nerve trauma to the left optic nerve such that the visual evoked response to flash stimulation is grossly reduced over both hemispheres of the brain when the left eye is stimulated. This finding, therefore, is entirely consistent with indirect trauma of the left optic nerve. There has been no penetrating wound. (*a*) Right eye; (*b*) left eye

An example of such damage can be seen in *Figure 3.14*. As can be seen in both these conditions, the amplitude is markedly reduced and in some cases may be entirely absent if the optic nerve has been entirely severed.

Toxic conditions

Toxic conditions affecting the optic nerve include tobacco/alcohol and ethambutol. Surprisingly few patients who suffer from tobacco/alcohol poisoning show tobacco/alcohol amblyopia and the electrodiagnostic findings reflect this pattern. Only in patients where the visual deficit is clearly apparent, is there a reduction and delay in the VEP. Ethambutol toxicity, on the other hand, appears to have a much more profound effect even when the visual symptoms are clinically not apparent. This is most important because patients who are treated for pulmonary tuberculosis very frequently are immigrants and language and subjective assessment may be a problem. In almost 25% of these patients without visual symptoms, the visual evoked response is both reduced and delayed even when they are treated at the recommended dose level. When this dose level is exceeded and the patient shows clinical symptoms, the changes in the VEP are most marked and, even when the drug is stopped, the symptoms persist for a long time.

Atrophies

Hereditary optic atrophies produce marked effects on the VEP. Both Leber's X-linked optic atrophy and the autosomal dominant optic atrophy tend to produce an exaggeration of a negative wave at approximately the same latency of the P_2 component. The PNP or positive–negative–positive type response gives a classic 'W'-shaped format and is easily recognizable (*Figure 3.15*). It is suggested by some authors that these responses are associated with central scotoma in the visual fields (Halliday, 1976), but in a study of 27 members of six families with dominant optic atrophy the PNP type, response was not associated with central scotoma (Harding and Crews, 1982).

Space-occupying lesions affecting either orbit and producing either compression or extension of the optic nerve, or optic gliomas, all produce similar effects. Pattern-reversal and pattern-appearance of responses are affected first and tend to disappear while the flash response is still preserved though often delayed (Halliday and Mushin, 1980).

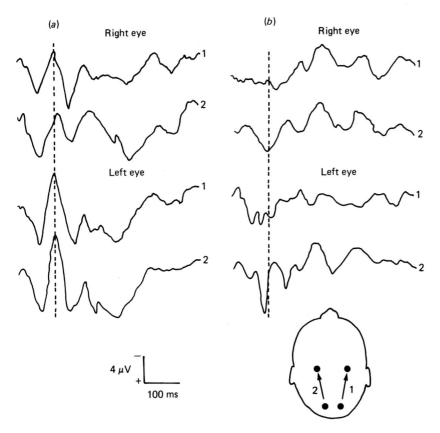

Figure 3.15 The VEP to flash stimulation in hereditary optic atrophy often shows a 'PNP' type waveform with the negative occurring at 100 ms, i.e. where the P_2 component would be expected. This response is usually more clearly seen on flash stimulation than on pattern reversal. (*a*) Flash; (*b*) pattern reversal

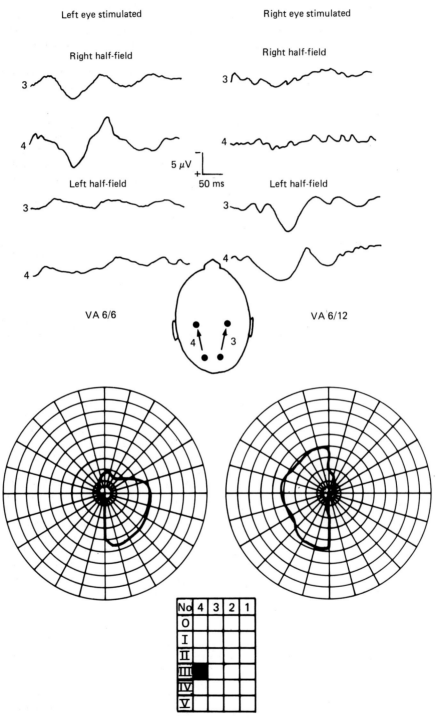

Figure 3.16 The VEP elicited by half-field stimulation in a patient with bitemporal hemianopia. When the left eye is stimulated in the preserved right half-field a clear response is elicited which is of greater amplitude over the left visual cortex than the right. When the left half-field is stimulated there is no response. When the right eye is stimulated over the preserved left half-field, a clear response is observed which is of greater amplitude over the right visual cortex. When the absent right half-field is stimulated there is no response. In this case the stimuli were reversing checker-boards

Chiasmal and postchiasmal lesions

Chiasma

Chiasmal lesions are classically those of bitemporal hemianopia. In these patients on binocular stimulation, relatively normal VEPs are recorded fairly symmetrically over the two cerebral hemispheres. However, when one eye is stimulated, the crosslateral hemisphere receives practically no visual input and the evoked response becomes markedly asymmetrical. Unfortunately, due to the complexities of field size, check size and electrode placement and linkage, the electrode under which the signal is apparently reduced is often difficult to predict. It would appear that if wide-spaced occipital electrodes are used with common reference recording to the midfrontal electrode, F_Z, the signal is reduced over the opposite hemisphere to that which one would expect from an anatomical model. Thus, when the right eye is stimulated, the signal is apparently missing over the right cerebral hemisphere. This is so long as a 0-15° radius, 50' checkerboard stimulus is used. If the checks are smaller and, if the field is smaller than this, asymmetry may vary (Harding, Smith and Smith, 1980). When electrodes are placed directly over the occiputs and are referred to other 'inactive' references (such as the central rolandic region), the pattern that one would expect from the anatomical model is observed. Thus, when the right eye is stimulated with any size of checks or with flash, the response is reduced over the contralateral hemisphere. It is probably not without significance that these two differing electrode placements, the first as used by Halliday and his co-workers and the latter by Harding and the Birmingham group, have a vector difference of around 45°. It is therefore essential that clinical workers recognize this problem and standardize on one or other electrode placement, and at least one of the standard stimulators to provide a datum point for their studies.

An example of a patient with bitemporal hemianopia is shown in *Figure 3.16*. As can be seen the asymmetry of the VEP reverses as each eye is stimulated. In addition, the figure shows the use of half-field stimulation which is always a most worthwhile technique in any patient with a suspected hemianopia. It can only be performed with pattern-reversal or pattern-appearance, but the elegance of having the response disappear when the 'missing' half-field is stimulated, compared to a large response from the preserved half-field, helps to reinforce the significance of the clinical finding.

Postchiasmal

Postchiasmal lesions are difficult to localize, although lateralizing them is easy. Needless to say, the response from a hemianopic patient is similar to that when one eye of the patient with bitemporal hemianopia is stimulated. In this case, whichever eye is stimulated, the response is always asymmetrical and according to the placement of electrodes and the type of stimulus used will follow the pattern discussed earlier. It is at present not possible to localize the lesion to the optic tract, or the lateral geniculate bodies, the optic radiations or the visual cortex. The use of the visual evoked subcortical potential (Harding and Rubinstein, 1980) does allow differentiation between cortical and subcortical responses. The technique is not as yet suitable for regular clinical use. In some cases, the presence of cortical abnormality can be confirmed by the use of the *electroencephalogram* (EEG) and certainly, if a cortical lesion is considered probable, this technique should always be used to supplement the VEP.

In all those conditions not involving the globe, the ERG and EOG will usually be entirely normal. It is this ability of clinical neurophysiology to locate lesions in differing areas of the visual pathway that is its greatest contribution to optometry and ophthalmology.

The complementary nature of the various measures cannot be stressed too much; clinics which only record the ERG or the EOG or the VEP are losing more than two-thirds of their diagnostic capabilities, since it is often the combination of the techniques that makes the diagnosis certain.

References

ARDEN, G.B., BARRADA, A. and KELSEY, J.H. (1962) New clinical test of retinal function based upon the standing potential of the eye. *Br. J. Ophthalmol.*, **46**, 449–467

ARDEN, G.B., CARTER, R.M., HOGG, C., SIEGAL, I.M. and MARGOLIS, S. (1979) A gold foil electrode: extending the horizons for clinical electroretinography. *Invest. Ophthalmol. Vis. Sci.*, **18**, 421–426

ARMINGTON, J.C., GOURAS, P., TEPAS, D. and GUNKEL, R. (1961) Detection of the electroretinogram in retinitis pigmentosa. *Exp. Eye Res.*, **1**, 74–80

ARMINGTON, J.C., JOHNSON, E.P. and RIGGS, L.A. (1952) The scotopic 'a' wave in the electrical response of the human retina. *J. Physiol.*, **118**, 289

BABEL, J. STANGOS, N., KOROL, S. and SPIRITUS, M. (1977) *Ocular Electrophysiology: A Clinical and Experimental Study of Electroretinogram, Electro-oculogram and Visual Evoked Response.* pp. 1–172. Stuttgart: George Thième Publishers

BURIAN, H.M. and BURNS, C.A. (1966) A note on senile cataracts and the electroretinogram. *Doc. Ophthalmol.*, **20**, 141–149

CHATRAIN, C.E., LETTICH, E., NELSON, P.L., MILLER, R.C., McKENZIE, R.J. and MILLS, R.P. (1980) Computer assisted quantitative electroretinography. *Am. J. EEG Technol.*, **20**, 57–77

COBB, W.A. and MORTON, H.B. (1954) A new component of the human electroretinogram. *J. Physiol.*, **123**, 36–37

CREWS, S.J., THOMPSON, C.R.S. and HARDING, G.F.A. (1978) The ERG and VEP in patients with severe eye injury. *Documents Ophthalmologica Proceedings Series No. 15*, pp. 203-209. The Hague: Junk

DAWSON, G.D. (1951) A summation technique for the detection of small signals in a large irregular background. *Physiol.*, **115**, 2–3

DAWSON, W.W., TRICK, G.L. and MAIDA, T.N. (1981) Evaluation of the DTL corneal electrode. *Documenta Ophthalmological Proceedings Series No 31*, The Hague: Junk

FULLER, D.G., KNIGHTON, R.W. and MACHEMER, R. (1975) Bright flash ERG, for evaluating eyes with opaque media. *Am. J. Ophthalmol.*, **80**, 214

FRANCESCHETTI, A., FRANCOIS, J. and BABEL, J. (1963) *Les Heredo-degenerescences Chorioretiniennes*, Vol. 1, pp. 226–306. Paris: Masson

GRANIT, R. (1933) The components of the retinal action potential in mammals and their relation to the discharge in the optic nerve. *J. Physiol.*, **77**, 207–239

HALLIDAY, A.M. (1976) Visually evoked response in optic nerve disease. *Trans. Ophthalmol. Soc. UK*, **96**, 372–376

HALLIDAY, A.M. and MUSHIN, J. (1980) The visual evoked potential in neuro-ophthalmology. In *International Ophthalmology Clinics, No. 20: Electrophysiology and Psychophysics: Their Use in Ophthalmic Diagnosis*, edited by S. Suckle, pp. 155–183. Boston: Little Brown

HARDING, G.F.A. (1974) The visual evoked response. *Adv. Ophthalmol.*, **28**, 2–28

HARDING, G.F.A. and CREWS, S.J. (1982) The VER in hereditary optic atrophy of the dominant type. In *Clinical Applications of Evoked Potentials in Neurology*, edited by J. Courgon, F. Maughuiere and M. Revol, pp. 21–30. New York: Raven Press

HARDING, G.F.A. and RUBINSTEIN, M.P. (1980) Components of the visually evoked subcortical potential (VESP) to flash stimulation in man. In *EEG and Clinical Neurophysiology*, edited by H. Lechner and A. Aranibar, pp. 464–474. Exerpta-medico International Congress Series No. 256

HARDING, G.F.A., SMITH, G.S. and SMITH, P.E. (1980) The effect of various stimulus parameters on the lateralisation of the visual evoked potential. In *Evoked Potentials*, edited by C. Barber, pp. 213–218. Lancaster: MTP Press

JEFFRIES, D.A. (1977) The physiological significance of pattern visual evoked potentials. In *Visual Evoked Potentials in Man: New Developments*, edited by J.E. Desmitt, pp. 134–136. Oxford: Farendon Press

KRISS, A. and HALLIDAY, A.M. (1980) A comparison of occipital potentials evoked by a pattern onset offset and reversal by movement. In *Evoked Potentials*, edited by C. Barber, pp. 205–212. Lancaster: MTP Press

SHAGASS, C., AMADEO, M. and ROEMER, R.A. (1976) Optical distribution of potentials evoked by half-field pattern reversal and pattern onset stimuli. *Electroencephalogr. Clin. Neurophysiol.*, **41**, 609

THOMPSON, C.R.S. and HARDING, C.F.A. (1978) The visual evoked potential in patients with cataracts. *Documenta Ophthalmological Proceedings Series No. 15*, pp. 193–201. The Hague: Junk

VAN LITH, G. and BALICK, J. (1970) Variability of the electro-oculogram. *Acta Ophthalmol.*, **48**, 1091–1096

WRIGHT, C.E. (1983) Clinical studies of spatial and temporal aspects of vision. *PhD. Thesis*, The University of Aston in Birmingham

Further reading

Electroretinograms and electro-oculograms

GALLOWAY, N. (1981) *Ophthalmic Electrodiagnosis*, 2nd edn. London: Lloyd and Luke

BABEL, J., STANGOS, N., KOROL, S. and SPIRITUS, M. (1977) *Ocular Electro-physiology: A Clinical and Experimental Study of Electroretinogram, Electro-oculogram, Visual Evoked Response*. Stuttgart: George Thième Publishers

Visual evoked potential

HALLIDAY, A.M. (Ed.) (1982) *Evoked Potentials in Clinical Testing*. Edinburgh: Churchill Livingstone

Part 2

Clinical optometry

4

Aims of examination

Deryck Humphriss

How to handle the patient

When a patient attends for eye examination, the prerequisite for a successful outcome is the identification of the patient's main and secondary problems, an assessment of their expectation of the outcome of the consultation (even if this is misdirected or unreasonable), detection of ocular or systemic abnormality if present and an accurate refractive result.

The scope of the examination will be determined by these factors and by any constraints or responsibilities placed on the practice of optometry by legal or contractual obligations.

The presenting symptoms, when considered in the light of previous history, will give a general indication of the likely causative factors. Where refractive, visual difficulty will provide clues, particularly when the distribution of refractive errors and their variation with age, gender and ethnic background are considered. General and ocular pathology will often present with signs or symptoms which must be detected during examination or will at least give results suggestive of further or supplementary tests. In addition, there is a responsibility to screen for insidious, treatable conditions which would not produce symptoms until late in their progression.

The refractive result must be prescribed in a way that meets the patient's visual requirements, taking into account occupational and recreational needs while minimizing or eliminating any objectional limitations or adaptive effects. Time must be spent explaining the purpose, scope and limitations of the correction and alerting the patient to potential adaptational problems before they occur. In this way non-tolerance problems will be minimized. It should be remembered that, at the very least, every consultation is an exercise in 'self-promotion' by the practitioner which, when successful, will enhance rapport and aid patient satisfaction. The practitioner must recognize the effect that personality has on the application of, and the response to, tests.

Experimental psychologists have applied their knowledge of testing procedures to the process of refractive examination and have criticized much of what is done as unscientific, leading to errors as a result. Hence an examination can be improved if the practitioner is aware of these criticisms and of the changes recommended to mitigate them.

Psychological method is a procedure which has been established scientifically to give the best possible results when two people, the tester (practitioner) and the testee (patient), are involved in a process of human measurement. This includes refractive assessment.

The basic psychological knowledge required is that there are personality types which tend to behave in a similar way in test situations; there are traits which have a marked effect on performance and states which detract from the results. A psychological state differs from a trait in that the former is dynamic — a condition of the person, such as agitation, which will change normal behaviour. A trait is a unitary part of a personality which can be isolated and measured separately, such as a fast reactor or a slow reactor. A pattern of traits produces a psychological type, such as a neurotic.

One psychological type which may be recognized before the refraction takes place, is the extrovert, whose opposite is the introvert. The extent to which a patient is extroverted or introverted can be judged partly during the interview when the case history is being taken. The extrovert will talk readily, describe symptoms in detail, and answer questions with little hesitation. He will be fast and perceptually flexible. A slight lack of cooperation may be suggested in an attitude of impatience.

Extroverts are very willing to 'have a go'; they will guess happily at tests which they cannot perform and are not disturbed if their answers are incorrect. Introverts are disinclined to begin a test which they cannot complete and have to be encouraged to start and keep going. An emmetropic extrovert, given the same instructions, will record a higher visual acuity than an introvert because of the willingness to guess.

Introverts are careful, meditative and cautious, are slow and over react to stress situations. They will be persistent and cooperative, must be encouraged to talk and details may not easily be elicited. They will wish to cooperate but may seem uncooperative because of their slowness and disinclination to incriminate themselves with any answer which is not factually precisely correct. A psychological trait found in the introvert is perseveration which is defined as 'a tendency to continue an activity' or 'difficulty in shifting from one task to another'. In popular parlance this patient has a one-track mind. One of the methods of measurement of perseveration will make this latter definition clear. The subject is asked to look at the drawing known as Rubin's goblet (*Figure 4.1*). This is usually seen first as a vase, but then it suddenly changes to two faces looking at each other. Again, without any apparent reason, it changes back to the vase. This does not occur with the perseverator, who having once seen the vase, refuses to accept that there is an alternative perception. This type of patient, on being given a duochrome refraction, and having in three consecutive tests seen that the circle on the red was clearer than that on the green, will continue to say that red is clear irrespective of how much minus is placed before that eye.

This recognition of the type of patient before the refraction has started is therefore a great help in

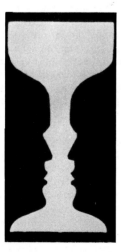

Figure 4.1 Rubin's goblet: this may be seen as a vase or as two black faces looking at each other

determining how to manage the patient during the visual tests.

The anxious patient

Of all the psychological states which might affect the results of a refraction, anxiety is the most important because anxious subjects do not perform so well in test situations. They are likely to make mistakes and very anxious subjects undergoing perceptual tests may not actually see items. Hence, an anxious patient may see no difference between two positions of a cross cylinder while the same patient when relaxed will notice that one position is clearer than the other.

Anxiety is probably present to some degree in every patient who is refracted. Many years ago Munn (1957) suggested that human beings have the capacity to anticipate all sorts of dangers and to worry about them, an opinion supported by Gray (1978) who concluded that no one today is entirely free from anxiety. Anxiety is the rule with children, the precocious child being anxious to show off by doing well. An additional cause of anxiety in children and young adults could be the need to wear spectacles as a result of the examination (Terry, 1981). It is also likely that a visitor from a foreign country, or a migrant worker from a different cultural background, will be more anxious than a member of the local population.

A high degree of anxiety in a patient must be detected by the practitioner because this type of patient may seek consultation with symptoms which are not of ocular origin, in particular parietal or occipital headache.

There are many physiological changes resulting from anxiety which are mainly consistent with a general pattern of innervation of the sympathetic nervous system. This can result in a dilatation of the pupils and possibly introduce more myopia in eyes with a large positive spherical aberration. Anxious patients often find fault with themselves or their own answers; they can also overelaborate them, introducing irrelevant aspects of the test in which the practitioner is not interested.

It is wrong to condemn the anxious patient for any lack of cooperation. The patient who has grown up in an atmosphere of controlled long-suffering patience in the face of difficulty will be cooperative, while the patient who has been brought up in an environment characterized by panic and uninhibited behaviour may well prove to be demanding, complaining and difficult. A patient tends to identify with a happy and peaceful atmosphere and the practitioner should attempt to provide this.

If a human ability is to be measured, it is clearly advisable to reduce anxiety to a minimum by establishing the best possible rapport with the patient. Failure to reassure the anxious patient results in an inefficient refraction. While a patient is being assessed, that patient is also assessing the practitioner. Psychological experiments on the reactions of a subject to a testing situation have shown that the patient prefers nothing extreme, an atmosphere of quiet efficiency being the ideal. The room should be clean and neat and the desk tidy. The furniture and any pictures on the walls should be pleasing rather than striking. Everything that the practitioner needs should be immediately at hand so that time is not wasted and a poor rapport created by searching for equipment which has been mislaid.

Practitioners should avoid extreme dress or any suggestion that they are not 'normal' people. While this enforces a degree of conservatism, it will contribute to building up the practice. The patient should always be greeted pleasantly suggesting that the practitioner is happy to see them.

Rapport

The relationship which is established between the patient and the practitioner is known as *rapport* and nothing is more important to a refraction than the establishment of good rapport, which is a state of cooperation between two people. In a testing situation it is understood that the patients will do their best to give accurate and honest answers to questions put to them and that the practitioners will so handle the testing procedure that this type of answering by patients is encouraged.

Maintaining rapport is necessary if the subject is to do well: the patient must feel that he wants to cooperate with the practitioner. No firm rules can be given for the establishment of rapport, but the person who proceeds coldly and scientifically to administer tests without convincing the patient that he is being regarded as a human being will frequently find it is difficult to maintain the patient's cooperation. Poor rapport is evidenced by inattention, restlessness and finding fault with the tests.

In particular, rapport can be a problem with young children who are not accustomed to doing tests or to undertaking tasks which call for sustained attention.

It may be assumed that the practitioner is unemotional and impartial like the physical scientist or engineer who measures an object with a technical tool. The 'object' in this case, however, is a person and testing involves a psychological relationship with that person. Shafer (1954) emphasized that the practitioner's personality influences the patient and brings its own hopes, fears, assumptions, demands and expectations to the testing situation, responding personally and often intensely to what goes on. Establishing good rapport may be difficult for inexperienced practitioners who are themselves anxious, but it should be remembered that the slightly anxious student is probably a better practitioner than one who is over-confident.

The establishment of good rapport begins as soon as the patient is met when a friendly welcome will be reassuring. This may be provided by the receptionist and by the practitioner when seating the patient in the consulting room. It will be supplemented by taking the case history in a firm but sympathetic attitude.

Taking the case history

The recording of an accurate case history is an art for which three attributes are necessary: knowledge relative to the patient's answers so that their significance can be correctly judged, the correct approach to the patient and the formulation of questions so that essential information is not lost because the questions which would have revealed it are not asked, and finally the ability to control the situation so that the introvert is persuaded to talk freely, while the extrovert is restricted to the essential answers.

Hence the patient should be given an amicable greeting, asked the recorded questions and finally questioned about particular visual problems.

At the core of the case history are the facts defining the reason for which the patient is seeking consultation. A patient will often misinterpret a question about the sort of work he does so that the question is better put in terms of the nature of his work. If the answer is vague, clarification can be gained by asking in what ways the eyes are used at work. The answer will usually indicate the area of vision which must be most carefully assessed or may reveal the fact that the patient is only concerned with leisure reading, with a problem concerning a hobby or with difficulty threading a needle.

A question which enquires about the particular things that are difficult to see clearly will often indicate the nature of the optical defect, while enquiring about what things are seen double will indicate if the practitioner has to deal with generally blurred vision (often described as double) or a state of diplopia. The patient who has genuine diplopia will describe targets which contrast sharply with the background.

There will be occasions when the answers to questions are so unhelpful that no clear picture of the patient's visual troubles can be created. It is then better to abandon further questions, proceed with the examination and, when the problem becomes clearer, to interrupt the refraction and ask the more pertinent questions which will reveal the true symptoms.

Anxiety in children can be avoided by taking a part of the case history from the child and not the parent; while some parents will object to this, it is wise to advise them that it is preferable to talk first to the child, and for the parent to listen carefully to the answers and to subsequently comment on them. In this manner it is often possible to obtain the cooperation of the child and the parent before the refraction is started.

Reducing anxiety

When the patient has been seated comfortably in the chair, instruction should be given to him which will set him at ease and will avoid the belief that if one wrong answer is given, he will be given the wrong prescription. Experience has shown that it is useful to give a preliminary explanation to patients as this helps the rapport between the patient and the practitioner. It should be emphasized that in modern methods all answers are cross-checked. An answer should not be changed if the patient thinks that it is wrong, since the test will be repeated and the answer confirmed. Small differences in clarity are unimportant and, if alternatives look alike, they should be reported as being the same.

It should be explained that all questions are asked twice and all the tests, where necessary, given twice. If at first unsure of an answer, the patient should be instructed to give it after the test is repeated. In particular, the patient should be assured that the vision testing is very easy, interesting and he should relax and hopefully enjoy it.

Phobias

The only phobia which the practitioner is likely to meet is claustrophobia, a condition aggravated by the use of a refractor head. The patient may become distressed, break out into a sweat and possibly thrust the refractor head away. If there are signs of distress when the patient sits in the refracting chair, he should be asked if a refractor head will worry him. If it does, a trial frame should be used without a head rest and the consulting room door should be left slightly open. Most claustrophobic patients will then be comfortable and the refraction can be performed normally.

Scientific methodology is aimed at obtaining the best possible result from a patient undergoing any type of test and, for this, rapport is essential. It is created by providing a warm-up so that the patient knows what is required of him and can do this part of the test without difficulty, by the design of instructions so that the patient continues to do what is required of him and the motivation is maintained. All of this is required in a scientifically conducted refraction.

The warm-up

There is a difference in intent between taking the uncorrected vision and taking the visual acuity. It is most important for future comparison in the case of early pathology to have an exact record of the latter, while the precise measurement of vision may not be so important, because the amount of blur induced by a refractive error varies considerably from one patient to another (Humphriss, 1958).

The taking of uncorrected vision may be used as a psychological warm-up, as it is a simple test which the patient can do easily. Therefore, the patient should not be pressed to try another line when he has stopped or hesitated. As soon as there is hesitation or an inability to see a smaller line, the other eye should be assessed. Nothing gives rise to better rapport than encouragement and the use of encouraging comments and indications of how well the patient is doing will be helpful.

The choice of retinoscopy target is important. The green square of the duochrome test is very suitable, directing the attention to the light which will relax accommodation. The use of letters is not recommended because the patient may be worried when they become blurred. Whatever target is used, the patient should be advised that it may become blurred or double. (For further discussion of the warm-up, *see* Chapters 5 and 8.)

Questioning techniques

Psychologists class questions as two types: open and closed. The open question has no definite answer: a good example might be the opening gambit when taking the case history in the form 'What is your problem?'. The closed question is used to obtain precise information: care must be taken in framing it, because the practitioner must present the patient with all the answers to the question, in such a form that he can choose between them.

One of the most common errors made by practitioners is the giving of incorrect instructions to the patient, or asking them the wrong, or carelessly worded, questions. This is particularly so in the use of the cross cylinder and the duochrome test. If the patient is asked whether position 1 or 2 of a test lens is clearer, it would seem that 1 and 2 are the only possible answers, but this is not so since they may look alike. The question should therefore be framed to include this possibility.

In duochrome refraction the correct instruction is even more important. It is essential to direct the patient's attention to the clarity of letters and not the clarity or brightness of the coloured lights.

When asking such questions, practitioners should be on their guard against the predictable behaviour of the perserverator. These patients have a one-track mind, easily getting into a groove and sticking there. When tested, they persist in making the same response when the stimulus has changed. For example, if asked to name four coloured lights which flash on consecutively, the first three being red and the fourth pink, all four will be called red. The same applies to a red–green test. It is equally remarkable how easily the individual with the one-track mind sees a track and gets into it. If the first three answers to the question are that red is clearer then the track is already laid down: it is that red is clearer. The individual with a one-track mind does not like making decisions, particularly when the choice is difficult, and prefers to make a decision and stick to it. Such patients must be given clear reversals.

The bracketing technique ends when the brackets are determined and acts as a safeguard against the behaviour of the perserverator.

The principle of bracketing

If the end-point of a test is required within known limits, then it can often be measured more accurately and with more ease for the patient, by using the method of bracketing. The principle is to establish the size of the bracket in relation to the accuracy of the method being used and to place that bracket symmetrically either side of the point to be measured. The advantage of this method in refraction is that it eliminates the question of whether a lens is better or worse.

If a patient has some diffuse opacities in the lens lowering the visual acuity to 6/12, and is 1.00 D myopic, he can indicate that a −0.50 sphere is clearer than a +0.50 sphere. If a −2.00 lens is placed before the eye, he can then indicate that the plus lens is clearer than the minus lens. Similarly, if retinoscopy gives −2.00 axis 180°, and if the cross cylinder is used in this position and the answer given that there is no difference between the two positions, this may confirm the axis. Alternatively, if the correct axis is 178°, the answer may only indicate that the patient is a poor observer. If the cylinder is rotated to 178° and to 182° and the patient indicates a rotation towards 180° in the one case and no change in the other, then the practitioner is made aware that axis 180° is not the best position.

Using the bracketing method the patient with a low visual acuity can be refracted by finding the power of lens to which he will respond and to establish the bracket with it. A method of refracting a patient with a low acuity due to irregular astigmatism is described by Humphriss (1984a). The essential principles in using bracketing for measuring human performance are: to establish a bracket so that the correct measurement is known to be within the bracket and not outside it; to reduce the size of the bracket until the patient cannot say which of two choices is the better. Tests are given so

that the bracket straddles the measurement symmetrically and the correct measurement is known to be the centre of the final bracket.

One of the essentials in assessing the ability of a patient to be accurately refracted is to know to what extent they are accurate observers. Their accuracy will depend on two factors: their personality and their visual acuity (V/A). A patient with a V/A of 6/60 cannot give accurate answers if tested on a 6/12 line. Alternatively a patient who is not motivated, is uncooperative and does not care if his answer is accurate or not, may have 6/6 V/A and still give inaccurate answers on a 6/12 test target.

Using a bracketing method, the size of the bracket is adjusted to the limit of accurate observation of the subject and, within these limits, the centre of a symmetrical bracket will give the correct measurement.

Establishing the correct limits

Refraction is usually carried out to a one-quarter of a dioptre (0.25 D) of sphere or cylinder. Some optometrists and ophthalmologists refract to one-eighth of a dioptre (0.125 D), but it is doubtful whether this degree of finesse can be supported scientifically.

Test–retest reliabilities on refraction have not been reliably established and it is very debatable whether statistical reliability would be found at the 0.12 level. It has been established that many patients undergo refractive variations of 0.25 D of sphere and cylinder, so that the additional 0.12 carefully worked out on Monday may be in the opposite direction at a subsequent refraction on Wednesday (Humphriss, 1958).

Research has been carried out in Benoni to indicate that the average patient can observe tests to an accuracy of 0.12 D, i.e. that they can establish a bracket of 0.25 D, so that a refraction can be carried out accurately to 0.12 D. This information may be of value when deciding what modification to make to the prescription obtained by the refraction against that to be prescribed for the patient.

The determination of astigmatism

In most schools of optometry, the procedure taught in testing for a cylinder is to use a random selection of position in which the lens is placed before the eye. It is questionable if this use of a random procedure can be justified in a scientific examination. A routine in applying the crossed cylinder is preferable and the following is suggested:

(1) *When there is no cylinder in the trial frame or refractor head.* The crossed cylinder is placed with the minus axis at 180°. It is rotated and the

patient asked which is clearer or whether they are equal. The minus lens is then placed at axis 45°, rotated and the same question asked. Whatever the two answers, the position of the first cylinder to be tried is known from the answers.

(2) *When there is a cylinder in the trial frame or refractor head.* The axis is checked before the power. The axis of the minus cylinder is placed so that it increases the axis measurement, i.e. if this position were chosen the minus cylinder would be rotated anticlockwise. After establishing the axis, the power is checked. The axis of the minus cylinder is placed along the axis of the trial frame or refractor head lens and using this as position 1, it is rotated so that it is at right angles to the cylindrical lens — position 2. Position 1 will always increase the power of the minus cylinder, and position 2 will always reduce the power.

If this procedure is used with a bracketing technique, it will be found to be both quicker and more satisfactory than a random method. If the patient selects the 180° position with certainty and the 45° position with doubt, the cylinder should be placed 10° nearer to 180°. Similarly, if the patient has accepted the vertical position with certainty and the 135° position with doubt, the lens should be set at axis 102°, i.e. 10° nearer 90 than the midpoint between 90° and 135°.

If a trial frame is being used, time can also be saved by using the cross cylinder as a moderating lens. When an increase in minus cylinder is indicated, instead of changing both the cylinder and the sphere, the cross cylinder is placed with the minus axis in line with the prescription and the patient asked if the vision is better with the lens or without it. This will indicate if the increase required is 1.00 D cylinder or more, or less than 1.00 D cylinder. The research leading to the design of a set of test lenses which minimize trial case lens changes is described by Humphriss (1984b). If further cross cylinder is indicated, then the trial frame prescription should be increased by +1.00/−2.00 and the test repeated.

Unsatisfactory refractions

There will be occasions when a refraction does not proceed satisfactorily and the patient's behaviour while being tested is not consistent with the apparent wish to cooperate, observed when the case history was taken. Only experience can determine when to terminate an unsatisfactory refraction. The indications are that the subjective results disagree considerably with the retinoscopy, or different tests of the same part of the prescription do not agree.

There may be a lack of response with long pauses before answering questions, and uncertainty in choosing between testing lenses which is out of proportion to the patient's visual acuity — this may be subnormal with no pathology to account for the lowering. There may be several genuine reasons for this. The patient may be unwell but did not wish to cancel the appointment. For the same reason, patients suffering from severe psychological trauma, such as a recent bereavement, may keep an appointment when it is impossible for them to concentrate on the testing procedure.

Uncooperative patients

If the patient is being uncooperative and not doing his best, it is part of the competence of the practitioners to improve his performance. This is rarely achieved by being cross or authoritarian. Kindly persuasion generally produces a response, as does a statement which implies that the practitioner knows that the patient could do better. An instruction which emphasizes that a difference can be seen or that letters can be read will often stimulate a better response.

Motivation

A refraction of an unmotivated patient cannot result in a wholly satisfactory conclusion. Unless he cares about the result, his visual state cannot be satisfactorily measured. It is essential to obtain ego involvement, i.e. the patient must desire to maintain self-respect and the respect of the tester or an observer. Effort may be stimulated by the interest in the testing procedure itself.

Some patients will ask the practitioner, during the course of the examination, why they are applying a particular test. It is unwise to interrupt the examination with a detailed explanation and equally wrong to reply that you cannot explain now. It is wiser to indicate that this is a most interesting question, hence building up the ego of the patient, and that if the question is repeated after the examination is completed, an explanation will be given.

The malingering patient

The malingering patient is the one who wishes to do badly. The practitioner is usually alerted to this during the taking of the case history. Answers are not readily forthcoming and the patient will contradict himself or be unnecessarily vague. A child with a severe recurrent headache can tell you the location of the headache in the skull, and the last time that the headache occurred. A child with genuinely blurred vision can describe particular things which he is unable to see. The malingering patient, when reading the letter chart, will make out difficult letters on one line and state that he cannot see the easy letters on the next smaller line.

There are two types of malingering patients: those who malinger consciously and those who malinger unconsciously. The latter patients usually suffer from hysterical amblyopia and their lack of sight is a means of avoiding a situation which is intolerable to them. They may, for example, exhibit a near normal distance acuity and a grossly subnormal near acuity to avoid having to work with figures which are going to reveal dishonesty or financial failure. There may be a lack of distance acuity with normal near acuity in a patient who wishes to discontinue driving a car. The consciously malingering child is likely first of all to say that the blackboard is blurred and, subsequently, that it is reading books that is difficult.

In general these patients will perform all the tests required of them except the reading of small print. The level chosen by the malingerer is usually between 6/12 and 6/24. The practitioner will be alerted to the probability that the patient is malingering by various responses: the retinoscopy results may not produce an improvement in the visual acuity or the patient may see the reversal of the red–green targets in a duochrome test with +0.25 and −0.25 spheres which is out of proportion to the visual acuity recorded. If there is a refractive error, the improvement in the VA through the lenses may be out of proportion to their power. The patient can be placed at 4 metres (13 ft) and the visual acuity taken and again at 2 metres (6.5 ft) and this repeated. The improvement is generally not in proportion to the shorter distance. A reading test can then be given and again the acuity is out of proportion to the size of type read.

Having established that the patient is malingering, the problem is how to handle the patient. If a child, the patient should be sent to the waiting room and the parent alerted to the possible cause. A visit to the family doctor together with a note explaining the situation may be appropriate in some cases.

If the patient is an adult, it is sometimes appropriate to refer the patient to the doctor with a note of the findings. It should be borne in mind that, with an adult, the patient may be attempting to obtain compensation through some sort of insurance policy and that a legal action may follow.

Hence, as always, a copy of the letter to the doctor must be filed with the patient's card which must have the details of the tests given recorded on it. In many cases, it is best simply to reassure the patient that all is well, and to suggest that this be reconfirmed in 2–3 months, thereby reinforcing the assurances.

Difficult patients

Some anxious patients may have drunk sufficient alcohol to make their responses to a refraction technique unreliable. When a refraction is clearly unsatisfactory, it is a waste of time to continue with it, it is better to tell the patient that their difficulty is evident, and to indicate what is the matter. The truth may then come pouring out. It is then better to terminate the appointment and re-examine at a later time.

In conclusion, the practitioner may be confronted with many types of difficult patients, but, while being sympathetic to them, must never lose control of the situation and allow the patient to dictate what tests are used. Sympathy must be tempered with firmness, the practitioner making it clear to the patient that the situation is under control and that the routine will deal with all the problems the patient may have.

References

GRAY, M. (1978) *Neuroses*. New York: Van Nostrand Reinhold

HUMPHRISS, D. (1958) Periodic refractive fluctuations in the healthy eye. *Br. J. Physiol. Opt.*, **15**, 30

HUMPHRISS, D. (1984a) *Refraction Science and Psychology*, p. 75. Cape Town: Juta & Co.

HUMPHRISS, D. (1984b) *Refraction Science and Psychology*, p. 70. Cape Town: Juta & Co

MUNN, N.L. (1957) *The Evolution and Growth of Human Behaviour*. London: George G. Harrap

TERRY, R.L. (1982) The psychology of visual correctives. *Optom. Monthly*, **73**, 137–142

5

Symptomatology

Geoffrey Ball

The majority of patients who attend for optometric examination present one or more of the following symptoms.

(1) Visual blur at some distance.
(2) Discomfort in, or around, the eyes.
(3) Headache.

These common complaints fittingly illustrate the three distinct categories of eye-related symptoms presented by patients: *visual symptoms, symptoms related to the eyes or adnexa*, and *referred symptoms*.

Many other problems are reported by individual patients, but with lower frequency. Nevertheless, some less commonly presented symptoms have a diagnostic significance such that the examiner must always be alert to their presence in a patient's history: the temporary visual loss and transient diplopia of multiple sclerosis; photopsia associated with commencing retinal detachment; reduced mesopic or scotopic vision as an early indicator of retinitis pigmentosa; and the classic coloured haloes around lights of chronic angle-closure glaucoma — these and many other specific symptoms must be recognized, noted and their importance weighed in the final assessment based on all the examination data. But, none of these symptoms alone are pathognomonic of the particular state.

In a single, short chapter it is possible only to indicate the rich variety of problems and symptoms presented by patients in the course of eye examination (*Table 5.1*) and to enlarge on some of those which have special significance to the process of clinical decision-making in optometry.

Clinical data

The information to be obtained and recorded for all patients, which represents defined data or the basic examination protocol, is a continuing topic for discussion. There can be little dispute on the details necessary for patient registration and identification, or on clinical matters such as visual acuities and subjective examination results. There will, however, be differences of opinion on the value of obtaining data for every patient on, for instance, monocular measures of accommodation, keratometry (ophthalmometry), colour vision tests or dynamic retinoscopy.

The development of 'minimum examination routines' for optometry such as the long-standing 21 point routine or standardized data bases (Heath, 1981; Ruskiewicz, 1982) has had much attention. These generalizations on the information to be collected for all patients are of most use if regularly updated and regarded as recommendations, so that account can be taken not only of changing concepts of the purposes of optometric examination but of clinical judgement based on the individual patient.

Whatever system of examination is decided upon the discussion and recording of patients' problems, symptoms and history is an essential part of any eye examination.

Where time is limited, there is merit in reducing the emphasis given to collecting basic information and using the time released for pursuing maximum details on the problems which concern the patient most (problem-specific data), then investigating and analysing that information by a problem-oriented approach.

Table 5.1 Some problems and symptoms presented by patients during optometric examination

Visual	*Ocular and adnexa*	*Referred or other problems*
Blurred vision	Discomfort (ache, pain)	Headache
Focusing problems	Red eyes	Near work held 'too close' or 'too far away'
Loss of vision	Watering eyes	Dizziness
Visual unease	Dry eyes	Vertigo
Colour vision deviations and chromatopsia	Excessive or forceful blinking	Nausea
Photopsia	Fibrillar twitch of lids	Drowsiness from visual tasks, e.g. reading, television
'Floaters'	Ptosis, partial or total	
Coloured haloes		
Metamorphopsia		
Diplopia Binocular Monocular		
Words 'running together' in reading		
Photophobia		

These lists are not exhaustive but include the symptoms dealt with in the text.

Nevertheless, concentrating the main effort on the patient's immediate concerns has to be balanced with the wider responsibilities of practitioners. These include seeking early warning at the time of examination of symptomless, but treatable, conditions such as diabetes or open angle glaucoma and of screening for congenital-type colour vision defects, particularly in young male children. Individual examination routines must take into account these community health-care responsibilities.

Clinical recording

The method used for recording the elements of eye examination for the individual practitioner is a matter for personal preference. These methods range from the traditional printed record card or sheet to microcomputer systems using disk storage, access by keyboard and with information on print-out or display.

It is convenient in any written account to distinguish between symptoms and history but this distinction is undesirable in record systems. If a patient suffers from headaches and has done so for 5 years, then it would be inefficient to record that information under two distinct headings.

Whatever system is used, there should be ample scope for entering details of the patient's symptoms, problems and history so that sufficient notes can be made whatever the depth of information presented. Some printed records give only minimal space to this important part of the examination. Practitioners

working single-handed, if using record cards, are well advised to experiment with and use their own design, so that it can be tailored to their own preferences and practice.

The history and symptom interview

The identification, through discussion, of patient's problems is an early part of examination and normally precedes the application of objective or subjective tests. It conveniently takes place after the formal registration details have been recorded — full names, addresses, date of birth, sex, occupation, and other relevant information of a routine nature.

The intimate face-to-face discussion of the patient's problems which follows, during which concise notes are written by the examiner, is a most important part of eye examination. It is important for several reasons. Not only does it develop the examiner's rapport, powers of communication, observation and interpretation, but it enables tentative judgements to be made on such matters as patient reaction, reliability, motivation and personality. By astute questioning, and especially by listening intently to the patient's words, expressions and descriptions, hypotheses evolve to account for the presented problems. In turn, these suggest techniques to be emphasized later in the examination. The discussion also gives unique patient satisfaction in that their concerns about eyes, vision, spectacles and related problems are conveyed to the examiner early on.

When this initial discussion has taken place, the

question of history, problems and symptoms is not concluded. Significant observations may be made by patients at any time so that this part of the examination must be seen as an open-ended exercise.

How the interview commences and develops will vary but, in general optometric practice, it is best to start with a general open-ended question (for example, 'Are there any special reasons for having your eyes examined?'). There should always be some measure of order to the history and symptom discussion, so that all the essential basic data are obtained together with specific information on the patient's problems (*Tables 5.2* and *5.3*).

The examiner must heed any interesting, even alarming, reports but should avoid being led into assumptions merely on the basis of patient's observations.

When a myope casually mentions occasionally seeing flickering lights out of the 'corner' of his eye, the examiner should be alerted because of the possibility of retinal detachment, but that complaint might also arise from other conditions such as migraine. Further questions must be posed on related indicators, such as headaches, trauma, 'floaters', and then the appropriate objective and subjective investigations made, before making an assessment.

It is useful to summarize the patient's problems as determined during the examination and to record these as a *subjective problem list*.

Table 5.2 Information required from patients in the history and symptom interview

---

(1) *Patient histories*
  Optical: last examination; prescriptions; glasses; contact lenses, including dates
  Visual and ocular: past vision/eye problems; state of vision, distance, near (patient's opinion).
  Medical: General health (e.g. allergies, illnesses, operations); present and past medications
  Family: eye-related problems (e.g. strabismus, myopia, glaucoma, colour vision defects)
  Occupational and recreational: visual tasks at work and in leisure

---

(2) *Patient problems and symptoms*
  Reasons for examination including, where determined:
    Main (primary) symptom or chief complaint
    Subsidiary (secondary) symptoms or minor complaints
    Summary of patient problems (subjective problem list)

---

(3) *Examiner's initial observations*, including:
  Motivation, personality, reliability

---

(4) *Personal information*
  Habits, idiosyncrasies, hobbies, recreations

Table 5.3 Symptom-specific data

Origin: date and time; sudden, gradual, previous indications or attacks

Location: unilateral, bilateral, ocular, adnexa, other

Association: event- or activity-related, pain, photophobia, or other problems

Duration: transient, persistent, variable

Prevention/relief: effect of medication, work, rest, sleep

Previous investigations/treatment

Personal information on the patient

Good history notes should not be restricted entirely to patient's problems. They serve other purposes. The busy practitioner in a large town or city will rarely be able to recollect individual patients at will, unless there was some obvious identifying factor, for instance, an unusual prescription. Personal notes on matters such as mannerisms, idiosyncrasies, interests, hobbies and recreations will help call that patient to mind should this be necessary at some future time. These notes also give the examiner some immediate points of contact when the person next visits.

A form of individual shorthand or code is advisable for recording sensitive information as a safeguard against a card record being lost or unauthorized access being made into whatever record system is being used.

Visual symptoms
Blurred vision

Uncorrected ametropia causing distance blur, or advancing presbyopia giving indistinct near vision, will be determined during the normal course of examination. Myopia and myopic astigmatism are the usual ametropic offenders for poor distance vision, with the visibility of bus numbers and writing on chalkboards being among the prime sources of difficulty for the patient.

School or college students who complain about blurred vision may also report difficulty in changing focus from one distance to another ('jump' accommodation/convergence), usually from near to a far-off projection screen or blackboard. This apparent lag sometimes indicates commencing myopia or a spastic state of accommodation from a near work position that is too close, but could also arise from uncorrected hypermetropia or from convergence inadequacy.

The magnitude of a patient's complaint will depend on many factors including the degree of defect, the types of visual task being undertaken, and also on the psychological make-up of the patient. Decisions on whether there is a need to correct any existing defect will be made in accordance with good clinical practice.

Sometimes a patient, often young, will express concern about blurred vision in one eye after comparing the performance of each eye in turn when viewing critical distance detail such as the time on a clock tower. In optometric terms, the blur is usually quite marginal and commonly found to be due to a minor degree of regular astigmatism sometimes as low as 0.12 D and needing no correction. For normal objects in the environment, the blur is more pronounced when the astigmatic principal meridians are oblique.

The practitioner must ensure that blurred vision is not arising from some simple spectacle dispensing anomaly such as misalignment of bifocal segments or from scratches on the front surfaces of toric or meniscus lenses which have been habitually placed convex surface downwards. Spectacle blur on removing contact lenses and visual blur following the instillation of cycloplegics are well-known phenomena.

Blurred vision in pathological states

Any loss of transparency in the ocular media may lead to symptoms of visual blur, but in general optometric practice the commoner causes are age related and include cataract, especially in nuclear sclerosis and vitreous haze. Changes in one eye only will not always be noticed if visual acuity in the other remains at an acceptable level for the individual. Peripheral lens opacities are more likely to affect vision in reduced illumination if the pupil has a reasonable dilatation.

Episodes of blurred vision either at distance or near occur when corneal mucus or vitreous opacities drift into and across the central field. The visual effects of migraine may sometimes be reported in terms of blur. Ciliary muscle spasm and other causes of acquired myopia (Roy, 1975(i)) — amblyopia from toxic conditions, the adverse effects of drugs, insufficiency of accommodation, central retinal oedema, and chronic angle-closure glaucoma — are but a few of the numerous other pathological states which give rise to the symptom of blurred vision along with general medical conditions such as diabetes and multiple sclerosis.

Bilateral relative central scotomata of low intensity which marginally reduce visual acuity, as in the early stages of some forms of toxic amblyopia, may be described by the patient as haziness of vision. This type of scotoma is more readily demonstrated under reduced illumination (Verriest, 1979) and with other special methods of perimetry.

Loss of vision

A patient's complaint of 'loss of vision' in one eye may sometimes merely indicate reduced vision from uncorrected ametropia, or maybe a long-standing amblyopia which reduces visual acuity but which has only recently been brought to the patient's notice. The individual performance of the two eyes fails to register with many people until special circumstances highlight any disparity. This often comes about when a temporary obstruction interferes with binocular vision so that vision in the 'bad' eye comes to be emphasized.

Occasionally, a patient will maintain that vision has been 'lost suddenly' in an eye which subsequently proves to have long-standing amblyopia ex anopsia or macular degeneration. The usual clinical methods of examination will have to be used for investigating and analysing the claim.

Sudden loss

If the loss complained of has taken place suddenly and is demonstrable at the time of examination, then foveal vision will normally have been affected such that visual acuity is greatly reduced or lost. Where the patient is not already undergoing medical or ophthalmological treatment for the condition, then the practitioner's responsibility will be to refer the patient taking into account the relative urgency assessed from normal investigative procedures, and the legislation which governs practice.

Conditions which give sudden loss of vision in one eye include: optic neuritis (other than chronic varieties), central retinal artery occlusion with no cilioretinal sparing, and haemorrhage of the macula or into the vitreous humour. Loss of vision in retinal detachment may be reported as sudden depending on the moment at which macular function begins to be greatly affected. Ophthalmoscopy and other objective methods (Ball, 1982(ii)) will be applied in the decision-making process.

In cases of real and sudden loss of vision, the practitioner's role is clear in the need to refer the patient for medical/ophthalmological investigation. It is when the complaint refers to a temporary loss (amaurosis fugax) occurring some time in the past and not present on examination that the closest attention to the history and symptoms is needed.

The possible causes are numerous. It may have been a transient 'greying out' on rising quickly from a stooping position or the effect of a dense vitreous opacity floating into the line of vision and just as quickly moving away. It could have arisen from the visual field disturbances of migraine or be a transient visual loss due to vascular insufficiency from some cause. Chronic angle-closure glaucoma, papilloedema and the optic neuritis of multiple sclerosis are some of the other many explanations.

The history and symptom discussion assumes even greater importance in these patients. As much information as possible must be obtained about the episode. Only rigorous attention to the history and to the later relevant objective parts of the examination will enable the examiner to make judgements on whether the reports should be of concern at that point in time. Where there is any reasonable doubt, then advice on a general health-care check is a wise precaution.

Partial loss within the visual field

Small peripheral scotomata are rarely noticed by patients. Even when close to the central area, minor, relative, monocular defects may not be appreciated due to the binocular overlap of a normal fellow eye. Such relative defects become noticeable subjectively as the general level of brightness of the surrounds reduces. Paracentral positive scotomata, even when small and particularly when overlapping binocularly, are a great source of trouble to those affected, and more so in reading if they lie horizontally to the right of the fixation point.

Gradually increasing peripheral depressions and contractions of the visual field can be extensive before coming to a patient's attention, as in open angle glaucoma. Any complaint of colliding with objects or people should alert the examiner to the possibility of some considerable field loss, although there are simpler explanations.

Vertical hemianopic defects such as left homonymous hemianopia might be assumed as a 'left eye' loss by a patient. Types of scotomata, depression and contraction are covered elsewhere (Chapter 22) and in special texts on visual field examination.

Visual unease

This symptom is distinct from discomfort in or around the eyes in that it refers only to the patient's *vision*. It is, therefore, a visual rather than an ocular type of symptom. Visual unease (Ball, 1982(i)) is less often complained of than blurred vision, eye discomfort or headache, and yet it is still reasonably common particularly amongst spectacle wearers. The patient reports 'not feeling comfortable' with his glasses or of having to 'stare' or 'peer' to see properly. Vision generally seems clear, however, and not blurred.

This kind of visual unease is typically seen in corrected myopes who need a small change of distance prescription for one eye only. It often occurs in minor amounts of unilateral, uncorrected ametropia. Vision of the affected eye is slightly blurred under certain conditions yet not noticed as such by the individual. The good vision of the other eye overrides the marginally blurred image so that the patient's vision binocularly remains normal.

The sense of unease probably arises from unilateral central suspension in the ametropic eye when attempting to fuse the blurred with the clear image.

Other minor stresses in the binocular fusion reflex give rise to this symptom, even if there are no complaints of eye discomfort. It can also be a result of close work when accommodation is just becoming overtaxed, as in patients who require their first small presbyopic reading additions. Neurosis and the performance of exacting visual tasks, such as prolonged driving, are other possible explanations for the symptom.

Complaints similar to visual unease have been reported (Arden, 1978) in conditions which cause loss of contrast sensitivity as in demyelinating disease.

Colour vision problems

Few patients make spontaneous complaints about the colour confusions resulting from male-orientated, congenital-type colour vision defects, of which deuteranomalous trichromatism is the most common. Under questioning, these patients may hint at mistaking the colours of everyday objects (wools, ties, snooker balls, pullovers) or admit to vocational problems, but they rarely present these as unprompted symptoms. An unsolicited complaint about colour vision is unusual and could suggest the possibility of some acquired anomaly. Occasionally, a patient remarks about 'seeing colours differently with each eye' or notices apparent brightness differences between the two eyes. This type of comment can be the result of unimportant contrast observations, but could indicate desaturation of colours or shifts in spectral values from a pathological state affecting one eye only. Alternatively, both eyes could be involved with the condition more advanced on one side. Oedematous maculopathies, retrobulbar neuritis, cataract, macular degeneration and diabetic retinopathy are but a few of the many abnormal states in which such symptoms might occur.

If the cause is obscure, then ophthalmoscopy, visual acuity measurements and visual field examination, especially under reduced illumination, are desirable conventional methods of examination. Of the various colour vision tests available, the Farnsworth–Munsell 100-hue test and some form of anomaloscope are useful for the investigation of colour perception in acquired anomalies of colour vision (*see* Chapter 26).

Coloured vision (chromatopsia) arises from selective absorption or scattering of light by the optic media or from the effects of toxins or disease on the retina or visual pathways. It is an uncommon symptom in optometric practice. It may precede later changes in colour vision demonstrable by conventional colour vision tests.

Photopsia

The appearance of light flashes within the visual field is best known for the association with migraine or with commencing retinal detachment. The photopsia of early detachment of the retina is often seen and described as a shower of sparks, flashes or arcs of coloured or white light. The visual aura of migraine is best likened to zig-zag flickering lights, commencing paracentrally as a small flickering disturbance just to one side of the fixation point, then expanding towards, then out of, the periphery of the visual field over a time period of around 20 minutes.

The presence of associated, often unilateral, headache in migraine, a history of trauma or myopia, similar symptoms previously in the history and the results of the relevant later objective tests (Ball, 1982) will provide some of the necessary information on which to form an opinion on the course of action. Retinal detachment calls for urgent ophthalmological attention and must be treated as an emergency in optometric practice.

Isolated flashes of light or points of light moving within the visual field occur in several other states (Roy, 1975(ii)), among which are myopia, mechanical traction on the retina from trauma, and a gravitational phenomenon on rising quickly from a bending position.

'Floaters'

Affected patients may not always use the word 'floaters' in their description of symptoms, but the term is in fairly common use by the lay public, especially among myopes who have heard the word in previous eye examinations. The complaint is often of 'spots in front of the eye', strings of beads, threads or tiny bubbles which float about, often downwards and the patient 'can't keep pace with them'.

Non-pathological embryonic remnants in the posterior vitreous humour are a frequent explanation for the symptom. These remnants are usually invisible on objective examination as they merely delineate areas of differing refractive index. Near-opaque remains of the hyaloid system are sometimes seen by ophthalmoscopy, but if these lie very close to the posterior surface of the crystalline lens they do not cast distinct retinal images except under special viewing conditions, but act more to reduce overall retinal illumination.

Vitreous opacities also occur in degenerative and inflammatory states, such as in uveitis and retinal detachment among many others. Positive scotomata, especially when close to the fixation area, may be reported as floating spots. The usual methods of visual field investigation will be applied.

Haloes

The appearance of coloured rings around lights, especially at night, is so emphasized in its relation to chronic angle-closure glaucoma that it is worth noting that coloured haloes could be observed in any state which causes corneal oedema or media haziness. The symptom must not, therefore, be considered pathognomonic of that type of glaucoma. It is unusual for an optometric patient to mention coloured haloes without special questioning. Normal diffraction haloes are brought about by the radial structure of the crystalline lens (Mellerio and Palmer, 1970) but are rarely remarked upon. White lights seen through steam-covered windows are surrounded by coloured haloes.

If a patient, under questioning, complains of this symptom then there should be special attention to such methods as tonometry, ophthalmoscopy, examination of the ocular media and visual field analysis in the later examinations.

Metamorphopsia

Micropsia with recently prescribed myopic corrections and macropsia from new presbyopic reading additions are well known, if simple, cases of 'spectacle metamorphopsia'. Prismatic elements incorporated into spectacle lenses also cause visual distortion for a time.

Pathological metamorphopsia, which is of peripheral origin and usually irregular, arises when the central region of the retina has been affected by oedema, degeneration, exudates or inflammation. It is demonstrable subjectively as areas of irregularity in line charts used for the examination of the central field. It is unwise to emphasize these central distortions to patients by too great an insistence on plotting and replotting their distribution. Where the fellow eye is normal in the binocularly superimposed area, then small unilateral defects can usually be ignored by the patient and it is best if they can be encouraged to do so.

Irregularities in the optical media also cause metamorphopsia. Metamorphopsia of central origin is seen in migraine and in drug intoxication as, for example, that from hallucinogens. Tumours of the parietal or occipital lobes and epilepsy are some other causes.

Diplopia

Patients sometimes comment about 'double vision' resulting from the effect of blurring of the retinal image. Such an observation is common during subjective examination when blurred fan chart lines or letters are described as double. The effect disappears when suitable correcting lenses are in place.

Mere blurred imagery must first, therefore, be eliminated if there are no obvious indicators for the symptom. Occasionally, when carrying out prolonged close work, convergence becomes relaxed and transient near double vision, probably also with blurring of print, occurs as a normal phenomenon.

The very many pathological states which give rise to true binocular diplopia cannot be dealt with here but are covered in the binocular vision chapters (Chapters 13–16) or in the relevant chapters of ophthalmology textbooks. Some indications only are given in *Table 5.4*.

Table 5.4 Some causes of binocular diplopia

Decompensated heterophoria

Paresis or paralysis affecting extraocular muscles,
    e.g. vascular, neural lesions, trauma

Displacement of one or both eyes,
    e.g. thyrotoxicosis, neoplasms

Neurological or muscular disease,
    e.g. multiple sclerosis

Psychoneurosis

The presence of true binocular diplopia of sudden origin will be apparent from the demeanour of the patient and from diplopia testing. The resultant deviation of the eyes will be demonstrated by the usual methods of objective examination, such as the cover test and 'nil-movement' observations on major amblyoscopes.

Binocular diplopia of sudden onset suggests a muscular, neural or centrally located lesion and calls for referral of the patient with some urgency. Complaints of transient diplopia in the history must be viewed with suspicion because of the possible association with demyelinating disease.

From an assessment of all the examination data, where there are reasonable grounds for suggesting that any transient double vision complaint referred to true binocular diplopia, then the patient should be sent for medical review. Physiological diplopia is hardly ever noticed unless the person has been associated in some way with orthoptic treatment, or has an underlying neurosis.

Monocular diplopia

In normal individuals, the prismatic effect of tear fluid or faulty positioning of bifocal segments sometimes precipitates complaints of double vision in one eye. The symptom can be merely the result of visual blur, but could also point to crystalline lens changes such as senile-type cortical cataract. Less commonly, pupil anomalies and psychoneurosis result in monocular diplopia.

Reduced mesopic or scotopic vision

Inability to see in the dark is the classic early symptom of primary pigmentary retinal dystrophy (retinitis pigmentosa), yet in the consulting room of the average practitioner, that condition and other retinal dystrophies are rarely seen. In this kind of practice, an unprompted report from a patient about visual difficulty out of doors in dim illumination is much more likely to arise from the simple need for a change in spectacle prescription or from media irregularities. Normal examination techniques confirm these states.

The smaller pupils of advancing age give reading problems for older patients in artificial lighting, such as the tungsten filament illumination often found in homes. Higher local illumination is desirable. Certain forms of glaucoma have been reported to give the symptom also and it is a wise precaution to check for these conditions in that type of patient.

True lack of scotopic function is found in the group of diseases commonly known as retinitis pigmentosa and in congenital night blindness. Hereditary linkages are well documented and electrophysiological investigations assist in early diagnosis. Reduced scotopic function also takes place at some stage of vitamin A deficiency through nutritional lack or faulty absorption, as in liver disease. Indeed, any abnormality affecting the retina or visual pathway may cause changes in the normal patterns of photopic, mesopic and scotopic vision.

Photophobia

The real 'fear of light' suggested by the word photophobia is rarely encountered and patients who are deemed to be suffering from photophobia exhibit varying degrees of discomfort, pain and intolerance to normal light levels.

Where an acute inflammatory condition of the anterior segment of the eye exists as in keratitis, then marked photophobia, intense pain, irritation and blepharospasm are presented. Such signs and symptoms are rare in general optometric practice and would necessitate immediate referral of the patient after any emergency measures have been taken.

Mild intolerance to normally encountered light levels is found in contact lens wear, myopia, migraine, chronic conjunctivitis and hay fever, among many identifiable conditions. Where there is no organic disease, then clinically significant refractive and binocular vision anomalies should be corrected. Often the cause is obscure and reflects a functional origin.

The symptom of photophobia must be distinguished from the objective condition of glare through excess light, particularly from small, intense sources which contrast highly with their background and in which situations quite normal individuals suffer considerable discomfort.

Ocular symptoms

Discomfort associated with the eyes or adnexa

Discomfort felt in or around the eyes is an everyday symptom presented in the consulting room. It may be described as occurring within or behind the eyes or in the surrounding structures, but often the complaints are vague and open to differing interpretations.

At the simplest level, the patient reports his eyes as feeling 'heavy, sore, itchy, burning, stinging', but the descriptions range from the ordinary to the ponderous and grandiose. If the word 'pain' is used then it is usually qualified by some adjective such as nasty, dull or sharp. The neurotic patient will be found to use more spirited accounts.

These descriptions serve more as pointers to personality and vocabulary rather than having any firm reliability as sound diagnostic indicators. Patients who, to the examiner, appear to be suffering from similar conditions voice their feelings in very different ways, one patient accepting a degree of discomfort with composure, another suggesting almost total incapacitation.

Discomfort arises in a wide range of abnormal states including ametropia, binocular vision disorders and neurosis, but it could also signal the retrobulbar neuritis of early multiple sclerosis or chronic angle-closure glaucoma.

Where, on examination, the reason for the complaint is obscure, it is good practice first to examine for, and eliminate, high frequency causes. Optical conditions which precipitate discomfort include uncorrected hypermetropia and hypermetropic astigmatism, early presbyopia, hyperphoria and relative esophoria at near. Similar complaints come from stress responses to life problems such as seen in college students preparing for important examinations, from the use of visual display units in industry or from other visual tasks requiring lengthy concentration, such as television viewing. (The uncorrected simple myope will have distance blur, but rarely complains of discomfort or headaches.)

There must be adequate clinical grounds for prescribing correcting glasses where the sole complaint is of vague eye discomfort or headache particularly for young persons and for minor errors. Apart from the responsibility for referral in suspected eye and related disease, a small correction will probably relieve the symptoms for a time from the placebo effect where the cause is non-optical, but then they usually recur.

The prescribing of optical corrections for ametropia and heterophoria involves much conventional wisdom and, although that experience is valuable, there needs to be further exhaustive research studies into the complex factors involved.

When correcting glasses are prescribed, it is wise to advise the patient about subsequent visits so that the long-term effect of the prescription can be assessed and whether there is a necessity for other investigations. Where the cause of persistent eye discomfort is unresolved the patient should be referred for medical attention.

Watering and 'dry' eyes

In cases where there is a reduction of tear fluid to the conjunctival sac, a patient might report the feeling of a dry eye but it is more likely that the sensations will be described as a hot, itchy or generally uncomfortable eye state. Lacrimal secretion reduces with age so that older patients are prone to the condition. Hay fever sufferers on antihistamine preparations sometimes experience dry eye symptoms and Sjögren's disease or syndrome is a well known example of glandular dysfunction with pronounced dry eye signs and symptoms.

Watering eyes are also common in older patients from the effects of cold winds or misplacement of the punctum. Accompanied by pain and discomfort, watering is also associated with corneal abrasions, irritants, allergies, corneal ulceration and loose or embedded foreign bodies.

Red eyes

Some of the very many reasons for a patient presenting with a red eye or eyes are listed in *Table 5.5*.

Most patients exhibiting red eyes will not find their way to the average optometric practice in view of pain often being the main symptom. An exception to this general rule would be cases of subconjunctival haemorrhage which usually present no discomfort.

The ultimate differential diagnosis of the red eye lies outside the existing sphere of activity of practitioners. If a patient does present such an appearance, then there is a responsibility to form an opinion on the urgency with which the patient needs other than emergency attention. Some factors to be considered are: the patient's history particularly if this indicates previous occurrences, the presence of ciliary injection, anisocoria and other pupil irregularity, exudates in the anterior chamber, reduction of visual acuity, photophobia and pain.

The patient would be referred for medical/ophthalmological attention taking into account the relative urgency for investigation.

Table 5.5 Discomfort and 'red' eyes

WHITE EYE(S)		RED EYE(S)
With no significant hyperaemia in uncomplicated cases	*With superficial hyperaemia in uncomplicated cases*	*With marked hyperaemia superficial and/or deep*
Minor psychological stresses	Irritants	Subconjunctival haemorrhage (commonly without discomfort)
Uses of eyes in prolonged exacting visual tasks	Lack of sleep	
Ametropia, presbyopia	Climate: cold, wind, sun	
Binocular vision anomalies	Contact lenses	
Sinus/nasal problems	Ametropia, presbyopia	
Contact lenses	Binocular vision anomalies	'Dry eye(s)'
Glaucoma — open angle (often symptomless)	Eyelash in punctum or in conjunctival sac	Age changes
Early retrobulbar neuritis	Other minor foreign bodies	Allergies
Glaucoma — chronic angle-closure	Allergies including conjunctival mucus (as in hay fever)	Toxins, drugs
Hysteria	Pinguecula	Anomalies of lacrimal/conjunctival glands
Malingering	Styes	Some forms of conjunctivitis
	Reduction in tear flow or lack of fluid reaching conjunctival sac	Nutritional deficiencies
	Minor trauma	Infrequent blinking
	Sinus/nasal infections	Some systemic diseases
		Rare syndromes
	Concretions	
	Trichiasis	Loose or embedded foreign body
	Glaucoma — chronic angle-closure	Corneal abrasions
	Nutritional deficiencies	Conjunctivitis: chronic/acute in its many forms
	Malingering (self-administered drugs/ chemicals)	Allergies
		Excess exposure to ultraviolet radiation
		Sinus/nasal infections
		Other corneal afflictions: ulceration, keratitis
		Trauma
		Blepharitis: chronic/acute in its many forms
		Acute iridocyclitis
		Infections of lacrimal apparatus
		Acute glaucoma
		Scleritis and episcleritis
		Tumours
		Malingering

Note: Discomfort may, or may not, be described in terms of 'pain'.
From Ball, 1982.

Other problems related to the eyes and adnexa

Excessive or forceful blinking occurs in conjunctival or corneal irritation and as a habit in children, but ametropia, heterotropia and clinically significant heterophoria must be excluded.

Myokymia or twitching of lid muscle, usually confined to the lower lid of one eye, is a frequent irritation to patients. Sometimes there may be an associated refractive error, but usually the condition is seen as an indicator of fatigue or the life habits of the individual — overwork and other stressful situations.

Patients complain less often of having to shut one eye in a visual task such as reading. This problem can be a result of clinically significant heterophoria and especially hyperphoria at the near distance, unilateral refractive error or monocular anomaly of accommodation.

The 'diplopic winking phenomenon' may be demonstrated in some cases of extraocular muscle paresis. The affected eye is partly closed as a means of avoiding diplopia in the main direction of action of the affected muscle.

Referred symptoms

Headache

The causes of head pain are legion and it is a regular symptom presented to all those involved in eye examination as well as in general medical practice. Headache may reflect an individual response to some tension-producing life situation but it could be a forewarning of some grave cerebral crisis. Head pain presents a challenge to the practitioner and there is no greater satisfaction for both examiner and patient than measures which provide lasting relief from the symptom.

How frequently headaches arise from ametropia or similar disorders is debatable — probably far less than is sometimes claimed, but acceptable statistical data are rare. No form of headache is specific to eye disorders; indeed descriptions of 'characteristic ocular headaches' must be treated with considerable caution. That point having been made, then where headaches do arise from refractive, binocular vision, accommodation or convergence anomalies, they will probably be described by the non-neurotic individual as a dull, steady ache around the brows, temples, 'behind' the eyes or maybe in the occipital region. There might be some association or latency of onset relative to the visual tasks in which the patient is involved. Patterned glare due to successive lines of text may cause discomfort and headache in reading (Wilkins and Nimmo-Smith, 1984).

But similar headache complaints could be recounted resulting from tension or neurosis. Guarded weight only should be placed on a patient's description of their headache experiences in terms of suggesting an origin. Decisions on courses of action must be reserved until the data collected during the whole examination have been analysed.

Conclusion

An opinion has to be formed, based on the integrated data of that examination, as to whether the findings uphold a reasonable suspicion of some alternative origin even in the presence of a correctable optical or binocular vision disorder.

General textbooks or any written account can provide limited help only in that process.

Sound decisions are encouraged by astute questioning of the patient, from listening and observing as the patient describes his experiences, by critical observation and analysis in the application of relevant examination techniques and from learning acquired in the sharing of experience with others working in the same field. If there is a significant optical-type error judged on sound clinical prescribing principles, and there are no indications which suggest some other cause, then correcting that error is justified in the presence of the headache symptom but only lasting relief will indicate whether this was the likely cause.

Where symptoms or signs suggest some origin outside the responsibilities of optometric practitioners, then the patient would normally be referred to a registered medical practitioner. In the UK, this is usually to the patient's own doctor but, in an emergency, referral could be direct to the medical personnel in hospital.

The practitioner working single-handed is at some disadvantage in lacking opportunities for mutual discussion with colleagues, on topics such as clinical decision-making in the presence of symptoms such as headaches and vague eye discomfort. Data banks and computer-type links have the potential to revolutionize that isolation.

References

ARDEN, G.B. (1978) Visual loss in patients with normal visual acuity. *Trans. Ophthalmol. Soc. UK*, **98**, 219–231

BALL, G.V. (1982) *Symptoms in Eye Examination*, pp. (i) 58–60, (ii) 96–99. London: Butterworths

HEATH, G.G. (1981) Representative important questions in clinical optometry. *Am. J. Optom. Physiol. Opt.*, **58**, 289–295

MELLERIO, J. and PALMER, D.A. (1970) Entoptic halos. *Vision Res.*, **10**, 595–599

ROY, F.H. (1975) *Ocular Differential Diagnosis*, 2nd edn, pp. (i) 353, 516–517, (ii) 526. Philadelphia: Lea Febiger

RUSKIEWICZ, J.P. (1982) Development of a standarized data base. *Am. J. Optom. Physiol. Opt.*, **59**, 494–499

VERRIEST, G. (1979) Modern trends in perimetry. *Br. J. Physiol. Opt.*, **33**, 24

WILKINS, A.J. and NIMMO-SMITH, I. (1984) On the reduction of eye-strain when reading. *Ophthal. Physiol. Opt.*, **4**, 53–59

Further reading

BALL, G.V. (1982) *Symptoms in Eye Examination*. London: Butterworths

CARR, R.R. and SIEGEL, I.M. (1982) *Visual Electrodiagnostic Testing. A Practical Guide for the Clinician*. Baltimore: Williams & Wilkins

HARRINGTON, D.O. (1981) *The Visual Fields. A Textbook and Atlas of Perimetry*, 5th edn. St Louis: C.V. Mosby

LANCE, J.W. (1982) *Mechanism and Management of Headache*, 4th edn. London: Butterworths

NEMA, H.V. (1973) *Ophthalmic Syndromes*. London: Butterworths.

PAU, H. (1978) (Translated by G. Cibis) *Differential Diagnosis of Eye Disease*. Philadelphia: W.B Saunders & Co.

PERKIN, G.D. and ROSE, F.C. (1979) *Optic Neuritis and its Differential Diagnosis*. Oxford: Oxford University Press

PORKORNY, J., SMITH, V.C., VERRIEST, G., and PINKERS, A.J.L.G. (1979) *Congenital and Acquired Colour Vision Defects*. New York: Grune & Stratton.

ROY, F.H. (1975) Ocular differential diagnosis, 2nd edn. Philadelphia: Lea & Febiger

STEIN, H.A. and SLATT, B.J. (1983). *The Ophthalmic Assistant. Fundamentals and Clinical Practice*, 4th edn. St. Louis: C.V. Mosby

TREVOR-ROPER, P.D. and CURRAN, P.V. (1984). *The Eye and its Disorders*, 2nd edn. Oxford: Blackwell Scientific

WOLFF, H.G. (rev. Dalessio, D.J.) (1980) *Wolff's Headache and Other Head Pains*, 4th edn. Oxford: Oxford University Press

6

Retinoscopy

Stephen Taylor

Retinoscopy is an objective technique for the investigation, diagnosis and evaluation of the refractive errors of the eye. Fundamentally, although two methods of retinoscopy exist, a static method in which accommodation is suppressed and a dynamic method in which accommodation is permitted, the basic optical principles involved in the two methods are the same. Essentially, light in the form of a cone, a cylinder or a streak is projected into an eye using a mirror with a central aperture through which the examiner can observe the pupil of the eye. The light entering the eye forms a small illuminated patch on the retina which acts as a secondary light source. It is the light from this secondary source which the examiner uses to assess the refractive state of the eye. Depending upon the ametropic state of the eye, the light emerging from the pupil will either converge or diverge.

It is obviously important to know from which layer of the retina the light is actually reflected so that an allowance, if necessary, can be made for the difference between the retinoscopic refraction and the subjective refraction (Freeman and Hodd, 1954; Emsley, 1955). Present research puts the reflecting surface at the boundary between vitreous and retina and would suggest a retinoscopic result slightly more hyperopic than the subjective result (Glickstein and Millodot, 1970; Millodot and O'Leary, 1978).

The optics of retinoscopy

To perform retinoscopy, the examiner uses movement of the 'reflex', i.e. the illumination in the pupil of the eye under examination which is derived from the secondary light source produced on the retina. The aim of the examiner is to neutralize the observed movement and so reach a point of *reversal* which will only occur when the far-point of the eye under test corresponds to the nodal point of the examiner's eye. Movement of the reflex is produced by tilting the mirror used to introduce light into the eye under test; this induces movement in the secondary light source on the retina. The direction of movement of the reflex will depend upon the refractive state of the eye, the examiner's viewing distance, and the vergence of the light leaving the mirror. Neutralization of the movement may be produced by either altering the viewing distance or the vergence of the light leaving the mirror, or by using supplementary trial lenses placed between the examiner and the test eye along the visual axis. In general, the use of a retinoscope with a slightly divergent beam and supplementary lenses placed along the visual axis close to the test eye is the accepted technique. The optics of neutrality, or the point of reversal, are shown in *Figure 6.1*, where the far-point of the test eye corresponds to the nodal point of the examiner's eye.

From *Figure 6.1* it can be seen that light from point O forms an image (i) at N_o and the observer sees the reflex. Light from point O' forms an image (i') in the plane of N_o and if construction of the image of i' formed by the examiner's dioptric system is attempted, a vertical line is produced in the plane of N_o such that no image is formed by the examiner's eye. The examiner interprets this visually as a loss of illumination of the test eye pupil with no apparent movement of the reflex. This is the point of 'reversal'.

The reflex in hypermetropia

The point of reversal or neutral point, however, is an unique point and for all other optical conditions the reflex will appear to move with movements of the primary light source. The direction and the speed of the observed movement of the reflex will

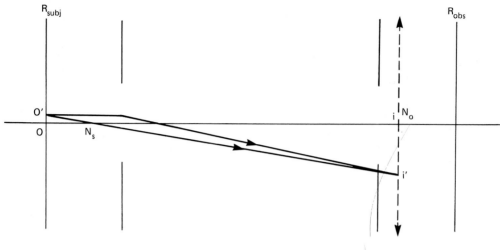

Figure 6.1 The optics of neutrality where reversal occurs
in retinoscopy

depend upon the type and degree of ametropia,
respectively. The optics for the case of hypermetropia are shown in *Figures 6.2* and *6.3*, representing a
low degree and a high degree of error. In hypermetropia, the far-point of the test eye will lie at some
point behind the retina. Therefore, if the secondary
light source on the retina moves from O to O', as a
result of tilting the primary light source, the image
O' formed by the dioptrics of the test eye will be
situated at i'. The secondary light source has therefore moved upwards in *Figure 6.2*. It is this image i'
that now acts as a source for the dioptrics of the
examiner's eye forming an image I' on the examiner's retina. This movement of the image on the
examiner's retina from I to I' is interpreted visually

as an upward movement of the reflex in the pupil of
the test eye. Hence the movement seen by the
examiner is in the same direction as the movement
of the secondary light source and this is called a
'with' movement.

The reflex movement for low degrees of hypermetropia is shown in *Figure 6.2* and for high degrees of
hypermetropia in *Figure 6.3*, both being in the same
direction and both therefore being described as
'with' movements. A difference does exist in the
speed of the movement observed. This can be
demonstrated by a comparison of the angles formed
at the intersection of the visual axis by a line joining
point i' to point I' in *Figures 6.2* and *6.3*. The angle
'a' formed in *Figure 6.3* is smaller than the angle 'b'

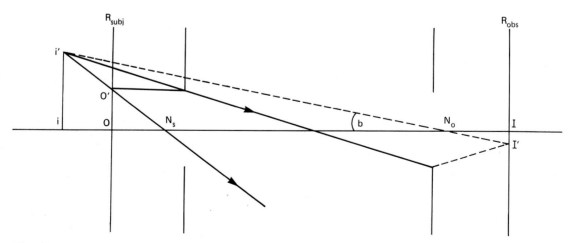

Figure 6.2 The optics of hypermetropia in retinoscopy
for low refractive errors

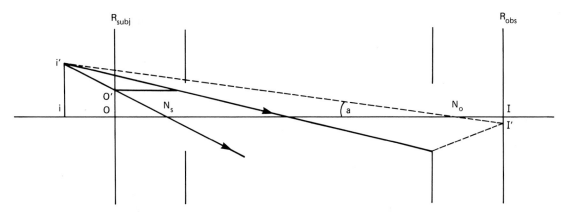

Figure 6.3 The optics of hypermetropia in retinoscopy for high refractive errors

formed in *Figure 6.2*; the rate of movement of the reflex is therefore less for angle 'a', i.e. the speed of the reflex decreases as the refractive error increases.

The reflex in myopia

The case of myopic refractive errors is not quite as straightforward as that of hypermetropic errors. The direction of the reflex displacement in myopia will depend upon the degree of refractive error and the working distance. In myopia, the far-point of the eye lies in front of the eye and three situations can therefore arise optically:

(1) In low degrees of myopia, the far-point of the test eye will lie beyond the nodal point of the examiner's eye as shown in *Figure 6.4*.
(2) For high degrees of myopia, the far-point of the test eye will lie in front of the nodal point of the examiner's eye as shown in *Figure 6.5*.

(3) For one specific set of circumstances where the far-point of the test eye is coincident with the nodal point of the examiner's eye, the reflex will appear to be at the point of reversal without a working distance lens, and occurs when the refractive error of the test eye is equivalent to the dioptric value of the working distance. This situation is the same as that shown in *Figure 6.1*.

In the first condition, the far-point of the test eye is behind the examiner's nodal point and upward movement of the primary light source causes the image on the retina to move from O to O'; the image of O' formed by the test eye is then situated at i' and i' becomes the source for the dioptrics of the examiner's eye, forming an image I' on the examiner's retina. This movement of the image on the examiner's retina is again interpreted as a 'with' movement.

In this case, the angle 'c' produced by drawing a

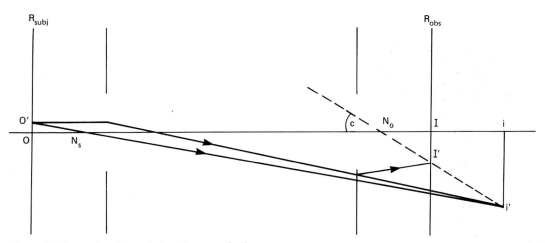

Figure 6.4 The optics of myopia in retinoscopy for low refractive errors

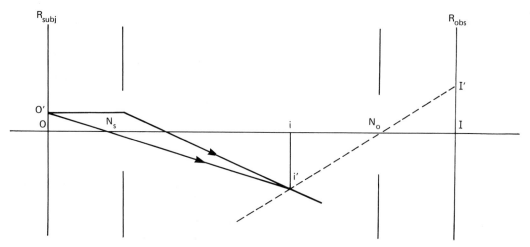

Figure 6.5 The optics of myopia in retinoscopy for high
refractive errors

line to join i′ and I′ and extrapolating this line to
intersect the visual axis is greater than either 'a' or
'b' found in the case of hypermetropia. This means
that the movement of the reflex observed is faster
than that in hypermetropia.

In the second condition, the far-point of the test
eye lies between the test eye and the examiner.
Upward movement of the primary source produces
a movement of the patch of light on the retina of the
test eye from O to O′; the image of O′ formed by
the dioptrics of the test eye is now situated at i′, and
this acts as the source for the dioptrics of the
examiner's eye, an image of i′ being formed at I′ on
the examiner's retina. The movement of the image
on the examiner's retina is interpreted as a downward movement of the reflex in the test eye pupil.
This is in the opposite direction to the direction of
movement of the primary and secondary light
sources and is, therefore, called an 'against' movement. If the working distance correction lens is
applied before retinoscopy commences, all myopic
reflexes will move 'against'.

The reflex in astigmatism

The previous sections have dealt with the optics of
retinoscopy for spherical refractive errors, and the
case of non-spherical refractive errors must now be
considered. In an astigmatic eye, the rays will be
refracted differently as they enter the eye and the
degree of refraction will depend upon the meridian
at which they enter, and the degree of the astigmatism. Two meridians will provide the 'sharpest' images, and these are the meridians of greatest and least
refractive power; in all other meridians the image
will be out of focus. The out-of-focus image on the
retina will, as in the case of spherical errors, act as a
secondary light source for the examiner's eye. There

is no single far-point plane in this case, but two
planes of 'brightest' and 'sharpest' focus will occur
and, in general, the two far-point planes will lie at
right angles to each other. It is necessary for the
examiner to neutralize these two planes separately
by using either spheres or, more probably, by using
a spherocylindrical correction.

If it is assumed that the far-point planes lie along
90° and 180°, by moving the primary source initially
horizontally and then vertically, it will be seen
whether the movement is of the same type in both
directions. If the movement is 'with' in both meridians, one of the movements, corresponding to the
lower refractive power, should be faster than the
other. If negative cylinders are used in the spherocylindrical correction (the choice of cylinder will be
considered later), it is necessary to correct the most
positive meridian with positive spheres first. This
induces an 'against' movement in the opposite meridian, which can then be corrected with negative
cylinders. At the neutral point for the first meridian
the situation shown in *Figure 6.1* will exist along the
neutralized meridian. If the primary light source is
moved in a direction at 90° to this meridian, then an
'against' movement will be seen and at any point
between the two meridians a reflex will appear
which will move obliquely to the direction of movement of the primary light source. The 'against'
movement seen in the second meridian may now be
neutralized by placing negative cylinders in front of
the test eye with the axis of the cylinder lying in the
plane of the neutralized meridian. When both meridians have been neutralized, then in all directions of
movement of the primary light source, the reflex will
disappear without any apparent movement as represented by the optics of *Figure 6.1*.

While the foregoing description relates to astigmatism with the meridians at 90° and 180°, the same

theory is applicable to all meridians and simply requires some initial evaluation by the examiner to determine the axis of one meridian. The precise method to determine the axis will, to some extent, depend upon the type of instrument to be used. As a guide, the astigmatism will distort the reflex seen from a round spot (if a spot retinoscope is used) to give two ovals corresponding to the greatest and least refractive powers. The major axes of the ovals indicate the axes of the astigmatism. As an added aid, if the primary light source is moved in a direction which is not along one of the two major axes, then the movement of the reflex will appear to be oblique to the movement of the light source.

Obviously, astigmatism is much harder to assess than spherical errors when the retinoscope is first used. Experience, however, soon enables the examiner to accurately determine the point of reversal of cylindrical corrections to 0.25 D and 2.5° giving an excellent start to the refractive routine.

General technique of static retinoscopy

Retinoscopy is carried out generally at a distance which allows a good view of the reflex and access to supplementary lenses for changes of power, but far enough away to prevent errors due to small changes in the working distance. These conditions tend to lead to a working distance of approximately arm's length or two-thirds of a metre. This is, however, only a conventional working distance and there is no reason why this cannot be adjusted to suit particular requirements, providing the implications of such a change are known. The working distance affects the final correction determined and an allowance needs to be made to account for this. In the case of a 0.66 metre working distance, the allowance is 1.50 D, i.e. the reciprocal of the working distance in dioptres.

Normally, the examiner's right hand and right eye are used to view the patient's right eye, and the examiner's left hand and left eye to view the patient's left eye. This is useful for two reasons: the examiner needs to work along the visual axis of the test eye without blocking a view of the fixation target and, in addition, it means that the examiner and patient are not breathing directly at each other. Although already mentioned, it is worth stressing the need to work along the visual axis of the test eye horizontally and vertically, if aberrations are to be reduced and an accurate refraction attempted.

When moving the retinoscope as the primary light source, a couple of short sweeps across the pupil should be sufficient to allow a decision on the direction and speed of the movement. Continuous rapid sweeping of the light source across the pupil causes discomfort for the patient, and may induce accommodative changes in the test eye that will complicate the apparent movement seen in the pupil.

It is important before starting retinoscopy to fit a trial frame phoropter accurately to the patient. If this is not centred correctly, in the horizontal and in the vertical, and if not fitted square to the patient's face, aberrations will be induced when attempts are made to work along the visual axis.

When using supplementary lenses, it is an advantage to always over plus or under minus the test eye. This means that for a hyperopic correction, when adjusting the positive sphere, the next trial lens should be placed in the trial frame before removal of the original trial lens and the reverse for a myopic correction, one trial lens being removed before the next lens is used. This procedure will minimize the accommodative stimulus and, therefore, prevent spasm of the ciliary muscle.

Frequently, it is stated that positive cylinders must never be used in spherocylindrical correction in retinoscopy. In fact, with a streak retinoscope positive cylinders give a clearer, more easily neutralized image. However, if positive cylinders are to be used, then the spherical correction is inevitably going to be under positive or over negative, in both cases stimulating accommodation. With the accommodation active, it is possible to achieve an apparent final correction when, in fact, the eye is accommodating to give a false neutral point. To overcome the problem, it is necessary to constantly assess the movement in the already corrected meridian, i.e. the sphere meridian, when any changes due to accommodation will cause a loss of neutrality in this meridian.

Once the neutral point has been reached, a simple check of the result is to move backwards and forwards slightly and watch the movement of the reflex. On moving forward, the working distance is effectively reduced and, therefore, if the neutral point is accurate, a 'with' movement should appear in all directions; on moving backwards, the working distance is effectively increased and an 'against' movement should appear in all directions.

The final refraction from retinoscopy is calculated by allowing for the working distance used to achieve neutrality. In most situations, a comfortable working distance will have been approximately 0.66 metre and an allowance of −1.50 D is added to the result in the trial frame phoropter.

Difficulties in retinoscopy
Scissors movement

This is a situation in which, instead of one reflex, two bands of light are seen in the subject's pupil. As the retinoscope moves, the two bands of light tend to move in opposite directions giving an opening and closing effect similar to the action of scissors, hence the name. It has been suggested that the effect is produced by non-alignment of the optical elements of the subject's eye, the retinoscope and the examiner's eye (Bennett, 1951). There are no clear-cut ways to deal with the 'split reflex' which may still be apparent after careful alignment. Whatever the course of action, it is essential to try and pick out the very central area of the reflex for neutralization. A technique that is useful in these cases is to increase the positive power in front of the subject until an 'against' movement is obtained in all directions, as normal. The spherical power is now reduced until the scissors movement first appears—this indicates the sphere power. The examiner then moves forward until the central reflex is clearly visible and then back to the original working distance, watching the movement of the central reflex. While at the close working distance, the different speeds of the movement are noted and an attempt made to determine the main axes. When back at the original working distance, a negative cylinder is placed along the 'probable' axis and the reflex viewed. It should be remembered that the appearance of the 'split-reflex' suggests that the neutral point is near.

Media changes and opacities

Media effects generally fall into two main categories: simple changes in the refractive index and opacification of the media. The effect of localized refractive changes in the media is to produce marked fluctuations and variations in the retinoscopic reflex. The direction, speed and brightness of the reflex may change and a satisfactory 'approximation' of the true refraction is often all that can be achieved.

In the case of opacification of the media, the brightness of the reflex is reduced and various odd patterns may appear corresponding to the areas of opacification. In extreme cases, it may be that the opacification is so great that no reflex at all is visible within the pupil. However, opacities may be dealt with satisfactorily in most cases and the technique used will depend upon the type of opacity.

Dense central opacification

It is often possible in these cases to work off-axis and thereby obtain a satisfactory, if imprecise, measure of refraction.

General opacification

The effect of general opacification is to reduce the brightness of the reflex. In many cases, reducing the working distance will produce an increase in brightness and allow assessment of refraction. It may be

necessary to approach to within 10 cm to obtain a workable reflex and, while this reduces accuracy because of errors in working distance, it may yield a retinoscopic result.

Irregular opacification

In this case, it is necessary to search the opacification choosing one particular area to neutralize. The area chosen should lie as near to the visual axis as possible and again it may be useful to reduce the working distance. It is essential that all reflexes, other than that to be neutralized, are ignored.

Total opacification

There is little that can be done in this situation where the reflex may appear black or white. If it is essential to obtain a result, then it may be possible to use a mydriatic in an attempt to increase the diameter of the pupil, allowing a view through any peripheral area beyond the opacification.

Differences in pupil size

It is unusual to find a patient with pupils so small that retinoscopy becomes impossible. There may, however, be occasions where a patient is on drug therapy which produces miosis making it difficult to obtain a precise result. If the patient has naturally small pupils then it may be possible to improve the reflex by dimming all room lights and reducing the retinoscope intensity. Sometimes, it is enough for the patient to sit in a darkened room prior to examination. As a final resort a mild mydriatic may be used.

The opposite situation of large pupils, either through the use of a cycloplegic or from natural causes, is less of a problem. The effect of a large pupil is to produce marked aberrations in the peripheral reflex in the pupil. If it is not possible to isolate and concentrate on the central bright part of the reflex, a pinhole disc of 3 mm diameter can be placed in the back cell of a well-centred trial frame and retinoscopy carried out as normal.

Infants

The most difficult part of retinoscopy on infants is controlling the fixation and the accommodative effort. It is for this reason that many practitioners automatically require an infant to be under cycloplegia when refracting. While this is quite understandable, there is no reason why an attempt cannot be made to refract initially without cycloplegia. Using one of the parents or the receptionist as a fixation target and a lens bar in 0.50-D steps, an approximate measure can be made. It should take very little time to carry out, no trial frame is used and cylinders are estimated from the lens bar observations. Alternative methods using a form of dynamic retinoscopy have also been proposed as a useful way of dealing with an uncooperative infant patient (Mohindra, 1977; *see also* Chapter 12).

Sight hole effects

The size of the sight hole of the retinoscope determines, to some extent, the precision of location of the neutral point (Saishin *et al.*, 1979). The larger the sight hole, the less precise the measurement of the refractive error. This effect is due to the optics of the system at the neutral point as described in the first part of this chapter. If the subject's far-point coincides with the sight hole as the examiner swept the light across the subject's pupil, small movements of the retinoscope will cause the bundle of rays to fall off the sight hole aperture and the image is lost. If the sight hole were made larger, then a greater sweep could be made before the image was lost. There is, therefore, an optimum sight hole size. A further problem associated with a reduction in the size of the sight hole is the subsequent loss of brightness of the reflex whenever the far-point plane lies outside the plane of the sight hole, since the aperture would restrict the amount of light entering the examiner's eye. One answer to the problem is to have an instrument with a variable size of sight hole, using a larger aperture for initial assessment then reducing the size as the neutral point is approached.

A second effect due to the sight hole is dependent upon the way that the sight hole is produced. If the hole is made by drilling into the mirror itself, then a dull patch corresponding to the area of the sight hole will appear in the reflex. While this patch is still present with a semisilvered aperture, it is less noticeable. The induced patch does not influence the optics of the system but may produce some confusions in the examiner's assessment of the movement.

Fixation and accommodation

There is little consensus on the ideal fixation target for static retinoscopy. The target should preferably have no stimulus to accommodation, should be situated at least 6 metres or 20 feet from the patient, should be small to minimize eye movements and well defined enough not to be confused with any other distance objects. The targets used range from the spotlight on the test chart to the rings on the green block of the duochrome (Cockerham, 1957; Borish, 1975) and each has its own relative advantages and disadvantages. There is little information available on the effect of different targets in retinoscopy, but it has been shown that fixation on a black target on a red background gives a more negative correction than fixation on a black target on a green background (McBrien and Taylor, 1986). This effect is, however, quite small and within the limits of accuracy discussed later in this chapter. The differences between results increase when the lights are turned out, probably due to the increase in chromatic aberration when pupil size increases, and all of these give a more consistent result than a light with no superimposed target, whatever its colour (McBrien and Taylor, 1985). If colour were to be used to control accommodation, then it is likely that it would need to be provided across the whole field to give a complete chromatic image, and then an allowance made for the chromatic aberration in the eye.

One of the aims of the fixation target is to maintain a constant state of no accommodation. In practice, the control of accommodation is extremely important throughout not only the retinoscopy, but also the subjective refraction (*see* Chapter 8). This control is particularly important when examining young patients and those with a tendency to accommodative spasm. Apart from the use of an adequate fixation target, there are two possible avenues open to control accommodation—using fogging lenses or cycloplegia.

Use of fogging lenses

It is always advisable to start retinoscopy with a lens in the trial frame that is more positive or less negative than that expected for the final correction. When performing retinoscopy, the accommodation in the visual system will be controlled by the fixating eye and not the eye under examination and it is, therefore, important to ensure that the fixating eye is over plussed or under minussed by obtaining an 'against' movement in all directions. However, care must be taken not to over correct by too much, because an over correction of more than about 1.50 D will actually stimulate the accommodation. The routine of retinoscopy should, therefore, be carried out in two stages: approximating the result in each eye by reducing the positive power or increasing the negative power until the eye appears to be approximately neutral, and then checking that small changes in one eye to achieve a precise neutral point do not affect the reflex in the other eye. In this way the neutral point is always approached from a fogged position while not allowing the degree of fog to be enough to interfere with the result by stimulating accommodation.

Cycloplegia

Retinoscopy in children is often carried out under cycloplegia. Peripheral aberrations visible through the dilated pupil may make the reflex more difficult to interpret and care must be taken to concentrate on the central patch. (For a review of available preparations *see* Chapter 29.)

It is to be remembered that cycloplegia is one of the tools open to the optometric practitioner in practice, but not the only tool. Despite the suggestion in much of the literature (Abrams, 1978), it is not always 'essential' to use cycloplegia on all children. The cases where it is useful to use a cycloplegic in practice are:

(1) On children where it is difficult to obtain a result because fixation is not steady, although a non-cycloplegic examination should be attempted first.
(2) In all cases where the patient presents with a convergent squint.
(3) In cases where the patient has a significant or unstable esophoric muscle balance.
(4) In cases where the retinoscopy result varies markedly during retinoscopy suggesting spasm of the ciliary body.
(5) In cases where the retinoscopy and the subjective result are markedly different.

In all cases where a cycloplegic examination is to be undertaken a precycloplegic or a post-cycloplegic examination should always be made prior to prescribing.

Dynamic retinoscopy

Dynamic retinoscopy differs from the static technique in that the subject is asked to fixate a target at near in order to stimulate accommodation. The reflex, however, appears the same and is neutralized in the same way. Lens racks are often an advantage for speed of neutralization. The aim of the method is not to produce a measure of the distance refractive error, but rather to provide an objective assessment of the optical condition of the eye focused for near vision. It is essentially designed to evaluate the near requirements and to assess the accommodation/convergence relationship. A breakdown of the differential diagnoses and treatment derived from dynamic retinoscopy was given by Swann (1939) and this is shown in *Table 6.1*.

The technique requires the assessment of two characteristics of the optical system at near: the low neutral (sometimes called the objective lag) and the high neutral (also called the dynamic neutral).

Low neutral

It is normally accepted that, when an observer directs attention to an object, the object is fixated prior to the visual system being focused. Because there is no need to focus precisely for most tasks, and possibly because of the effect of chromatic

aberration changes in the accommodated eye, there is normally a lag of accommodative effort behind convergence. The lag approximates between 0.50 D and 0.75 D at a 33-cm viewing distance. This lag is termed the 'low neutral' and represents the amount of sphere required over and above the distance correction to first produce neutralization of the reflex.

High neutral

Also called the dynamic neutral, this characteristic represents the amount of positive power that can be added to the low neutral before an 'against' movement appears. The high neutral is said to represent the negative relative accommodation, i.e. the amount of accommodation that can be relaxed while convergence remains fixed and, for normal subjects, this has a value of approximately 1.25 D at 33 cm but it decreases with age.

Accuracy and reliability of retinoscopy

It is not easy to assess the accuracy of a retinoscopy technique because it is the examiner who produces the greatest variability. The purpose of retinoscopy is to measure the power of the optical system required to place the image of distant objects on the retina and the greatest variable in the execution of this function is the judgement of the examiner. Obviously, the eye under observation also plays a part in accuracy, as does patient cooperation, but the more skilful practitioner should produce a more repeatable result even in these cases.

There are few reported studies of reliability and accuracy of retinoscopy in the published literature. Probably the most widely quoted and best controlled studies were carried out in the early 1970s by Safir and his co-workers (Safir, Hyams and Philpot, 1970; Hyams, Safir and Philpot, 1971). The study used a panel of five ophthalmologists and 10 cooperative young adults with refractive errors of less than 3.00 D and normal acuity and pupil reactions. In terms of reliability, statistics showed that there was a 50% probability of two consecutive measures of the sphere power differing by 0.40 D. It was also found that there was a three-fold difference in reliability comparing the most precise with the least precise practitioner. Surprisingly, perhaps, it was found that retinoscopy, according to Safir, was most sensitive for the cylinder axis, followed by cylinder power, followed by sphere power.

Reliability is, therefore, not good. Accuracy requires a study in which the true refractive state of the eye is known and to which retinoscopic findings can be compared. This is difficult to achieve: the subjective refraction is not of any real use as a

Table 6.1 Differential diagnosis and treatment in dynamic retinoscopy

Age	Normal dynamic neutral	Unequal dynamic neutral	Higher dynamic neutral	Lower dynamic neutral
<30	+ 1.25 D to + 1.50 D convergence tests normal; static prescription correct for all purposes	Distance prescription may be incorrect; difference not likely to be greater than 0.25 D. Revert to static prescription, try difference on distance test type and check on infinity balance test Difference of 1.0 D or thereabouts is often found if vision of one eye does not exceed 6/24 Unequal accommodation may be present if above does not account for difference If, for instance, static prescription is R + 4.50 D, L + 1.0 D, the right eye may need an addition of + 0.50 D for intensive near vision because of effectivity Convergence is most likely to be normal; check with convergence tests Hyperphoria can cause an unequal DN if not corrected	If 0.25 D higher, static prescription will suffice if it is the first prescription prescribed. Indicates necessity for re-examination at early date If DN is 0.5 D in excess of normal, a reading addition of + 0.50 D is required. If addition is not accepted for distance in, say, 6 months, the accommodation is subnormal. If it is accepted, the 0.50 D was latent hypermetropia May be due to effectivity if static prescription exceeds + 4.0 D both eyes sphere cylinder, or in combination Convergence is most likely to be normal; check with convergence tests Convergence may be weak if accommodation is subnormal through a nuclear lesion	If 0.25 D or 0.50 D lower, tendency to either convergence weakness or excessive accommodation. If convergence tests normal, DN will correct itself after prescription has been used for a time If DN is + 0.75 D or less, convergence may be weak. Confirm convergence tests. If weakness proven, give convergence orthoptics and produce stability. If successful, DN should reach normal If convergence tests are normal, case is excessive accommodation. Prescription is as follows: lowest plus; weak base-in prisms; slight absorption If no prescription has been used, and prescription required exceeds + 1.50 D, excessive accommodation is secondary Prescribe static prescription and the excessive accommodation will correct itself
30–35	+ 1.0 D – + 1.25 D	As in previous age group	As in previous age group	As in previous age group. Excessive accommodation is likely to be present in this age group
35–40	+ 1.0 D	As above	As above	As above
40–45	+ 0.75 D *If this amount is found, presbyopia is not present*	As above A true unequal accommodation may be due to early presbyopia in one eye. This is possible if one eye has suffered a pathological process, even though distance acuity of vision has been restored to normal. Treat as unequal accommodation if considerable close work is performed Use of convergence tests to prove condition of convergence Rule out hyperphoria	The dioptric amount above + 0.75 D is due to presbyopia. Senility is setting in early. Study symptoms and history for possible cause. Reading addition required. Use convergence tests to prove condition of convergence	Rare finding Accommodation is not likely to be excessive at this age unless hysterical element exists Convergence may be normal. Prove with convergence tests Indicates that presbyopia is not present
45–50	After reading addition at 33 cm has been found, DN is + 0.50 D. If addition is for 50 cm DN will be + 0.25 D	If distance prescription is needed re-check distance test. If present correction suffices, check inequality on Comparator Card 3 or Turville near balance test. Convergence tests Hyperphoria must be corrected	DN is not likely to exceed + 0.75 D or + 1.0 D Be sure that present addition is sufficient. If it is, case is senile and physique is good. Observe this factor Convergence tests	Convergence may be weak. Use convergence tests If convergence is normal, senility is advanced for age. Study history and symptoms. Insist on use of distance prescription if it exceeds + 0.75 D
50–55	As above, but DN is + 0.25 D	As above	As above, but DN is not likely to exceed + 0.50	As above
>55	DN is + 0.25 D to nil	As above	Not likely to be higher	Hardly applies

Additional notes. If esophoria exists at near vision in excess of that at distance, a reading addition of approximately + 0.75 D to both eyes will be required unless a course of abduction orthoptics can be undertaken. Convergence test No. 1 is used to diagnose this condition and is followed by the FL test. If E is seen, convergence is stable and correction by orthoptics is likely: if FL convergence is unstable and a reading addition is certainly required, although orthoptics may also be prescribed. If esophoria in near vision does not exceed that in distance vision, the static correction may suffice. This also applies if the static correction exceeds + 2.50 both eyes and has not been used previously. Its use will most probably render convergence normal in a short time.
If in presbyopia convergence is weak, orthoptics can be prescribed unless a definite toxic condition is present. If prisms are prescribed, do not exceed 3 Δ base-in divided between the eyes unless the case is markedly toxic. In these cases, 6 Δ base-in divided between the eyes can be tried. Prisms and orthoptics may prevent the case from getting entirely out of hand. DN, dynamic neutral; D, dioptre; R, right; L, left. From Swan, 1939.

comparison because so many factors other than the pure optical system influence the result. Instrumentation is also of limited value because there is a need to presuppose some way of assessing the instrument. There is no simple way of overcoming this difficulty and it is therefore necessary to think of retinoscopic accuracy only in terms of repeatability; if a particular examiner is obtaining highly repeatable results, but the results are always 0.50 D different to the subjective result, then the examiner learns to make an allowance for this, and there is probably some inherent inaccuracy in the routine. The problem, in practice, is that examiners rarely see patients frequently enough to be able to assess their own repeatability and are not, therefore, in a position to pick up any problems. Essentially, retinoscopy must be seen as a method of approximating the refractive power of the eye, which is likely to provide a result that is within 0.5 D of any subsequent retinoscopy 50% of the time. Doubtless there will be practitioners who can repeat the same result, but by the same reasoning there will be those whose successes are substantially poorer than 0.50 D, 50% of the time. The above considerations, however, only relate to young cooperative subjects; accuracy may decline with uncooperative children or cataractous patients. It is therefore important that the practitioner is aware of the shortcomings in human judgements and realizes that retinoscopy is not an infallible technique.

Additional non-refractive uses of retinoscopy

(1) The ability to detect certain types of pathology with the retinoscope should not be undervalued. Among many practitioners, routine retinoscopy is carried out prior to ophthalmoscopy and is, therefore, the first objective view of the internal structure of the eye. A number of pathological and physiological changes show up in the appearance of the retinoscopy reflex, the most common being: cataract—the presence of a cataract or indeed any media opacity or index change is easily seen with the retinoscope and, in some cases, the change may be more apparent in the reflex than it appears on ophthalmoscopy; keratoconus, which produces distortion of the corneal curvature, has the effect of causing a swirling of the reflex in the pupil such that neutralization is particularly difficult; retinal detachment in the central area will produce a loss of the redness of the reflex and a grey reflex is seen.

(2) Assessment of the fit of soft contact lenses. It has been suggested that the retinoscope is an extremely sensitive method of assessing whether a soft contact lens is too tight. A tight fitting lens causes the apex of the lens to misalign with the apex of the cornea producing a distortion in the central portion of the retinoscope reflex (Hales, 1978).

(3) Indirect ophthalmoscopy can be carried out with a retinoscope and a high plus sphere providing the illumination from the instrument is adequate (*see* Chapter 9).

Choice of instrument

There are three basic instruments on the market at present for retinoscopy.

The original type which is still available provides a spot of light reflected from a silvered mirror with a central aperture. The disadvantages are that the light intensity may be high and, to prevent constriction of the pupil, the rheostat control may have to be adjusted; in addition, a central shadow is produced corresponding to the central aperture which may interfere with the reflex.

An advance on this type is the retinoscope using a piece of plane flint glass in place of the silvered mirror. The flint glass has a high reflection factor so that light is still illuminating the subject's pupil area, but being transparent it allows the examiner to view the pupil. This instrument, therefore, removes the problem of the central shadow and also reduces the illumination level by virtue of its reduced reflectance.

The third instrument available in the streak retinoscope. Unlike the previous two instruments a streak of light rather than a spot of light is produced; this is said to have the advantage of improving the accuracy of determination of the cylinder axis, a point with which many spot retinoscopists have disagreed. Recently, the halogen bulb has been introduced into the retinoscope. This provides an extremely high power source which can be run at low power on the rheostat for normal patients, but can be boosted up to provide a much higher illumination in cases of opacities in the media. It is available for both streak and spot retinoscopes.

In conclusion, it is advisable to consider the following:

(1) A spare bulb should be kept in the practice and in a domiciliary kit.

(2) Keeping spare batteries or remembering to recharge the handle every evening is a sensible precaution.

(3) The mirror on the instrument should be cleaned periodically.

(4) All trial lenses should be cleaned regularly, it being much easier to see a reflex through a clean lens.

(5) The mirror of the retinoscope should never be poked with a finger, as this tends to produce misalignment of the system which, in turn, produces difficulty in use.

References

ABRAMS. D. (1978) *Duke-Elder's Practice of Refraction*. London: Churchill Livingstone

BENNETT. A.G. (1951) Oblique refraction of the schematic eye as in retinoscopy. *The Optician*, **121**, 553

BORISH. I.M. (1975) *Clinical Refraction*, 3rd edn. New York: Professional Press Inc.

COCKERHAM. D. (1957) Research in streak retinoscopy. *Br. J. Physiol. Opt.*, **14**, 236–247

EMSLEY. H.H. (1955) *Visual Optics*, Vol. 1. London: Hatton Press

FREEMAN, H. and HODD. F.A.B. (1954) A comparative analysis of retinoscopic and subjective refraction. *Optician*, **128**, 262

GLICKSTEIN. M. and MILLODOT. M. (1970) Retinoscopy and eye size. *Science*, **168**, 605–606

HALES. R.H. (1978) *Contact lenses—A Clinical Approach to Fitting*. Baltimore, Maryland: Williams & Wilkins Co.

HYAMS. L., SAFIR A. and PHILPOT. J. (1971) Studies in Refraction. ii. Bias and accuracy of retinoscopy. *Arch. Ophthalmol.*, **85**, 33–41

McBRIEN. N. and TAYLOR. S.P. (1986) Effect of fixation target on objective refraction. *Am. J. Optom. Physiol. Opt.*, **63**, 346–350

MILLODOT. M. and O'LEARY. D. (1978) The discrepancy between retinoscopic and subjective measurements; effects of age. *Am. J. Optom. Physiol. Opt.*, **55**, 309–316

MOHINDRA. I. (1977) A non-cycloplegic refraction technique for infants and young children. *J. Am. Optom. Assoc.*, **48**, 518–523

SAFIR, A., HYAMS, L. and PHILPOT. J. (1970) Studies in refraction. i. The precision of retinoscopy. *Arch. Ophthalmol.*, **84**, 49–61

SAISHIN, M., MINE, K., MATSUDA, T., NAKAO, S. and NAGATA, R. (1979) Exact clinical application of retinoscopy. *Jap. J. Ophthalmol.*, **23**, 31–37

SWANN. L.A. (1939) *Recent Advances in Objective Refraction*. London: Raphaels

7

Computerized refractive examination

Ivan Wood

Fifty years ago, Collins (1937) conceived and designed the first infrared refractionometer. This pioneering instrument used a measuring head to focus an oscillating invisible near infrared measuring beam (*Figure 7.1*) by a Badal system optometer lens, through the optics of the eye, onto the electro-optics of selenium photocells. These detectors were connected via the electronics — in this case a differential valve amplifier—to the output device — a cathode ray tube (Charman, 1976). The three components were: optical measuring head; electronic detection, servocontrol and amplification; output. These form the basic design criteria of all the currently available objective autorefractors.

The electro-optical principles of autorefractors

The infrared source

The source of the infrared light of an autorefractor can either be a conventional incandescent bulb surrounded by a Kodak Wratten 87 filter or a gallium arsenide light-emitting diode (LED). Both these sources produce an emission spectrum in the near infrared at 820 nm. Around this wavelength, approximately 40% of the incident infrared light is reflected (*Figure 7.2*; Geeralts and Berry, 1968) from the sclera (Charman, 1980). These near

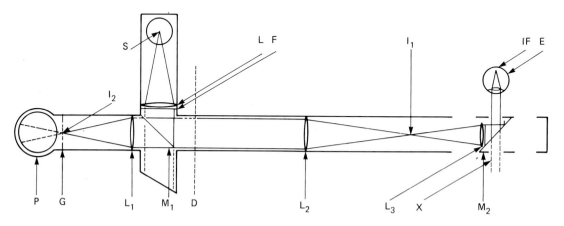

Figure 7.1 Collins' electronic refractionometer.
S = source; P = photoelectric cell; I_1 = image of filament which is caused to move by sliding L_2 towards or away from L_3, thus providing focusing adjustment to enable refraction to be measured; I_2 = final image upon grating; IF = fundus image; L = condenser for light from source; L_1 = condenser for light returning from eye; L_2 = focusing lens; L_3 = refractionometer lens;

G = grating; M_1 = vibrating mirror (transparent); M_2 = infrared reflector; E = eye being refracted (emmetropic); F = filter; D = dividing plane, for determining astigmatism — portion to the left of this line is rotatable through 180°. (Redrawn from G. H. Giles, 1965, *Principles and Practice of Refraction*, Hammond and Hammond, London)

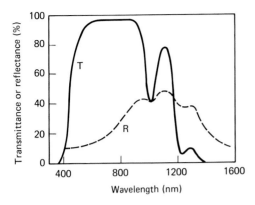

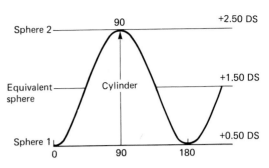

Figure 7.3 Graph of sin θ^2 of *Rx* +2.50/–2.00 × 90

Figure 7.2 Transmittance (T) of the ocular media and reflectance (R) of the retina, choroid and sclera. (After Geeralts and Berry, 1968)

infrared wavelengths render any refractive measurement spuriously myopic which, together with the longitudinal chromatic aberration of the eye, necessitates a systematic correction of about –0.50 DS for visible light.

The target

The infrared light usually passes through a chopper wheel to be focused by the optical components of the measuring head as an oscillating low spatial frequency image (2 cycles/deg) on the patient's retina (Charman, 1985).

Badal optometer and sine-squared function

Most of the measuring heads use a Badal optometer lens system which allows the dioptric power of an eye in a given meridian to be determined by calibrated linear movements of the test target or optometer lens and/or the photodetector by Newton's equation (Emsley, 1963; Bennett, 1978). The variation in dioptric power of an astigmatic eye is achieved by rotating the test target through 360° while moving the Badal optometer lens along the astigmatic pencil. The locus of the image of least blur or maximum visibility resulting from the motion of the test target is best described by the sine-squared function (*Figure 7.3*; Keating and Carroll, 1976). Bennett (1960) and Brubaker, Reinecke and Copeland (1969) have shown that, by analysing the meridional power in three chosen meridians, it is possible to determine the spherocylindrical correction for an astigmatic eye. Consequently, the calibration of the Badal system and the meridional positions of the measuring head are stored along with the sine-squared analysis in the microcomputer read-only memory (ROM).

Digital electronic alignment and measurement system

Alignment

To effect a measurement, the optical head of a given autorefractor must be properly aligned to gain the maximum signal for the photodetectors of the measuring system at a set vertex distance. To centre the pupil and set the vertex distance, the Dioptron V autorefractor uses a decentred direct viewing system. This viewing system is, however, closed during the measurement cycle which means that the patient's eye cannot be recentred if fixation wanders during the measurement. This can affect the reliability of the refractive measurement.

Recently developed autorefractors have a TV alignment system which is electronically interlaced with the electro-optics of the measurement system. In this interlaced system there is a servo-loop between the target, the Badal optometer lens and central processing unit (CPU). Coarse alignment of the measuring head is usually achieved by the operator by sighting a mire on the two catoptric images of two angled lights thereby setting the vertex distance.

This technique is illustrated by the Nidek 2000 system which interlaces the output of the receiving alignment demodulator with the demodulator of the measurement system. *Figure 7.4* shows the pair of light emitting diodes (LEDs) driven by the LED drive board C. the pulsed infrared beam produced by these diodes will only reflect off the cornea to the alignment photodiodes when the measuring head is correctly aligned with the patient's eye. The reflection of the alignment LEDs, amplified via a pre-amplifier, saturates the alignment demodulator D, which in turn signals to the microswitch M to open the measurement phase discrimination circuit E which drives the CPU. The measurement part of the program is then executed by the CPU after the starter button is pressed.

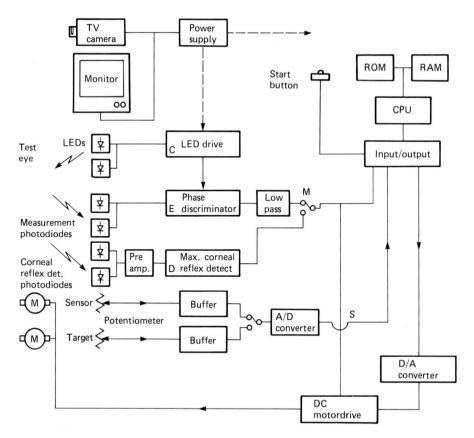

Figure 7.4 Block diagram of Nidek 2000 autorefractor

The measurement cycle

The CPU then reads the digital signal from the phase discrimination circuit E via the analogue-to-digital converter and drives the servomotors F and G of the measuring head via a digital-to-analogue converter. The measurement is made by focusing and scanning the measuring beam through the dioptric range of the instrument, while rotating the scanning beam through 360° to check for variations in the incoming signal from the phase discriminator circuit, the latter denoting the variation of dioptric power in astigmatism. The position of the maximum signal from the phase discriminator circuit E is matched via a servoloop with positional signal S obtained from the digitized target and the sensor potentiometer signal by the CPU. The resultant interaction between these signals is stored by the CPU as the refraction measurement.

As will be appreciated the interaction between the optics of the measuring head and the program stored will vary with the principles on which the instrument was designed. Therefore, in the following section, the operating principles of the currently produced autorefractors will be outlined.

Operating principles

Quality of retinal image analysis

In direct and indirect ophthalmoscopy, the clarity of the retinal image will alter with the varying vergence of a beam of light at the eye from a target placed in front of it. The vergence of light which gives the sharpest image (*Figure 7.5*) corresponds with the ocular refraction of that eye. This technique of measurement integrates the refractive error over the complete pupil area of the patient's eye and appears to be relatively immune to positioning errors of the optical measuring head (French and Wood, 1981). However, it has been suggested that eyes with larger pupils produce a more myopic correction (−0.5 DS)

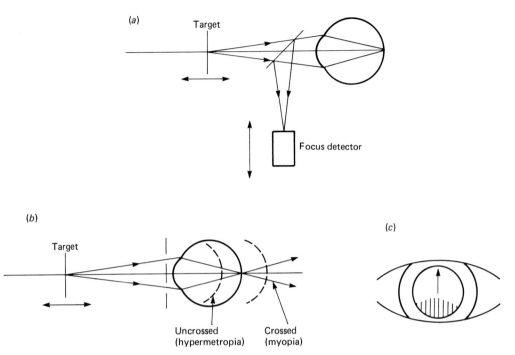

Figure 7.5 Basic methods for objective refraction in both visible and infrared light. (*a*) Quality of retinal image; (*b*) coincidence method; (*c*) retinoscopy

when using an image analysis infrared refractor (Charman, Jennings and Whitefoot, 1978; Wong *et al.*, 1984). In 1986 there were three autorefractors on the market using image analysis: Dioptron V (Cooper Vision), the Canon AutoRef 10 and its clone the Hoya Autorefractor.

These refractors image a moving circularly polarized, high contrast, square wave grating through a Badal lens into the patient's eye (*Figure 7.6*). In general, the resultant retinal image is blurred. The plane of the circularly polarized blurred retinal image changes phase by 90° when it is reflected from the sclera, enabling the returning infrared beam to pass through the Badal lens onto a fixed mask consisting of a similar square wave grating of equal period to the target. The modulation of the returning beam is recorded as the blurred retinal image is focused by the Badal lens. The dioptric position of the Badal lens will correspond to the patient's refraction in the plane perpendicular to the grating bars when these are sharply focused on the patient's retina and their conjugate point on the mass in front of the photodetector. The information about this dioptric position is then stored while the position of the peak signal is stored in five other meridians in turn. The six values of the meridional refraction are then fitted to a sine-squared curve by the microprocessor.

Coincidence methods

These date back to the invention of the double pinhole by Scheiner (1573–1650). If an image of a target (*see Figure 7.5*) is formed through two different portions of the patient's pupil, the resultant, possibly blurred, retinal images will only be coincident if the target and the retina are conjugate. If the line target is used in conjunction with an 'optometer' lens, then the amount of refractive error can be determined as demonstrated by Porterfield (1696–1771) and later by Young (1773–1829). The Nidek and the Topcon Autorefractors rely on a coincidence method of measurement.

These refractors image the two LED sources into the plane of the patient's pupil to give a Scheiner double pinhole effect (*Figure 7.7*). Any ametropia leads to a double image of the target on the retina; uncrossed if the patient is hypermetropic and crossed if myopic. To determine if these retinal images are crossed or uncrossed, the photodetectors of the optical head are split into two independent halves and the LEDs are switched alternately at 500 Hz. The reflected double retinal image in the presence of ametropia will fall on one half of the detector thereby being in phase with the LED if uncrossed or 90° out of phase for crossed images. Thus, the phase of the signal generated by the receiving photodiodes will indicate the type of

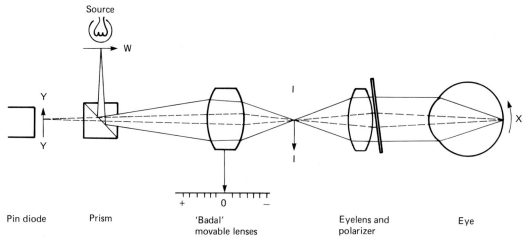

Figure 7.6 The illumination system and detection system of the Dioptron autorefractor

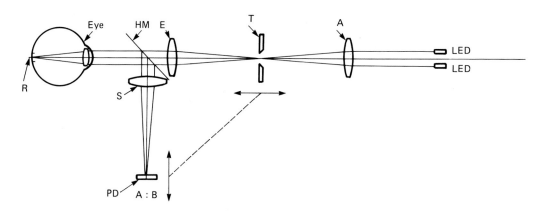

Figure 7.7 Diagram of measuring head of Nidek autorefractor. LED = light source for measurement; T = small aperture; HM = semisilvered mirror; PD = photodetector (divided into A and B); A = condenser lens; E = objective lens in optical emitting system; S = objective lens in optical receiving system; R = retina. (Redrawn from Wood *et al.*, *Ophthalmic and Physiological Optics*, 1984, Vol. 4, pp. 169–178)

ametropia and the sign of the refractive correction via filter and phase discriminator logic. This signal will then drive the LEDs as the target until coincidence at the retina is achieved, when both halves of the photodiode will receive equal amounts of light. The target vergence must then correspond to the ametropia present. The distance travelled by the LEDs can be monitored by a potentiometer, the voltage value of which can be stored in the microcomputer as dioptric measurement.

In the presence of astigmatism, the two retinal images will separate both vertically and horizontally. Thus four sources are used and the photodetector is divided into four quadrants; opposite quadrants form a pair and enable the system to measure the refraction along a particular meridian and at right angles to it.

To avoid the problem of radial astigmatism, it is necessary to centre the 'Scheiner disc' in the pupil plane and align the photodetectors correctly. In the Nidek autorefactor, this critical alignment is achieved by centring the image of a flashing infrared spot on the mires of the TV monitor. When alignment is achieved, the flashing cursor is detected by another infrared detector which opens the measuring circuit. The detection and observation systems work in antiphase enabling both critical alignment and coincidence to be achieved.

Retinoscopy

In retinoscopy, a scanning beam of collimated light moves across the patient's pupil plane and the resultant speed of the 'with' and 'against' movements of the retinal reflex indicates the refractive state of the patient's eye. The far point of the eye is located by nulling or 'neutralizing' the retinal reflex with lenses and this principle was used in the Ophthalmotron, the first microchip automated infrared autorefractor. The Ophthalmotron has been extensively reviewed (Safir *et al.*, 1970; Bizzel *et al.*, 1974; Floyd and Garcia, 1974; Mohrman and Hogan, 1977; Guillon, 1986). Current instruments, such as the Nikon 2000, 5000 and 7000 autorefractors are based on measuring the speed of the reflex.

This type of autorefractor illuminates the eye with an infrared streak image generated by an infrared LED passing a very coarse (i.e. low spatial frequency) chopper wheel, as shown in *Figure 7.8.* The streak image is rotated by the reflecting prism which is driven by the infrared stepping motor. The rotation of the infrared image is monitored by an axial reference potentiometer, an analogue-to-digital interface and the CPU of the control board. After passing through the dichroic mirror which reflects the fixation target into the patient's eye, the

convergent beam of light is brought to a focus on the patient's cornea. Thus the image of the LED is conjugate with the LED source. This reduces the reflected infrared light from the cornea and increases the signal-to-noise ratio of the observation system (compare indirect ophthalmoscopy). The image of the rotating chopper wheel forms a secondary defocused image at the patient's sclera (*Figure 7.9a*).

The vergence of the reflected streak image in this type of autorefractor (Nikon) is not altered by a servo-controlled optometer lens as in the Ophthalmotron (Mohrman and Hogan, 1977). The reflected beam of infrared light is refracted by the patient's eye to emerge as parallel in emmetropia, convergent in myopia and divergent in hypermetropia. The reflected beam, as shown in *Figure 7.9a*, retraces the same light path of the incident beam through the dichroic mirror, the image rotating prism and the half mirror to be condensed by an objective lens O onto a stop T.

This stop T (*Figure 7.9b(i)*), then forms a knife edge which is conjugate with the retinal image of the emmetrope. Similarly, *Figure 7.9b(ii)* shows the stop T in front of the projected retinal image of a myopic eye and *Figure 7.9b(iii)* shows the stop T in front of the projected retinal image of a hypermetropic eye. As a consequence, the motion of the

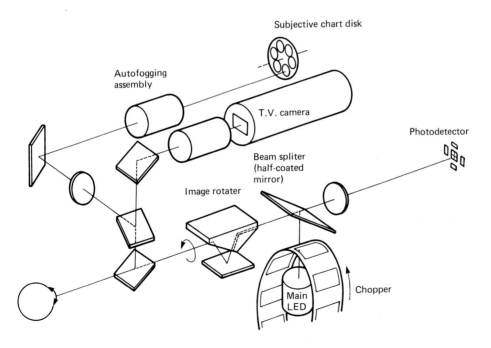

Figure 7.8 Nikon autorefractometer NR 7000 (objective and subjective). (Redrawn with permission of Nikon Instruments UK)

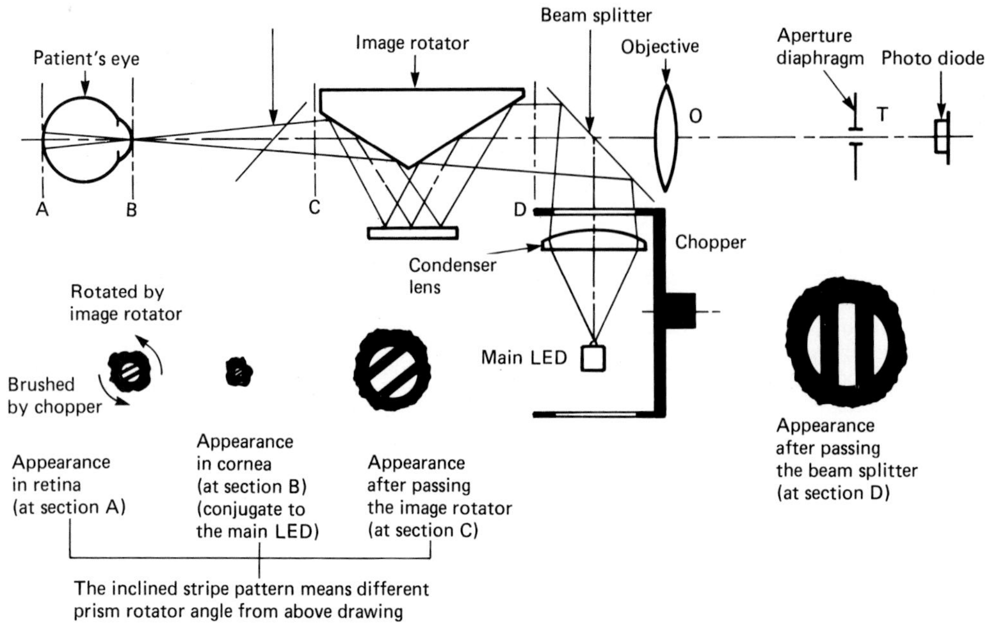

Figure 7.9 Principle of the Nikon autorefractor. (*a*) Illumination and optical system.

bars of the retinal image produces a neutral reflex on the photodiode in emmetropia, a 'with' motion in myopia and an 'against' motion in hypermetropia. The motion of the reflected streak image is detected by four photodetectors which, by phase difference, measure both the speed and direction of the reflex. In this respect, the detection system is similar to the Humphrey Autorefractor described by Bennett and Rabbetts (1984).

Detection of refractive power by the photodetector/phase discriminator circuitry

Even though the speed and direction of the chopper wheel is constant, the speed and direction of its image on the photodiode, as shown by the cross-hatched area on the diagram (*Figure 7.10*), will depend on the refractive power of the patient's eye. The photodetectors P1 and P2 in the diagram are shown as being set orthogonally to the direction of movement of the chopper wheel image. P1 and P2 produce an AC signal from the alternating movement of the light/dark bars of the incident chopper wheel image. If P1 signals before P2, the combined output is interpreted as a 'with' (hypermetropic) movement. If P2 signals before P1 then the combined output is interpreted as an 'against' (myopic) movement. The phase difference (the time interval

$\triangle t$) between the AC signals from P1 and P2 gives a measurement of the spherical component of refractive error.

Detection of the astigmatic axis by the photodetector/phase discriminator circuitry

During the measurement cycle, the photodiode is rotated together with the chopper wheel through 360°. The speed of the chopper wheel reflex is determined by measuring the phase difference of the AC output between P1 and P2 and separately between P3 and P4 at 0.5° intervals. As shown in the lower part of *Figure 7.10*, when the plane of the chopper wheel image does not coincide with the astigmatic axes of the patient's eye, the photodetectors P3 and P4 will be stimulated unequally. This produces a smaller phase difference in the combined output of P3 and P4 than when these photodiodes are orthogonal to the chopper wheel image. Over the 360° measurement cycle, the phase difference of the two pairs of the photodiodes varies as a sine-squared curve. The planes of the astigmatic axes are determined when the phase difference between the combined output of each pair of photodetectors P1–P2 and P3–P4 is zero!

The results from the output of the phase discriminator are then compared with an ideal sine-squared

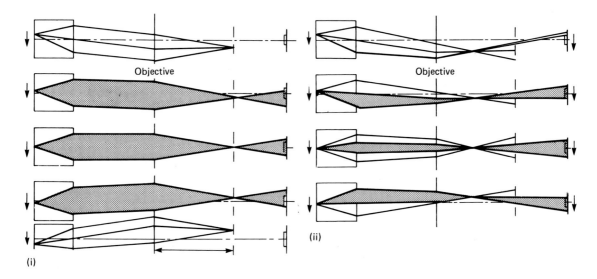

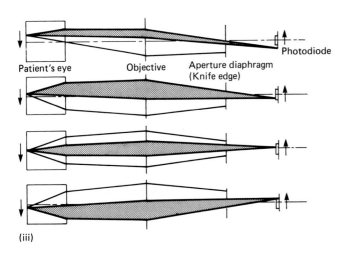

Figure 7.9 (*b*) Pupil reflex (i) in emmetropia — the 'knife edge' is conjugate to the patient's eye; the movement of the pupil reflex is stopped on the photodiode — neutral. (ii) In myopia: the patient's retinal conjugate lies in front of the 'knife edge'. The pupil reflex projected on the photodiode moves in the same direction of the 'brushed beam' — 'with' motion. (iii) In hyperopia: the patient's retinal conjugate lies behind the 'knife edge'. The pupil reflex projected on the photodiode moves opposite to the direction of the 'brushed beam' — 'against' motion. (Redrawn with permission of Nikon Instruments UK)

curve stored in the read-only memory of the microcomputer to produce the final autorefraction measurement.

Problems of infrared refractors

Whatever the underlying principle of measurement chosen for a particular autorefractor, the instrument will use near infrared light (800–900 nm). This is because the transmission and reflection through the optical media of these particular wavelengths of electromagnetic radiation light is high (Geeralts and Berry, 1968).

The amount of light transmitted and reflected will depend on the pupil size of the patient, a pupil size below 3 mm reducing the reflected light to a point where it will become undetectable in the normal background radiation. On the other hand, a blink of the patient's eyelids will produce an oversaturated infrared signal.

The ocular longitudinal chromatic aberration produces a shift between the ocular foci for infrared and visible light rendering the eye hypermetropic under infrared light. (Charman, 1985). The reflectance layer for this longer wavelength infrared light appears to be in the deep layers of the choroid or the sclera (Charman, 1980). Thus an empirical correction must be applied to the problem of the dioptric calibration of the infrared optometer for visible light. However, the use of 'invisible' infrared light

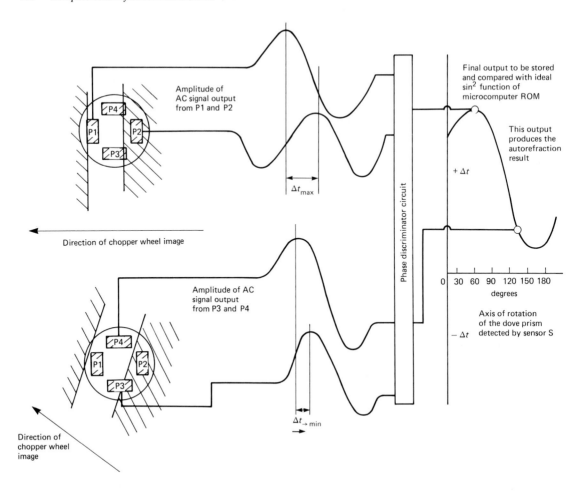

Figure 7.10 Determination of the refractive power in the Nikon 2000 autorefractor. $\triangle t_{max}$ = maximum phase difference between P1 and P2 = speed of reflex for spher- ical ametropia. $\triangle t_{min}$ = near minimum phase difference between P3 and P4 = speed of reflex which sets plane of the astigmatic axes

does help to overcome the problem of patient accommodation. Proximal accommodation is also reduced by steady fixation of a blurred target (Reese and Fry, 1941; Heath, 1956).

General specification of infrared refractors

The optical specification

In spite of the differences in operating principles, all the current autorefractors cover the spherical (±15 DS), cylindrical (±6 DC) and axis (0–180° in 1° steps) range of refractive error. Most of these autorefractor specifications claim to over-refract

soft contact lenses, spectacles, hard contact lenses and intraocular lens implants (IOLs). To overcome the problem of proximal accommodation by the patient, all of the current autorefractors present the patient with a fogged target. This usually takes the form of a blurred star target although the Canon Autorefractor presents the patient with a pleasant country scene which is much appreciated by patients.

However attentive the patient is to the fixation target, blinks will always occur. With the saturation of the photodiodes due to the increased reflectance of the patient's lids, the infrared refractor re- executes the measurement cycle or prints an error message.

It is expected that the current generation of autorefractors will have facilities to contend with the above mentioned problems; however, the only way to assess these instruments is to compare the results of repeated autorefraction measurements with those obtained conventionally.

Accuracy of autorefractors

Accuracy can be defined in different ways, resulting from the different ways of measuring it. It is best to separate accuracy into two elements: reliability and validity. Reliability is the consistency with which measurements are made, i.e. their repeatability. Therefore an autorefractor's reliability can be obtained by repeating the measurement, preferably on separate occasions.

Validity, on the other hand, is the degree with which tests measure what they claim to measure. In order to assess the reliability and validity of autorefractors, a blind study of the patient's refraction has to be carried out using both autorefraction and conventional retinoscopy, and subjective refraction techniques. It has been pointed out (French and Jennings, 1974; French and Wood, 1981; Wong *et al.*, 1984) that these conventional refraction techniques are prone to bias and error. However, at present they are the norm and it is only natural that they should be the main criteria against which these autorefractions should be validated.

Reliability studies of autorefractors

The reliability of the currently available auto-refractors is shown in *Tables 7.1* and *7.2*. These results have been produced from two autorefraction measurements taken on two separate occasions, the statistics used being the Pearson product moment correlation coefficient, the standard error of measurement (*Table 7.1*) and the more familiar frequency dioptre difference table (*Table 7.2*).

The correlation coefficient (Rxy) describes how close a linear relationship exists between the repeated spherical power and cylindrical power and axis measurements. Complete agreement between these measurements plotted graphically would produce a straight line at 45° to the ordinate and the abscissa. Both the slope, the Pearson product moment coefficient (Rxy) and the index of reliability $[(Rxy)^2]$ will be 1. The index of reliability, formed by squaring the reliability correlation coefficient Rxy, indicates the percentage agreement between repeated refraction measurements.

These reliability statistics, Rxy and $(Rxy)^2$, of the studies listed in *Table 7.1* show there is at least a 90% agreement between the first and second spherical autorefraction measurements. An example of the close agreement between the spherical equivalent data for the repeated measurements of the

Table 7.1 Reliability of autorefractors and conventional refractive techniques

Study	*Reference*	*Refractive component*	*Pearson product moment correlation coefficient*	*Index of reliability (%)*	*± s.e.m.*
Dioptron II	French and Wood (1981)	Sphere Cylinder Axis	0.99 0.91 0.99	0.99 0.82 0.98	0.17 DS 0.15 DC 6°
Nidek	Wood *et al.* (1984)	Sphere Cylinder Axis	0.97 0.82 0.93	0.82 0.68 0.88	0.37 DS 0.22 DC 15°
Canon RI	Wood (1982)	Sphere Cylinder Axis	0.98 0.79 0.54	0.94 0.62 0.29	0.34 DS 0.33 DS 19°
Nikon	Kaps (1980)	Sphere Cylinder Axis	Not available		0.37 DS 0.21 DC 22°
Duochrome, Simultan laser	Jennings and Charman (1973)	Equivalent sphere	0.98	0.97	0.32 DS
Subjective	French and Jennings (1974)	Equivalent sphere Sphere Cylinder Axis	0.98 0.98 0.60 0.91	0.96 0.96 0.36 0.82	0.23 DS 0.25 DS 0.17 DC 18°

Table 7.2 Cumulative frequency difference table of repeated autorefractor and conventional refractive measurements

Study	Number	Percentage difference (D)			
		Axis at 10°		Axis at 5°	
Dioptron II	249	Sphere	76	Sphere	92
(French and Wood, 1981)	249	Cylinder	82	Cylinder	97
	100	Axis	59	Axis	83
Nidek 2000	178	Sphere	76	Sphere	92
(Wood *et al.*, 1984)	169	Cylinder	75	Cylinder	97
	169	Axis	30	Axis	47
Nikon 1000	203	Sphere	84	Sphere	93
(Kaps, 1980)	193	Cylinder	89	Cylinder	97
	193	Axis	20	Axis	45
Humphrey Autorefractor	48	Sphere	90	Sphere	98
	48	Cylinder	92	Cylinder	98
(Wong *et al.*, 1984)		Equiv.			
	61	sphere	90	Sphere	98
	61	Cylinder	97	Cylinder	100
Canon RI	100	Sphere	85	Sphere	97
(Wood, 1982)	56	Cylinder	76	Cylinder	90
	56	Axis	74	Axis	90
Retinoscopy	420	Not available		Sphere	63
(Bizzel *et al.*, 1974)	420	Not available		Cylinder	77
Duochrome, Simultan and		Equiv.			
laser (Jennings and	8	sphere	56		
Charman, 1973)					
Subjective refractions		Equiv.			
(French and Jennings,	17	sphere	73		
1974)	17	Sphere	68		
	17	Cylinder	85		
Conventional refraction		Sphere	91	Sphere	99
(Perrigin *et al.*, 1984)		Cylinder	95	Cylinder	100
		Axis	71	Axis	88

Dioptron II autorefractor is shown in *Figure 7.11*. However, these reliability statistics for repeated cylinder axis and power autorefractor measurements show that there can be marked variation in agreement between each type of autorefractor.

An alternative measurement of reliability can be obtained from the standard deviation of repeated autorefractor or conventional refractive measurements and its derivative the standard error of measurement (s.e.m.). These statistics give an overall idea of the dispersion of the repeated measurements. Together these reliability statistics seem to indicate that, based on image analysis, the autorefractors seem to produce more reliable estimates of astigmatism than those based on coincidence or retinoscopy methods of measurement. The increased variance, shown by the index of reliability and the standard error of measurement statistics for

these machines, may be caused by the lack of control of accommodation (Wood *et al.*, 1984) or an error on the fitting procedure of the sine-squared function to the stored data in the microcomputer. For comparison, recent studies of repeated retinoscopy (Bizzel *et al.*, 1974) and repeated subjective measurements (Jennings and Charman, 1973; French and Jennings, 1974; Perrigin, Perrigin and Grosvenor, 1982; Grosvenor, Perrigin and Perrigin, 1984) should be reviewed. Perrigin *et al.* (1984) have pointed out that the repeatability of some of these studies is higher than would be expected in optometric practice, because their subjects were to some extent trained observers.

The cumulative frequency analysis of the repeated difference scores (*Table 7.2*) confirms that some autorefractors produce a result which is better than those gained by retinoscopy (Hirsch, 1956; Safir *et*

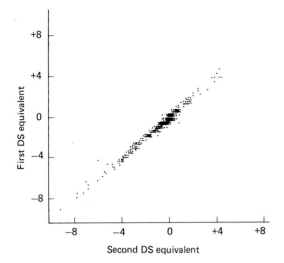

Figure 7.11 Open clinic data scattergram of reliability. $n = 249$; $Rxy = 0.994$

al., 1970) and subjective techniques (Jennings and Charman, 1973; French and Jennings, 1974; Perrigin, Perrigin and Grosvenor, 1982; Grosvenor, Perrigin and Perrigin, 1984; Perrigin *et al.*, 1984).

Validity of autorefractors

To determine the validity of autorefractors, blind autorefractor measurements are usually compared with the results obtained by conventional retinoscopy and subjective techniques using the Pearson product moment correlation coefficient and the magnitude of differences statistics. *Table 7.3* summarizes the results of these statistics derived from the various studies undertaken to date.

These studies show that there is over a 60% agreement between the sphere and cylinder power components of infrared refractors and conventional refraction measurements. However, there is a much lower level of agreement between cylinder axes measurements of the autorefractors and conventional refractive techniques. This is because both conventional and autorefraction techniques become less able to cope with detecting low-powered cylinder axis components, because of a decrease in the signal-to-noise ratio with cylinder powers below 1.00 DC. It is usual for validity studies of autorefractors to quote the percentage agreement between autorefractors and conventional techniques with cylinders above 1.00 DC. Most recent validation studies (Rassow and Wesseman, 1984; Wong *et al.*, 1984; McBrien and Millodot, 1985; Wesseman and Rassow, 1987; Wood, 1987) conclude that the autorefractive measurements are not valid measure-

ments of the final refractive data and, therefore, can only be used as preliminary refraction data. Unfortunately, these authors seem to ignore the reliability studies of the final conventional refractive findings described above.

Automated subjective refraction

Verification of the autorefraction through visual acuity

In a bid to improve the autorefractive measurement, most of the autorefractor manufacturers have recently added the option of a subjective check of the visual acuity to optimize the autorefraction measurement. This option is usually presented at the end of the monocular autorefraction measurement. If this option is chosen, the spherical component of the *objective* refraction is simply introduced by changing the position of the optometer lens stepper motor by -0.75 D, to compensate for the more 'myopic' infrared refraction. The cylindrical component of the infrared refraction is introduced by a stepper motor-driven Stokes lens. A Snellen visual acuity test chart is then presented in the light path of the measuring head. The patient then indicates the level of acuity obtained and this result is then punched into random access memory (RAM) of the autorefractor for the final printout.

Subjective modification of the spherical component of the autorefraction by increased visual acuity

Viewing these Snellen acuity targets, the patient then optimizes the spherical component of the autorefraction either by changing the position of a stepper motor-controlled movable mirror or a stepper motor-controlled optometer lens. The visual acuity of the subjectively modified *Rx* is then recorded for the final printout.

Modification of the cylindrical component of the autorefraction

The autorefractors of Japanese origin also include a cross-cylinder subjective test for the astigmatic components of autorefraction measurement. However, this procedure prolongs the examination in the headrest of the instrument and may cause visual fatigue.

Contrast sensitivity measurements of autorefraction results

A novel attempt to refine the spherical component of autorefraction measurement by contrast sensitivity was used in the now defunct Dicon autorefractor.

Table 7.3 Validity of autorefractors

Autorefractor	Study	Refractive component	Rxy	$(Rxy)^2$	Mag. of differences		
					>0.25 D 5° (%)	>0.50 D 10° (%)	>1.00 D 20° (%)
Dioptron II	French and Wood (1981)	Sphere	0.994	0.99	78	96	99
		Cylinder	0.912	0.83	82	95	100
		Axis	0.998	0.99	59	83	99
Nidek	Wood *et al.* (1984)	Sphere	0.976	0.95	30	59	92
		Cylinder	0.827	0.68	60	89	98
		Axis	0.939	0.88	20	31	50
Canon RI	Wood (1982)	Sphere	Not available		49	72	95
		Cylinder			59	83	90
		Axis			58	76	84
Nikon	Kaps (1980)	Sphere	Not available		54	74	Not quoted
		Cylinder			46	74	
		Axis					
Nova (Coherent)	Perrigin *et al.* (1984)	Sphere	Not available		53	74	Not quoted
		Cylinder			81	91	
		Axis			57	78	

Instead of viewing a conventional Snellen chart in the light path of the measuring head, the patient was told to observe a very small sinusoidally moving LED display (Optical Science Patent No. 3992087). The sinusoidal fixation eye movement was monitored using an infrared detector. As *Figure 7.12* shows, the luminance of the LED was logarithmically attenuated until the patient lost fixation. This loss of fixation was taken as the detection threshold of the spotlight which in turn was calibrated in terms of static visual acuity. This formed the end-point of the visual acuity measurements (Adams *et al.*, 1984). These workers claim that the reliability correlation coefficient is 0.83–0.85 and the validity correlation coefficient is 0.75, the latter correlation comparing the contrast sensitivity with Snellen acuity.

Errors in subjective refraction

The standard deviation of various subjective testing methods is about 0.30 D (Jennings and Charman, 1973). This standard deviation, coupled with the 0.1 D depth of focus of a 3-mm pupil (Emsley, 1963), will result in a non-optimal subjective refraction. Thus patients are likely to accept ±0.25 DS variation in the final *Rx*, i.e. prescribed to the nearest 0.50 DS. Thus an erroneous modified autorefraction result and associated visual acuity measurements can be printed out alongside the objective

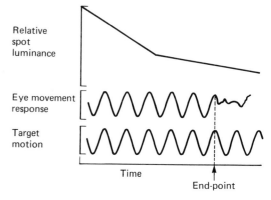

Figure 7.12 Schematic of test conditions: upper solid line shows spot luminance ramps during the test. The centre trace indicates an example of eye movement response to target motion shown in the lower trace. When the spot is no longer visible (end-point), eye movement tracking ceases. (Redrawn from Adams *et al.*, 1984)

results of the autorefractor. The error in subjective refraction may be compounded by large amounts of proximal accommodation; up to 8 D in young children can be induced in autorefraction measurements (Helvaston *et al.*, 1984).

Erroneous or not, this output can be transmitted to automated subjective refractors or with personal microcomputer and mass storage devices via an appropriate interface.

Automated subjective refractors

The stepper motors of each lens race in automated refractor heads are controlled by stepped potentiometers, e.g. Nidek 1100, or a calculator keypad, e.g. Rodenstock Phoromat, Hoya Refractron linked via an input/output chip to the CPU. This digital output, showing the dioptric value of the refractor head lenses, can be displayed on dedicated cathode ray tube (CRT; Hoya), liquid crystal display (LCD; Nidek), LED (Rodenstock) displays.

Retinoscopy can be replaced by the autorefractor result being transmitted to the automated refractor head via the communicating RS 232C line. On receiving the transmitted data in an input buffer, the digital data will be fed by the CPU controlled input/output chip to the stepper motors of the lens discs.

Of particular interest is the automated version of the cross-cylinder lens. In the Phoromat, either 0.50 DC or 0.25 DC cross cylinders can be locked in place. The correct power and axis are then deter-mined by a pre-programmed procedure. In the Hoya subjective automated refractor, the cross-cylinder measurement is made by an autocross cylinder test which is similar to the Simultan test (Beissels, 1967). The associated and dissociated phorias at distance and near, and the near reflex tests are not automated in these refractors. At the end of the refractive examination, the refractive data from these automated subjective devices can be printed out and stored on disk. In spite of the innovation of stepper motors, the results of the refraction derived from these automated subjective refractors is based on conventional refracting techniques. However, recent development of remote and direct imaged refracting systems of the Humphrey Vision Analyser has shown that digital electronics can be married to new refractive techniques.

Imaged subjective refractors

Humphrey Vision Analyser

The Humphrey Vision Analyser (*Figure 7.13*) presents the practitioner with perhaps the most innovative and expensive remote refracting systems cur-

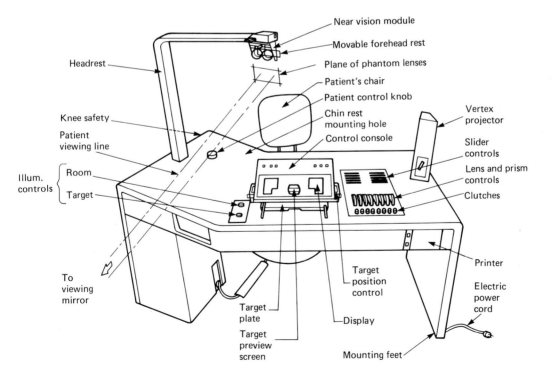

Figure 7.13 Diagram of Humphrey Vision Analyser. (Redrawn with permission of Allergan Humphrey Inc. USA)

rently produced. As shown in *Figure 7.14*, the vision analyser projects two separate test targets through the corrective lens system A and a concave mirror B to be viewed remotely by the patient at C. Each projector light path can be used separately for monocular testing, e.g. visual acuities, cylinder estimation, or together for binocular testing, e.g. dissociated and associated phorias, reading additions and random-dot stereopsis measurement, by using the correct test targets.

The vergence of these projected test targets is altered by the Alvarez/Humphrey lens system. These aspheric lenses are remotely imaged by a concave mirror of 3 m centre of curvature into the approximate spectacle plane of the patient. With no corrective power added by the Alvarez/Humphrey lens system, the test target, e.g. Snellen chart, is focused by the projection system at the anterior focal point of the concave mirror M (*Figure 7.15*). The vergence of the light incident upon the patient's eye is therefore parallel and the test target is seen at infinity.

The variable power lenses of the vision analyser

The Alvarez lens (Alvarez, 1978) is formed from two unique aspheric surfaces which move laterally to form a continuously variable air lens of zero power (*Figure 7.16*, position A) to +7.00 DS or −7.00 DS. This lateral movement is brought about by a lens wheel linked via a linear potentiometer to the microcomputer. For refractive powers greater than −7.0 and +7.0 D an auxiliary ±10 D lens can be placed in each projector light path.

Similarly, the Humphrey variable astigmatic lenses (VAL) (Humphrey, 1976) can alter the meridional power and hence the meridional vergence of the projected beam which is used to cancel out the patient's astigmatism. The Humphrey VAL system acts like two pairs of cross cylinders: the axes of the first VAL being set horizontally (180°) and vertically (90°) and the axes of the second VAL being set obliquely at 135° and 45°. Consequently, the first VAL changes the meridional power obliquely at

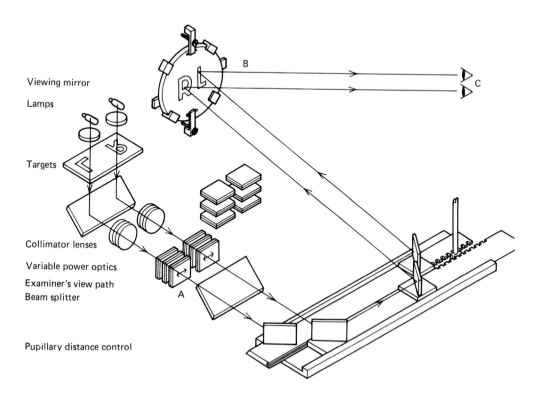

Viewing mirror

Lamps

Targets

Collimator lenses

Variable power optics

Examiner's view path

Beam splitter

Pupillary distance control

Figure 7.14 Vision analyser optical schematic. The basic optical assemblies are shown in simplified form. (Redrawn with permission of the Society of Photo-Optical Instrumentation Engineers and Allergan Humphrey Inc. USA)

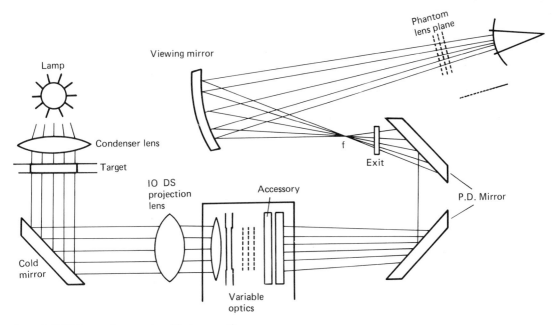

Figure 7.15 Vision analyser optics. (Redrawn with permission of Allergan Humphrey Inc. USA)

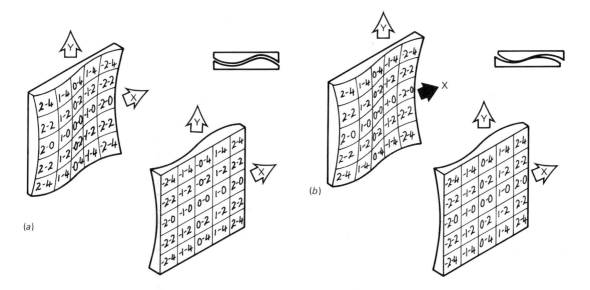

Figure 7.16 Power maps of variable power sphere elements. Sphere and astigmatism powers over the surface of the variable power sphere elements are tabulated in a form such that the combined power of an element pair may be summed for the untranslated (*a*) and translated

(*b*) positions. In actual use, the elements are located much closer together than shown here. (Redrawn with permission of the Society of Photo-Optical Instrumentation Engineers and Allergan Humphrey Inc. USA)

135° and 45° and the second VAL lens changes the meridional power horizontally (180°) and vertically (90°). As shown by Humphrey (1976), Yager (1982), and Saunders (1980, 1982), these meridional powers can be combined together to form an appropriate sphere/cylinder at a given axis.

Fortunately, the use of these variable power lenses in the subjective routine is simplicity itself. The change of the spherical power introduced by the Alvarez lens can be carefully monitored by the patients observing the projected visual acuity targets, while slowly changing a thumb wheel connected to the Alvarez lens. Similarly, both the 90/180 and 135/45 Humphrey astigmatic lenses are used in conjunction with the same thumb wheel to equalize the contrast of the outer two fan lines of each of the precision astigmatic measurement (PAM) targets. These targets are projected with a 4 DC lens (PAM lens), the axis of which is set at 45° for the 90/180 VAL lenses and at 90° for the 45/135 lens. In the presence of ocular astigmatism, both the 90/180 and the 135/45 PAM target lines are likely to vary their contrast. The patient, therefore, reduces the blur ellipse for each PAM target consecutively, so that the contrast of the outer limbs of the three-line target is equal.

Electronics of the vision analyser

The output voltage of the linear potentiometers is monitored by the associated analogue-to-digital interface of a conventional eight-bit computer. The derived digital information is relayed through the registers of the CPU and an output chip on an eight-bit bus to separate right and left LED displays mounted above the dual projection system (*Figure 7.17*). Thus, altering the position of any of the variable focus lenses changes the dioptric value of each LED display. The resultant voltages of the three potentiometers subserving the Alvarez and the two Humphrey variable astigmatic lenses are combined together into a final sphere cylinder combina-

tion which is displayed on the LEDs. This result is stored in the memory of the computer which can be retrieved and dumped to the printer at any time. It is also interesting to note that the CPU of the vision analyser computer can receive on-line data from the Humphrey lens analyser via a RS 232C connector.

The reliability and validity of the Humphrey Vision Analyser

The validity of the refractive measurements of the Humphrey Vision Analyser has been carried out in a study by Kratz and Flom (1977). The results of this study show that the reliability of vision analyser measurements was in reasonable agreement. The validity of this instrument's measurement appeared to be of the same magnitude as those of the auto-refractors, namely 80% of the spherical component was within ±0.50 DS and 79% was within ±0.50 DC of the cylinder power. These values are very similar to those found in a recent validation study by Woodruff and Woo (1978) of the AO SRIII — a monocular, technician-assisted subjective refractor (*see* Bennett and Rabbetts (1984) for further details of the AO SRIV subjective refractor).

These differences should also be viewed in the context of other recent studies of subjective refraction (Jennings and Charman, 1973; Jennings and French, 1974).

Future developments

The use of microprocessors is likely to increase as the unit cost of the semiconductor devices decreases and demand increases. Within the next 10 years, the average ophthalmic practice is likely to acquire an autorefractor, a digitized fundus/slitlamp camera, and an automatic field screener. An optometric computer will correlate and store ophthalmic and

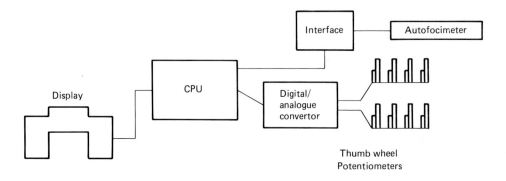

Figure 7.17 Block diagram of vision analyser electronics

optometric data gathered from this instrumentation on optical disks. The accuracy of these measuring devices depends on the increase in the signal-to-noise ratio of the detecting devices (Charman, 1985).

References

ADAMS, T. HAEGERSTROM-PORTNOY, G., BROWN, B. and JAMPOL-SKY, A. (1984) Predicting visual resolution from detection thresholds. *Am. J. Optom. Physiol. Opt.*, **61**(6), 371–376.

ALVAREZ, L.W. (1978) Development of the variable focus lenses and a new refractor. *J. Am. Optom. Assoc.*, **49**(1), 24–29

BENNETT, A.G. (1960) Refraction by automation. *Optician*, **139**, 5–9

BENNETT, A.G. (1978) Methods of automated objective refraction. *Ophthal. Opt.* **18**, 8–15

BENNETT, A.G. and RABBETTS, R.B. (1984) *Clinical Visual Optics*. London: Butterworths

BIESSELS, W.J. (1967) The cross-cylinder simultans test. *J. Am. Optom. Assoc.*, **38**, 473

BIZZEL, F.W., HENDRICKS, J.C., GOLDBERG, F., PATEL, M. and ROBINS, G.F. (1974) Clinical evaluation of an infra-red refracting instrument *Arch. Ophthalmol.*, **92**, 103–108

BRUBAKER, R.F., REINECKE, R.D. and COPELAND, J.C. (1969) Meridional refractometry. *Arch. Ophthalmol.*, **81**, 849–852

CHARMAN, N. (1976) A pioneering instrument. The Collins electronic refractionometer. *Ophthal. Opt.*, **16**, 345–348

CHARMAN, W.N. (1980) Reflection of plane polarised light by the retina. *Br. J. Physiol. Opt.*, **32**, 78–93

CHARMAN, W.N. (1985) Editorial — Infra-red refractors — here to stay? *Ophthal. Physiol. Opt.*, **5**, 237–239

CHARMAN, W.N., JENNINGS, J.A.M and WHITEFOOT, H. (1978) The refraction of the eye in relation to spherical aberration and pupil size. *Br. J. Physiol. Opt.*, **32**, 78–93

COLLINS, G. (1937) The electronic refractionometer *Br. J. Physiol. Opt.*, **11**, 30–42

EMSLEY, H.H. (1963) *Visual Optics*, 5th edn, Vol. 1, p. 39. London: Hatton Press

FLOYD, R.P. and GARCIA, G. (1974) The Ophthalmotron: a clinical trial of accuracy. *Arch. Ophthalmol.*, **92**, 10–14

FRENCH, C.N. and JENNINGS, J.A.M. (1974) Errors in subjective refraction — an exploratory study. *Opthal. Opt.*, **14**, 797–806

FRENCH, C.N. and WOOD, I.C.J. (1981) The Dioptron — in practice. *Optician*, **181**, 18–30

GEERALTS, W.J. and BERRY, E.R. (1968) Ocular spectral characteristics as related to hazards from lasers and other light sources. *Am. J. Ophthalmol.*, **66**, 15–20

GROSVENOR, T., PERRIGIN, D., and PERRIGIN, J. (1984) A three way comparison of retinoscopy, subjective and Dioptron Nova refractive findings. *Am. J. Optom. Physiol. Opt.* **62**, 63–65

GUILLON, M. (1986) Automated refraction in aphakia II. Its repeatability and accuracy compared to conventional techniques. *Ophthal. Physiol. Opt.*, **6**, 85–89

HEATH, G.G. (1956) The influence of visual acuity on the accommodative response of the eye. *Am. J. Optom. Arch. Am. Acad. Optom.*, **33**, 513–524

HELVASTON, E.M., PACHTMAN, M.A., CADERA, W., ELLIS, F., EMMERSON, M. and WEBER, J. (1984) Clinical evaluation of the Nidek AR autorefractor. *J. Pediatr. Ophthalmol. Strab.*, **21**, 227–230

HIRSCH, M.J. (1956) Variability of retinoscopy measurements when applied to large groups of children under visual screening conditions. *Am. J. Optom. Physiol. Opt.*, **32**, 410–416

HUMPHREY, W.E. (1976) A remote subjective refractor employing continuously variable sphere–cylindrical corrections. *Opt. Eng.*, **15**(4), 286–291

JENNINGS, J.A.M. and CHARMAN, W.N.C. (1973) A comparison of errors in some methods of subjective refraction. *Ophthal. Opt.*, **6**, 8–18

KAPS, S.E. (1980) *Report of Nikon Autorefractor*. Nikon Publications

KEATING, M.P. and CARROLL, J.P. (1976) Blurred imagery and the cylinder sine-squared law. *Am. J. Optom. Physiol. Opt.*, **53**, 66–69

KRATZ, L. and FLOM M. (1977) The Humphrey Vision Analyser: Reliability and validity of refractive error measures. *Am. J. Optom. Physiol. Opt.*, **54**, 653–659

McBRIEN, N. and MILLODOT, M. (1985) Clinical evaluation of Canon Autoref R-1. *Am. J. Optom.*, **62**, 786–792

MOHRMAN, R.C. and HOGAN, J.G. (1977) Automatic retinoscopy. *Ophthal. Opt.*, **17**, 22–28

PERRIGIN, J., PERRIGIN, D. and GROSVENOR, T. (1982) A comparison of clinical refractive data obtained by three examiners. *Am. J. Optom. Physiol. Opt.*, **59**, 515–519

PERRIGIN, D., GROSVENOR, T., REIS, A. and PERRIGIN, J. (1984) Comparison of Dioptron Nova refractive data with conventional refractive data. *Am. J. Optom. Physiol. Opt.*, **61**, 497–483

RASSOW, B. and WESEMANN, W. (1984) Automatic infrared refractors 1984. *Ophthalmology*, **91**, *Instr. Book Suppl.* 10–26

REESE, E.E. and FRY, G.A. (1941) The effect of fogging lenses on accommodation. *Am. J. Optics Arch. Am. Acad. Optom.*, **18**, 9–16

SAFIR, A., HYAMS, L., PHILPOT, J. and JAEGERMAN, L.S. (1970) Studies in refraction 1. The precision of retinoscopy *Arch. Ophthalmol.*, **84**, 49–61

SAUNDERS, H. (1980) A method of determining the mean value of refractive errors. *Br. J. Physiol. Opt.*, **34**, 1–11

SAUNDERS, H. (1982) The mean value of refractive error. *Ophthal. Physiol. Opt.*, **2**, 88–90

WESEMANN and RASSOW (1987) Automatic infrared refractors — A comparative study. *Am. J. Optom.*, **64**, 627–638

WONG, E.K., PATELLA, M., PRATT, M., MYERS, S., GASTER, M. and LEOPOLD, L. (1984) Clinical evaluation of the Humphrey Automatic Refractor. *Arch. Ophthalmol.*, **102**, 870–875

WOO, G. and WOODRUFF, M.E. (1978) The AO SRIII Subjective refractor system: A comparison with phoroter measures. *Am. J. Optom. Physiol. Opt.* **55**(8), 591–596

WOOD, I.C.J. (1982) A comparative study of autorefractors. *Ophthal. Opt.*, **22**, 221–225

WOOD, I.C.J. (1987) A review of autorefractors. *Eye*, **1**, 529–535

WOOD, I.C.J., PAPAS, E., BURGHARDT, D. and HARDWICK, G. (1984) A clinical evaluation of the Nidek autorefractor. *Ophthal. Physiol. Opt.*, **4**, 169–178

YAGER, A.S. (1982) The mean value of refractive error. *Ophthal. Physiol. Opt.*, **2**, 87–88

8

Subjective refraction

Daniel O'Leary

In subjective refraction, tests are performed for two reasons: to determine the optimum optical correction and to ensure that visual functions are normal.

While a variety of test targets are used during a refraction, the most useful from an optical and diagnostic consideration is the letter chart used to measure visual acuity.

Visual acuity charts

Tauber designed the first apparatus intended to measure visual acuity (Levene, 1977). It is likely that letters of different sizes were employed in refraction prior to this (Jurin, cited in Smith, 1738); however, credit for the popularity of visual acuity measurement is due to Snellen (1862) who made the test systematic and easy to apply.

Snellen advocated the use of a chart containing graded letter sizes, each constructed on a grid. He uses grids either 5 or 6 units wide and 5 units high, where the strokes on the letters were the size of 1 unit of the grid.

Present letter charts are constructed in much the same way, and either 5 × 5 or 5 × 4 grids are used.

Although there are several ways to specify the size of letters on the chart, the most widely used system is the Snellen notation. This gives the letter size in terms of the distance at which one element of the construction grid subtends 1′ of arc. Thus a letter which is 17.5 mm high is built on a grid of unit size 3.5 mm. At a distance of 12 metres, 3.5 mm subtends 1′ arc, hence the Snellen size of a letter 17.5 mm high is 12 metres (*Figure 8.1*).

The basis of visual acuity

Visual acuity is a broad term covering the ability of the visual system to detect spatial changes. In clini-

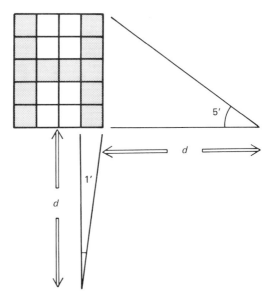

Figure 8.1 Principle of construction of Snellen letters. Letters are constructed on a grid, 5 units high and 4 or 5 units wide. The Snellen size of the letter is measured by the distance (*d*) which one unit of the grid subtends 1′, or at which the letter height subtends 5′

cal usage it means the visual ability to resolve separate points and recognize shapes.

The optical and neural processes preceding perception may each impose their own limits on visual acuity. The optics of the eye do not form perfect images; performance is limited by diffraction at the pupil, aberration from the refracting surfaces and by intraocular scattering of light. Neurally, the limitation of acuity depends at first on the size of the retinal receptors, and later on the fidelity with which their signals are processed.

Optical basis of resolution

Instead of forming point images of object points, the eye forms blur circles. The diameter of the blur circles depends on the size of the pupil, the extent of any aberrations and the state of focus. For an in-focus eye, the blur circle size is controlled by pupil size. Very small pupils introduce large blur circles by diffraction (the Airy disc), but they minimize the contribution of spherical aberration. As pupil size is increased, the Airy disc diameter decreases, but the blur due to spherical aberration increases.

If the blur circles from two object points do not overlap, then as far as the optics of the eye are concerned, the two points can be resolved. If the object points are brought closer together, then eventually the blur circles will overlap (*Figure 18.2*). The amount of overlap that is required to prevent resolution is assumed to be about half a blur circle diameter. With this separation there is only a small change in intensity of light between the blur circle centres. The separation of the two object points represents the resolving power of the optics of the eye. It is usually expressed as the angle between the two objects at the eye, i.e. separation of objects/distance from eye. It should be noted that, although the gap between the objects is not resolved by the optics of the eye beyond the resolution limit, the light pattern on the retina is not the same as for a single point or a bar; the retinal image still contains some 'information' indicating the presence of two point objects.

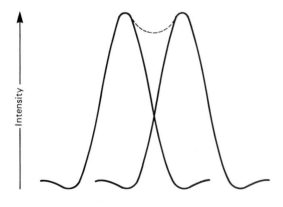

Figure 8.2 The Rayleigh limit of resolution. The light distribution in the images of points (the Airy disc) is shown. When the maximum of one Airy disc falls on the minimum of another, the two are just resolvable. The overall intensity is shown by the dashed line; at the assumed resolution limit there is a small dip in the intensity between the two maxima

Neural basis of resolution

At the fovea, cones have a diameter of about 1.5 μm. If two objects were imaged on adjacent cones, then it would not be possible for the visual system to separate them — the gap between them would not be resolved. On anatomical grounds alone, then, the separation of the two image points must be at least 1.5 μm, corresponding to an angular separation of 20″. With extended objects this argument has only limited validity.

Performance of the visual system

In measuring visual acuity clinically, the results are influenced by both optical and neural performance. For a normal observer under optimum conditions, resolving power is often less than 1′, and occasionally values of 30″ may be found. Snellen letters are usually used, the chart being read so that the smallest discernible letters can be found. For the letters to be recognized the detail that must be resolved is the size of 1 unit of the 5×4 grid used in their construction.

Clinical notation

There are several different ways of specifying the resolving power of the eye. Clinically the most widely used notation is the Snellen fraction, D/d. The numerator (D) indicates the distance between observer and chart, and is usually 6 metres or 20 feet. The denominator (d) is the Snellen size of the letter, i.e. the distance at which 1 unit of the construction grid subtends 1′. Thus if the test is conducted at 6 m and the 9-m line is the smallest that can be read, the result is recorded is 6/9.

It is becoming more common to record the result as the minimum angle of resolution (MAR notation). Since a Snellen letter requires 1′ resolution at d metres, it requires d/D in minutes resolution at the test distance. An acuity of 6/9 in the Snellen notation gives an MAR of 1.5′ (9/6).

Others prefer to record acuity in decimal notation, by dividing the Snellen fraction. Here, 6/9 acuity becomes 0.67 (decimal).

The Snellen notation is almost universally understood, and is not open to confusion. This makes a very strong case for preferring it. It contains all the information required to calculate either the MAR or decimal values, but it cannot be derived from these. Additionally, it is difficult to confuse the value of the result with anything else.

Ancillary notes

When a special chart is used in measuring performance, this is usually recorded. Thus if the chart consists of Cs, the result is written as 6/6(c).

It is good practice to note whether all the letters on a line were read or where one or two extra letters on a smaller line could be seen. This could be recorded as 6/6 +2 or 6/9 −1.

Vision and visual acuity

In the clinic, these two terms have precise meanings. Vision (V) means the performance reached without any correction, and visual acuity (VA) is used to indicate the corrected performance.

Sometimes visual performance may be poorer than the minimum recordable using the chart at its normal distance. In these cases the test may be performed at a reduced distance. Where a precise value is not needed or where vision is much impaired, then a rapid evaluation can be made based on:

(1) The ability to count the examiner's fingers, usually at 1 or 2 m. This is recorded as CF, 1 m etc. (resolution of fingers, when widely spread, corresponds roughly to resolution of the 36-m letters).
(2) Where finger counting fails, a hand movement may be seen. This is usually performed at 1 m, but may be repeated at further distances. The result is recorded as V = HM (1 m).
(3) Where hand movements are not seen, the ophthalmoscope is held close to the eye. If the position of the light can be made out, the result is recorded as light perception with projection or LP if the light is seen without its position being located.

Construction of visual acuity charts

The grid system of constructing letters is used in most modern charts, but other important features of the charts are less well standardized. These features include the selection of letters, the spacing of letters and lines, the grading of letter sizes and the luminance of the chart. Variations in these parameters between charts may result in different measurements of visual acuity under otherwise identical conditions.

Some letters are easier to recognize than others. According to Sheard (1921), L, T, U, V and C are the easiest to recognize, and S, G, H and B are the most difficult. The variation can partly be explained by the complexity of the letters (L is simple whilst B is complicated) and partly by their confusability (F and P are easily confused, as are D and O). Some charts consist of letters of nearly equal legibility while others include letters of varying difficulty. There is something to be said in favour of both types of chart; the former tend to give 'all-or-nothing' measurements, the patient reading all the letters on a line, or none, while the latter give graded measurements — being able to read one or two easy letters, but not the more difficult ones. For standardization, letters of equal legibility are more appropriate.

Letter and line spacing have a measurable effect on visual acuity. Flom, Heath and Tagahashi (1963) found that the ability to resolve the gap in a C was affected by the position of surrounding contours. Resolving power was maximal when the surrounding contours were separated from the C by at least five times the gap size. It may be deduced that letter charts should be constructed with controlled letter spacing (*Figure 8.3*).

In general practice all charts contain 6-m letters and 60-m letters, with an assortment of intermediate sizes with one or two smaller lines. Letters larger than the 60-m size are rarely included because they take up too much space — it is better to move the patient and the chart closer together when it is important to investigate low visual acuity. Bennett (1965) described three ways in which the letter sizes could be determined:

(1) A geometrical progression in the denominator.
(2) An arithmetic progression in vision — a decimal notation.
(3) An arithmetic progression in the denominator.

The selection of a letter chart based on one or other of these progressions may affect measurement of visual acuity, because they force acuity into discrete (and different) categories, where acuity actually occupies a continuum. The step size also limits the ability to detect changes in performance produced by changing the optical correction.

Most letter charts have one 60-m letter, and an increasing number of letters on lower lines. Bailey and Lovie (1976) consider this to be a deficiency, suggesting that conditions should be kept as near constant as possible from line to line, so that size (and hence resolution) is the only significant variable. The letter chart they designed controls several important factors (*Figure 8.4*): letters are of nearly equal legibility and are spaced by one letter width. Each row consists of five letters; rows are separated by a gap equal to the letter height in the smaller row. The progression chosen is a geometrical progression in the denominator, where the ratio of the progression is 1.26 (0.1 log unit steps). The use of a logarithmic step is claimed to facilitate conversion from Snellen notation to decimal acuity when non-standard test distances are used. It has a further benefit at non-standard distances in the constancy of the visual task; reading the 48-m line at 6 m is equivalent to reading the 24-m line at 3 m. This makes it particularly suitable for assessing the visually disabled, where the test distance is often governed by their visual acuity.

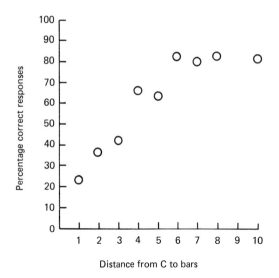

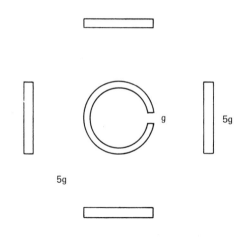

Figure 8.3 The effect of adjacent contours on visual acuity. The test target configuration is shown on the right. The distance between the C and the bar was varied from g up to 10 × g. The position of the gap in the C was varied, and the number of correct responses for each test configuration is shown in the graph. (Subject G.Hi, from Flom, Heath and Tagahashi, 1963)

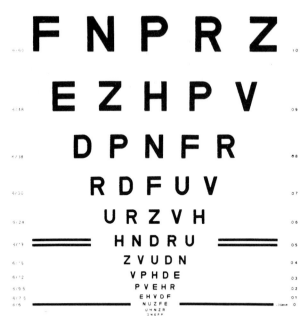

Figure 8.4 The Bailey–Lovie chart. (Courtesy of the authors and the NVRI)

Single optotype charts

When the visual acuity chart consists of a single optotype (either a 'C' or an 'E'), the orientation of the letter is varied. Usually only four orientations are used: the gap in the C or the open side of the E is located on the left, right, top or bottom. It is possible to use oblique orientations, but this detracts from the simplicity of the charts.

These charts are most useful for patients who are unfamiliar with the alphabet (hence they are sometimes called 'illiterate' charts) and so most consulting rooms are equipped with one. They are rather tedious to use and it is sometimes difficult to identify which line or character is being referred to— requiring the practitioner to point to them individually. For these reasons, single optotype charts are not widely used for assessing visual acuity.

Despite their limited application during the routine refraction, there is a case for considering these charts in the final measurement of visual acuity. During a refraction, it is necessary to determine whether acuity is improving or decreasing, and frequent reference is made to the test chart for this reason. The final assessment of visual acuity is recorded for future reference, so that any deterioration or improvement may be ascertained. It is clearly desirable that charts for making this assessment should be as standard as possible, so that valid comparison of data from different clinics may be made. Single optotype charts are not subject to bias due to either relative legibility of letters or cultural factors, and so satisfy some of the basic requirements of a standard test (Enoch, 1971).

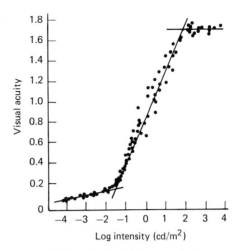

Figure 8.5 The relationship between luminance and visual acuity (Koenig). The ordinate gives visual acuity in decimal notation; the lines through the data were added by the author. (Data from *Textbook of Physiology*, edited by John F. Fulton, 1949, Philadephia, W. B. Saunders Co.)

Luminance and contrast

Luminance has a profound effect on visual acuity. In the dark, detection of large objects such as houses and trees is difficult until they are very close. Acuity increases with luminance. It can be seen (*Figure 8.5*) that there are three phases to the increase: first acuity increases slowly until the luminance reaches about 10^{-2} cd/m^2, then acuity increases more rapidly from 10^{-2} cd/m^2 up to 10^2 cd/m^2 and finally acuity hardly changes for luminances above 10^2 cd/m^2. Over the second phase acuity increases linearly with log luminance.

The form of the acuity–luminance function has led to the suggestion that a minimum luminance of 120 cd/m^2 should be adopted for test charts; there is little point setting an upper limit (BS 4278, 1968).

Contrast

Contrast refers to the relative luminance of the test target and the background. If the luminance of the target is T, and of the background is L, then contrast is expressed as $(L-T)/L$. The relationship between contrast and visual acuity has been investigated by Ludvigh (1941) (*Figure 8.6*). As contrast is increased from zero, acuity increases very rapidly at first. For contrasts of between 0.3 and 1.0, the increase in acuity is much slower. In clinical measurements, Sloane (1951) considered that 0.84 was the minimum acceptable contrast level while BS 4274 (1968) stipulates a minimum contrast level of 0.9. In practice, it is difficult to achieve contrasts very much higher than this.

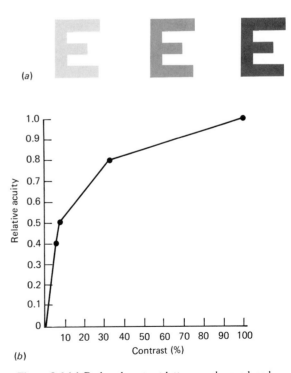

Figure 8.6 (*a*) Reduced contrast letters can be produced using Letratone or similar art material. These letters were made from 10%, 30% and 60% tints. (*b*) Visual acuity measured with reduced contrast letters. (Data from Ludvigh, 1941)

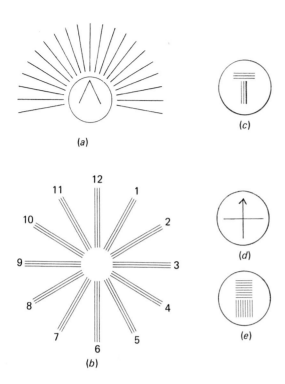

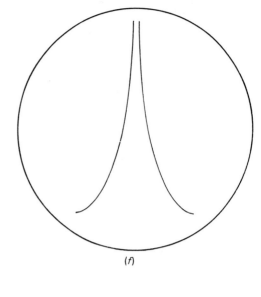

(c)

(d)

(e)

Figure 8.7 Astigmatic charts: (*a*) Fan chart, with rotating 'V'; (*b*) clock dial; (*c*) rotating T; (*d*) rotating cross with arrowhead; (*e*) blocks; (*f*) Raubitschek arrow (paraboline)

Other test targets

Duochrome tests

These consist of black targets on red and green backgrounds. Because the focal length of the eye is longer for red light than for green, the two sets of targets are focused in different planes. If the red targets are seen more clearly than the green, the eye is myopic and if green is clearer, the eye is hypermetropic. It is assumed that the eye is correctly focused when the two sets of targets are equalized.

Targets for astigmatic analysis

These consist of two types (*Figure 8.7*): fixed targets and rotatable targets.

(1) Fixed targets — these are made up of radial lines, evenly spaced at either 10° intervals or 30° intervals.
(2) Rotatable targets — these may consist of lines at right angles to each other (rotating cross, blocks, T), lines at an acute angle to each other (V or arrowhead) or curved lines (paraboline). They are used to refine the axis, and to determine the correct cylinder power.

Effect of defocus on resolution

The resolving power of the out-of-focus eye can be predicted reasonably well by blur circle theory. Typical values for acuity are shown in *Figure 8.8*, together with a theoretical function of blur circle size. According to this theory, the minimum angle of resolution should double when the pupil size is

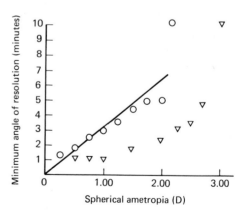

Figure 8.8 The vision found in different amounts of spherical ametropia (data from Peters, 1961). Myopes (○); hyperopes aged 45–55 (▽). The line through the data is the theoretical resolving power of a reduced eye with a 2-mm pupil

doubled, but the change is actually smaller than this for pupil sizes over 4 mm (Tucker and Charman, 1975). This is probably another manifestation of the Stiles–Crawford effect.

During a refraction, the level of visual acuity provides a useful guide to the extent of the uncorrected ametropia. However, for many of the tests, the primary concern is not with the resolving power but with contrast; changing focus may alter contrast and it is this alteration which must be seen.

The contrast of the retinal image depends on the contrast of the object as well as on the optical performance of the eye. It will be recalled that when the contrast of the test type is reduced, visual acuity is depressed. It is possible to establish a threshold acuity level for any contrast. For low contrast objects it is easiest to control contrast with an oscilloscope and the targets of choice are grating patterns. Usually the size of the grating is kept constant during a measurement and the contrast is increased until the grating is seen. The test is then repeated for different grating sizes. Very high contrast is required for the finest gratings to be detected, but for coarser gratings, threshold may be as low as 0.05. Typical data are shown in *Figure 8.9* together with equivalent data for Snellen letters. Over the range where measurements are available, it seems that there is reasonable agreement between the two sets of data. The performance of the eye on clinical tests can therefore be deduced from the performance on gratings.

As the eye is defocused, contrast is reduced. In order to detect a grating, the contrast in the object must be increased accordingly. The reduction in image contrast is less for coarse gratings than for finer ones (Campbell and Green, 1965) (*Figure 8.10*).

The change in contrast is not a linear function of the amount of defocus. If the eye is defocused in 0.25-D steps, the initial changes in contrast are smallest. This means that the eye is relatively insensitive to small changes of focus when it is in focus, and much more sensitive when it is out of focus. This was demonstrated by Campbell and Westheimer (1958) using a Badal optometer. The target was moved back and forth by increasing amounts until subjects noticed a change in the target. Typical results are shown in *Figure 8.11*. The eye is most sensitive to change in focus when it is out of focus by 1–2 D.

Denieul (1982) noted that it was difficult to find the best focus directly by locating the position of highest contrast. He suggested that sensitivity is improved if the eye is defocused with positive and negative lenses and the blur compared. The position of best focus is midway between the lenses which produce equal amounts of blur (*Figure 8.12*).

In refraction extensive use is made of this principle, and in many tests the end-point is found by

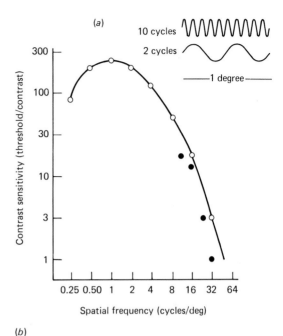

(b)

Figure 8.9 (*a*) Grating size is specified by the number of cycles/deg visual angle. (*b*) Contrast sensitivity function, for different gratings (open circles). The closed circles are taken from *Figure 8.4*, and show the sensitivity for Snellen letters

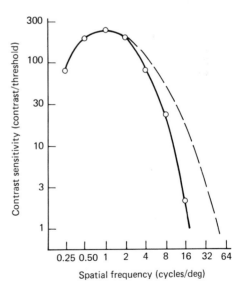

Figure 8.10 Effect of defocus on contrast sensitivity for different gratings. The dashed line shows the in-focus function for comparison; 0.75 D defocus was used (author's data). Note that course gratings have the same threshold as previously, but now gratings finer than 20 cycles/deg are not seen even at maximum contrast

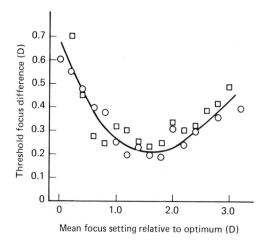

Figure 8.11 Sensitivity of the eye to differences in focus with induced hypermetropia (○) or myopia (□). The line through the data was fitted by eye. (Data from Campbell and Westheimer, 1958)

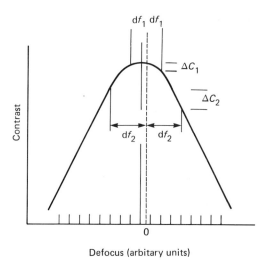

Figure 8.12 The relationship between contrast and defocus. Contrast is maximum at the optimum focus (0). A small amount of defocus (vertical dashed line) results in a very small decrease in contrast. If the contrast is examined on either side of this position (df_1), the contrast difference is increased ($\triangle C_1$). If bigger steps are used (df_2) the contrast difference is increased further. (After Denieul, 1982)

equalizing blur, rather than by locating sharpest focus directly.

Subjective refraction

The first steps in subjective refraction are determined by the level of vision, measured with a standard acuity chart. Vision is recorded for each eye in turn, and then one eye is occluded while the other is refracted. It is assumed below that the subjective refraction does *not* commence with retinoscopy findings.

It is usually possible to make a tentative diagnosis of the likely refractive state at this stage by considering the vision together with the case history. In children, a history of deteriorating distance vision usually indicates myopia, while near vision problems are more commonly found with medium to high degrees of hypermetropia. Astigmatism may produce symptoms of blur or asthenopia associated with distance vision or near vision, although the recorded vision is often near normal.

In adults, the gradual loss of accommodation causes distance vision problems for the hypermetrope and near vision problems for everyone. Usually the deterioration of distance vision is so insidious that it remains unnoticed until measured in an acuity test. Occasionally, myopia develops in adults, sometimes with visible lens changes but possibly with no obvious cause, producing symptoms of deteriorating distance vision with normal near vision.

Although any diagnosis can only be tentative at this stage, some conditions can be positively excluded. For example if vision is 6/5, moderate to high degrees of myopia and astigmatism can be ruled out in all subjects, as can high hyperopia in presbyopes. If vision is reduced to 6/9 or beyond then moderate hyperopia in young subjects cannot be excluded. Peters (1961) produced tables giving typical values for uncorrected vision in a wide range of refractive states (*see Figure 8.8* and *Table 8.1*)

Reduced vision — the pinhole test

When vision is reduced to 6/18 or beyond, it is useful to see whether vision is improved with a pinhole. This is a standard accessory in all trial cases and refractor heads. Although the size of the pinhole has has not been standardized, it is usually about 1 mm diameter.

When vision is reduced substantially by a refractive error, it will be improved by a pinhole. When such an improvement is not achieved, it must be concluded that ametropia is not the major factor, but that some other factor is also present. In high ametropia, vision may be outside the range of the chart. In cases where vision is less than 6/60, pinholes are exceptionally useful. Where they do not improve vision to at least 6/60, it may be assumed that either the refractive error is high — probably greater than 5 D — or that the condition is pathological.

The best vision sphere

Where vision is 6/60 or better

Initially, positive spheres are added. Vision may improve, remain unchanged or decrease.

If vision improves then the eye is hypermetropic, with or without astigmatism. If vision gets worse then the eye is myopic.

In the hyperope, adding plus may continue to improve vision, or at least leave it unchanged. Eventually if plus continues to be added vision starts to deteriorate. In the absolute hyperope — where there is no accommodation — it is safe to assume that all the hypermetropia has been revealed. In other cases this may not be so. Theoretically, it is assumed that accommodation relaxes as far as possible when plus is added and is active when plus is reduced. In practice, the accommodative response is idiosyncratic (Reese and Fry, 1941; Heath, 1956; Millodot and Newton 1981), and depends on a multitude of stimuli. The clinician must be alert to the possibility that accommodation is not completely relaxed when vision starts to deteriorate. The most consistent clue to this behaviour is fluctuating vision. Following an increase in plus, vision is at first blurred but gradually improves if sufficient time is allowed. Often following an improvement, vision then deteriorates again. The only skills needed here are patience and a suspicious nature.

In seeking out hypermetropia the routine is tailored to find the recalcitrant. After an increase in plus, the best vision achieved is noted, and then more plus added in small steps allowing ample time in between. It will be recalled that an increase in defocus of 1.00 D should produce a reduction in resolution of about 3′ — from 6/5 to 6/18 or from 6/12 to 6/30. If much more than 1.00 D is needed to produce this reduction, then fogging has probably caused accommodation to relax.

In the myope, adding plus always reduces vision, and accommodation is usually well behaved. In astigmatism, the disposition of the focal lines may allow some letters on several lines to be read while other letters on the same lines remain illegible.

Whatever the refractive state, plus is increased until a measurable reduction in vision is produced. A report that a lens has made the letters 'worse' is not a sufficient indicator of blur; if fogging is stopped at this stage hypermetropia may remain undetected. Where vision is good many practitioners add plus until vision is fogged to 6/18. If vision is initially 6/12 or worse, a reduction of one or two lines is often adequate, especially if the other indications point to the presence of myopia.

Once a measurable blur has been established, plus lenses are removed (or minus added) in small steps until vision shows no further improvement. The maximum positive lens (or minimum negative lens) that allows this level of vision is the best vision sphere (BVS).

During this procedure vision is determined with increasing blur and then with decreasing blur. Often the lens required for a particular level of vision is more positive on the decreasing run than on the increasing run. This indicates that fogging has relaxed accommodation. Care must be taken on the decreasing run to avoid excessive reduction of fog. The criterion used to decide whether vision is improved is an increase in the number of letters read, not an improvement in clarity. Adjustments for clarity are made at a later stage in the refraction when the sphere is refined. The decrease in fog should also be commensurate with the improvement in vision; if it seems too great then overaccommodation is suspected.

Where vision is worse than 6/60

First a pinhole is placed in front of the eye. If vision improves to 6/60 or better then the patient probably has a spherical error of less than 7 D, high astigmatism or an irregular refraction due, for example, to keratoconus. If vision is less than 6/60 with the pinhole, the patient has a refractive error of greater than 5 D or some complicating pathology.

Initially spherical lenses are added in large steps; when vision with the pinhole is 6/60 or better, 2-D steps are appropriate. Where vision is worse than 6/60 with the pinhole, steps of 3 or 4 D are better. With the phoropter, it is easiest to change power using the coarse sphere adjustment which gives 3- or 4-D steps in most cases. Except in aphakic patients, hyperopia of greater than 12 D is extremely rare in general practice; however, myopia of over 20 D is occasionally encountered. In this test it is important to exhaust all the possibilities; if necessary the full range of lenses available should be tried before myopia or hypermetropia are excluded as the major cause of the reduced vision.

When the reduced vision is mainly due to a spherical error, it will eventually be improved by this technique. Once the approximate range of the error has been determined and vision is 6/24 or better, the normal techniques for determining the BVS may be applied.

Where vision cannot be measurably improved with any spherical lens, the condition is either high astigmatism or pathological. In high astigmatism, the BVS may be determined with the pinhole. The accuracy of the procedure is very limited but a rough evaluation to the nearest 1 or 2 D is sufficient at this stage.

Measuring the astigmatism

The maximum likely amount of astigmatism may be evaluated from vision with the BVS (*Table 8.1*), This estimate is the starting point for lens manipulation. As a rough rule of thumb:

$$A = L/9$$

where A is the estimated astigmatism, and L is the letter size (in metres, Snellen notation).

Table 8.1 Maximum amount of astigmatism from vision with the BVS

Vision with BVS	Assumed astigmatic error (D)
6/5	0.50
6/9	1.25
6/12	1.75
6/15	2.00
1/18	2.50
6/24	3.00
6/36	4.00

After Peters, 1961.

The fogging method

With this technique, it is assumed that the BVS places the circle of least confusion on the retina. If the clock dial or fan is viewed, all the lines should be equally blurred. Adding positive spheres moves both astigmatic foci forward; the posterior focal line is now closer to the retina than previously and the anterior focal line is further away. This procedure makes the posterior focal line clearer and the anterior focal line less clear.

The aim of the fogging method is to place both focal lines in front of the retina using positive spheres, and then to move the anterior focal line back using cylindrical lenses. The first problem is the amount of positive sphere to be added to the BVS, the added positive sphere being called the fogging lens (*Figures 8.13–8.16*).

The power of the fogging lens (S) may be calculated from:

$$S = \tfrac{1}{2} A + 0.5 \ (D)$$

where A is the assumed astigmatic error. For example, if vision with the BVS is 6/18, then $A = 2.50$ D, and $\tfrac{1}{2} A = 1.25$ D and from this $S = 1.75$ D. A lens of power +1.75 D is therefore added to the BVS. If all the assumptions are correct, the posterior focal line is now 0.5 D in front of the retina, and the anterior focal line is 3.00 D in front of the retina.

The axis of the correcting cylinder

With the fogging lens added to the BVS, some lines on the fan chart or clock dial should be clearer than the orthogonal lines. The clear lines are used to find the meridian of the posterior focal line, the anterior focal line being at 90° to this meridian. The clock dial has its lines drawn at 30° intervals; if one set of lines is clearest, and the lines 30° on either side are equally blurred, then the direction of the clearest lines indicates the direction of the posterior focal line. Where two or three sets of lines are clearer than the others it is sometimes possible to extrapolate the meridian. For example, if the 1 o'clock and 2 o'clock lines are equally clear, and the 12 o'clock and 3 o'clock lines are equally blurred, the meridian lies half-way between the clear lines; if the 12 o'clock lines had been clearer than the 3 o'clock lines, then the meridian would have been closer to the 1 o'clock position than to the 2 o'clock position. Thus, it is sometimes possible to determine the cylinder axis to better than 10°; however, the clock dial cannot be relied upon for accurate axis determination. Charts with more meridional lines may give more accurate axis position.

Refinement of the axis with a 'V' chart

Many astigmatic charts have a rotating central disc on which two lines are drawn to make a V-shape (or arrowhead). As the disc is rotated the V points to the different meridional lines.

The acute angle formed by the arms of the V may be between 30° and 90° depending on the chart, but most charts use a 60° configuration. When the V is pointing to the in-focus meridian, the two arms of the V are equally blurred. If the V is incorrectly orientated then one arm will be clearer than the other and the V is then rotated away from the clearer arm until both arms are equally blurred. By approaching the clearest meridian from the two sides, the range of positions where the V arms are equally clear may be determined rapidly. The orientation of the posterior focal line is taken as the midpoint of the range.

The V test for axis is an accurate method of refining the position of the posterior focal line. It is superior to the fan because axis position is continually variable, it employs blurred rather than in-focus lines and places the defocused lines close to each other for easy comparison.

The correcting cylinder is placed at 90° to the meridian marked by the V. On many charts the fan lines adjacent to the V are marked with the correct position of the negative cylinder. The vertical line is marked 180; when the vertical line is clearest, this indicates that a negative cylinder axis 180° is required.

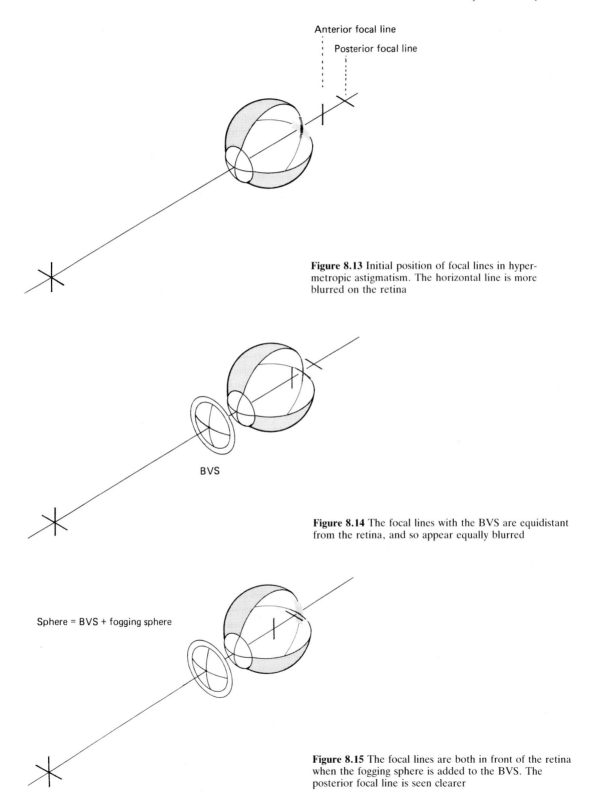

Anterior focal line

Posterior focal line

Figure 8.13 Initial position of focal lines in hypermetropic astigmatism. The horizontal line is more blurred on the retina

BVS

Figure 8.14 The focal lines with the BVS are equidistant from the retina, and so appear equally blurred

Sphere = BVS + fogging sphere

Figure 8.15 The focal lines are both in front of the retina when the fogging sphere is added to the BVS. The posterior focal line is seen clearer

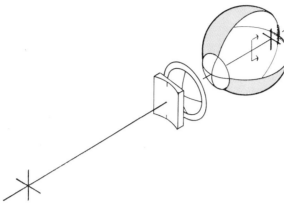

Figure 8.16 Correcting the astigmatism with a cylinder. The cylinder axis is parallel to the anterior (vertical) focal line. Its effect is to move this focal line back towards the posterior focal line. When the cylinder power is correct, both focal lines are the same distance in front of the retina, and so vertical and horizontal lines are seen equally blurred

Determining the power of the correcting cylinder

Negative cylinders are added at the correct axis until all meridians are equally clear. Where an excess of power is added, the lines parallel to the cylinder axis will be clearer than the others. This test may be carried out using the clock dial or the fan chart, but specialized targets are often available. These all consist of two sets of lines at right angles to each other; they are often located with the V so that one set points along each of the principal meridians when the V test has been completed. Because of the proximity of the two sets of lines, judgement is easier than for the widely spread lines of the fan chart.

Checking for errors in the fogging routine

Power
If the fogging lens used at the start of this procedure was of insufficient power to place both focal lines in front of the retina, then the cylinder power may be too low. If, for example one focal line had been left behind the retina when the fogging lens was added, then the cylinder power to equalize the chart would have left the anterior focal line in front of the retina. To exclude this possibility, a check test is employed after the chart has been equalized. A +0.50 D sphere is added. If the lines on the chart are still equal then the cylinder is correct. If the lines marked by the V are now clearer, then the cylinder power is too low; the chart must again be equalized. Rarely, it is discovered that the lines parallel to the cylinder axis are clearest, in which case the cylinder has been overcorrected. In the case of undercorrection, the test must be repeated after equalization to ensure that a final value for the correcting cylinder has been determined. Failure to make this repeated check is the most common cause of undercorrected astigmatism with the fogging routine.

Axis
The axis determination with astigmatic charts is only approximate, although the V test allows considerable refinement in some cases. If the cylinder is off axis, this will become apparent as the cylinder power is increased. Instead of the lines delineated by the V remaining clearest, lines at about 40–50° to this position gradually become clearest.

It is important to remember that only a small axis error is needed to produce this picture, although a large error may be present. To correct the error, the cylinder power should be neutralized as near as possible using the T or blocks. The clearer lines will have apparently moved either clockwise or anticlockwise from the originally clear position. The correcting cylinder is rotated in the same direction. (Care must be taken when using a direct chart; the direction that appears clockwise when the examiner looks at the direct chart is anticlockwise when the patient is viewed.)

Final power check
This is required only if the axis has been modified.

When the cylindrical correction has been checked, the spherical part of the correction is modified by reducing the fog until best vision is achieved. Similar precautions must be taken in refining the sphere as were taken for determining the BVS.

Rationale of cylindrical determination

Several other approaches can be used to determine the astigmatic error with fog. The technique described here is intended to make maximum use of the information gained from determining the BVS, and to maximize the contrast in determining the cylindrical correction. The maximum contrast in astigmatism is reached when one focal line is slightly in front of the retina and the other is further in front;

this follows from a consideration of the effects of defocus on modulation.

Other less rigorous techniques have been suggested (Borish, 1970). These include:

(1) Fogging to 6/12 and then using an astigmatic dial.
(2) Reducing fog with the patient viewing the fan chart until one focal line is clearer than the other lines.
(3) Fogging with a +1.50 DS, and reducing fog if one line on the fan is not clearer than others.

In addition to these, some prefer to add +0.50 DS to the BVS, and proceed to the fan chart.

Very often all of these techniques will end up giving similar starting points for axis determination, but none makes maximum use of the information available from determining the BVS. Of the other techniques, only Borish's (2) will consistently give contrast approaching the maximum. Provided the proper checks are carried out, all of these other methods are capable of producing the correct results, although the sensitivity may be less than optimum.

The Raubitschek arrow test

With the fogging method of determining astigmatism, separate charts are needed to locate and refine the axis position and to determine the power of the correcting cylinder. The lines on a clock dial or fan chart are too far apart to allow precise location of the axis, and so a V chart is used to refine axis — the V chart does not indicate axis position initially because its sides show only two directions. Cylinder power is most accurately determined with the T chart or blocks because of the close proximity of the blurred lines to the clear ones.

Raubitschek (1928, 1958) proposed an elegant simplification of astigmatic analysis that allowed axis and power to be determined with a single target, the arrow. The arrow consists of two wings, each of which is a portion of a parabola. It is drawn on a disc which can be rotated to any meridian. Whatever the orientation of the arrow, the posterior focal line of the eye will be tangential to a point on one or other wing. Provided the eye is slightly fogged, this point will appear blacker than the rest of the arrow and provide the initial indication for axis determination.

The test is conducted under a small amount of fog after the BVS has been found. The black portion of the arrow (called 'the shadow') is identified on one wing or the other, and the arrow is rotated away from this wing. This causes the shadow to run up the wing in an easily discernible way. When the correct axis location is approached the shadow starts to run down the other wing, and when the shadows on the two wings are of equal length the arrow points to the

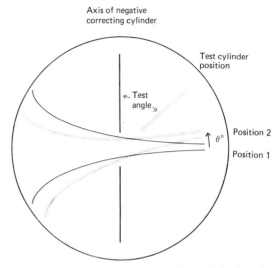

Figure 8.17 The Raubitschek method of finding the cylinder. Position (1) of the arrow gives the axis of the correcting cylinder (−cylinder axis is at 90° to position 1). A cylinder of known power is placed at the test angle (usually 50° from the correcting axis) and the arrow rotated through θ° to equalize the shadow again (position 2). The power of the correcting cylinder can be found from tables (*see Figure 8.18*)

in-focus meridian. Raubitschek claims that the test is the most precise method of locating cylinder axis.

Determining the power of the correcting cylinder with the Raubitschek arrow is more complicated than with T charts. Several techniques have been suggested: Raubitschek originally proposed that the arrow should be used with a 'bias' cylinder (*Figure 8.17*). After axis determination, a cylinder is inserted at a predetermined angle to the meridian. The combination of the ocular astigmatism and the bias cylinder produces a new astigmatic state. The resultant astigmatism will vary in amount and axis, depending on the two components. Raubitschek suggested that the axis of the resultant astigmatism should be measured with the arrow; from the theory of obliquely crossed cylinders, the ocular astigmatism may be calculated, or tables may be consulted—the important parameters are the power of the bias cylinder, and the subsequent rotation of the arrow. *Figure 8.18* shows a range of these values, and the calculated ocular astigmatism.

Later, Raubitschek produced an arrow test incorporating a nomograph which allowed a direct estimation of the astigmatism; the essential method was the same, however. These methods have not proved to be popular for two reasons: the accuracy with which astigmatism can be determined is limited by the sensitivity of the axis determination, and error of about 1° in determining the posterior principal meridian and the neutral point when the bias cy-

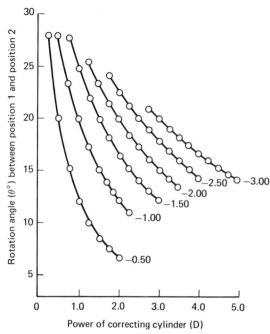

Figure 8.18 Nomograph for calculating correcting cylinder power. The test cylinder power is indicated at the bottom of each curve. The test angle in this case is always 50°. When the rotation angle, θ, has been determined, the correct cylinder power is read off from the abscissa. For example, if the test cylinder power is −1.50°, and the rotation angle, θ is 13°, then the correct cylinder power is −2.75 D. (After Eskridge, 1958)

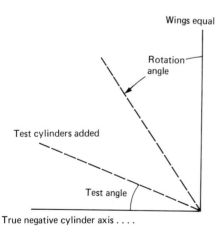

Figure 8.19 Pascal's method for determining cylinder power: (1) Locate position where wings are equal (90° in diagram); (2) true cylinder axis is at 90° to this position (180° in diagram); (3) the test angle is chosen (20° in diagram); (4) the paraboline is moved through the rotation angle (90° − test angle)/2; (5) cylinder power is increased at the test angle until the wings are equalized; this cylinder power is correct; (6) the correct cylinder power is positioned at the correct axis

linder is included together can produce a 1.00 D error in the calculated ocular astigmatism; other methods are, however, available to determine the astigmatism and these do not require interpolation from tables—these other methods (due to Pascal, 1953 and Heath, 1958) are more widely used.

Pascal's method is based on the theorem that two cylindrical lenses of equal power produce a resultant cylinder with an axis exactly midway between them (*Figure 8.19*). If the two cylinders are unequal then the resultant lies at some other angle. Treating the ocular astigmatism as a negative cylinder, it is exactly neutralized by a negative cylinder of equal power placed at 90° to the axis of astigmatism. If the correcting cylinder is placed at any other axis, a resultant cylinder is produced with an axis midway between the two.

Once the axis of astigmatism is determined with the arrow, the correct orientation of the negative correcting cylinder is known. A position for the correcting cylinder is chosen at some angle (the 'test' angle) away from this position; for small amounts of astigmatism a test angle of 30° may be used, while for larger errors smaller test angles are used. The arrow is now rotated to bisect the acute angle between its original position and the test angle. The power of the correcting cylinder is now increased until the two sides of the arrow are equalized in this new position; because the resultant of the ocular astigmatism and the correcting cylinder must lie along this direction, the power of the correcting cylinder must now equal the ocular astigmatism. It is now placed at the previously determined axis.

Heath (1958) and Eskridge (1958) have suggested that the arrow should be moved from the 'axis' position for power determination, but the correcting cylinder should be placed at the principal meridian rather than be rotated through a test angle. In Heath's method the arrow is rotated through 20°, while Eskridge suggested that a rotation of 90° should be used. When a 20° rotation is used the two sides of the arrow have unequal shadows. As the correct cylinder power is approached the sides tend to equalize. With Eskridge's method the two sides of the arrow are always equal, but the two tips are blurred. As cylindrical power is introduced the shadow moves along the wings. In all these techniques the end-point is reached when the shadow disappears.

The cross-cylinder technique for determining astigmatism

A cross cylinder is a lens with a positive cylinder on one surface and a negative cylinder of numerically equal power on the other surface, the axes of the two cylinders being at right angles to each other.

They are dioptrically equivalent to a sphero-cylindrical lens—for example, a cross cylinder composed of a +1.00 DC on one surface and an orthogonal cylinder of power −1.00 D on the other surface is equivalent to a spherocylindrical lens of power +1.00 DS combined with a −2.00 DC, the axis in this case coinciding with the axis of the negative component of the cross cylinder. They are used to determine both the axis and power of the correcting cylinder.

The cross cylinder is used in this text with the circle of least confusion on the retina—the principal foci of the astigmatic eye are equally defocused, one meridian lying behind the retina, and the other an equal (dioptric) distance in front of the retina. When the eye is in this state, the cross cylinder always leaves the circle of least confusion on the retina, no matter what its power or how its axes are disposed.

The concept of the circle of least confusion is an optical one rather than a visual one. When any other part of the image space is considered, one meridian is always more blurred than the other, but between the principal foci the total area of the blur is actually maximum at the circle of least confusion. There are no sound physiological reasons for assuming that any special visual preference exists for the circle of least confusion, but the assumption is made in the absence of indications to the contrary.

The correct sphere

Before the cross cylinder is used, the spherical correction is manipulated. Initially, the BVS is determined using the letter chart. It is useful at this stage to note vision, because it provides a clue to the extent of the astigmatic error.

A further reduction in plus is usually required before the circle of least confusion is on the retina; this is because of the finite depth of focus of the eye for letter-type targets. It is difficult to estimate the depth of focus in the young because any accommodation will cause an overestimate. One solution to this problem is to add an arbitrary negative lens to the BVS; Borish (1970) suggested that the BVS should be modified by −0.25 D before commencing the cross-cylinder test. In moderate to high amounts of astigmatism, this will probably leave the circle of least confusion in front of the retina and a larger modification may be required.

Freeman suggested that the duochrome test should be used to determine the starting point for cross-cylinder analysis. The spherical power is modified so that targets on red and green backgrounds are equally distinct, at which point the circle of least confusion may be assumed to lie on the retina (Freeman, 1955). This approach works well in most cases, but difficulty is often encountered when best vision is 6/9 or worse with spheres. This may be due to the large amount of blur imposed by the ametropia in comparison with the chromatic difference in focus between the red and green targets.

Usually, an approximately correct sphere can be found by one method or the other. Cross-cylinder analysis is now started with an investigation of the axis of astigmatism. Because the astigmatism is nearly always corrected with negative cylinders during a refraction, it is the axis of the negative component of the cross cylinder that is considered. First, the cross cylinder is introduced with its axes along 90° and 180°. When the cross cylinder is twirled the axes are transposed, so that if the negative axis was initially along 90°, twirling places it along 180°.

The patient views a target with the cross cylinder in the two positions, and indicates whether the first or second position gives the clearer view. The preferred orientation of the negative axis is noted. The cross cylinder is now rotated so that its axes lie along 45° and 135°, and the process is repeated.

If the correct axis for the negative cylindrical correction is 70°, in the first presentation of cross cylinder (with axes vertical and horizontal), the vertical orientation of the negative cross-cylinder axis is preferred to the horizontal, because it is closer to the correct axis. Similarly, with the 135°/45° presentation, the negative axis is preferred along 45°. It may be deduced that the correct axis lies between 45° and 90° and, if a negative cylinder is placed midway in the preferred quadrant, it should be within 22° of the correct axis. In the above example a −0.25 DC, axis 67° is introduced which is called the working cylinder.

Refinement of axis position

With the working cylinder in place, the cross cylinder is always positioned with reference to the working axis, in this case 67°. To refine the axis, the cross cylinder is located with its axes 45° on either side of the working axis. In this position, the handle of the cross cylinder lies along the working axis (or at 90° to it) which serves as the easiest way to position it. As before, the patient views a target while the two positions of the cross cylinder are presented, and indicates which position gives the better view.

In both positions of the cross cylinder, its negative axis is at 45° to the working cylinder; the resultant combination of the working cylinder and the cross cylinder has the same power in the two positions, but the axis of the resultant changes. The axis of the resultant (negative) cylinder always lies between the axes of its negative components. When the working axis is 67°, the cross cylinder axes lie along 112° and 22°. When the negative cross cylinder axis is along 112°, the resultnat axis lies between 112° and 67°; in the other position it lies between 22° and 67°. The position preferred by the subject indicates whether the correct axis lies between 112° and 67° or between 67° and 22°; in the example where the correct axis is 70°, the first position is preferred. This indicates that the working cylinder should be rotated twoards the preferred position of the cross-cylinder negative axis.

There is no indication of how much to change the axis of the working cylinder from the response of the subject. It is usual to use 10° steps until the correct axis is past, and then to use smaller steps employing a bracketing method (*see* Chapter 4). In the example the working axis is altered to 75–80°, the cross cylinder adjusted accordingly, and the two positions are again offered. (With a working axis of 80°, the cross-cylinder axes will be 35° and 125°) This time the 35° position of the negative axis is preferred to the 125° position, indicating that the correct axis has been passed; thus the axis may be refined to the limit, where no difference between the positions is detected, the twirl of the cross cylinder merely placing the resultant axis equally incorrectly on each side of the correct axis (*Figure 8.20*).

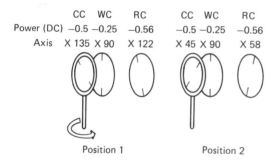

	CC	WC	RC	CC	WC	RC
Power (DC)	−0.5	−0.25	−0.56	−0.5	−0.25	−0.56
Axis	X 135	X 90	X 122	X 45	X 90	X 58

Position 1   Position 2

Figure 8.20 Axis determination with the cross cylinder. In position 1 the working cylinder is −0.25 DC axis 90° (WC). The cross cylinder (CC) has a total cylinder power of −0.50 DC axis 135°. The resultant cylinder is −0.56 DC axis 122° (RC). In position 2 the working cylinder is unchanged, the cross cylinder is now −0.50 DC axis 45°, and the resultant cylinder is −0.56 DC axis 58°. Whichever resultant is nearer the correct axis is preferred

Cylinder power

Once the correct axis has been located, the power of the correcting cylinder is determined. The cross cylinder is rotated so that the handle lies at 45° to the working cylinder axis. The two cross-cylinder positions now place either the plus cylinder or the minus cylinder axis along the working cylinder axis. If the plus cylinder gives better vision than the minus cylinder, then the power of the working cylinder is too great, but the minus cross cylinder is preferred, then the working cylinder undercorrects the astigmatism. The power of the working cylinder is adjusted appropriately.

To keep the circle of least confusion on the retina, the sphere power must be changed when the working cylinder power is changed. For each −0.5 D increase in the working cylinder, +0.25 D must be added to the sphere. This rule may only be applied where the initial sphere was accurately determined; where the cylinder power is 1.00 D or greater it is good practice to check the sphere at intervals using the duochrome or letter chart (*Figures 8.21–8.23*).

Time may be saved, and considerable repetition avoided, by changing the cylinder power in the correct step. This may be calculated from the initial estimate of astigmatism. As a general rule, the initial step should be about half the estimated amount of astigmatism deduced from vision with the BVS. When the cross cylinder shows that the working cylinder power exceeds the correction, the step size may be reduced, and power is eventually refined to 0.25 D.

Targets used with the cross cylinder

With the circle of least confusion on the retina, the cross-cylinder aims to influence the size of the retinal blur circle while its shape remains unchanged. In principle, any test which is constructed for the detection of blur may be used here. However, the cross-cylinder test has certain deficiencies which may alter the suitability of some targets under particular circumstances.

The test alters the magnification of the retinal image as well as the blur circle size. When the cross cylinder is twirled from one position to the other, the shape factor is changed from being greater than unity to less than unity. In addition, the meridional magnification due to the cylinder will change, giving a 'scissors' rotation.

In addition, the cross-cylinder test requires the circle of least confusion to be on the retina. When this condition is not met, the shape of the retinal blur circle changes, as well as its size.

These deficiencies do not invalidate the test, but make it more complex; judgements of clarity may be coloured by the distortions of the test as well as by the blur circle size. The optical distortions may be minimized by optimizing the cross cylinder (Haynes, 1957), but such lenses are not in commercial production at present. The aim must be to minimize distortion by other means. One precaution is to use the lowest power cross cylinder, other factors being equal. The influence of the visual target on the effect of the distortions and blur circle shapes must be considered.

Four target configurations will be considered here, although others may be as useful. The four configurations are: letter charts, ring shapes, a cross and dots.

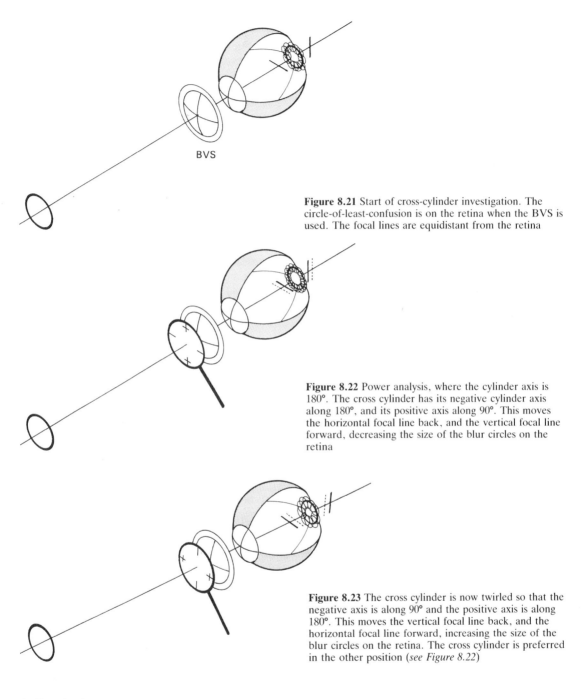

Figure 8.21 Start of cross-cylinder investigation. The circle-of-least-confusion is on the retina when the BVS is used. The focal lines are equidistant from the retina

Figure 8.22 Power analysis, where the cylinder axis is 180°. The cross cylinder has its negative cylinder axis along 180°, and its positive axis along 90°. This moves the horizontal focal line back, and the vertical focal line forward, decreasing the size of the blur circles on the retina

Figure 8.23 The cross cylinder is now twirled so that the negative axis is along 90° and the positive axis is along 180°. This moves the vertical focal line back, and the horizontal focal line forward, increasing the size of the blur circles on the retina. The cross cylinder is preferred in the other position (*see Figure 8.22*)

Letter charts

These are widely used in cross-cylinder analysis. A line above the smallest which can be read is viewed. The clarity of the line is assessed through the alternate positions of the cross cylinder. While the optical distortions of the cross cylinder will influence the appearance of the letters, they do not affect their legibility to any extent. People are generally familiar with many typefaces from italic through roman, with or without serifs etc. The essential quality of any letter remains unaltered and recognizable, and so the distortions are easily integrated into the percept of the subject. Subsidiary benefits of letter charts are the ease with which the benefit of one position over another may be verified from the patient's reading and the large range of target sizes available to cover a range of astigmatic blur.

There are two disadvantages in the use of letter charts. It takes slightly longer to scan a line of different letters and verify legibility than to perform a simpler visual task, and (more important) the chart may incorporate a bias towards one position of the focal lines over the other, in contradiction to the criterion for minimal astigmatism (Williamson-Noble, 1943). This generally only occurs when the circle of least confusion is not on the retina; here there may be a preferential bias to have the vertical focal line nearer the retina than any other configuration. In practice this usually produces the comment that some letters are clearer for one position of the cross cylinder while the second position shows other letters to be clearer; however, this cannot be relied upon as an indication to adjust the sphere, because often the sign is ignored by the subject.

Ring shapes

Freeman and Purdom (1950) considered the letter chart to be a confusing target in comparison to the Landolt C chart, which was the preferred presentation. This opinion was probably based on the legibility difference produced when the circle of least confusion is not on the retina, because no other contradiction has been shown to depend on the use of letter targets. In this case there can be no bias in preferred orientation with ring targets, because there is no preferential position for focal lines.

Some test charts include two pairs of rings for cross-cylinder analysis; these were originally designed for use with a septum in binocular refraction, so that each eye saw one pair of rings. The rings seen by each eye are arranged concentrically (Verhoeff rings).

While these targets may be less susceptible to misinterpretation when the sphere power is incorrect, any departure from a circular image is easily seen. In the author's experience, the problems due to distortion are more prominent with these targets than with letters, and outweigh the advantages. A further disadvantage of the circular targets is that it is more difficult to interpret clarity and blur; the targets should be used as acuity tests but it is hard to do this with short presentations. Where circular targets are to be used, the Landolt chart gives a greater range of sizes and so may be preferable.

Cross target

Haynes (1958) suggested that a target composed of an orthogonal pair of lines can be used to reduce problems of distortion. With these targets, patients distinguish changes in contrast; there is no acuity task, and the response may only be verified by repeating the presentation. Unless lines of different thicknesses are available, this test may also be insensitive for some astigmatic errors.

Dot targets

Dot targets are simple to construct and are found in many clinics including the London Refraction Hospital and the eye clinic at the University of New South Wales. They have the advantage of incorporating an acuity limitation due to the spacing of the dots, but otherwise they have the same advantages and limitations as a cross target.

Further notes on the use of letter charts

Cross-cylinder analysis gives a transiently distorted view of the letter chart, and so careful instruction of the visual task is important. Borish (1970) suggested that several lines should be read with the cross cylinder in one position, so that the smallest discernible letters are identified. The cross cylinder is changed to the second position, and the patient identifies whether he/she can read further down the chart with the first presentation or the second. Grosvenor (1982) found this technique to work well.

Inexperienced patients should be instructed at the start of the test that the cross cylinder will make the chart a little blurred and distorted; a common clinical approach is to ask which position is the worse (rather than the better) which seems to reassure people that the chart is supposed to be blurred.

The sensitivity of the cross-cylinder technique

The rationale of axis determination with the cross cylinder presented earlier considered the combination of the cross cylinder with the working cylinder. For the two positions of the cross cylinder (each at 45° to the working cylinder axis), the resultant cylinders were of the same power but of different axis. The resultant axis closer to the correct axis is preferred. This analysis provides a simple way of remembering how to manipulate the working axis; however, a more powerful analysis is available that reveals much about the sensitivity of cross-cylinder analysis. This has been investigated extensively by Carter (1966, 1981), and O'Leary (1985).

The eye does not look to see which axis of the resultant cylinder is closer to the correct axis; the blur seen by the eye results from the combination of three cylinders at oblique axes. These components are the cross cylinder, the working cylinder and the ocular astigmatism. It is the size of the resultant of

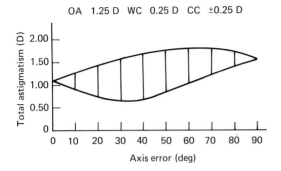

OA 1.25 D WC 0.25 D CC ±0.25 D

Figure 8.24 The total resultant cylinder in the two positions of the cross cylinder (CC) when the working cylinder (WC) is off-axis (OA) by different amounts. In this example, the ocular astigmatism is 1.25 D, the working cylinder power is 0.25 D, and the cross cylinder is a ±0.25 D cross cylinder (total astigmatic power of cross cylinder 0.50 D). The top line shows the resultant cylinder in the worse position, and the bottom line the resultant cylinder in the better position. The vertical separation of the two lines at any axis error is the difference in blur between the two positions

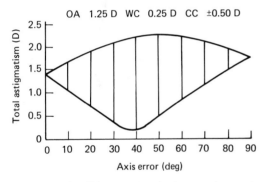

OA 1.25 D WC 0.25 D CC ±0.50 D

Figure 8.25 Conditions are exactly the same here as in *Figure 8.24*, except the size of the cross cylinder has been increased to ±0.50 D (total astigmatic power of cross cylinder 1.00 D). Note that the difference between the two positions (top line − bottom line) is greater in this case than in the previous figure, indicating a bigger difference in blur

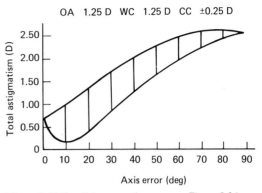

OA 1.25 D WC 1.25 D CC ±0.25 D

Figure 8.26 Conditions are the same as *Figure 8.24*, except the working cylinder is now 1.25 D. Note that the separation of the two positions (top line − bottom line) is greater than in *Figure 8.24* for small axis errors

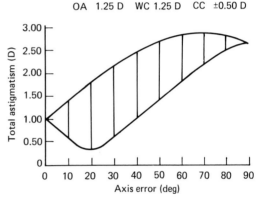

OA 1.25 D WC 1.25 D CC ±0.50 D

Figure 8.27 The working cylinder is 1.25 D, and the cross cylinder is ±0.50 D (total astigmatic power of cross cylinder is 1.00 D). Note that for axis errors greater than 25°, the differences between the two positions (top line − bottom line) is less than in *Figure 8.25*, where the same cross cylinder was used with a smaller working cylinder (WC). For small axis errors, the differences between the two positions are similar to those in *Figure 8.26* where the working cylinder power was the same; however, the overall level of blur is less in *Figure 8.26* than in *Figure 8.27*

these three components that determines the amount of blur seen by the eye. When the cross cylinder is presented in the two positions, the size of the overall resultant is less in one position than in the other, and it is this difference which allows one position to appear clearer than the other.

For any one eye the ocular astigmatism is fixed; however, the working cylinder may be of any power, and the working axis may differ by any amount from the correct axis. In addition, different cross-cylinder powers may be used. The axis of the cross cylinder is determined by the working axis; the two positions are 45° on either side of the working axis.

Whatever the combination of working cylinder power and axis all cross cylinders produce a total resultant cylinder (ocular astigmatism + working cylinder + cross cylinder) of lower power when the negative cylinder axis is closer to the correct axis. However the difference in power between the two cross-cylinder positions varies greatly with the conditions of the test.

If an eye with 1.25 D astigmatism were considered, then in the early stages of the investigation, a working cylinder of −0.25 D may be used with different cross cylinders. *Figures 8.24* and *8.25* show the total resultant astigmatism for different axis errors of the working cylinder. For large axis errors, the larger cross cylinder gives appreciably bigger differences between the two positions than the smaller cross cylinder. The ideal cross cylinder to use here is one whose power is equal to, or slightly less than, the ocular astigmatism.

After the approximate axis of the cylinder is found, and the power determined, the axis is further refined. The effect of the different cross cylinder is shown in *Figures 8.26* and *8.27*. When the axis error is small, the smaller cross cylinder gives the same power difference between the two positions, but the overall level of blur is less. It should be noted that the power differences when the axis error is large are not so great as in the previous examples.

These considerations lead to the following conclusions:

(1) When the cylinder axis is unknown, the power of the cross cylinder should be equal to or slightly less than the estimated astigmatic error.
(2) The axis should be refined using a +0.25 D cross cylinder after the power has been determined.
(3) With small amounts of astigmatism where the axis is difficult to determine with a −0.25 D working cylinder, it is better to leave out the working cylinder altogether. The cross-cylinder should be no greater than ± 0.25 D.
(4) With large astigmatic errors, when the axis location is suspected e.g. from retinoscopy) confusing answers may be given using a small cross cylinder. In this case, it is best to reduce the power of the working cylinder and increase the cross-cylinder power in line with (1).

Effect of excess cross-cylinder power

It may be noted that, for small axis errors, the power differences offered by a cross cylinder, in its two positions does not vary much with the power. However the absolute amount of blur does depend on cross-cylinder power, and so the 'better' position of the cross cylinder becomes increasingly defocused as the power is increased. If defocus were the only determinant of cross-cylinder sensitivity, this would not make any difference to the ability to discriminate between the two positions; it would be as easy to see the difference produce by the large cross cylinder as that produced by the small cross cylinder. When the distortion introduced by the large cross cylinder is considered, it must be more difficult to discern the change in blur when it is accompanied by the distortional effects than when these are minimized. As a general rule for selecting cross-cylinder power, this means the lower power should be preferred to minimize distortion.

Special considerations in correcting astigmatism

It is sometimes found that the fogging technique for estimating astigmatism gives results at variance with the cross cylinder—either may differ from retinoscopy results. Some of these differences may be accounted for as resulting from technical differences between the tests, and it is possible that some people may find one or other subjective method easier to understand (Borish, 1970). However, the possibility should also be considered that the eye is suffering from meridional bias. There are two examples of this: Freeman, Mitchell and Millodot (1972) have shown that some people with large astigmatic errors show a difference in resolving power between the principal meridians termed 'meridional amblyopia', a form of ametropic amblyopia; Freeman (1975) has also demonstrated that this type of amblyopia produces a marked accommodative preference for the clearer meridian.

When the fogging technique is used, meridional amblyopia may cause incorrect equalization. In the myopic eye the anterior focal line may be amblyopic. After fogging, the anterior focal line must be closer to the retina than the posterior focal line to equalize the T chart or blocks, and so astigmatism may be overestimated. The reverse applies to the hypermetropic case. Of course, in either case it may not be possible to equalize the chart.

It is less simple to predict the behaviour with the cross cylinder; however, uncorrected astigmats often reject cylinder with this test (Grosvenor, 1982). Since visual preferences seem to be controlled by the non-amblyopic meridian, it may be assumed that this meridian lies closer to the retina when the BVS is found. If the normal cross-cylinder procedure is employed — the sphere being adjusted by +0.12 D for each increase of −0.25 D in the working cylinder — then the better focal line will be moved to the inappropriate side of the retina before the cylinder is correct. Take for example an eye requiring a correction of ±1.50 DC: the best vision sphere may be incorrectly assessed as −0.25 D, and even here the eye may accommodate to bring the posterior focal line closer to the retina (Freeman, 1975). When the cylinder is adjusted to −0.75 D, the sphere will be +0.12 D. In this situation the cross-cylinder position which places the posterior focal line closer to the retina, while being worse on blur circle considerations, may give better vision, leading to rejection of cylinder.

Arriving at an appropriate cylindrical correction is rather difficult in these cases. Where the retinoscopy results are rejected with the cross cylinder, then the fogging technique may give more reliable results. It may also be appropriate in these cases to consider overcorrecting the subjective cylinder slightly if all considerations indicate that meridional amblyopia is unduly influencing the subjective tests, and the retinoscopy cylinder can be repeatedly verified.

Refining the sphere

There is generally a range of lenses compatible with maximum acuity, due to the depth of focus of the eye. The size of the range depends on the maximum acuity reached, and on the pupil size (Tucker and Charman, 1975). With small pupils and poor acuity the range of lenses may be several dioptres.

Although any lens within this range gives the same resolving power, contrast is not constant. It can be assumed that there is a unique value for the correction which gives maximum contrast. (Where accommodation is active, maximum contrast may be maintained through several lenses; in this case the most positive lens that gives maximum contrast corresponds to the optimum correction.)

Where the range is small (less than 0.50 D), the optimum correction is the lens that gives maximum resolution. A change of 0.25 D in either direction will cause a measurable decrement in the number of letters read. In other cases, this criterion cannot be applied. Here the judgement must be one of relative contrast or, in clinical terms, sharpness and blackness.

As Denieul (1982) pointed out, it is more sensitive to probe the effects of defocus than to try to locate the optimum focus directly: the following routine is used by the author.

First vision is fogged slightly, and then plus is reduced to find the lowest line that can be read. The first lens that gives this resolving power is kept in place. Freeman twirl spheres are now used.

The plus sphere is shown first, and time is allowed for the blur to be assessed. Generally 2 or 3 seconds is sufficient. Next the twirls are flipped so that the minus lens is shown; the sphere is adjusted in the direction giving the clearer view, and the process repeated.

With non-presbyopes, care must be taken to avoid accommodation influencing the results. If the minus lens is left up too long, the eye may adjust to the second presentation. Since the reaction time of accommodation is slightly less than 0.5 s (Campbell and Westheimer, 1960), it is sometimes necessary to keep the minus presentation brief. To compensate for this, two or three presentations of the alternative views may be required. In addition advice that the second presentation must be kept short, but further views still shown, does much to help avoid the impression that the answer is being hurried.

Although the Freeman twirl spheres are convenient to use, they are not essential. The spherical power can be increased by +0.25 D, and a −0.50 D trial case lens can be used to give the second presentation.

In some cases the depth of focus of the eye is so large that the ± 0.25 D twirls are of no use. A ± 0.50 D twirl — or sometimes higher — is then used.

The duochrome test

With the duochrome the sphere is adjusted until the characters on the red and green are equalized. Where the characters are letters of different sizes the task depends on differences in acuity. Often only one character is available on each colour; in this case the contrast between the red and green sides is compared. O'Connor Davies (1957) compared the duochrome end-point with the sphere which gave maximum acuity on the letter chart. In most cases the characters on the red side were seen more clearly when the optimum lens for the letter chart was used; in over 76% of all subjects, a−0.25 DS produced either equality of the characters on the red and green, or made the green clearer than the red (*Figure 8.28*).

Jennings and Charman (1973) compared the correction found with the duochrome and the correction found with the letter chart using a ±0.25 D defocus (Simultan test). The two tests gave statistically indistinguishable results; the standard deviations were also similar (mean s.d. 0.20 D for the duochrome, 0.24 D for the Simultan test).

The duochrome and the letter chart give different information; the letter chart indicates the extent to which the eye is defocused, but the duochrome

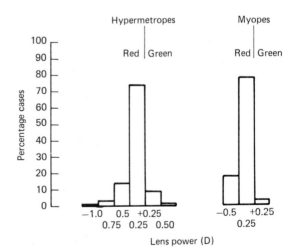

Figure 8.28 The duochrome preference of hypermetropes and myopes when the correct sphere (determined with a letter chart) is used. Beneath each bar is the lens power required to either equalize or reverse the duochrome. The height of the bar indicates the relative incidence

indicates the direction of defocus. It is sensible to use the two in conjunction rather than relying entirely on one or the other. However, when the sphere is checked during the cross-cylinder test the rapidity of the duochrome check offers a significant advantage.

The construction of duochrome tests is not standardized, and so the peak wavelengths transmitted by the red and green filters may vary from test to test, giving different dioptric intervals (Mandell and Allen, 1960). The relative brightness of the red and green also affects the reliability of the test (Murrell, 1955). These factors may make individual tests unreliable if the dioptric interval is too small or if one colour is very much brighter than the other. The dioptric interval decreases with age, because the chromatic aberration of the eye reduces quite markedly over the age of about 55 years (Millodot, 1976), and when the pupil is small the difference in blur circle size is further reduced. In these cases, the duochrome test gives results inconsistent with letter chart acuity — often it is difficult or impossible to obtain red and green equality — and here the duochrome results must be ignored.

Laser refraction

If the eye views a diffuse patch illuminated by a laser, a diffraction pattern is formed on the retina. The patch of laser light has a speckled appearance. If the diffusing surface is moved, the speckle pattern also moves in a direction depending on the refractive state of the eye. In hypermetropia, the speckles move in the same direction as the surface, while in myopia an 'against' movement is seen. Emmetropes may see a swirling pattern in which there is no preferred direction of movement.

Knoll (1966) suggested that the refraction could be determined using the speckle pattern, and several studies have applied the technique (Baldwin and Stover, 1968; Dwyer *et al.*, 1972; Jennings and Charman, 1973; see Whitefoot and Charman, 1980 for a review.) Generally the laser is shone onto a slowly moving drum, and the orientation of the drum is changed to refract different meridians.

In astigmatism, the movement of the speckle pattern is oblique unless the drum is rotating along one of the principal meridians. In determining the refraction of the principal meridians, any change in accommodation will give an error in cylinder power. This may be overcome by using two drums with their axes at right angles so that the neutrality of the principal meridians can be verified simultaneously (Whitefoot and Charman, 1980).

Laser refraction gives slightly more hypermetropic results than conventional techniques due to the chromatic aberration of the eye (Knoll, 1966).

When repeated measurements are made with this technique, the standard deviation is found to be about 0.3 D (Dwyer *et al.*, 1972; Jennings and Charman, 1973). However, while the spherical portion of the correction determined with the laser agrees well with other methods (correlation coefficient, $r = 0.988$) the cylindrical correction agrees less well ($r = 0.853$) which may reflect a disadvantage of meridional refraction over direct estimation of astigmatism (Whitefoot and Charman, 1980).

The laser technique offers several advantages over other methods: it indicates the direction of ametropia, including astigmatism; it can be used when the eye is so defocused that the letters on the test chart cannot be used — the speckle pattern is seen independent of the state of focus of the eye; it also depends on the detection of movement rather than changes in resolution; and it can be used in low illumination where other techniques may fail.

The disadvantages of the test include the fact that the equipment is cumbersome at present. In addition, although the direction of ametropia is indicated the amount of ametropia is not, and cylinder accuracy seems to be worse than with other methods — for example, the cross-cylinder test. These disadvantages suggest that the laser technique should be used in conjunction with other tests, such as the letter chart and cross cylinder. Its advantages in high ametropia, and when low illumination is indicated, are not offered by any other subjective method.

Further considerations of the sphere

Test distance

A correction which is ideal for 6 m (0.17 D) may require modification for general distance vision. In young people, duochrome equality at 6 m seems to give an adequate general correction. Presumably their accommodation is correctly adjusted for 6 m during the test and can relax slightly for more distant viewing. With presbyopes this is not the case, and the correct sphere for 6 m will be too positive. In deciding whether to modify the correction to account for this, there is much to recommend a conservative approach, taking into account the previous correction, symptoms and occupational needs. Thus if the previous correction overplussed for distance viewing, and in the absence of symptoms, there seems little point in reducing the test results to give better distance vision at the expense of intermediate vision. In other cases — for example where distance vision was previously underplussed — the test results may be modified.

Spatial frequency

An optical system only has a single correct focus when it is free of aberrations. In the presence of spherical aberration, the optimum focus depends on spatial frequency, and so the correct focus for fine (high frequency) targets will give reduced contrast for coarse (low frequency) targets (Green and Campbell, 1965; Charman, Jennings and Whitefoot, 1978) (*Figure 8.29*). In the normal young eye, the loss of contrast in coarse targets is not severe in relation to the overall performance. However, in eyes suffering from abnormal aberrations — for example in keratoconus, corneal scarring or lens pathology — the loss may be more important. Such

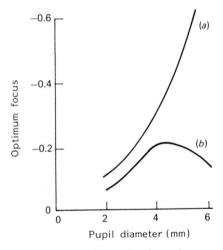

Figure 8.29 Dependence of optimum focus on spatial frequency for an eye with typical amounts of spherical aberration. (*a*) 5 cycles/deg; (*b*) 30 cycles/deg. (After Charman, Jennings and Whitefoot, 1978)

cases may complain that their correction does not give clear vision in general use, even where it gives optimum performance on the letter chart. In these cases it is foolish to insist that the letter chart is the only determinant of clear vision, and the refraction may have to be evaluated in the conditions where the correction is unsatisfactory.

Night myopia

In low illumination, the eye becomes relatively myopic due to several factors. Since fine detail is not visible under these conditions, and the pupil is dilated, the eye must be corrected for low spatial frequencies (Green and Campbell, 1965). In addition the eye accommodates by any amount up to 4 D, depending on the individual (Leibowitz and Owens, 1975). Refraction under low illumination

may be attempted (Richards, 1967), but this is a difficult procedure if conventional techniques are used. Owens and Leibowitz (1976) suggested that the refraction could easily be performed with a laser optometer as the target. They investigated the performance of subjects under simulated night driving conditions using (*a*) the normal correction, (*b*) the correction required in total darkness and (*c*) a correction midway between (*a*) and (*b*), and found that correction (*c*) was optimum in most cases. In a field experiment where nine subjects were given the three corrections to evaluate while driving at night, eight selected correction (*c*) while the ninth subject had only a small difference between the three corrections.

Meridional refraction

Conventional techniques of determining the correction for astigmatism utilize spherical and cylindrical lenses to neutralize the eye's refractive error. In meridional refraction, only spheres need be used and only one meridian is considered at a single determination. The final correction is formulated from the results of two or more meridians.

The stenopaic slit

At its simplest, meridional refraction is performed along two orthogonal meridians. These are isolated with a slit of width about 0.75 mm and length about 15 mm. In the meridian at right angles to the slit, the effect is similar to a pinhole; varying the lens in front of the eye has only a small effect on vision. Along the slit, the aperture of the eye is normal and varying the lens power will alter vision.

The stenopaic slit is placed in front of the eye after the best vision sphere has been determined in the usual way. If a refractor head is used, the slit should be located on the auxiliary cylinder holder. A two-step refraction is then performed (Long, 1975). First the eye is fogged, and the patient watches an acuity chart. As the slit is rotated vision may vary, indicating the presence of astigmatism. The slit orientation for maximum acuity is found (this orientation is the required axis of the minus cylinder).

Next the fog is reduced until vision no longer improves; the maximum acceptable sphere is the spherical part of the correction.

The slit is rotated through 90°, which reduces vision. The fog is again reduced until acuity no longer improves. The difference in the best spheres for the two positions of the slit gives the cylindrical portion of the correction.

During this procedure, Long (1975) recommends that 0.5 D steps should be used because smaller steps are not noticed; additionally, acuity should not be expected to reach the same level as without the slit. During the test a separate standard for best acuity is found. The accuracy of the technique is greater for axis than for power.

Applications

Stenopaic slit refraction may be considered when conventional methods fail. The principal causes of failure in which this technique may offer advantages are high ametropia, and confused responses.

In high ametropia, the slit may be used instead of a pinhole so that at least part of the chart is read; it offers the advantage of differentiating between an astigmatic error and spherical ametropia, and between an astigmatic error and a pathological condition. High astigmatic errors are among the more difficult to detect, and meridional refraction provides a simple way of checking for astigmatism. Even where an error of 1.00 D is present, the method is useful where people do not understand other astigmatic tests.

Borish (1970) suggested that the two meridians investigated may not be at right angles if the astigmatism were irregular. In these cases, the resultant refraction may be computed from the theory of obliquely crossed cylinders. Long (1974a) noted that there was an infinite number of spherocylinders that could produce any one combination of oblique refractions; he suggested that the resultant with the minimum cylindrical component should be taken as the spherocylindrical correction.

Multimeridional refraction

Rather than locating the principal meridian of an eye, and then refracting it, it is possible to investigate the eye along preselected meridians (Bennett, 1960). At these oblique positions the eye does not have foci, and so it is not possible to find a power for each meridian investigated. Bennett suggested that the prismatic effect along any meridian could be determined, however, and three such determinations (say along 180°, 45° and 90°) allowed the sphere power, cylinder power and axis to be determined. Reinecke *et al.* (1972) performed 'refractions' along three such meridians, isolated by a stenopaic slit.

Laser optometers may be used to evaluate the performance of oblique meridians (Phillips, Sterling and Dwyer, 1975). When the optometer drum rotates at any angle away from the principal meridians, the speckle pattern moves along some other direction. Long and Haine (1975) analysed the motion of the speckle pattern for oblique rotations of the drum. As the sphere is adjusted, the direction of movement of the speckle changes. For one lens,

the speckle pattern moves along the axis of the drum (at right angles to the rotation of the drum). This sphere corresponds to the notional ametropia of the meridian at right angles to the drum axis.

Once a number of meridians have been investigated, and the notional powers found, the spherocylindrical correction may be computed. Long (1974b) produced a complex computational routine that allowed the correction to be found from the notional powers of a number of arbitrarily selected meridians; in practice this requires a computer. Worthey (1977) has simplified the calculation by only considering evenly spaced meridians.

Accuracy of multimeridional refraction

The analysis of meridional data consists of finding the best fit of the general expression for notional meridional power. This is of necessity an approximation because data are accurate to only about 0.25 D. The inaccuracy of an individual datum can be compensated for by measuring more meridians.

Practical assessments of laser multimeridional refraction (Haine, Long and Reading, 1976; Whitefoot and Charman, 1980) suggest that the technique gives results of comparable accuracy to conventional subjective methods, provided that six meridians are considered. Even then, if the error cross cylinder is considered, the error in the Whitefoot and Charman study is greater than 0.25 D in nearly 50% of cases.

Where a laser optometer is not available, multimeridional measurements may be made using the stenopaic slit. The orientations at which the slit will be placed should be decided in advance; they should be evenly spaced to allow calculations by Worthey's method. Either letter charts or line targets may be used, the line targets being orientated at 90° to the slit (if the 'blocks' or T chart are used, the lines parallel to the slit act as the in-focus comparison target). The eye is fogged, and the blur reduced for clearest vision.

Binocular balancing

Since the level of accommodation may fluctuate during the monocular refraction, a final check is made to ensure that the correction refers to the same level of accommodation in the two eyes. The procedure was popularized by Turville, who named the technique infinity balancing (Turville, 1951).

The Turville Infinity Balance (TIB) technique is used with an indirect chart, viewed through a mirror. A small area of the mirror is covered by an occluding strip 3 cm wide (the septum). This ensures

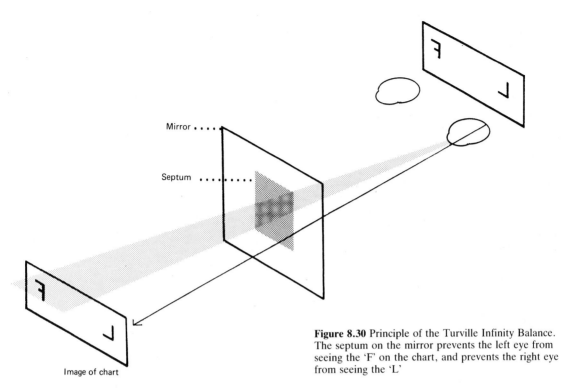

Figure 8.30 Principle of the Turville Infinity Balance. The septum on the mirror prevents the left eye from seeing the 'F' on the chart, and prevents the right eye from seeing the 'L'

that a small area of the chart, 6 cm wide, is blocked off from each eye. Within this area, the other eye can see the chart. Targets within the occluded areas are seen monocularly, allowing the refraction of each eye to be checked under quasibinocular conditions. The targets may consist of small letters, or duochrome tests (*Figure 8.30*).

Other techniques of separating the targets seen by the two eyes include prism dissociation and cross polarization. With prism dissociation, a small vertical prism is placed before each eye so that targets are seen in diplopia. The room is usually darkened to minimize rivalry from the surrounds. Horizontal prisms may be used; however, the separation achieved must be greater to exceed the fusional reserves, and this is a disadvantage. The target is usually a horizontal line of letters, although duochrome targets may also be used. In both these cases, ambient conditions are hardly binocular.

Several slightly different methods are available to dissociate the two eyes using polarizing filters. The major variant is whether the target itself or the background is polarized. In either case the two eyes view through crossed polarizers so that each sees only part of the target (Borish, 1970).

The eyes may also be equalized using successive viewing. Each eye in turn is occluded while the other looks at the targets, and then the occluder is removed keeping the sequence of occlusion the same (e.g. R, L, remove occluder) for a repeat of the presentation.

Methods

Duochrome targets

The correction is adjusted for the same end-point in the two eyes. Where one side of the duochrome is preferred, the targets on the other colour should be equally blurred to the two eyes, and the same sphere added to each eye should equalize or reverse the duochrome.

Letter targets

The eyes are fogged by equal plus spheres, and the clarity of the letters seen by each eye is compared. If one eye sees clearer than the other, the fog is increased on that side until vision is equalized. The fog is then reduced by 0.25-D steps binocularly, and vision is checked at each stage to ensure that equality is maintained.

Flom and Goodwin (1964) found that asymmetries between the two eyes in aberrations, fixation accuracy, or neural response could all give rise to an inequality of the perceived blur even where the initial spheres were correct. Equalizing the eyes under fog does not, therefore, necessarily equalize the accommodation. Goodwin suggested that the fog should be kept to a minimum; initially the two eyes should be blurred by 0.25–0.50 D. If acuities were unequal, a +0.25 DS is added to the better eye. If this fails to equalize the acuity it is removed. Now a −0.25 DS or, if necessary, a −0.50 DS is added to the worse eye. If the acuities cannot be equalized, then the monocular findings are probably in error (Goodwin, 1966).

While these criticisms must be kept in mind, blurring is a very sensitive method of detecting small differences in defocus. The author employs Humphriss' method of refraction (*see* Chapter 9 for detailed explanation), where the eye not under test is fogged with a +0.75 DS. At the end of the refraction a +0.75 DS is added to the eye under test, and the vision is checked for equality. Where acuity is unequal, the duochrome end-point is re-checked while the other eye is fogged. Thus the fogging procedure is used as a screening test rather than as the final arbiter of the sphere.

Gentsch and Goodwin (1966) compared several techniques for equalization with a haploscopic test (*Figure 8.31*). They found the Turville Infinity Balance gave the most consistent results, confirming earlier results from Morgan (1949). Surprisingly, they found the duochrome to be a relatively poor test, however, as Goodwin (1966) noted this might well be a reflection of the test conditions. Other studies of the duochrome have shown it to have a similar sensitivity to other subjective techniques (Jennings and Charman, 1973), and earlier comments on its reliability are relevant here.

The precision of subjective refraction

Power determination

When a measurement is repeated a number of times, the standard deviation of the measurements provides an index of the sensitivity of the method. This analysis could be applied to refractive data if the eye under consideration had remained optically unchanged during the tests. In other cases, it is possible that fluctuations in the refraction contribute to the variance of the measurements.

Humphriss (1958) selected 132 subjects on the basis of the consistency and exactness of their responses during refraction. A second refraction was performed between 1 and 90 days after the first, and the results of the two were compared. In 78% of eyes a change in the correction was found. Analysing the data as differences in mean sphere and cross cylinder, the standard deviation of the spherical determination was 0.254 D, and of the cylinder 0.214 D. If only presbyopes were considered, the standard deviation of the sphere would be 0.208 D (88 eyes), while for pre-presbyopes the standard deviation would be 0.275 D. It may be assumed that the difference between the two groups can be accounted for on the basis of more active accommodation in the latter group; where the optical state of the eye is more constant, precision appears to be improved. Humphriss used the duochrome to determine the sphere, and crossed cylinders to measure the astigmatism. The Turville Infinity Balance technique was used throughout.

Jennings and Charman (1973) used duochrome, Simultan test and laser refraction on eight subjects. The overall standard deviation of the techniques was 0.32 D, and there was no significant difference in the precision of the tests. Refractions were all carried out monocularly. There was considerable intersubject variation in the standard deviations (the range was from 0.06 D to 0.63 D) and older subjects tended to be more precise.

Perrigin, Perrigin and Grosvenor (1982) each refracted 32 young subjects using carefully defined techniques and end-points. Their results are compared in *Table 8.2*.

The results for anisometropia and cylinder power are very similar, indicating that the less concordant

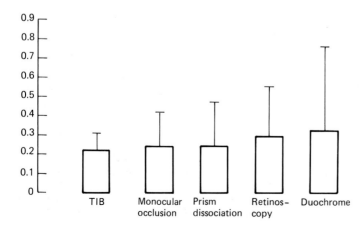

Figure 8.31 The mean difference between binocular balancing using different clinical methods, and a laboratory haploscopic technique (reference methods – clinical method). The columns show the mean deviation of each technique from the reference, and the vertical bars equal one standard deviation

Table 8.2 Comparison of results of three optometrists

	No deviation (%)	Within ±0.25 D (%)	Within ±0.50 D (%)
Spherical equivalent	27	86	98
Cylinder power	51	93	99
Anisometropia	44	95	100

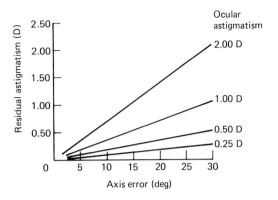

Figure 8.32 The residual astigmatism caused by off-axis error for different amounts of ocular astigmatism

results for spherical equivalent are possibly due to accommodative fluctuations. The standard deviations of the results are not given in this study but it may be deduced that for the sphere it must be less than 0.20 D, and even smaller for cylinder power.

It may be concluded from these studies that a change in cylinder power of 0.50 D or more is probably not due to experimental error, while a change of 0.25 D may be found if the refraction is repeated. More caution is required in assuming that a 0.50-D change in sphere power is not due to chance fluctuation, but it seems that in older people who are good observers, a 0.50-D change is probably significant.

In deciding whether a change in correction should be prescribed, other factors must be taken into account: the reliability of the observer may indicate that a 0.25 D change is easily appreciated, and the incidence of symptoms which can be explained by the change in refraction indicate that the correction should be updated. If spectacles are to be replaced in any case, the latest refraction is most likely to be correct, even though this is without great certainty.

Cylinder axis

Carter (1981) suggested that axis errors should be considered in terms of the residual astigmatism induced. If a value for what power change is significant can be assumed, then the axis error that gives this amount of residual astigmatism is also significant. *Figure 8.32* shows the residual astigmatism produced by axis errors. For example, a 10° axis error in a 1.00 DC gives a residual error of 0.17 D. The general formula is:

$$RA = 1.414A(1 - \cos 2\phi)^{-1/2}$$

where RA is the residual error, A is the correcting cylinder and ϕ is the axis error.

Generally, the cross cylinder allows the axis to be refined considerably more precisely than is needed from a consideration of residual error, and so axis errors are rarely a problem from this source. However it should be noted that there is little point in trying to achieve great accuracy in axis for small cylinders.

With larger cylinders there are two sources of problems: if the refractor head or trial frame is not levelled to the same reference as the correction, the axis error may be important, and the meridional magnification of the cylinder alters axis when the cylinder is changed, and in practice this may cause more problems than the residual error. As in all refractive procedures, it is best to determine the end-point as precisely as possible for the individual eye and then decide whether a change is warranted.

Acknowledgements

The author is grateful to Jan Lovie-Kitchin for supplying a copy of the Bailey–Lovie chart, and to Philip Anderton for supplying *Figure 8.2*.

References

BAILEY, I. L. and LOVIE, J. E. (1976) New design principles for visual acuity letter charts. *Am. J. Optom. Physiol. Opt.*, **53**, 740

BALDWIN, W. R. and STOVER, W. B. (1968) Observation of laser standing wave patterns to determine refractive status. *Am. J. Optom. Physiol. Opt.*, **45**, 143

BENNETT, A. G. (1960) Refraction by automation? New applications of the Scheiner disc. *Optician*, **139**, 5

BENNETT, A. G. (1965) Ophthalmic test types. *Br. J. Physiol. Opt.*, **22**, 238

BORISH, I. M. (1970) *Clinical Refraction*, 3rd edn, Chap. 19. Chicago: Professional Press

BS 4278 (1968) Specification for test charts for determining distance visual acuity. British Standards Institution, London

CAMPBELL, F. W. and GREEN, D. G. (1965) Optical and retinal factors affecting visual resolution. *J. Physiol*, **181**, 576

CAMPBELL, F. W. and WESTHEIMER, G. (1958) Sensitivity of the eye to differences in focus. *J. Physiol.*, **143**, 18P

CAMPBELL, F. W. and WESTHEIMER, G. (1960) Dynamics of accommodation response of the human eye. *J. Physiol.*, **151**, 285

CARTER, J. H. (1966) Sensitivity variations in the Jackson crossed cylinder axis test. *Optom. Weekly*, **57** (28), 29

CARTER, J. H. (1981) Some variations in methodology for crossed cylinder astigmatic tests. *Optom. Monthly*, **72** (2), 15

CHARMAN, W. N., JENNINGS, J. A. M. and WHITEFOOT, H. (1978) The refraction of the eye in relation to spherical aberration and pupil size. *Br. J. Physiol. Opt.*, **32**, 78

DENIEUL, P. (1982) Effects of stimulus vergence on mean accommodation response, microfluctuations of accommodation and optical quality of the human eye. *Vision Res.*, **22**, 561

DWYER, W. O., KENT, P., POWELL, J., McELVAIN, R. and REDMOND, J. (1972) Reliability of the laser refractive technique for different refractive groups. *Am. J. Optom. Physiol. Opt.*, **49**, 929

ENOCH, J. M. (1971) The need for standards in tests of vision. *Am. J. Ophthalmol.*, **72**, 836

ESKRIDGE, J. B. (1958) The Raubitschek astigmatism test. *Am. J. Optom. Physiol. Opt.*, **35**, 238

FLOM, M. C. and GOODWIN, H. C. (1964) Fogging lenses: differential acuity responses between the two eyes. *Am. J. Optom. Physiol. Opt.*, **41**, 388

FLOM, M. C., HEATH, G. G. and TAGAHASHI, E. (1963) Contour interaction and visual resolution: contralateral effects. *Science*, **142**, 979

FREEMAN, H. (1955) An analysis of the crossed cylinder method in determining the axis of an astigmatic correction. *Optician*, **130**, 393

FREEMAN, H. and PURDOM, G. (1950) An analysis of the crossed-cylinder. *Optician*, **120**, (3108), 375

FREEMAN, R. D. (1975) Asymmetries in human accommodation and visual experience. *Vision Res.*, **15**, 483

FREEMAN, R. D., MITCHELL, D. E. and MILLODOT, M. (1972) A neural effect of partial deprivation in humans. *Science*, **175**, 1384

GENTSCH, L. W. and GOODWIN, H. (1966) A comparison of methods for the determination of binocular refractive balance. *Am. J. Optom. Physiol. Opt.*, **43**, 658

GOODWIN, H. (1966) Optometric determination of balanced binocular refractive corrections. *Optom. Weekly*, **57** (28), 47

GREEN, D. G. and CAMPBELL, F. W. (1965) Effect of focus on the visual response to a sinusoidally modulated spatial stimulus. *J. Opt. Soc. Am.*, **55**, 1154

GROSVENOR, T. P. (1982) *Primary Care Optometry: A Clinical Manual*, Chap. 8. Chicago: Professional Press

HAINE, C. L., LONG, W. F. and READING, R. W. (1976) Laser meridional refractometry. *Am. J. Optom. Physiol. Opt.*, **53**, 194

HAYNES, P. R. (1957) A homokonic cross cylinder for refractive procedures. *Am. J. Optom. Physiol. Opt.*, **34**, 478

HAYNES, P. R. (1958) Configuration and orientation of test patterns used with the homokonic cross cylinder for the measurement of astigmatism. *Am. J. Optom. Physiol. Opt.*, **35**, 637

HEATH, G. G. (1956) The influence of visual acuity on accommodative responses of the eye. *Am. J. Optom. Physiol. Opt.*, **33**, 513

HEATH, G. G. (1958) cited in Borish (1970)

HUMPHRISS, D. (1958) Periodic refractive fluctuations in the healthy eye. *Br. J. Physiol. Opt.*, **15**, 30

JENNINGS, J. A. M. and CHARMAN, W. N. (1973) A comparison of errors in some methods of subjective refraction. *Ophthal. Opt.*, **13**, 8

KNOLL, H. A. (1966) Measuring ametropia with a gas laser. *Am. J. Optom. Physiol. Opt.*, **43**, 415

LEIBOWITZ, H. W. and OWENS, D. A. (1975) Anomalous myopias and the intermediate dark-focus of accommodation. *Science*, **189**, 646

LEVENE, J. R. (1977) *Clinical Refraction and Visual Science*, Chap. 2. London: Butterworths

LONG, W. F. (1974a) A mathematical appraisal of meridional refractometry. *Am. J. Optom. Physiol. Opt.*, **51**, 91

LONG, W. F. (1974b) A mathematical analysis of multimeridional refractometry. *Am. J. Optom. Physiol. Opt.*, **51**, 260

LONG, W. F. (1975) Stenopaic slit refraction. *Optom. Weekly*, **66**, 1063

LONG, W. F. (1981) The accuracy of multimeridional refraction. *Am. J. Optom. Physiol. Opt.*, **58**, 1161

LONG, W. F. and HAINE, C. L. (1975) The endpoint of laser speckle pattern meridional refraction. *Am. J. Optom. Physiol. Opt.*, **52**, 582

LUDVIGH, E. (1941) Effect of reduced contrast on visual acuity as determined with Snellen letters. *Arch. Ophthalmol.*, **25**, 472

MANDELL, R. B. and ALLEN, M. J. (1960) The causes of bichrome test failure. *J. Am. Optom. Assoc.*, **31**, 531

MILLODOT, M. (1976) The influence of age on the chromatic aberration of the eye. *von Graefe's Arch. klin. exp. Ophthalmol.*, **198**, 235

MILLODOT, M. and NEWTON, I. (1981) VEP measurement of the amplitude of accommodation. *Br. J. Ophthalmol.*, **65**, 294

MORGAN, M. W. (1949) The Turville infinity binocular balance test. *Am. J. Optom. Arch. Am. Acad. Optom.*, **26**, 231

MURRELL, S. C. (1955) An evaluation of the bichrome test. *N. Carol. Optom.*, July–Aug., cited in Borish (1970)

O'CONNER DAVIES, P. H. (1957) A critical analysis of bichromatic tests used in clinical refraction. *Br. J. Physiol. Opt.*, **14**, 170

O'LEARY, D. J. (1985) Analysis of the cross cylinder and chevron techniques for finding the axis of astigmatism. *Aust. J. Optom.*, **68**, 144

OWENS, D. A. and LEIBOWITZ, H. W. (1976) Night myopia: cause and a possible basis for amelioration. *Am. J. Optom. Physiol. Opt.*, **53**, 709

PASCAL, J. I. (1953) The Pascal–Raubitschek test for astigmatism. *J. Am. Optom. Assoc.*, **25**, 491

PERRIGIN, J., PERRIGIN, D. and GROSVENOR, T. (1982) A comparison of clinical refractive data obtained by three examiners. *Am. J. Optom. Physiol. Opt.*, **59**, 515

PETERS, H. B. (1961) The relationship between refractive

error and visual acuity at three age levels. *Am. J. Optom. Physiol. Opt.*, **38**, 194

PHILLIPS, D., STERLING, W. and DWYER, W. O. (1975) Validity of laser refractive technique for determining the cylindrical error. *Am. J. Optom. Physiol. Opt.*, **52**, 328

RAUBITSCHEK, E. (1928) Neue subjektive untersuchungs-methoden. *Klin. Monatsbl. Augenheilkd.*, **81**, 164

RAUBITSCHEK, E. (1958) The Raubitschek arrow test for astigmatism. *Am. J. Ophthalmol.*, **35**, 1334

REESE, E. E. and FRY, G. A. (1941) The effect of fogging lenses on visual acuity. *Am. J. Optom. Physiol. Opt.*, **18**, 9

REINECKE, R. D., CARROLL, J., BEYER, C. K. and MONTROSS, R. T. (1972) An innovation in eye care. *Sight Saving Rev.*, **42**, 35

RICHARDS, O. W. (1967) Night myopia at night automobile driving luminance. *Am. J. Optom. Physiol. Opt.*, **44**, 517

SHEARD, C. (1921) Some factors affecting visual acuity. *Am. J. Physiol. Opt.*, **2**, 168

SLOANE, L. L. (1951) Measurement of visual acuity. *Arch. Ophthalmol.*, **45**, 704

SMITH, R. (1738) *Compleat System of Opticks: Supplement; Essay on Distinct Vision.* Cambridge

SNELLEN, H. (1862) *Scala tipografica measurae il visus.* Utrecht

TUCKER, J. and CHARMAN, W. N. (1975) The depth of focus of the human eye for Snellen letters. *Am. J. Optom. Physiol. Opt.*, **52**, 3

TURVILLE, A. E. (1951) Some recent experiments on infinity balance. *Trans. Int. Opt. Congress*, British Optical Association, London, 299

WHITEFOOT, H. D. and CHARMAN, W. N. (1980) A comparison between laser and conventional subjective refraction. *Ophthal. Opt.*, **20**, 169

WILLIAMSON-NOBLE, F. A. (1943) A possible fallacy in the use of the cross cylinder. *Br. J. Ophthalmol.*, **27**, 1

WORTHEY, J. A. (1977) Simplified analysis of meridional refraction data. *Am. J. Optom. Physiol. Opt.*, **54**, 771

9

Binocular refraction

Deryck Humphriss

Binocular refraction techniques appear to have developed through a series of chance discoveries, and because of the development of polaroid filters and analysers. The Turville Infinity Balance method resulted from a chance observation of Turville's assistant optometrist, while the psychological septum was discovered during very academic research into the relation of personality difference to binocular performance (Humphriss, 1979). From these early researches, a number of binocular techniques have been developed which are commercially available today and it is these clinical procedures which will be considered in some detail. In all of these techniques binocular refraction is made possible by the elimination of a foveal or macular area of vision of one eye while retaining peripheral fusion. Hence, all vision is binocular except for the small central area. This is achieved by one of three methods: a small central occluder, a fogging lens or polaroid filters.

The first commercially produced system was that of Turville (1946) which is reviewed in Chapter 8.

British practitioners soon adapted the Turville method by using a strip of metal hung from the top of the mirror to act as a septum. Binocular refraction can also be effected by the blurring of one eye so that the visual impressions for the sharpness of the image are taken from the clearer eye (Humphriss, 1979). The method has the advantage that no special equipment is necessary. It can be undertaken with various levels of blurring, the minimum being the flipper technique of Calder Gillie (1957) in which the patient can recognize a state of better binocular acuity when small changes of plus and minus lenses are presented to one eye with the other eye open and unfogged.

The Humphriss immediate contrast (HIC) method of refraction requires fogging of one eye with a +0.75 or 1.00 DS, while the method of Cooper is carried out with fogging by a +2.00 DS. According to research on the stability of binocular vision with one eye blurred (Humphriss, 1979), this greater level of fogging would produce unstable binocular vision which tends to break down into diplopia.

The use of polaroid filters and analysers allows all the vision to be binocular except for targets which are monocular and seen by the eye being refracted. The eyes can be refracted separately with both open by separating the images vertically with a base-down prism, but this condition is not truly binocular being a state of simultaneous vision.

The advantages of binocular refraction

The objection to monocular refraction is that, when an occluder is placed before an eye, several changes take place which can affect the refraction significantly — variations which can be predicted as an outcome of the patient's change from binocular to monocular vision. The pupil enlarges and, if the cornea has any asymmetry, the refractive error may be altered; the accommodation–convergence relationship is destroyed, allowing the ciliary muscles to become active and the eyes to accommodate, and the eye behind the occluder is required to suppress over a wide area. If this eye happens to be strongly dominant, the attention of the patient to the chart seen by the non-dominant eye is difficult to maintain. In fact some patients may find they cannot do this and close the other eye.

In both normal and abnormal patients, there is an improved accuracy of observation in binocular vision. This can be observed clinically in most cases and may be very marked in nystagmus.

Conditions for binocular refraction

There is agreement, on the whole, among those who have researched the requirements for ideal binocular refraction about the conditions required. Grolman (1966), in his introduction to the use of the polarization and vectogram system of binocular refraction, suggested that a refraction technique which engages both eyes simultaneously provides a more realistic format for clinical investigation. Such a binocular test should enable the practitioner to observe and determine the performance of each eye as it actually contributes to the binocular act and the motor and sensory efficiency with which the two eyes function together. The demands of the test on the patient and the environment should minimally influence or derange the patient's normal binocular posture.

Cowan (1959), arguing in favour of a simplified clinical routine, indicated that a requirement of binocular vision refraction is that conditions correspond as nearly as possible to those in which the eyes are normally used. There must be a fusional lock and the testing procedure must be simple and accurate, using simultaneous comparisons of targets, allowing the test to be reversed within known limits, being repeatable and being confirmable by an alternative method. Cowan suggested that a foveal lock covering no more than 1° and capable of revealing fixation disparity is a fundamental requirement of binocular refraction.

The psychological septum

The existence of the psychological septum, i.e. the ability of one fovea to be inhibited in favour of the sharper image presented to the other, was first deduced and subsequently confirmed from a long programme of research which established that psychological rigidity exists in binocular vision; this varies with the personality of the subject and produces marked changes in binocular behaviour. The research which led to the deduction of the psychological septum and the subsequent steps taken to develop the Humphriss immediate contrast method of refraction are described by Humphriss (1984). This research demonstrated that:

(1) The positive fusional reserve is reduced very little by placing a +1.00 DS before one eye. If the sphere is increased to 1.50 DS, then binocular vision begins to collapse.
(2) The effect of the blurring by the sphere causes the central fovea to be inhibited so that, although there is binocular vision, all answers relating to the perception of edge sharpness are removed from the unfogged eye.

(3) It was subsequently demonstrated that the inhibited area could be extremely small, as little as 0.5° or the area of the fovea centralis necessary to recognize letters with a visual acuity of 6/9.

This effect can also be effected by lowering the illumination of one eye (Lyons, 1962) or by fogging one image with a cross cylinder (Mallett, 1964).

Establishing the psychological septum for near refraction

The psychological septum can be established for near vision testing by adding +0.75 DS to the reading prescription of the right eye of the patient and shortening the distance of the reading test by 3 cm. If the patient is slightly presbyopic, the right eye will now be clear and the left eye will be blurred. As the left fovea centralis will now be suspended the right eye can be refracted.

Alternatively, it can be achieved by adding plus to one eye only in steps of 0.50 D until the right–left difference causes more blur than the monocular sharpness, produced by the increased plus. It is important to note that in distance HIC binocular refraction, the eye not being refracted is fogged with the plus sphere.

The method of binocular refraction selected will depend on the equipment available. If the consulting room is equipped in typically British style, then refraction will be carried out with reverse letters seen in a mirror, and with a septum or similar device, and the prescription will be finalized using a trial frame. It is likely that the chart will be internally illuminated and used with normal room lighting. If the equipment is based on American practice, then refraction will be direct in a 6-m long room, the targets will be produced by a projector which will be polarized, and the refraction carried out with a phoropter equipped with analysers from beginning to end.

While other binocular refraction systems have been investigated, only Grolman's vector slides offer a complete refraction using polaroid slides under binocular conditions. All other polaroid systems are end tests following a monocular refraction. The HIC binocular system can be used following retinoscopy, while a complete refraction can be carried out using the Turville Infinity Balance, although a prior monocular refraction is preferable.

Polaroid

The American optometric practitioners were experimenting with binocular refraction using Polaroid many years before the vector system was introduced. At that time its disadvantage lay in the low level of illumination and hence poor contrast in the tests provided. This was overcome by a new technique developed by Grolman (1966), who explained the improved system as follows: 'Polarized or vectographic symbols and characters are formed by a high resolution printing process which involves the deposition of a dichroic dye on a stretched polyvinyl alcohol (PVA) film. The stretching causes the straightening of the long chains of gross PVA molecules in a single direction which, in turn, provides for a similar unidirectional orientation of the dichroic dye crystals. Since a dichroic crystal transmits light along one axis or plane and absorbs at right angles to the first, a symbol, printed thusly, will appear (through appropriately oriented analyzers) densely opaque to one eye while the other views an even, bright, unpatterned background in that same area. The test targets afford visibility which is subjectively comparable to that of an orthodox photographic test slide.'

Using this method Grolman produced a complete binocular refractive method. The procedure has now been altered to a series of slides which take the patient through the Grolman technique in individual steps.

A monocular acuity test under binocular conditions is provided in a new vectographic distance projection slide which presents to one eye high contrast test letters ranging from 20/100 (6/30) to 20/16 (6/45) Snellen size. Hence the practitioner may carry out the normal monocular routine, under binocular conditions.

An astigmatic clock of radial lines is presented with the right half of the clock seen by the right eye and the left half by the left eye. The lines are only spaced at intervals of 15° so that the test is a coarse one. Fusion is maintained by the two black dots and a short vertical bar, serving as strong macular fusion stimuli. By directing the patient's attention to first one half and then the other, the same questioning that is used in an orthodox monocular far chart technique will lead to the determination of the gross astigmatic axis of each eye under binocular conditions. Refinement of astigmatic axis and amount, using a cross-cylinder technique may also be executed within the framework of binocular vision using alternate composite targets.

Determination of an equal or balanced, minimal, binocular accommodative effort and a balance of acuity in each eye may be achieved using composite test target figures. Two similar sets of high contrast letters (20/40 to 20/25 or 6/12 to 6/75) are presented, one to each eye. The central vertical bar, projected aperture and the room itself provide strong macular and extensive peripheral fusion stimuli. The balancing procedures employed in the Turville Infinity Balance (TIB) techniques are applicable with this vectographic target, as are any of the techniques described for balancing the accommodative effort.

The binocular refraction of presbyopia

Infrequently, cases are found where, having balanced the accommodative efforts in distance viewing, and with equal acuity of the two eyes, there remains an inequality in both the visual acuity and the accommodative effort at the near distance. This difference will only be uncovered by carrying out a near binocular refraction.

The differences may be due to a variety of causes. The refraction, both sphere and cylinder power, may be altered by the reduction of the pupil diameter which accompanies convergence, or the cylinder axis may rotate due to a cyclophoria which is present in a small degree with convergence and looking downwards.

Rabbetts (1972) compared the refractions of the same patient for monocular and binocular conditions for distance and near vision. To do this he investigated refractive methods which were similar for distance and near refraction, deciding to use the HIC system for distance. For near, Rabbetts first investigated the method recommended by Mallett of fogging one eye with a 0.50 D cross cylinder and then experimented with neutral filters as recommended by Lyons (1962). With a 30% filter he found that peripheral binocular vision at near remained, but that the lower illuminated fovea was suspended.

Using the +0.75 DS for distance fogging, and the neutral filter for near, he found that 25% of eyes showed cylinder axis variations in any of the four changes: distance to near monocularly or binocularly and monocular and binocular at distance or near, but few of these can be regarded as significant. The power changes recorded were similarly slight, 0.25 DC variations being three times as common (18%) as changes of 0.50 DC or more (6%). The change from distance to near fixation produced about three times as many variations as the alteration from monocular to binocular fixation.

Cylinder power changes from monocular to binocular refraction occurred in 13% of the eyes examined, but only 3% by 0.50 D or more. Cylinder power changes from distance to near refraction occurred in 35% of the eyes examined, but only 10% by 0.50 D or more. Axis variations occurred in about 25% of the refractive alterations, but were mostly of less than 7° and were rarely significant.

It is important that in binocular balancing, the eyes must be in the fuctional position of rest. This is particularly important in the refraction of presbyopia. The patient should be asked to sit slightly forward, and to drop the head well forward to the normal reading position. The trial frame must be positioned so that the patient's optic axes pass through the centres of the lenses. In this position, holding the book at the normal reading distance, there is a strong psychological innervation to convergence and probably equally to pupillary constriction. It is doubtful if this is similarly achieved with a phoropter.

The sphere is balanced by matching the polarized duochrome red and green targets which are presented monocularly with the peripheral vision binocular. It has been the experience of the present author using this technique that the balanced spherical correction using duochrome results in an overcorrection and has to be modified as follows: with addition up to 2.00, deduct binocularly 0.50 DS, with additions 2.25–2.75 deduct 0.25 DS.

The cylinder may be refined using a cross cylinder and a polarized target such as that provided in the Mallett Hamblin near vision test. A circle on the duochrome test may be used by adjusting the sphere so that the green-backed target is sharp. As in the case of distance binocular tests, any prism which is to be prescribed should be in place when the near vision binocular tests are carried out.

In cases where there is doubt as to the correct balance, dynamic retinoscopy can be performed after the final presbyopic correction has been given to the patient. In most cases, as with the red–green near tests, plus has to be added to give reversal, and this should not be prescribed. The near retinoscopy will indicate whether the accommodative effort of the two eyes is equal and whether the cylinders are correct both in axis and power for near vision.

Two methods of binocular refraction for presbyopia have been developed using the HIC technique and these are described later.

Table 9.1 has been drawn up from pamphlets and booklets obtained from the manufacturers and their agents, the literature being extremely difficult to obtain. It is therefore possible that there may be omissions of equipment that is available for binocular refraction.

Advantages of HIC binocular refraction

The process of Humphriss immediate contrast (HIC) refraction is based on three hypotheses which have been substantiated with scientific research. The events which led up to the development of the technique are:

(1) That in a state of normal binocular vision, if one eye is slightly blurred, a very small central area, possibly covering only the fovea centralis is inhibited (Humphriss, 1979).

(2) That this inhibition has little or no effect on the normality of binocular vision (Humphriss, 1979).

(3) That when accommodation takes place, it does so equally in the two eyes.

The principle of immediate contrast can be applied monocularly. The binocular system of HIC refraction is an end check on the prescription under binocular conditions. It is very similar to the Turville Infinity Balance method except that it makes use of a natural psychological septum. The HIC test is not a balancing technique and measures the point at which a patient begins to accommodate for each eye separately, under conditions of normal binocular vision.

Rabbetts, comparing various methods of binocular refraction suggests: 'The obvious advantage of binocular refraction is that the eyes are visually in a more natural state than in monocular routines, provided single macular vision can be maintained without undue effort. Most importantly, the eyes are held in a state of normal convergence, at least as far as Humphriss' technique is concerned.' He also maintains: 'This has the advantage that the +0.75 DS fogging sphere in front of the eye not under examination tends to relax the patient's accommodation and allows parafoveal vision to be used. Since a +0.75 DS produces a fog to about 6/12, the central 3/4° radius circle of the fovea is rendered relatively insensitive, allowing the patient's attention to be concentrated on the image in the tested eye. The parafoveal and outer regions of the retinae provide a binocular lock for fusion. A second advantage of this method is that no special apparatus is required and, unlike the TIB, is applicable in exophoria.'

When the HIC technique is applied binocularly, it has a number of unique advantages, which are not available with any other method:

(1) The suspension of accommodation with a plus sphere, and the tying of the accommodation to convergence, greatly increase the accuracy of the HIC method when the duochrome is used with children.

(2) In the normal eye, the sphere can be cross-checked to a certain accuracy of 0.25 D in each eye in conditions of normal binocular vision.

(3) No septum as in TIB or polaroid analysers is necessary. The system uses the suspension of the central cones, a process which takes place normally whenever one eye is slightly blurred.

(4) The method reveals if there is a macular suppression or if binocular vision is grossly normal, without carrying out special tests to determine this.

(5) The use of a plus fogging lens before the eye not being refracted produces maximum suspension of accommodation hence releasing more latent hypermetropia for measurement than other methods (Lim, 1967).

(6) Patients find the HIC method more comfortable than other routines; in particular they are not in doubt as to the answer to be given to the questions put to them by the practitioner.

Table 9.1 Manufacturers, in alphabetical order, of polarized equipment for distance and near refraction

Name of manufacturer	Country of origin	Polarized projector or illuminated slides	Polarized phoropter
American Optical Co.	USA	Vectographic Slides	Analysers
Archer Elliott	UK	Cowan subjective unit	Archer Bobes
		Freeman unit	
Bausch & Lamb	USA	Polaroid only by request	
Hoya	Japan	Hoyatron	Analysers
Magnon	Japan	Numbers	Analysers at 45°
Nikon	Japan	Numbers	Analysers
Takagi	Japan	Binocular numbers	Analysers at 45° or 90°
Topkon	Japan	Letters, numbers Landlodt rings Duochrome	Analysers at 45°
Zeiss	Germany	Polar Test Letters Duochrome	Built into trial frame

Near vision refractors

Name of manufacturer	Country of origin	Chart	Analysers
Archer Elliott	UK	Freeman Archer	Clip onto trial frame
Hoya	Japan	Lumichart	Hand-held analysers
Keystone	USA	Binocular reading chart	Keystone viewer
Mallet Hamblin	UK	Near vision test with duochrome and individual targets	Visor
Zeiss	Germany	Polar Test	Built into trial frame

(7) In most cases of nystagmus, the method can be used binocularly when the nystagmus is usually minimized.

(8) The method can be used when the patient is wearing his own glasses to check the difference between the lenses and the refractive result. This is particularly valuable when the prescription is high and the exact effectivity is difficult to determine.

(9) The use of the 12 testing and moderating lenses, mounted on the four handles, almost eliminates the need to change trial case lenses.

HIC refraction has the disadvantage in comparison with the TIB system that it does not reveal any retinal slip. A method for the estimation of a relieving prism has been developed depending on the ability of the patient to recover from a position of diplopia and not on the retinal slip towards it (Humphriss, 1984).

The binocular HIC technique

Use can be made of the selective action of the psychological septum early in the refraction. It is particularly of use with suspect retinoscopy results or in cases of ciliary spasm.

After retinoscopy has been performed the working distance correction is left in place. The patient's vision would then be fogged and the binocular visual acuity should be between 6/36 and 6/24. The recording of this visual acuity alone may indicate an error in the retinoscopy, with poorer vision indicating more myopia and better vision indicating that there is more hypermetropia, perhaps in one eye only.

It is quite possible that the visual acuity recorded comes from the one clearer eye because the spheres are not correctly estimated. A binocular technique can now be used to estimate whether this is so. Plus is reduced in 0.50 D steps until a visual acuity of 6/12 is reached and the plus is then reduced in two 0.50 D steps from the right eye only until 6/6 is achieved.

The psychological septum has now come into operation, and the cones of the fovea centralis of the left eye have been suspended, so that the answers regarding clarity relate only to the right eye. An add of +1.00 D is now added back to the right eye so that it is again fogged and the plus before the left eye is reduced in 0.50 D steps until 6/6 is achieved. If the retinoscopy result were correct and the spheres balanced, then 6/6 would be reached in each eye with the same adjustment of the sphere. If it were in error, then more plus would have to be removed from one eye than the other.

If either eye cannot achieve an improved visual acuity, one of three conditions applies: the eye may be inhibited, hence the binocular refraction will not work; the retinoscopy result may have been grossly inaccurate, or there may be ocular pathology.

If the visual acuities were normal, the binocular technique could be applied after any type of monocular refraction either using a trial frame or a refractor head. The author would like to stress that it is his opinion that better results are obtained with a trial frame.

Having arrived at this stage in the refraction when the binocular HIC check is to be undertaken, it is important to give the correct instruction to the patient. The author recommends that the patient look at a letter (usually a 6/12 H). The patient is told that two lenses will be placed before the eye and that he should indicate which lens makes the edge of the letter clearer or if they are equally clear.

If the timing of the use of the HIC lenses is carefully applied, then the test may be used with patients of any age.

Testing for the sphere with a trial frame

The monocular refraction is left so that the patient is slightly myopic, i.e. red is better if the duochrome is used. A +0.75 DS is placed in the front cell of the left side of the trial frame. The 0.75 fogging lens is sometimes inadvertently prescribed if it is not placed in the front cell of the trial frame. The correcting sphere should be placed in the back cell of the trial frame, the cylinder in the back of the front rotating cells and the fogging 0.75 lens in the front cell of this part.

A +0.25 test lens is placed before the right eye. It is held in place for a full second and then replaced by a −0.25 lens. This is held in place for 0.5 s and then replaced with the plus lens for a full second, followed by the minus lens for a further 0.5 s. It is then removed. There may be one of four responses:

(1)   If the patient is not accommodating, the minus lens will be chosen immediately as the clearer lens. If the patient is accommodating there may be one of the following answers.
(2)   That the plus is clearer.
(3)   That after a hesitation they do not know which is clearer.
(4)   That the minus lens is clearer, but makes the letters blacker or smaller.

In almost all cases any answer other than the immediate rejection of the plus means that the patient is accommodating.

If the plus lens is accepted the test may be repeated with the addition of a +0.25 DS to the eye being tested provided that the other eye is fogged with a +1.00 D lens. If the eye is only fogged with a +0.75 D lens then this must be increased. Whenever plus is accepted by the eye being tested, accommodation is relieved binocularly; the amount of fogging may have been reduced to a level where it is not effective.

The rejection of the minus lens due to accommodation may be due to its effect on the eye not being refracted, but contributing to the binocular perception. The reasoning is based on the principle that, if the eye being refracted is made to accommodate, then the fogged eye will accommodate by the same amount and the fogging will be increased accordingly.

If a patient were emmetropic and the left eye open and fogged with a +1.00 DS, when −0.50 DS was placed before the right eye, both eyes would accommodate by 0.50 D. The patient is then asked to choose between the clarity of two lenses: a +0.50 and a −0.50 DS placed successively before the right eye. The +0.50 DS will neutralize the +0.50 DS and will make the right eye emmetropic. With the minus lens before the right eye, the accommodative effort will increase from 0.50 to 1.00 D in order to achieve clear vision. The left eye will accommodate by a similar amount so that this eye is now relatively fogged by 2.00 DS and binocular vision will have become unstable. The binocular reactions to these lens changes are illustrated in *Table 9.2*.

The comparison made is not, therefore, between the clarity of vision with a + and −0.50 DS lens, but

Table 9.2 The binocular reactions to the addition of minus and plus lenses to the right eye

Condition	Right eye	Left eye
(1)	Emmetropic	Fogged 1.00 D
(2) Add −0.50 to	Accommodated 0.50 D	Accommodated 0.50 and therefore fogged 1.50 D
(3) Place +0.50 before right eye	Emmetropic	Fogged 1.00 D
(4) Place −0.50 before right eye	Accommodated 1.00 D	Accommodated 1.00 and therefore fogged 2.00 D

between binocular conditions (3) and (4). This may explain why many young persons with adequate accommodation prefer the plus to the minus.

Hence, if a patient is slightly myopic and is moved in steps from myopia to hypermetropia by placing increasingly larger minus lenses before that eye, the point at which the patient begins to accommodate can be located by the change from an immediate rejection of the plus lens to hesitation or an acceptance of the plus lens. It is important to stress this principle. The HIC method of refraction is not a balancing technique, it is a method of determining when a patient is no longer myopic or emmetropic, but is accommodating and this point is measured for the right and the left eye in a state of normal binocular vision.

Furthermore, the activity of the psychological septum suggests that visual acuities should not be balanced. This mechanism exists so that, under any one brief set of circumstances, the best visual acuity of the right or left fovea comes to the conscious level. Hence, if for any reason one eye has a higher visual acuity than the other, it should not be reduced and balanced with the second eye.

Duochrome using HIC

The prescription can be cross-checked using red–green refraction binocularly. The effectivity of the method has been proved in thousands of refractions but the exact mechanism of the perceptual result has not been confirmed by research.

From a practical point of view it is known that it is essential to assure that the eye not being refracted is fogged by a full 0.75 DS, and if there is any doubt about this the eye should be fogged by +1.00 DS or even a +1.25 DS. The well known reaction of children who are refracted monocularly with duochrome targets of accommodating for any minus placed before the eye very rarely takes place.

If the arguments put forward in support of the HIC methods were correct, then the mechanism of duochrome HIC could be deduced. For ease of calculation it is assumed that the red-backed target will induce 0.25 of hypermetropia and the green 0.25 of myopia.

If the binocular vision is considered in relation to the red and green of the right and left eyes the following deductions may be made from *Table 9.3*.

(1) Condition 1: the left red and green targets will be inhibited in favour of the same targets seen by the right eye. These two targets will be seen to be equally clear.
(2) Condition 2: the red and green targets seen by the left eye will be inhibited in favour of the right targets. The red target will be seen as clearer than the green.

Table 9.3 Binocular conditions using duochrome refraction and a left +0.75 fogging lens

Condition of right eye	Right eye		Left eye +0.75 fog	
	Red target	Green target	Red target	Green target
(1) Plano	Blurred 0.25	Blurred 0.25	Fogged 0.50	Fogged 1.00
(2) Add +0.25 to right eye	Clear	Blurred 0.50	No change	No change
(3) Add −0.25 to right eye	Blurred 0.50	Clear	No change	No change

(3) Condition 3: both red targets will be blurred 0.50 D and will probably be fused. The left green target will be inhibited in favour of the right which will be seen to be clear.

The binocular effect is to produce an identical result compared with the use of the duochrome test monocularly, except that the accommodation is tied to the convergence. In general, even when refracting young children, the method works easily, with increasing accommodation resulting in red always being clear not occurring.

Comparison of the two methods

As the best sphere can be judged to 0.25 D by the HIC method, and can be similarly determined by the binocular duochrome method, these two refractive results should agree. It has been found in practice that one of two conditions applies: in a majority of cases the two methods agree to 0.25 D, in the other cases the HIC method results in the uncovering of 0.25 D hypermetropia more than the red–green method.

In a majority of refractions, the HIC method can be used with 0.25 spheres. The binocular HIC test should be used clinically with plus and minus 0.50 spheres instead of the 0.25 test lenses in those cases where these lenses give better results. They are:

(1) When there is a ciliary spasm.
(2) When there is an equally lowered acuity in both eyes.
(3) When the patient has difficulty in making a choice between the plus and minus lenses. This latter condition is mostly psychological.

Testing for the cylinder

When the duochrome HIC test has been completed, the right eye should be left with the green target clearer and, as this represents a small amount of accommodation of 0.25 D, the condition is ideal for cross-cylinder refraction. The left eye is fogged with the +0.75 DS and the cylinder of the right eye can now be checked with a cross cylinder in the usual manner.

When the cylinder has been corrected, the sphere is again checked and left red better. The +0.75 fogging lens is removed from the left eye, placed before the right eye and the whole procedure repeated on the left eye. Finally the +0.75 is removed from the right eye.

HIC testing at the reading distance

When plus and minus lenses are presented to a presbyope, the factors deciding which lens is clearer

are different from the distance refraction because the patient may do one of two things: he may relax accommodation and choose the plus lens, or he may accommodate and choose the minus.

For many years, attempts to make the HIC technique effective when the patient was accommodating proved fruitless. Finally it was discovered that it required a special target. The principle of design is the same as the distance test. A letter which can be recognized easily is needed as the point of fixation, but a relatively larger fusional lock is required, particularly if there is any appreciable amount of exophoria causing an eye to wander.

Since this target has been available, the application of the HIC method of near vision testing has been the subject of considerable research. The principle remains the same — that the patient is presented with two alternatives one of which disturbs his binocular vision and the other, not quite as sharp monocularly, is preferable binocularly.

If the choice between the lenses depends on which binocular state gives the best vision, then the test gives an indication of whether the low plus prescription should be given or not. The HIC test can be used at the reading distance to give the following information:

(1) Whether one eye is under- or overprescribed for a plus sphere in relation to the other.
(2) In doubtful cases, whether the early presbyopia should be corrected or whether the practitioner should wait a little longer before prescribing the first pair of reading spectacles.
(3) In doubtful cases of young hypermetropes, particularly monocular hypermetropes, whether a prescription should be given or not.

Checking the sphere

To check the sphere, it should be assumed that a patient aged 50 has been correctly refracted and the reading prescription is before his eyes. The HIC near sphere target, the H, is then placed at the reading distance. No plus lens is added to either eye and the reading test is held at the usual distance. The +0.50 D lens is placed before the right eye and held there for about one second. The minus lens is then placed before the eye for a similar length of time and the patient asked to choose between them: most patients choose the plus lens, although the reason for this is not known. It may be due to the precise distance of accommodation being a little further than the distance of the reading test resulting in a small accommodative lag. This would be corrected by the +0.50 lens and aggravated by the minus lens. The +0.50 is now added to the right eye and the test repeated. If the presbyopic addition is correct, the second +0.50 is rejected in favour of the minus.

The second test offers the patient a choice between the relief of accommodation giving a sharp image, but with one eye blurred and inhibited, and both eyes in equilibrium but with the accommodation possibly under strain. It has been found that, in those cases where a full plus prescription is required, the second plus lens is preferred to the minus. With practice, an inequality of the two focusing efforts is easily detected, as is the need for a higher reading addition and these may be prescribed.

Checking the cylinder at near

To achieve this the HIC near test is placed 7 mm closer than the best reading distance and +0.75 is added to the right eye. This eye will then be sharp but the left eye will be fogged by 0.75 D of uncorrected presbyopia.

The cylinder of the right eye can now be checked with a cross cylinder for axis and power. While the test is very sensitive, it does appear that most patients on whom the technique has been used respond better to a 0.50 cross cylinder than to a 0.25. However, this has not yet been adequately investigated, particularly in regard to axis change, and the technique may have to be modified.

The HIC near vision test has been found to be particularly useful in deciding whether to prescribe in cases of low monocular errors, particularly those of hypermetropia. An example would be a patient complaining of slight difficulty in close work whose refraction is: R: Pl; L: +0.75 DS. The practitioner has to decide if to prescribe the correction for near vision or not.

The clarity between ±0.50 spheres can be checked with the H target at the normal reading distance. The patient who requires the plus lens gives an immediate response of better vision with the plus. The patient who hesitates will probably not derive any advantage from them. The same test may be applied if one eye is myopic and similar results are obtained, the minus sphere being accepted as giving improved binocular vision by those patients who require the prescription.

The method has also been used to determine if a worn prescription should be altered in one eye only by 0.50 DS. Those who appreciate the improvement in their binocular vision are anxious to have the change; those who see no difference are probably as well off with their old prescription. The test is carried out wearing their own spectacles, which is particularly valuable in high prescriptions where it is difficult to assess the precise effectivity of the lenses.

The near fixation test can also be given to determine if a first presbyopic correction should be given. With an early emmetropic presbyope who requires a low add (e.g. +0.75), it is often difficult to determine whether the prescription will offer any advantages over a longer working distance. The influence of fatigue is unknown. If the near test is conducted with the add in place at the usual working distance, +0.50 will usually be preferred to −0.50. If a further +0.50 is accepted, this suggests that the relaxation of accommodation is preferred to the increased relative blur of the left eye and the prescription should be given with the add as found (in this case +0.75).

It must be stressed that these near vision reactions were only developed recently and much further research is required, but only those effects which have been repeatable on many cases are described here.

When binocular HIC does not work

It is a feature of the HIC technique that, when applied to a patient during a refraction, it either works perfectly or it does not work at all. There may be several reasons for failure:

(1)   The plus fogging lens may add to an existing binocular instability and break fusion causing diplopia and/or suppression of one of the images.
(2)   There may be no heterophoria, but the macular image of one eye may be permanently inhibited, such as in a suppression amblyopia.
(3)   The second eye may not be properly fogged.

In clinical practice, when there is no reaction to the plus and minus lenses, or no change in the red–green test, the best procedure is first to check that the failure to use the test is not due to under fogging of the second eye. Grolman (1966) reports cases when the binocular plus sphere was 1.00 D higher than the monocular. Hence fogging should be increased to +1.50 and even to +2.00 and the HIC test repeated. If the HIC test can now be carried out, then the practitioner knows that a considerable amount of hypermetropia remained latent during monocular refraction.

The HIC test, in addition to being an end test on the refractive state, is also a very sensitive test on the activity of the fovea in the binocular state. If there is a strong macular dominance which is not reversible then the fogging of the dominant eye will not result in its suspension and, since the answers regarding clarity will be taken from this eye, the patient will be unable to respond to tests on the other eye.

In order to establish the existence of this condition, the best simple test is to fog the one eye with a +1.00, add −0.50 to the other and use duochrome.

A normal patient will see the green more clearly and since the red target behind the fogging 1.00 must be clearer than the green, this means that the unfogged eye has selected the green as clearer by inhibiting the foveal image of the fogged one. If the patient is unable to do this, it indicates an inability to inhibit the fovea of the fogged eye. The practitioner must now investigate the state of the binocular vision by any of the standard tests for macular suppression. Tests not requiring any special equipment for this are described by Humphriss (1984).

Charts and targets

A chart for binocular refraction must meet certain requirements which are not necessary in monocular refraction. Fusion must be stable and therefore there must be a peripheral or perimacular fusional lock to achieve this. Turville used a black rectangle 10 cm wide on a white background. Goersch stated that the edge of the Polar test chart was a sufficient lock. Grolman (1966) in designing his vectogram slides, placed his tests inside rectangular boxes. If the test is conducted in normal room lighting then a perimacular lock has been found to be effective.

As the patient has been instructed to judge the clearer lens by the sharpness of the edge of the letter, a small letter such as 6/6 (20/20) is unnecessary and, testing with the larger letter has proved more comfortable for the patient, e.g. 6/12 or 6/15.

If a projector is used, a single letter can be selected by crossing the vertical and horizontal line selectors. If the practitioner is unable to present a single letter, then an H for spherical test, and an O or C for the cylinder testing should be indicated in a 6/12 line and the patient asked to concentrate on that particular letter.

References

CALDER GILLIE, J. C. (1959) The flipper technique. *Optician*, November 6

COWAN, L. (1959) Binocular refraction. A simplified clinical routine. *Br. J. Physiol. Opt.*, **16** (2), 60–82

GROLMAN, B. (1966) Binocular refraction. A new system. *New Engl. J. Optom.*, **17**, 5

HUMPHRISS, D. (1979) Non visual variables in binocular performance. *PhD Thesis*, University of Witwatersrand

HUMPHRISS, D. (1984) *Refraction Science and Psychology.* Cape Town: Juta & Co.

LIM, K. T. (1967) A comparison of the Humphriss binocular technique with a similar monocular technique for the subjective determination of the spherical refractive error in the human eye. *Masters thesis in Optometry*, University of Indiana

LYONS, J. G. (1962) Refraction and the binoculus. *Optician* July 6, 663–666

MALLETT, R. F. J. (1964) The investigation of heterophoria at near and a near fixation disparity technique. *Optician*, **148** 547–551, 574–581

TURVILLE, A. E. (1946) *Outline of Infinity Balance*. London: Raphaels

RABBETTS, R. B. (1972) A comparison of astigmatism and cyclophoria in distance and near vision. *Br. J. Physiol. Opt.*, **27** (3), 161–189

Further reading

ESKRIDGE, J. B. (1973) A balancing refractive procedure. *Am. J. Optom. Physiol. Opt.*, **50**, 499

GROSVENOR, T. (1978) Balancing tests and overfogging techniques. *Optom. Monthly*, August

LAYTON, A. (1975) A supplementary technique for balancing refraction. *Am. J. Optom. Physiol Opt.*, **52**, 125

10

Near point testing

Rogers Reading

One of the earliest uses of convex spectacles was to extend the productive years by allowing near work to be performed beyond the fourth decade of life (Levene, 1977). An ever increasing emphasis on close detailed tasks due to evolving occupational demands has been augmented by continued interest in avocational activities that also require near point precision. The simple remedies to this rather benign result of the gradual processes of ageing constitutes a major element of optometric work, and determining the proper solution for patients' problems with accommodation consumes some proportion of every practitioner's time.

It is well known that there is a steady decline with age in the maximum obtainable change in focus by accommodation up to the age of about 60 years (Donders, 1864). At this latter stage, measurements of emmetropic eyes show that the near point of clear vision is almost always beyond 1 m and represents only a manifestation of the depth of field (*Figure 10.1*). It signals the end of the ability to change focus by way of the accommodative mechanism (Alpern, 1969).

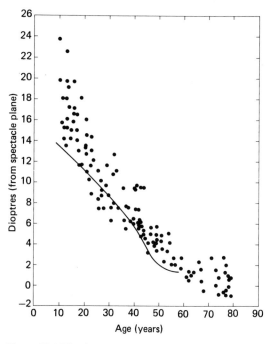

Figure 10.1 The decrease in the amplitude of accommodation with age. The points represent the data of Donders; the line represents the average values of Duane. Note the essentially linear trend up to the age of 60 years

Measurement of accommodation

Measurement of the accomodative amplitude is usually accomplished by presenting a patient, wearing the best correction for distance seeing, with a test card at some convenient distance and then slowly moving the card toward the spectacle plane while the patient attempts to keep the print as clear as possible. When the card passes inside of the patient's near point (punctum proximum), a blur will be reported. The reciprocal of this distance in metres is the dioptric value of the amplitude of accommodation.

The technique is applied to measurements involving each eye separately and both eyes together in order that certain comparisons can be made. This implies that the two monocular amplitudes should be equal, within the allowances of the measurement error. The binocular amplitude is slightly larger than either of the two monocular values (Duane, 1912). A unilateral deficiency can be a sign of neurological involvement and occurs along with oculomotor nerve paralysis (Leigh and Zee, 1983) or intraocular disease processes such as glaucoma and other inflammatory processes involving the uveal tract (Duke-Elder, 1949). In these cases, other symptoms and signs will serve to guide the practitioner to the correct causes, although the reduction in amplitude should be one of the effects that prompts the clinician to investigate these possibilities. Amblyopia (*see* Chapter 13) also gives rise to a difference between the two monocular amplitudes (Hokoda and Ciuffreda, 1982).

The amplitude is frequently compared to the usual values for people of the same age, in order to judge whether or not it is within normal limits. This can be done by utilizing the values of Donders (1864), Duane (1912) and Sheard (1917), or the more recent values of Turner (1958). Some of these are collected in *Table 10.1*. Because the relationship between age and amplitude is well characterized by a straight line, Hofstetter (1950) has suggested the use of simple linear formulae based upon the data of Donders and Duane:

Maximum amplitude (D) = 25.0−(0.4 × age in years)

Probable amplitude (D) = 18.5 − (0.3 × age in years)

Minimum amplitude (D) = 15.0 − (0.25 × age in years)

Table 10.1 Decreasing amplitude with increasing age*

Age (years)	Amplitude (D)			
	Donders (push-up)	Duane (push-up)	Turner (push-out)	Sheard (minus lenses)
10	19.75	13.50	—	—
15	16.00	12.50	10.50	11.00
20	12.75	11.50	9.50	9.00
25	10.50	10.50	8.00	7.50
30	8.25	9.00	6.50	6.50
35	6.25	7.25	5.75	5.00
40	5.00	6.00	4.50	3.75
45	3.75	3.75	2.50	—
50	2.50	2.00	1.50	—
55	1.75	1.25	1.00	—
60	1.00	1.00	0.75	—

* Extrapolated from values reported by various investigators and rounded to the nearest 0.25 D.

An unusually low amplitude at any age may result from certain systemic disease processes, from a loss of accommodative facility in an otherwise normal visual system, as discussed below, or possibly from some environmental factors, for example those implied by the continuing appearance of reports of the relatively early onset of presbyopia for people living in the tropics (*see*, for example, Coats, 1955; Kragha, 1985).

The technique described above is known as the Donders or push-up amplitude. It requires the use of a target with small enough detail so that a slight defocus is easily detected. When a just noticeable blur occurs, the test object should be moved in further to see if it becomes worse, then moved back until it clears. The midpoint between first blur and first clear positions then represents the near point of distinct vision (Morgan, 1960). A variation involves the so-called push-out method of starting the target in a position close to the spectacle plane and then slowly moving it away until a small line of print can just be successfully read. This alternative produces systematically lower values for the amplitude than does the simple push-up method (Fitch, 1971).

Tests of the amplitude of accommodation require suitable illumination of the test card and are usually preceded by a measurement of the visual acuity (Dismuskes, 1980) at near (40 cm). The acuity check assures that visual performance is adequate at this distance and thus allows the examiner to detect those patients in need of an additional near correction. If the patient cannot correctly identify letters on a line of type that is at a near acuity level equivalent to that obtained at distance with their best correction, plus (convex) lenses should be added until this refractive condition is met. Then the target can be moved slowly in as before and the near point measured. In these instances, the actual amplitude is determined by subtracting the amount of add in place from the measured value.

Minus lens method

An alternative approach involving the use of minus (concave) lenses was proposed by Sheard (1917). A near point card is placed at 40 cm (Sheard used 33.3 cm) and minus lenses introduced in 0.25-D increments until the patient reports the first noticeable blur that cannot be cleared by further conscious effort. The total amplitude is equal to the amount of negative lens power in place plus the 2.50 D of vergence power required to clear the near point object. The test is performed both monocularly and binocularly. However, the latter can be reduced due to a relatively low amplitude of negative fusional vergence, in which case it does not represent a true amplitude determination (Hofstetter, 1983).

In presbyopia where the amplitude is frequently less than 2.50 D, plus lenses are added to just clear a small line of letters and the total power used subtracted from the dioptric value of the test distance. For example, if characters subtending 5′ at 40 cm are just cleared by adding +0.5 D to the distance correction, the amplitude is 2.00 D.

This technique is referred to as the concave-at-near amplitude (Sheard, 1917), the positive relative accommodation amplitude (Hendrickson, 1980), or the minus-lens amplitude (Hokoda and Ciuffreda, 1982). Advocates suggest that it is superior to the technique of Donders because, as a target approaches the eye, its angular size increases and the pupil constricts. These changes tend to cause an increase in the depth of field (Emsley, 1952) and might produce higher amplitudes for the push-up method.

Measurements of the depth of field indicate that it usually has a value of around ± 0.50 D under ideal laboratory conditions (Campbell, 1957). Yet the minus lens amplitudes are some 2.00 D lower than those found using the push-up method (*see Table 10.1*). Furthermore, Somers and Ford (1983) investigated the angular size effect under conditions that kept pupil size constant and found that a difference of only 0.60 D could be attributed to the magnification of constant linear sized details viewed at decreasing distances, such as occur during the push-up test. In addition, Hokoda and Ciuffreda (1983) have identified a proximal component in the accommodative response during push-up which is reduced for the concave-at-near approach. Such a factor is known to facilitate convergence responses to near objects (Hofstetter, 1951). In addition, the application of negative lenses produces a spectacle minification (Bennett and Francis, 1962) which could also reduce these findings slightly. Nevertheless, the minus lens test has proven useful as a partial basis for determining the power of the near point added lens requirements, as is discussed below.

Near vision retinoscopy

A useful method of determining the amplitude of accommodation, particularly where verbal communications are difficult, is provided by the patient fixating a near object while the examiner performs retinoscopy. It requires the use of test letters displayed on a near point card containing an aperture so that the retinoscopic reflex can be viewed from a plane at a distance beyond that in which the patient is to fixate and as close to the primary line of sight as possible. Several aspects of this are presented in *Figure 10.2*.

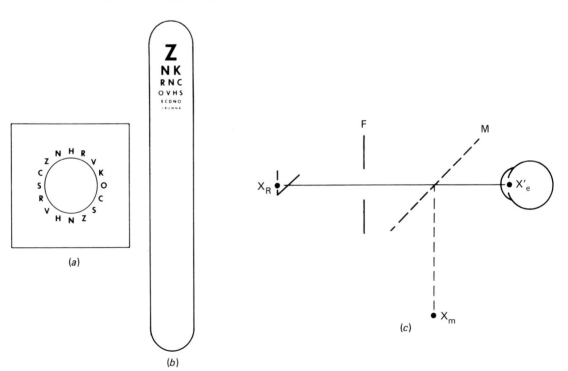

(a)

(b)

(c)

Figure 10.2 (*a*) Near acuity letters arranged around the rim of an aperture to allow dynamic retinoscopic measurements of the accommodative response. (*b*) A narrow near point card to be used during dynamic retinoscopy. (*c*) A schematic drawing showing the testing arrangement for dynamic retinoscopy. Dashed lines show an alternative using a half-silvered mirror: F is the fixation plane; M is the mirror; X'_e is the exit pupil of the eye being examined; X_R is the exit pupil of the retinoscope; and X_M is this same point when using the mirror

The reflex should show an against motion when viewed from a point somewhat beyond the plane of the near object (*see* Chapter 6 for an explanation of retinoscopic reflex motion). The examiner advances toward the card until this motion is neutralized. Then the card is advanced toward the patient. As long as this increase in accommodative demand is met with an increase in accommodative response, the 'against' motion will again be observed. The card is advanced and the reflex neutralized until the distance at which neutrality occurs ceases to advance with further advances of the test object. Accurate measurement of this distance then represents the datum from which the amplitude can be determined.

Dynamic retinoscopy is also useful for verification of responses elicited during the push-up procedure, as is illustrated by the following example. An appropriate near point card, initially displayed at 40 cm (2.50 D), is continually read by the patient. The examiner observes the retinoscopic reflex from a vantage point behind the card and locates the point of neutrality at 67 cm (1.49 D). Now the card is advanced and the neutral point tracked into a point located at 22.5 cm from the spectacle plane when the card is located at 18 cm. At this point, the patient first reports the presence of a noticeable blur. Advancing the card further produces the report of an increased defocus while the neutral point remains at 22.5 cm. The amplitude is then 5.56 D by the subjective criterion and 4.44 D by dynamic retinoscopy.

The technique is not without its drawbacks, since the bright light source can prove a powerful distractor to the patient. If the patient happens to fixate on this, rather than on the optotypes, accommodation will lag considerably, because the light source is a relatively crude accommodative stimulus, and a deceptively low amplitude will be recorded. Dimming the beam as much as possible minimizes this (Hokoda and Ciuffreda, 1982).

Cause of variations in measurements

When comparing amplitudes to age-related norms, it is important to remember that the various values are based upon different approaches. Thus, Donders and Duane used the push-up method, while Turner used push-out, and the values of Sheard are for the minus lens technique (*see Table 10.1*). Similar values do not appear to have been compiled for retinoscopy. However, these should agree with the push-up amplitudes to within about 1.00–1.50 D. Furthermore, if a value of about 1.00 D is taken as the dioptric interval due to chromatic aberration (Millodot and Sivak, 1973) and it is considered that at near the green region of the spectrum is in best focus (Bobier and Sivak, 1978),

then by measuring amplitudes using chromoretinoscopy, in which a green filter is placed over the light source, an even better agreement should be achieved.

All amplitudes reported here are with reference to the spectacle plane. While this is the usual clinical procedure, the corneal plane is used when accommodative issues are considered in cases of large amounts of ametropia and anisometropia (Obstfeld, 1978).

Other methods

Visually evoked cortical potentials can also be used to measure accommodative responses (Millodot and Newton, 1981), as can laser refraction (Owens and Leibowitz, 1975).

Determination of the near additions

Added lens power for near can be determined from the amplitude of accommodation by applying simple rules which are based upon the assumption that the normal individual can sustain accommodation at a level which represents only a certain portion of the amplitude (*see*, for example, Morgan, 1954). The most popular of these fixes the ratio at 0.5. The near power to be added is then determined by subtracting one-half of the measured amplitude from the dioptric power of the working distance (Bannon, 1955). For example, if the amplitude is 2.00 D and the working distance is 40 cm (2.50 D), then an add of +1.50 D is indicated. A variation of this approach calls for leaving one-third of the amplitude in reserve (Bennett and Francis, 1962), i.e. in the above example, the amplitude is multiplied by 0.67 and the add becomes +1.16 D, which would usually be rounded to the nearest 0.25 D step and result in an add of +1.25 D.

The success of this simple method depends upon an accurate measure of amplitude and a precise determination of the habitual working distance of the patient. Usually practitioners employ the indicated add as a starting point to be followed by measuring the linear range of distances over which the patient can see clearly, while a near point card is moved in and out. As the amplitude diminishes with age and the required power rises, the range of distances for clear vision shrinks so that the precision required becomes increasingly important to the success of the patients with their new spectacles. For higher adds, a multifocal lens can be considered. *Table 10.2* presents an example of the collapse of the range of clear vision with increasing add power.

As with the determination of amplitudes, add powers can be arrived at by fixing the test distance

Table 10.2 Ranges of clear vision through various adds

Amplitude	Add for 40 cm	Near point through distance portion (cm)	Range through near portion (cm)
	Full amplitude used (occasional seeing)		
3.00	+1.00	33	100–25
2.00	+1.50	67	67–29
1.00	+2.00	100	50–33
	Two-thirds of the amplitude used (casual seeing)		
3.00	+1.00	50	100–31
2.00	+1.50	75	67–35
1.00	+2.00	150	50–38
	One-half of the amplitude used (detailed seeing)		
3.00	+1.00	67	100–40
2.00	+1.50	100	67–40
1.00	+2.00	200	50–40

(here assumed to be at 40 cm) and altering lenses. This approach uses the concave-at-near finding in conjunction with a convex-at-near value to determine the add. The convex-at-near procedure consists of adding plus lenses, usually in 0.25-D steps, until the letters on the near point card are reported to begin to blur. The midpoint between these two values then constitutes a measure of the power needed to help optimize visual function at near (Grosvenor, 1982). For example, if the minus lens to blur finding is plano and the plus lens to blur finding is +2.50 D, then an add of +1.25 D is indicated. It is important to note that, when the amplitude is less than the demand of the near testing distance, both values will be in plus form. Thus, if the amplitude is 2.00 D, then when testing at 40 cm the minus lens finding will be +0.50 D.

The plus lens finding will be less than the dioptric equivalence of the near testing distance if the positive fusional vergence amplitude is lower than about 15 Δ (Hofstetter, 1983). It should never exceed this amount by more than 0.25 D since excesses indicate that the distance correction contains an insufficient amount of plus power, or an excess of negative power. Applying these principles, a plus lens finding of +1.50 D would indicate a relatively low positive fusional facility, whereas a +3.00 D plus lens value would suggest an undercorrection of distance by 0.50 D.

Cross cylinder method

Another approach to add determination utilizes the cross cylinder which introduces an astigmatic interval into the optical system being tested (Stokes, 1849). A test object, such as the one illustrated in *Figure 10.3*, is displayed to a patient who binocularly

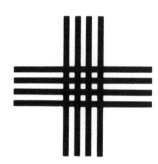

Figure 10.3 A multiple-line cross object used in conjunction with binocular cross cylinders to determine the power of the near point add in presbyopia

views it through cross cylinders oriented with the minus cylinder axes in the vertical meridian. Because the white-light response of accommodation will usually be less than the stimulus, this will cause the horizontal lines of the target to appear darker. Plus lenses are added to balance the apparent contrast between the vertical and horizontal sets of lines. If precise equality cannot be established, reversal can be used. For example, if through an add of +1.50 D the horizontal lines are preferred and through an add of +1.75 D the verticals are reported to be better, then the indicated add is +1.62 D, which might be rounded up or down to the nearest 0.25 D step depending upon the particular needs of the patient.

The test assumes that the patient does not undergo a change in accommodation as the plus lenses are added (Westheimer, 1958). Dimming the illuminance (Goodson and Afanador, 1974) and applying the test only to presbyopes (Fry, 1940) produces quite useful results. It is important to use a sufficiently large astigmatic interval so as to create a strong enough difference between the clarity of the target components. A 0.50 D cross cylinder is recommended for routine application, with larger powers being applied in cases involving low vision. Because of the astigmatism introduced and the nature of the accommodative response in younger patients, it is possible to find +0.50 – +0.75 D of indicated additional near power on virtually all prepresbyopic patients (Morgan, 1960).

Certain cases of high astigmatism may require some increase in the cylinder correction to reflect the effective power change required to completely neutralize this form of ametropia at near (Bennett and Francis, 1962). This avoids introducing a possible bias into the patient's responses toward one or the other of the binocular cross-cylinder target orientations. The problem could be avoided by using target and cross-cylinder orientations that are 45° from the principal meridians; however, such oblique orientations tend to complicate the patient's response options.

Some practitioners apply the technique monocularly as well as binocularly. This has the advantage of detecting unequal accommodative demands such as occur in anisometropia and require the fitting of differing add powers for each eye. In fact, all of the tests described here can be applied both monocularly and binocularly.

Duochrome method

A near balance point can also be determined subjectively by using a duochrome method. As with the version of this used at distance, the near test utilizes the chromatic focal interval of the human eye by displaying optotypes on both red and green backgrounds (Giles, 1960). The filters used should be of equal luminance transmittance and with dominant wavelength foci at equal dioptric intervals from the yellow sodium line at 589.6 nm (Mandell and Allen, 1960). The test uses colour without depending upon colour perception as such. Thus colour anomalous patients can respond on the basis that the letters on one side are clearer, more blurred, or equal, to those on the other (Heath, 1970). Protan defects will cause the red side to appear dimmer (Wright, 1946).

The technique amounts to the addition of plus lenses until the two halves of the duochrome chart are balanced, although some practitioners prefer to stop 0.25 D toward a better focus for the green portion. Some workers do the test monocularly first, leaving the red letters as just better, and then perform the procedure binocularly with the end point in balance between optotypes displayed on the two colours. Work on chromatic aberration (Millodot and Sivak, 1973) suggests that prescrip-

tions based on adds that leave the green side in superior focus may be most acceptable (Wilmut, 1960).

Dynamic retinoscopic method

In addition, multifocal power can be determined by dynamic retinoscopy. As mentioned above, this consists of using a special near point card set at the usual working distance of the patient. Plus lenses are added until the reflex is neutralized, when observed from a plane behind the card. Again, chromoretinoscopy can be applied to assess the chromatic aspect of the accommodative response in the presbyopic patient, or the white light reflex neutralized in a plane that is about 0.50–0.75 D weaker in vergence power than the habitual working distance.

It should be emphasized that all adds determined by the above methods are to be considered as starting points only. The experienced practitioner soon learns that trial and error testing, involving the direct choice of the patient as to the exact add power to be applied to her/his usual working distances, is the most useful method of satisfying the patient's needs, provided that such a choice yields an adequate range of clear vision. Where the range through the patient's choice of adds is severely restricted, intermediate trifocal power should be determined by similar means (Kragha, 1985).

Accommodative dysfunction

Accommodative dysfunctions in prepresbyopic patients are not uncommon. While these problems are usually associated with school-age children, adults also show such symptoms. It is manifest either as spasm of accommodation or a loss of normal accommodative facility. In both instances, it is important to rule out associated conditions which would indicate that the anomaly is a symptom of a disease process, a result of a neurological lesion, or a side-effect of some pharmacological agent.

Symptoms include those associated with asthenopia, as well as blur upon reading or blur when looking up from near work (Duke-Elder, 1949). It is wise to fully correct hyperopic ametropia, utilizing the findings from a cycloplegic examination.

Spasms are believed to be associated with prolonged near work and can be relieved by plus lenses at near. It frequently remits with this sort of treatment in 4–5 weeks, providing no associated ametropia is left unattended (Donders, 1864).

Accommodative insufficiency, which is revealed by unexplained low push-up amplitudes, should be confirmed by dynamic retinoscopic measurements. Accommodation usually returns to normal by using simple home orthoptics procedures for 4–5 weeks. These consist of repeated push-ups, such as are used in the binocular Donders amplitude measurement technique, or jump-foci, either with alternate fixation distances, involving printed material as test objects, or viewing such objects through alternating ± 2.00 D lenses (Grisham, 1983). Moderate reductions in amplitude in which adults cannot alternately clear optotypes viewed through ± 2.50 D 'flipper' lenses 20 times in 60 seconds will also benefit from such training in terms of improving the time course of responses and the reduction of symptoms (Griffin, 1976).

References

ALPERN. M. (1969) Accommodation. In *The Eye*, edited by H. Davson, Vol. III, pp. 217–254. Academic, New York: Academic Press

BANNON, R.E. (1955) Physiological factors in multifocal corrections: I. Measurement of ocular functions. *Am. J. Optom.* **32**, 57–69

BENNETT, A.G. and FRANCIS, J.L. (1962) Ametropia and its correction. In *The Eye*, edited by H. Davson, Vol. IV, pp. 131–180. New York: Academic Press

BOBIER, C.W. and SIVAK, J.G. (1978) Chromoretinoscopy. *Vision Res.* **18**, 247–250

CAMPBELL, F.W. (1957) Depth of field of the human eye. *Opt. Acta*, **4**, 157–164

COATS, W.R. (1955) Amplitude of accommodation in South Africa. *Br. J. Physiol. Opt.*, **12**, 76–81, 86

DISMUSKES, K. (1980) Recommended standard procedures for the clinical measurement and specification of visual acuity: report of working group 39. *Adv. Ophthalmol.*, **41**, 104–148

DONDERS, F.C. (1864) *On the Anomalies of Accommodation and Refraction of the Eye*, pp. 173-235. London: New Sydenham Society

DUANE, A. (1912) Normal values of accommodation at all ages. *J. Am. Med. Assoc.*, **59**, 1010–1013

DUKE-ELDER, W.S. (1949) *Text-Book of Ophthalmology*, pp. 4415–4448. London: Henry Kimpton

EMSLEY, H.H. (ed.) (1952) *Visual Optics*, Vol. I, pp. 67, 98, 357–358. London: Hatton Press

FITCH, R.C. (1971) Procedural effects on the manifest human amplitude of accommodation. *Am. J. Optom.*, **48**, 918–926

FRY, G.A. (1940) Significance of fused cross cylinder test, *Optom. Weekly*, **31**, 16–19

GILES, G.H. (1960) *The Principles and Practice of Refraction*, pp. 193–202. Philadelphia: Chilton Book Co.

GOODSON, R.A. and AFANADOR, A.J. (1974) The accommodative response to the near point crossed cylinder test. *Optom. Weekly*, **65**, 1138–1140

GRIFFIN, J.R. (1976) *Binocular Anomalies: Procedures for Vision Therapy*, p. 123, Chicago: Professional Press

GRISHAM, J.D. (1983) Treatment of binocular dysfunctions. In *Vergence Eye Movements: Basic and Clinical Aspects*, edited by C. M. Schor and K. J. Ciuffreda, pp. 605–646. Boston: Butterworths

GROSVENOR, T.P. (1982) *Primary Care Optometry: A Clinical Manual*, p. 264. Chicago: Professional Press

HEATH, G.G. (1970) Color vision testing. In *Clinical Refraction*, pp. 585–614. Chicago: Professional Press

HENDRICKSON, H. (1980) *The Behavioral Optometry Approach to Lens Prescribing*, pp. 15-17. Duncan: Optometric Extension Program Foundation

HOFSTETTER, H.W. (1950) Useful age-amplitude formula. *Optom. World*, **38**, 42–45

HOFSTETTER, H.W. (1951) The relationship of proximal convergence to fusional convergence and accommodative convergence, *Am. J. Optom.*, **28**, 300–308

HOFSTETTER, H.W. (1983) Graphic analysis. In *Vergence Eye Movements: Basic and Clinical Aspects*, edited by C. M. Schor and K. J. Ciuffreda, pp. 439–464. Boston: Butterworths

HOKODA, S.C. and CIUFFREDA, K.J. (1982) Measurement of accommodative amplitude in amblyopia. *Ophthal. Physiol. Opt.*, **2**, 205–212

HOKODA, S.C. and CIUFFREDA, K.J. (1983) Theoretical and clinical importance of proximal vergence and accommodation. In *Vergence Eye Movements: Basic and Clinical Aspects*, edited by C. M. Schor and K. J. Ciuffreda, pp. 75–97. Boston: Butterworths

KRAGHA, I.K.O.K. (1985) Factors in the determination of the age of onset of presbyopia. *PhD thesis*, Indiana University, Bloomington

LEIGH, J.R. and ZEE, D.S. (1983) *The Neurology of Eye Movements*, pp. 166-181. Philadelphia: Davis

LEVENE, J.R. (1977) *Clinical Refraction and Visual Science*, pp. 35-88. London: Butterworths

MANDELL, R.B. and ALLEN, M.J. (1960) The causes of bichrome failure. *J. Am. Optom. Assoc.*, **31**, 531-533

MILLODOT, M. and SIVAK, J. (1973) Influences of accommodation on the chromatic aberration of the eye. *Br. J. Physiol. Opt.*, **28**, 169–174

MILLODOT, M. and NEWTON, I. (1981) V E P measurement of the amplitude of accommodation. *Br. J. Ophthalmol.*, **65**, 294–298

MORGAN, M.W. (1954) The ciliary body in accommodation and accommodative convergence. *Am. J. Optom.*, **28**, 3–10

MORGAN, M.W. (1960) Accommodative changes in presbyopia and their correction. In *Vision of the Ageing Patient*, edited by M. J. Hirsch and R. E. Wick, pp. 83–112. Philadelphia: Chilton Book Co.

OBSTFELD, H. (1978) *Optics in Vision*, pp. 138-190. London: Butterworths

OWENS, D.A. and LEIBOWITZ, H.W. (1975) The fixation point as a stimulus for accommodation. *Vision Res.*, **15**, 1161–1163

SHEARD, C. (1917) *Dynamic Ocular Tests*. Columbus: Lawrence, reprinted in *The Sheard Volume* (1957) pp. 90-112. Philadelphia: Chilton Book Co.

SOMERS, W.W. and FORD, C.A. (1983) The effect of relative distance magnification on the monocular amplitude of accommodation, *Am. J. Optom. Physiol. Opt.*, **60**, 920–924

STOKES. G.G. (1849) On a mode of measuring the astigmatism of a defective eye. British Association for the Advancement of Science, ninth meeting, report 1849, 10, cited by Levene (1977)

TURNER. M.J. (1958) Observations on the normal subjective amplitude of accommodation. *Br. J. Physiol. Opt.*, **15**, 70–100

WESTHEIMER. G. (1958) Accommodation levels during near crossed-cylinder test. *Am. J. Optom.*, **35**, 599–604

WILMUT. E.B. (1960) Bichromatic refraction: *The Optician*, **139**, 533–534

WRIGHT. W.D. (1946) *Researches on Normal and Defective Colour Vision*, pp. 73–104. London: Henry Kimpton

Part 3

Paediatric optometry

11

Visual development: acuity and binocularity

Jerry Nelson

'As children get older, they get better at things.' (McKee's First Law; *see* Teller, 1982; Teller and Movshon, 1986)

There are several reasons for trying to refine McKee's first law of child development:

(1) The paediatric practitioner requires norms against which pathology and its treatment can be judged.

(2) Methods developed for infant assessment benefit the paediatric practitioner, who requires early detection of abnormalities, lest undesirable sensory adaptations become irreversible, and better monitoring of visual function during early treatment.

(3) Things get better at different times. Separate stages in the maturational sequence show the separation of visual system functions, and suggest separate underlying brain mechanisms.

(4) Whenever clinical grading (e.g. Worth's grades of binocular vision) does not follow the sequence of infant development, more appropriate scale of performance assessment can be developed for the child patient.

(5) Development tells us something about susceptibility to damage. In a congenital esotrope of a certain age, visual deficits cannot occur in visual skills which would normally not yet have appeared at that age.

The maturation of spatial vision is emphasized. Clinical norms for children may be found in Chapter 12, and procedures of examination in Chapter 15. The levels of performance attainable with the laboratory techniques mentioned below do not represent norms for clinical tests.

Maturation of the visual pathways

Optics and retina

The optic media are clear at birth in man. Definitive quantitative data, requiring general anaesthesia, are not available. Such data can be obtained by a photoelectric scan of a line imaged on the fundus to measure its blurriness; Fourier transformation of this 'line spread function' gives the transfer function of the eye as an optical system (because the image suffers optical degradation on the way in and upon reflection outward, the square root of the Fourier transform must be taken; *see* Chapter 13 and Westheimer, 1986).

In the newborn, fixation precision may be limited by the incompletely developed state of the fovea (reviews: Amigo, 1972; Banks and Salapatek, 1983; Boothe, Dobson and Teller, 1985). Foveal receptor density and cone outer segment length both increase after birth, as foveal cones become longer and thinner. Amacrine, bipolar and especially ganglion cells migrate as the fovea develops a pit in the first 4 months. Because of cell migrations and growth of the eyeball, a fixed retinal image will fall on a changing array of cells. Growth of the head slowly magnifies disparity input for steropsis. Brain centres for spatial vision must have the plasticity to continually recalibrate themselves as the periphery matures. Pathology of these plastic mechanisms underlies anomalous correspondence.

In most respects, the retina has reached adult maturity at 11–15 months, in rough agreement with the best results for tests of monocular acuity (*see below*). However, the practitioner may find the reflex from the foveal pit absent in 2- to 4-year-olds (Amigo, 1978), while outer segment length and packing density are still half of adult values at 45 months (Yuodelis and Hendrickson, 1986). Acuity development is probably neurally, not optically, limited, but not all neural limitations are retinal.

Cortex

The full complement of adult cortical cells is present well before birth in the ventricular zones below the cortex. Neurones migrate radially outwards to assume their final positions by the time of birth. These migration trajectories may help to define the radial organization of the cortex. A blossoming of spines on the poorly arborized dendrites of the neonate's neurones reaches its peak at 2 months and dies back. Spines (little 'pepper grains' on the twiggy branches of a neurone) are often sites for synaptic input. The neurones may be reaching out to all possible neighbours as an aid in deciding which ones are worth connecting to. By the age of 6 months, the spine counts are down again while dendrites have become richly ramified.

Functionally, there is no binocular vision at 2 months when spines are in overabundance. Later, when the dendrites are in place, disparity discrimination is also present. Inputs from the two eyes also become segregated within the ocular dominance columns (*see* Chapter 13), which may be an aid in generating neurones with binocular disparity selectivity (*see* Chapter 14). During this time (1 month postnatal in the monkey; before 3–5 months in man), the cortex can better support pattern vision (and presumably contribute to monocular oculomotor control) than it can deal with binocular vision, disparity detection or vergence.

Myelination of the cortex follows myelination of the optic nerve (complete for all fibres by 3 months), but still makes dramatic increases in thickness for the first 2 years. This brings gradual changes in evoked potential latency, where the P_1 component for fine checkerboards has still not attained adult values at 5 years (Moskowitz and Sokol, 1983).

Basic visual skills

Accommodation

Accommodation occurs at 1 month of age, becomes more regular by 2–3 months (if large stimuli are used), and shows an almost adult-like range by 6 months (Atkinson and Braddick, 1979; Braddick *et al.*, 1979; Banks, 1980; *Figure 11.1*). Limits on the development of acuity after 6 months are, therefore, more likely set by neural (especially cortical) than by optical factors. Even when accommodation is inaccurate, the visual system benefits from a smaller eyeball's greater depth of field, just as a wide-angle lens (shorter focal length) has greater depth of field. The early perfection of accommodation suggests that vergence errors in the infant are fusional vergence errors (disparity processing inadequacies) and not accommodative vergence inaccuracies. These inadequacies would be tapped by both prism and stereopsis tests. It is likely that accommodation is primarily driven by W-stream-innervated, subcortical centres; subcortically mediated functions are thought to mature early.

Infants have largely against-the-rule astigmatism (greatest refractive power horizontal) which fades between the ages of 1.5 and 4.5 years (Dobson, Fulton and Sebris, 1984; Gwiazda, Scheiman and Held, 1984; Howland and Sayles, 1984; *see* also Chapter 12). Left uncorrected in the older child, appreciable astigmatism can cause meridional amblyopia to arise, an orientation-dependent acuity loss, neurally caused and not immediately correctable by refractive means (*see* Chapter 13). Meridional amblyopia has not been detected, however, until the third year of life and, at this time, it is still reversible, as shown by 3 months of continuous spectacle wearing (Mohindra, Jacobson and Held, 1983). Astigmatism and its related sensory (mal)adaptation have matched periods of development. Either the visual system or a refractive correction must get cylindrical refraction right only by some time after the second birthday.

Monocular acuity

Optokinetic nystagmus, pattern-reversal evoked potentials and preferential looking (*see below*) techniques, each employed with ever-finer stripes, provide means of assessing infant acuity. The acuity limit is reached when the stripes are too fine to elicit a nystagmus reflex, a scalp potential or looking at the target in preference to a blank screen. The acuity range reported in the literature from all methods at 3 months is 6/15 (12 cycles/deg) to 6/90 (2 cycles/deg; Dobson and Teller, 1978; *see also* Chapter 12, *Table 12.2*). Newer studies show better acuities.

Evoked potentials (EPs) have always shown the best acuity levels: 6/24 acuity at 2–3 months, and nearly adult acuity levels at 6–8 months. For behavioural testing, 6/60 (3 cycles/deg with gratings) is a 'classic' value at 3 months; 6/24 (7.5 cycles/deg) may be demonstrated at 4 months with recent improvements in techniques.

Evoked potential

The visual evoked potential (VEP) versus behavioural discrepancy has been cause for concern (Dobson and Teller, 1978), but when under cycloplegia adults are defocused, there is no discrepancy. Acuity loss measured psychophysically and electrophysiologically with the same *grating* patterns shows striking agreement (*Figure 11.2b*). The relationship between VEP results and *Snellen* acuities is more variable (*Figure 11.2a*); this variability stems from the complexity of the traditional Snellen test, which involves identification as well as discrimination, and requires segmentation of a crowded pattern.

Cortical evoked potential acuity estimates are probably more reliable than inferences from opto-

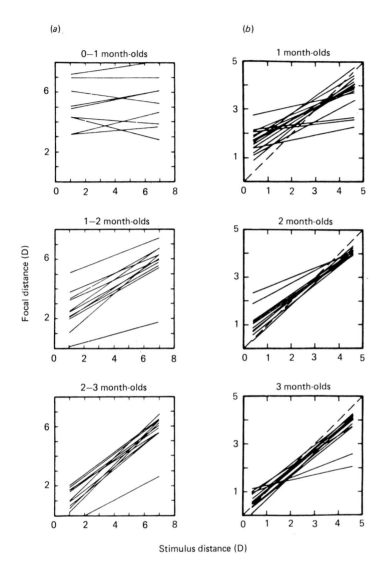

Figure 11.1 Accommodation in the infant measured by retinoscopy. Accommodation and the distance of the object being fixated are both expressed in dioptres (D). Perfect accommodation is described by a line of 45° slope, while fixed acommodation produces a horizontal line. (*a*) The same object was presented at 14–100 cm; (*b*) at greater distances larger targets were employed so that visual angle remained constant (range: 21–300 cm). Accommodation is better, and almost adult-like at 2 months. (Original data: Haynes, White and Held, 1965; Banks, 1980; reproduced from Aslin, 1987, courtesy of the Publisher, Academic Press)

kinetic nystagmus (OKN), which is not exclusively a product of cortical performance. Behavioural methods depend on infant motivation and are still being developed.

The VEP has its peculiarities, however: the 'well-behaved' data of *Figure 11.2* imply that the VEP would still be present in an observer with no form vision ('zero acuity'). Two sources of this anomalous response are: the presence of local flicker compon-

ents in the 'pattern' VEP (the VEP responds to luminance changes) and pathways from the secondary visual system to the cortex. These pathways are also implicated in preserved VEPs in blind subjects (Kupersmith and Nelson, 1986). This aside, the cortical evoked potential is the most sensitive assay of infant acuity, for which the striate cortex (a heavy contributor to the recorded response) is known to set the performance limit.

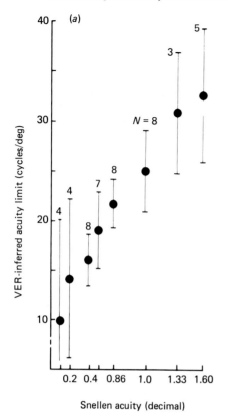

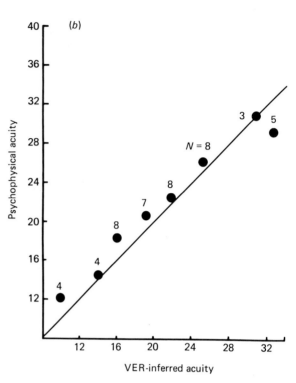

Figure 11.2 Acuity can be accurately measured from the visual evoked potential (VEP). (*a*) Acuity inferred from the VEP compared to Snellen acuity in the same subjects with cycloplegia at various levels of defocus. Vertical lines: 95% confidence limits; *N* = number of subjects tested. (*b*) The same VER inferred acuity versus grating acuity measured in the same subjects. Grating acuity is inherently less variable than Snellen acuity. In both graphs, a diagonal line through the origin implies perfect agreement between electrophysiological and subjective acuity determinations. (From D. E. Wiener, K. Wellish, J. I. Nelson and M. J. Kupersmith, Comparisons among Snellen, psychophysical and evoked potential visual acuity determinations, *Am. J. Optom. Physiol. Opt.* **62**, 667–679, © The American Academy of Optometry, 1985)

Gradual development

When acuity levels are immature, it is possible that fundamental cellular mechanisms are absent, or are present but lacking in refinement. In evoked potentials, one grating pattern does not begin to lower the potential elicited by another until 6 months of age (Morrone and Burr, 1986). This suggests that new cortical circuits are still emerging. Perhaps adult acuteness of vision depends on the sensory sharpening that these circuits achieve. Acuity matures gradually over an extended period because several mechanisms appearing at different times and places all contribute to it.

Rapid acuity and ocular dominance shifts during treatment

Acuity changes rapidly and must be monitored during treatment. In the kitten 12 hours' experience with either strabismus or monocular occlusion will nearly destroy cortical binocularity (six 2-hour periods of visual experience administered over 2 days with the animals otherwise in darkness; Van Sluyters and Malach, 1984). Visual deprivation in infants from any source (burns, infection, media opacity or occlusion therapy) can cause losses (or gains) of one line of Snellen acuity per week (Mohindra *et al.*, 1979; age, 10 months).

Monocular visual function testing is becoming a routine part of patient management in certain procedures. For example, following bilateral cataract surgery, behaviourally determined acuity deterioration in one eye may be the first sign that one contact lens has slipped or is ill-fitting (Jacobson, Mohindra and Held, 1981a).

Ocular balance is essential for preventing a shift in ocular dominance (*see* Chapter 13). Where there is any suspicion that one retinal image may be clearer than the other, or where surgery is late and the end of the critical period is near, monocular preferential-looking acuity testing should be considered. By taking a hand in balancing ocular dominance, the option of normal binocular vision may be reserved for the patient, even though conventional clinical binocularity tests (e.g. stereopsis tests or amblyoscope testing) can not be performed at this age.

Appearance of competition and occlusion effects

The need to perform corrective surgery *before* the critical period closes is widely recognized; however, there is no point in acting before plasticity has begun. New infant assessment techniques suggest the critical period does not begin at birth. For example, acuity will not respond to deprivation until 4 months of age (cataract: Taylor *et al.*, 1979), which also marks the sudden onset of stereopsis. This suggests that binocular interaction must appear in the cortex before amblyopia can develop (Held, 1984), and that amblyopia involves interocular competition and suppression (von Noorden, 1985). The necessary substrate for this binocular interaction is a system of well-separated ocular dominance columns, developing in part by retraction of retinogeniculate inputs in cortical layer IV. The left eye–right eye competition reflected in ocular dominance column width changes can then begin (*see Figure 13.6*, Chapter 13).

Contrast sensitivity

Contrast sensitivity increases, and the contrast sensitivity function's optimum shifts to higher spatial frequency, as acuity improves. The sensitivity roll-off at low spatial frequencies, seen in adults, is absent in 5-week-old infants. This decrease in contrast sensitivity first appears at 2 months (Atkinson, Braddick and Moar, 1977; Atkinson and Braddick, 1981). By implication, some kind of lateral inhibition is arising at this time, either a receptive field component (an inhibitory surround to cancel the centre response) or lateral inhibition from beyond the classic receptive field (Nelson and Frost, 1978). Such inhibition could cause the roll-off because stripes broad enough to stimulate opposing mechanisms would elicit a weaker *net* response. Without such spatially opposed mechanisms, acuity for spatial position suffers. The other side of the spatial acuity coin is a larger spatial summation area, three times larger at 1 month than in the adult. This summation permits absolute brightness sensitivity to come much closer to adult values when large diameter test flashes are used (Hamer and Schneck, 1984).

Oculomotor development

The five basic kinds of eye movement are *saccades* (rapid motions for refixation), *tracking* (pursuit) motions of moving targets, *vergence* or disjunctive movements responding to object depth (disparity) changes and also linked to accommodation, the *optokinetic reflex*, a stereotyped tracking motion elicited by movement of the visual field rather than a small object within it and *vestibulo-ocular reflexes*, present at birth, which stabilize the eye when the head assumes different static positions, or the body turns. At 3 months, infants can *inhibit* this type of reflex more accurately to maintain fixation. This implies that cortical centres interact with lower centres (brainstem and cranial nerve nuclei) and first gain ascendancy over them at this time.

For binocular vision, accuracy of tracking motion, fixation saccades and especially vergence are of concern; OKN, a lowly reflex which surprisingly reflects binocularity in the cortex, is discussed in Chapter 13.

Fixation saccades and tracking

The latency for fixation saccades is around 1 second at 1 and 2 months of age, about five times the adult value. At this time, the infant makes a series of fixed-amplitude saccades until the object of interest is reached, rather than releasing a measured command to the extraocular muscles calculated to flick the eyes to within 10% of the desired position. Back-to-back saccades are also observed up to at least 5 months of age. These occur in opposite directions without the characteristic 200–250 millisecond intersaccade interval of the adult and give the appearance of brief eye oscillations (Hainline *et al.*, 1984).

Tracking of isolated, fixated objects appears and shows rapidly increasing quality between 6 and 12 weeks (Aslin, 1981). Before this period, 'tracking' consists only of repeated saccade-and-hold sequences, although the oculomotor system itself can make smooth tracking motions when whole-field motion elicits an optokinetic nystagmus reflex. For low velocities (20° oscillation once every 3 seconds), tracking shows zero phase lag by 12 weeks. This implies anticipation of the oscillating moving target's position, a predictive ability found only in sophisticated control systems. Tracking, then, requires cortical machinery and it cannot be assumed that this machinery is available just because the subcortical accessory optic system and OKN reflex can move the eyes smoothly.

Vergence

Adult vergence has a latency of 130–250 milli-seconds (160 ms typical). Saccades are ballistic. After an initial burst of acceleration, the eyes coast accurately to their target; in so-called *main sequence saccades*, the peak velocity attained is proportional to the amount of rotation programmed. In contrast, vergence motions are under continuous visual control, running to completion only in about 1 second (Jones, 1983).

Angle κ/λ problems

There is a pitfall in vergence measurements to remember when reading the earlier literature or making observations of infants themselves; infants are not necessarily as exotropic as they may appear.

Early experimenters photographed the mid-pupillary axis and assumed coincidence between it and the foveal axis (Wickelgren, 1967, 1969; Maurer, 1975). This is not true; corneal reflections not centred in the pupils generally make the eyes appear more diverged than they really are. This misevaluation of photographic data occurs for several reasons:

(1) A parallax error arises because the virtual image of a corneal reflection does not lie in the plane of the iris.
(2) The sphericity of the cornea displaces the reflection in oblique positions of gaze.
(3) The angle λ is positive in infancy, i.e. the line of sight used for fixating passes on the nasal side of the pupil (*see Table 11.1* and Chapter 16).

Growth in the infant's eyeball causes a reduction in these errors which has been misinterpreted as growing out of an 'infantile exotropia'. Correction for these optical errors of measurement is straight-forward (Slater and Findlay, 1972). After correction, fixation in different parts of the visual field and vergence at different distances may be accurately read from eyeball photographs, but it has still not been established that the line of sight used for fixating really starts at the fovea (absence of fixation disparity, eccentric fixation).

The neonate

Binocular fixation can be demonstrated in newborns as young as 18 hours old (Slater and Findlay, 1975; 12 subjects, median age approximately 1 week). The problem of specifying absolute foveal position is side-stepped by measuring *changes* in vergence; the measurements show that convergence increases as fixation distance changes from 20 to 10″, but binocular fixation is lost at 5″. Like adults, infants are said to have a 'specific distance tendency', but assume a nearer object distance than adults in the absence of

Table 11.1 Ocular and fixation angles

Readily measured	*Difficult to ascertain*
(A) Midpupillary axis	(C) Optic axis; geometrical axis of eye (or retina)
Where the eyeball is	
	Where the fovea is
(B) Line of sight Fixation axis or line	(D) Visual axis Foveal axis Visual line

Angles between lines A, B, C, D

A–B: angle λ. If it were zero, a centred pupillary reflex would mean the subject were fixating the observer/camera, although not necessarily with his fovea. Angle λ is commonly read off photos and interpreted as an angle α; if not zero, then the person is strabismic. However, the interpretation is shaky insofar as axis A is not identical to axis C and B is not identical with D

A–D: angle κ; because these two axes do not coincide but instead form the angle κ with one another, the fovea isn't where you think it is by looking at the pupils. Angle κ is positive in infancy, pupillary axis temporal to foveal axis; eyes appear diverged

C–D: angle α, formed at first nodal point; if not zero, a person appears strabismic when he is orthophoric. Impractical to measure

B–C: angle γ

B–D: He's fixating this point, but is he using his fovea? This angle is non-zero in fixation disparity and eccentric fixation

Notes: Multiple terms in (B) and (D) are synonymous; optic axis and geometrical axis are not. Their specification is inexact, due in part to the non-spherical and scattered nature of the parts of the eye. The concept of optic axis hides problems in specifying and choosing among (1) the corneal axis (major axis of the corneal ellipsoid), (2) the lens axis, (3) the normal to the cornea at its geometrical centre and (4) the (approximate) line passing through the centres of curvature of all optical elements of the eye. The geometrical axis of the eye coincides with the optic axis if all refractive surfaces are symmetrically located within the eye. 'Refractive surface' is itself an abstraction; e.g. the refractive index of the lens varies continuously through its depth.
The *midpupillary axis* should pass perpendicularly through the cornea.
The *visual axis* from the fovea theoretically passes through posterior and anterior nodal points of the eye, as is a jogged (broken) line.
The *fixation axis* connects the external object of fixation to the centre of rotation of the eye.

cues to the contrary. Therefore, vergence testing at intermediate distance produces greatest accuracy; measurements will otherwise be disturbed by fixation disparity.

Although the above group of 12 newborns would change fixation from 20″ to 10″ with an *average* vergence accuracy of 0.5°, one individual's fixation will wander within an area 14° in diameter around a vertical line of interest. (Even if this is taken as a visual scan pattern rather than the best possible fixation, it is very loose.) Vergence changes may be jerky (Slater and Findlay, 1975). Responses to a 5 and even 10 Δ prism (base-out) occur on only about half the trials at 6 months, and almost not at all at 4.5 months (Aslin, 1977). Retarded response to disparity (prism) and a strong early monocular fixation reflex have been suggested as a preclinical stage of strabismus (Cogan, 1982).

Competition between monocular fixation and binocular vergence

Traditionally, increasingly strong and accurate fixation reflexes are assumed to be the basis for the development of motor fusion. However, Cogan (1982) suggests that monocular fixation and binocular vergence are in competition during development, a concept sometimes mentioned in connection with microtropia. Cogan points out that infants will often fixate with one eye. If the bilateral, monocular fixation responses develop precociously compared to binocular fusion, alternating strabismus develops. Improving acuity through careful refraction would then only exacerbate alternating monocular fixation; fogging should be practised instead. Fogging (not over-plussing) should be slight enough to leave pupillary response, vergence initialization and, if possible, accommodation unaffected while impeding foveal fixation. Cogan (1982) distinguishes two groups of strabismics in support of his aetiological model: strabismus onset before age 1 year, strong monocular fixation reflex, alternating tropia and high acuity in both eyes; and onset between 2 and 4 years of age (true vergence disorder), unilateral squint, amblyopia, possible anisometropia. The prevalence of alternation in congenital esotropia is generally acknowledged, but the pattern is more complicated than the Cogan model: for example, Lang (1971) characterizes congenital esotropia by vertical deviation, head turning, excyclorotation of the deviating eye and latent nystagmus (appears when one eye is covered).

This model reminds us that development is not a train timetable showing when stations along the line will be passed. Rather, various systems interact. All mutually assisting systems should be strengthened (trained). But where systems interact competitively, a precociously or unfairly successful component may need to be *hindered*, not assisted.

A co-variance principle for sensory-motor development

In infancy, poor oculomotor control is paralleled by loose single-unit (cortical) tuning, so that oculomotor fluctuations can be tolerated which would cause diplopia and suppression in the adult. Development is a *bootstrap* operation in which increasing refinement of the motor system (more stable fixation) fosters tuning of sensory systems, whose greater stimulus selectivity permits better control of fixation. A co-variance principle can be suggested: observed oculomotor variability is a measure of breadth and scatter of sensory neurones' tuning curves. Similarly, tuning curve widths and cell-to-cell scatter in the visual system limit the precision displayed by oculomotor control.

Stereoscopic depth

Early research measured the infant's gradual progress in navigating the rich visual environment of the everyday visual world. Total fixation time (Fantz, 1961) shows infant preference for three-dimensional spheres over two-dimensional discs. Crawling babies avoid a precipice in the visual cliff apparatus (Walk and Gibson, 1961); the aversion may be detected in 8- and 16-week-old infants by using the unconditioned heart-rate supression response (Campos, Langer and Krowitz, 1970).

The many cues available in these early studies were divided only into 'monocular' and 'binocular'. Recent work definitively isolates the emergence of binocular processing of interocular disparity. After one perceptual cue with one underlying neural-mechanism was isolated, it was discovered that stereopsis appears suddenly during development.

Line-drawing stereograms

Purpose of stereo testing

Testing with either line-drawing or random-dot stereograms seeks simultaneously to establish the existence of binocularity and the ability to discriminate disparity (perceived depth). Ideally, the threshold for disparity discrimination is determined, instead of merely making a go/no-go determination of performance. Sensory fusion has received little attention in work with children. One suspects that Panum's areas are exaggerated during infancy and narrow later. This would obviously free the developing binocular visual system from the danger of suppression during a time of poor oculomotor control.

Results

Suppression of heart rate or sucking reaction in response to the surprising appearance of stereoscopic depth ('dishabituation paradigm') places the emergence of gross stereopsis at a median age of 8.3 weeks (Appel and Campos, 1977; 40 infants). Preferential looking tests (*see* Chapter 12) with line-drawing stereograms show that most infants can detect disparities of 58′ arc at 4 months (Held, Birch and Gwiazda, 1980; six infants). A stereoacuity of 1′ arc was reached at a mean age of 21 weeks, with individual subjects improving from 58′ to 1′ arc in as few as 4 weeks.

Crossed disparity detection emerges earlier (Birch, Gwiazda and Held, 1982), perhaps because it plays a more important role in segregating objects of interest from the background. The earlier emergence implies that crossed and uncrossed disparity detection is served by separate mechanisms, which is known to be the case from cortical neurophysiology (*see* Chapter 14).

The early absence of disparity and correlation detection is not a reflection of vergence error because:

(1) Infants of this age make at least grossly appropriate vergence adjustments.
(2) There are different emergence times for detection of crossed versus uncrossed disparities and patterns defined by uncorrelated–correlated versus disparate random dots (in both cases, the former appears sooner).
(3) Tests with repeating-stripe patterns minimize the effect of incorrect vergence and show the same results.

Random-dot techniques

Random-dot stereograms (RDSs) are employed to prevent successful discrimination based upon monocular cues. RDSs typically have small elements, so that high monocular acuity as well as binocular depth detection is required. This makes such stimuli well suited for population screening. RDSs also require a high degree of cooperation in the clinic, so that with 2- to 5-year-olds, operant reinforcement techniques (e.g. payoff with pennies: Cooper and Feldman, 1978) may be necessary to obtain optimal performance (about 100′ arc: Reinecke and Simons, 1974). Children who do worse than optimally may have refractive problems, transient eye infections or, of course, strabismus. For clinical tests based on random-dot techniques, *see* Chapter 15 and Simons (1981).

To use RDS stimuli with *infants*, the evoked potential (*see* Chapter 13) or a semireflexive oculomotor tracking task (*see below*) must be resorted to.

Stereograms—behavioural

Making a square stand out in depth from the visual 'snow storm' of a dynamic random-dot stereogram is visually dramatic. Infants will follow this floating square when it is made to move sideways with a small microprocessor-based pattern generator. Forcing an adult observer to infer whether the square moved left or right based only on the infant's

response (blind two-alternative forced choice method) provides a sensitive behavioural test of global stereopsis in young infants (*Figure 11.3*). Global stereopsis emerges between 3 and 5 months (Fox *et al.*, 1980; 40 infants; *see Figure 11.4*).

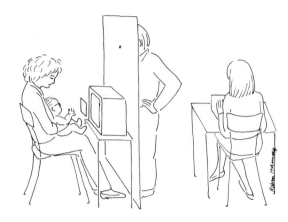

Figure 11.3 Behavioural testing with random-dot stereograms. Infant wearing red and green glasses views a random-dot stereogram portraying a square moving left or right. The examiner behind the screen must identify those trials on which a depth stimulus was presented and its direction of motion, based on the infant's head and eye movements. A second examiner (seated) runs the microprocessor-based stimulus control and data acquisition instrument. (Redrawn from Shea *et al.*, 1980)

Stereograms and correlograms—evoked potential

Evoked potential tests of binocularity in adults, some *not* involving random-dot stereograms, have been described in Chapter 13. Strong evoked potentials can be elicited when disparity is introduced into a random-dot stereogram, when anti-correlation is introduced into a binocular correlogram, or when random non-correlation is introduced into the same binocular correlogram (Julesz, Kropfl and Petrig, 1980). In the latter case, for example, a patch of dots is chosen to be black or white at random for each eye and on average half do not match, whereas, outside the patch, dots are all binocularly matched. All dots are picked anew at the frame rate of the display (e.g. 60 times a second—this is dynamic visual noise).

Correlograms are technically easier to produce than stereograms. Correlogram-evoked responses appear in normal infants between the ages of 2 and 4.3 months (Braddick and Atkinson, 1982), in good agreement with results from other methods.

Julesz, Kropfl and Petrig (1980) point out that with correlograms: 'The combination of three technological innovations permits the fast and objective determination of stereopsis in nonverbal subjects':

(1) Correlograms are as effective as stereograms in eliciting a visual evoked response (VER), but are much easier to generate.
(2) A correlogram is insensitive to head tilt, because uncorrelation (binocular rivalry) does not depend on the direction (horizontalness) of binocular disparity as is true with depth perception.
(3) Projection TV systems provide large screens which surround the subject so they cannot look away.

The waveform for a correlation change is different from that for a true disparity stimulus, but probably reflects the same brain mechanisms: neither occur in stereoblind children or adults, both are strong in stereonormal children and adults and, lastly, the growth of evoked responses to correlograms and to stereograms follows the same time course in infants.

Other binocularity tests

Symmetry of OKN

Optokinetic nystagmus produces tracking eye movements interrupted by fast return saccades identical in form to vestibular or labyrinthine nystagmus. It is an involuntary reflex which stabilizes the retinal image, and has long been employed to measure acuity (*see* Chapter 12).

The *monocular* OKN reflex to *temporalward* movement in the visual field is an effective test of binocularity. When it fails, cortical binocularity has been lost (e.g. adult stereoblindness, amblyopia). The same OKN asymmetry also occurs in the neonate; temporalward movement emerges later (3 months; Atkinson, 1979; Naegele and Held, 1982; 50 infants), at the same time or slightly earlier than stereopsis. The extrageniculostriate centres (nucleus of the optic tract and accessory optic system) involved in OKN and their dependence on the visual cortex for binocularity are described in Chapter 13.

Pupillary response

When a monocularly occluded eye is uncovered, the contralateral pupil shows a phasic contraction termed the 'consensual pupillary response', and then returns to a steady size which is smaller than it was with monocular viewing. The initial consensual response is present from birth; increased resting state contraction reflects binocular summation. The summation appears in infants at the same time as stereodepth sensitivity (16–24 weeks; Birch and Held, 1983). However, this form of binocular summation does not appear to be closely correlated with indicators of cortical binocularity (e.g. stereoblindness) in the adult.

The pupillary response is thought to be subcortically driven by nuclei receiving W-stream input

(Rodieck, 1979). Like the optokinetic nystagmus reflex, corticofugal input might reach the relevant nuclei during development, decreasing latency and conferring binocularity. The amblyopic eye of adults (Kase *et al.*, 1984) and infants too young to exhibit (cortically determined) stereopsis (Shea, Doussard-Roosevelt and Aslin, 1985) do both indeed have prolonged pupillary latencies (10% and 40% longer, respectively). Latency and not just summation should be tested as a sign of binocularity.

Depth perception from non-disparity pictorial cues (e.g. shading) is more cognitive and emerges later than stereopsis (5–7 months; Granrud, Yonas and Opland, 1985).

Conclusions

All infant tests suggest that binocular cortical function first emerges at 3–5 months (*Figure 11.4*). In the kitten (Timney, 1981), emergence of behaviourally demonstrable depth discrimination ability coincides with the maturation of depth-detecting binocular

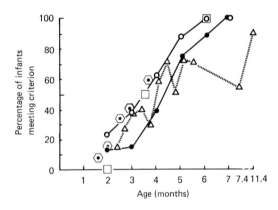

Figure 11.4 Sudden onset of disparity detection at age of about 3 months. Percentage of infants meeting criterion for detection is shown as a function of the infants' age. **Open circles:** behavioural, preferential looking, line stereograms; 58' arc disparities, 128 infants in all (Birch *et al.* 1982). **Filled circles:** as for open circles but 1' arc criterion (Birch *et al.*, 1982). **Large open squares:** evoked potentials, combined results for correlation–anticorrelation and random-dot stereograms, *N* = 13 (Petrig *et al.*, 1981). **Hexagons:** evoked potential, correlation–anticorrelation, 15 infants, median age of onset is 91 days (Braddick *et al.*,1983). **Triangles:** behavioural, forced choice preferential tracking, global stereopsis (random-dot stereograms) (Fox, 1981; approx. 142 infants, median age of onset, 127 days)

neurones, and the same is probably true in man. However, if an animal must be capable of running away from danger across rough ground when it is born, it will be born with functional disparity detectors; at least this is true in the newborn lamb (Ramachandran, Clarke and Whitteridge, 1977). In man, disparity detection and the oculomotor 'plant' to support it emerge suddenly at 3 months. Cortical maturation is responsible. Oculomotor improvement occurs at the same time in part because maturing visual cortical neurones gain access to subcortical oculomotor centres.

Onset of stereopsis or amblyopia

New neonatal testing methods show that sensory (mal)adaptations can first appear *after* the start of strabismus. This proves that esotropia is at least sometimes congenital and primary, while amblyopia and stereoblindness are secondary and, perhaps purely sensory adaptations. The oculomotor system, not the visual system, is the villain in this case.

It has been shown that stereopsis appears as usual at 3–5 months in a congenital esotropic infant, if the infant wears prism correction to bring disparities into the range of normal correspondence when tested (Birch and Stager, 1985). Without treatment, the infant immediately thereafter begins a descent toward stereoblindness. Monocular *acuity* loss takes longer to manifest itself, and was first detectable at 9 months (unilateral esotropes).

Other recent work (Jacobson, Mohindra and Held, 1981b) has demonstrated acuity differences between the eyes of neonatal strabismics at an average age of 5 months. In one infant whose esotropia emerged suddenly at 10 months, the ensuing deterioration in monocular acuity could be detected within 4 weeks. Rapid drops in acuity (and rapid recovery if sharp retinal images are restored) is the same for all causes of deprivation: eyelid closure from burns or infection, media opacities (e.g. cataract) and occlusion (Jacobson, Mohindra and Held, 1983).

There may be truth in the observation (e.g. Haase, 1984) that many infant esotropes are capable of enough alternation to keep acuity development on a normal course for a while. But the classic view that amblyopia is most likely to become manifest between the first and second birthdays must be re-examined with new acuity testing methods.

The vulnerability of stereopsis

In both the cat (Timney, 1984) and man, acuity improves more gradually, and over a longer time period, than binocular disparity processing. In both the cat and the monkey, stereopsis loss from stimulus deprivation is almost permanent, while acuity can be recovered. Stereopsis is most susceptible to damage from monocular deprivation when, in the cat, binocular neurones are most rapidly shaping their tuning curves to adult levels. This echoes

Scott's hypothesis (Scott, 1978) that plasticity occurs when growth is most rapid.

The simplest explanation for the vulnerability of stereopsis is the severity of the visual deprivation: strabismus greater than about 10° shifts disparity input completely out of its normal range, but does not greatly reduce the image quality of patterned visual input. Neurones can nurture their receptive fields in one eye or the other, even though coordination between the eyes is hopeless. Binocularity loss follows and is (along with spatial confusion, e.g. crowding and phase errors) a defining characteristic of strabismic amblyopia.

Special topics

Two visual systems

Several provocative suggestions for separating groups of neural structures and clusters of visual functions have been made. Within the limits in which these dichotomies are valid, the systems or skills involved may be expected to develop along separate timetables.

Primary and secondary visual systems

The primary system includes the classic retino-cortical pathways to higher centres of conscious perception. The secondary system is the tectothalamic system, dominated by the superior colliculus, which enjoys corticofugal as well as direct retinal innervation. This dichotomy (applied to infant development: Bronson, 1974; Karmel and Maisel, 1975) emphasizes the difference between the development of high-sensitivity, high-selectivity visual skills (acuities in central vision) and object identification versus the development of both oculomotor control (lower aspects of saccadic eye movements, tracking and vergence) and orienting reflexes, e.g. turning head and eyes toward a sound. There is some value in the generalization that the secondary system matures first. Today a third system would be added, the *accessory optic system*, including nuclei principally in the pretectal area responsible for optokinetic nystagmus and vestibulo-ocular reflexes. These are functioning at birth, but sometimes await input from the primary system to make them fast and binocular (*see* Chapter 13).

X and Y visual channels

This dichotomy distinguishes the acquisition of good temporal from good spatial resolution. Where both streams grow into the same area, competition can cripple the later arrival; the loss of Y cells in a monocularly deprived lateral geniculate nucleus of a cat is an example.

The functional and conceptual distinctions which have been suggested (*see below*) cut across the above neural dichotomies (*see* Chapter 13).

Central versus peripheral visual field development

A rule observed by the fovea but not generally otherwise is that central visual field functions develop later. This dichotomy echoes others: the Y system is more heavily involved in peripheral field processing, if not because of XY cell density differences at the retinal level, then because of the peripheral weighting given by cortical areas to which the Y stream provides an important input. Subcortically, the secondary and tertiary (accessory) optical systems lack the foveal dominance of the primary visual system, and are also nearly devoid of X input.

Where versus what

This dichotomy distinguishes the good alerting and orienting behaviours of the infant from his/her poorer ability to identify what he/she is seeing. The dichotomy evokes the primary/secondary distinction. The primary system, especially in inferotemporal cortex, is concerned with recognizing the pattern. Where to direct the head and gaze is the concern of the secondary visual system. Y and X systems may also be characterized as 'where' and 'what' systems, but the Y system also plays an important role in motion perception. A more apt Y/X dichotomization is: 'Quickly, where is it?' (with some advice about gross form) versus 'What colour and details does it have?'

The focal/ambient dichotomy

This is similar to 'what' versus 'where', and more closely tied to neurophysiological research (Schneider, 1967; Held, 1968; Trevarthen, 1968). It emphasizes the difference between deciding what one is fixating, and the many spatial orientation skills which are a prerequisite to getting the eyes and head turned toward the object. These include constructing an *allocentric map* of the external space (room) one is occupying, and maintaining an updated *egocentric map* of how the body is positioned in this space. The focal/ambient functional dichotomy was originally couched in terms of the primary (especially striate cortex) and secondary (superior colliculus) distinction, but sophisticated allocentric and egocentric map construction requires higher brain centres. The dorsal occipitoparietal projection of the primary visual system, relayed through the movement-sensitive mediotemporal cortex, is thought to be important in the construction of such maps.

The egocentric localization errors which occur in strabismus (e.g. past-pointing) arise here, in different cortical areas from the earlier ones where the angle of anomaly in binocular correspondence is set. Therefore, past-pointing errors often do not match the angle of anomalous correspondence (Sireteanu and Fronius, 1986). Little is known about these areas today. This will be tomorrow's frontier in strabismus research.

Local/global

The local/global distinction is narrower and closely tied to spatial frequency channel concepts (*see* Chapter 13). High acuity channels are important for local processing; global analysis (spread more widely across the visual field) can better begin with low spatial frequency channels. Used in this way, 'local versus *gross* analysis' would be more apt; globality is a narrower technical problem in random-dot stereograms. There is some truth in the generalization that grosser analysis develops earlier and occurs faster.

These dichotomies should not be regarded as absolute truths but should be used to provide a framework within which the facts that are known at present can be ordered.

Concluding remarks
Guiding the child out of the critical period

During early development, acuity is labile and the eyes compete for cortical access. Performance gains in one eye are matched by reciprocal losses in the other and binocular balance is in constant jeopardy. Management is delicate but rewarding, because changes are dramatic. In paediatrics today, increasing survival rates among infants born with low birthweights adds to the need for visual assessment tests (Morse and Trief, 1985) and treatment programmes capable of guiding the infant out of the critical period of visual development.

Treatment of aphakic infants with contact lenses can provide enough visual stimulation to keep acuity developing normally until 12–14 months. After bilateral cataract removal, however, preserving balance between the eyes requires repeated acuity testing and a partial occlusion regimen which is adjusted accordingly. Acuity loss may be the first sign of an ill-fitting or decentred contact lens (Maurer, Lewis and Brent, 1987). These are new procedures and new responsibilities for the practitioner. It is not yet known how long development can be kept on a normal course after 14 months or whether extraordinary means of stimulation can be found if development falters.

Cortical awakening at 3–5 months

Many important developments occur at 3–5 months:

(1) Monocular optokinetic nystagmus becomes symmetrical as the missing temporalward direction appears.
(2) Pupillary response shows binocular summation.
(3) Vestibulo-ocular reflexes can be inhibited to better maintain fixation.
(4) The contrast sensitivity function (CSF) begins to roll off at low spatial frequencies.
(5) Oculomotor tracking appears.
(6) Aversion to rivalrous stimuli appears.
(7) Stereopsis itself appears.
(8) Vernier acuity first becomes superior to grating acuity ('hyperacuity' appears).

Many of these changes reflect the ascendancy of the visual cortex. Lateral inhibition becomes available to sharpen neural selectivity and, partly because of this inhibition, better acuity is available to lock the eyes on target during tracking. Binocular neurones become available to support disparity processing for depth perception and vergence. Single unit tuning curves for disparity and orientation emerge (Braddick, Wattam-Bell and Atkinson, 1986) and become sharper. The cortex begins to contribute to and sometimes control lower centres: the nucleus of the optic tract gains binocularity from arriving corticofugal fibres (leading to OKN symmetry), the W-cell driven pupillary response (*see* Chapter 13) becomes faster, perhaps because of corticofugal input, and some helpful but gross vestibulo-ocular reflexes to body movement become able to be inhibited by higher centres so that more refined, visually locked fixation can prevail. This period also marks the point at which occlusion therapy begins to affect acuity, and is probably the start of the critical period.

It can be expected that future research will show that the familiar dendritic arborization story in visual cortex is the tip of an iceberg: functional architecture (e.g. ocular dominance columns) is also being refined postnatally, and the newest pathways in the brain, from neocortex *back* to older, distant subcortical centres, become active. At this time the practitioner, too, must be active, to be sure the congenitally disadvantaged infant has been identified and a treatment programme is ready.

Kinds of development

The philosopher's dichotomy between *nativist* and *empiricist factors* has not proved fruitful, because maturation involves the interaction of these factors. The role(s) of experience are better described as maintenance, facilitation and induction (Gottlieb, 1976). Gottlieb's refinement leads to the comprehensive scheme of Aslin and Dumais (1980), shown in *Figure 11.5*.

In terms of *Figure 11.5*, vestibulo-ocular reflexes, for example, are almost fully developed by birth, the development of optokinetic nystagmus is partial (temporalward movement is lacking) and stereopsis does not emerge until about 3 months. The emergence is a matter of a maturational schedule which even the congenital esotrope follows. Binocularity emergence is not *induced* by visual input from normally aligned eyes. After a scheduled emergence, experience facilitates the sharpening of binocular single-unit disparity tuning. If esotropia is present, binocularity and stereopsis will emerge and then be lost. 'Facilitation' understates the role of experience in providing guidance for maturation. Maturation with feedback from the environment draws upon uniformly and broadly capable neural resources and commits them to specific functions which they would otherwise never perform.

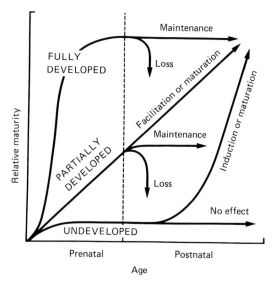

Figure 11.5 The role of experience in development may be induction, maintenance or facilitation. (Redrawn from Aslin and Dumais, 1980)

Acknowledgements

Preparation of the chapters by JIN was supported in part by NIMH grant 34793, the Naval Air Systems Command, and the Air Force Office of Scientific Research 83–0225. Linda Misa provided invaluable bibliographic help. I thank colleagues for generously sharing their work and comments, and Robin Hannay Nelson for drawing *Figure 11.3*.

References

AMIGO, G. (1972) Visuo-sensory development of the child. *Am. J. Optom. Arch. Am. Acad. Optom.* **49**, 991–1001

AMIGO, G. (1978) Fixation and its anomalies. *Aust. J. Optom.* **61**, 418–432

APPEL, M.A. and CAMPOS, J.J. (1977) Binocular disparity as a discriminable stimulus parameter for young infants. *J. Exp. Child Psychol.*, **23**, 47–56

ASLIN, R.N. (1977) Development of binocular fixation in human infants. *J. Exp. Child Psychol.*, **23**, 133–150

ASLIN, R.N. (1981) The development of smooth pursuit in human infants. In *Eye Movements: Cognition and Visual Perception*, edited by D. F. Fisher, R. A. Monty and J. W. Senders, pp. 31–51. Hillsdale, NJ: Erlbaum

ASLIN, R.N. (1987) Motor aspects of visual development in infancy. In *Handbook of Infant Perception*, edited by P. Salapatek and L. B. Cohen, pp.43–113. New York: Academic Press

ASLIN, R.N. and DUMAIS, S.T. (1980) Binocular vision in infants: a review and a theoretical framework. *Adv. Child Dev. Behav.*, **15**, 53–94

ATKINSON, J. (1979) Development of optokinetic nystagmus in the human infant and monkey infant: an analogue to development in kittens. In *Developmental Neurobiology of Vision*, edited by R. D. Freeman. New York: Plenum Press

ATKINSON, J. and BRADDICK, O.J. (1979) New techniques for assessing vision in infants and young children. *Child. Care, Health Develop.*, **5**, 389–398

ATKINSON, J. and BRADDICK, O. (1981) Acuity, contrast sensitivity, and accommodation in infancy. In *The Development of Perception: Psychobiological Perspective*, edited by R. N. Aslin, J. R. Alberts and M. R. Peterson, Vol. 2, pp. 245–278. New York: Academic Press

ATKINSON, J., BRADDICK, O. and MOAR, K. (1977) Development of contrast sensitivity over the first 3 months of life in the human infant. *Vision Res.*, **17**, 1037–1044

BANKS, M.S. (1980) The development of visual accommodation during early infancy. *Child Dev.*, **51**, 646–666

*BANKS, M.S. and SALAPATEK, P. (1983) Infant visual perception. In *Handbook of Child Psychology*, 4th edn, chief editor P. H. Mussen, Vol. II, *Infancy and Developmental Psychobiology*, edited by M. M. Haith and J. J. Campos, pp. 435–571. New York: Wiley

BIRCH, E. E., GWIAZDA, J. and HELD, R. (1982) Stereoacuity development for crossed and uncrossed disparities in human infants. *Vision Res.*, **22**, 507–513

BIRCH, E.E. and HELD, R. (1983) The development of binocular summation in human infants. *Invest. Ophthalmol. Vis. Sci.*, **24**, 1103–1107

BIRCH, E.E. and STAGER, D.R. (1985) Monocular acuity and stereopsis in infantile esotropia. *Invest. Ophthalmol. Vis. Sci.*, **26**, 1624–1630

*BOOTHE, R.G., DOBSON, V. and TELLER, D.Y. (1985) Postnatal development of vision in human and non-human primates. *Annu. Rev. Neurosci.*, **8**, 495–545

BRADDICK, O.J. and ATKINSON, J. (1982) The development of binocular function in infancy. *Acta Ophthalmol. Suppl.*, **157**, 27–35

BRADDICK, O.J., ATKINSON, J., FRENCH, J. and HOWLAND, H.C. (1979) A photorefractive study of infant accommodation. *Vision Res.*, **19**, 1319–1330

BRADDICK, O.J., WATTAM-BELL, J., DAY, J. and ATKINSON, J. (1983) The onset of binocular function in human infants. *Human Neurobiol.*, **2**, 65–69

BRADDICK, O.J., WATTAM-BELL, J. and ATKINSON, J. (1986) Orientation-specific cortical responses develop in early infancy. *Nature*, **320**, 617–619

BRONSON, G.W. (1974) The postnatal growth of visual capacity. *Child Dev.*, **45**, 873–890

CAMPOS, J.J., LANGER, A. and KROWITZ, A. (1970) Cardiac responses on the visual cliff in prelocomotor human infants. *Science*, **170**, 196–197

COGAN, A.I. (1982) Foveal fixation competing with binocular fusion? A developmental hypothesis. In *Functional Basis of Ocular Motility Disorders* edited by G. Lennerstrand, D.S. Zee and E.L. Keller, Wenner-Gren Symposium Series, Vol. 37, pp. 233–236. New York: Pergamon

COOPER, J. and FELDMAN, J. (1978) Operant conditioning and assessment of stereopsis in young children. *Am. J. Optom. Physiol. Opt.*, **55**, 532–542

DOBSON, V., FULTON, A. B. and SEBRIS, L. (1984) Cycloplegic refractions of infants and young children: the axis of astigmatism. *Invest. Opthalmol. Vis. Sci.*, **25**, 83–87

*DOBSON, V. and TELLER, D. Y. (1978) Visual acuity in human infants: a review and comparison of behavioral and electrophysiological studies. *Vision Res.*, **18**, 1469–1483

FANTZ, R.L. (1961) The origin of form perception. *Sci. Am.*, **204**, 66–72.(Reprinted *Frontiers of Psychological Research*, edited by S. Coopersmith San Francisco: W. H. Freeman, 1966, pp. 36–42 & 308)

FOX, R. (1981) Stereopsis in animals and human infants: a review of behavioral investigations. In *The Development of Perception: Psychobiological Perspectives*, edited by R. N. Aslin, J. R. Albert and M. R. Petersen, Vol. 2, pp. 335–381. New York: Academic Press

FOX, R., ASLIN, R.N., SHEA, S.L. and DUMAIS, S.T. (1980) Stereopsis in human infants. *Science*, **207**, 323–324

GOTTLIEB, G. (1976) The roles of experience in the development of behavior and the nervous system. In *Neural and Behavioral Specificity*, edited by G. Gottlieb, pp. 25–54. New York: Academic Press

GRANRUD, C.E., YONAS, A. and OPLAND, E. A. (1985) Infants' sensitivity to the depth cue of shading. *Percept. Psychophys.*, **37**, 415–419

GWIAZDA, J., SCHEIMAN, M. and HELD, R. (1984) Anisotropic resolution in children's vision. *Vision Res.*, **24**, 527–531

HAMER, R.D. and SCHNECK, M.E. (1984) Spatial summation in dark-adapted human infants. *Vision Res.*, **23**, 77–85

HAASE, W. (1984) Amblyopie aus der Sicht des Augenklinikers. In *Pathophysiologie des Sehens. Grundlagenforschung und Klinik der visuellen Sensorik*, edited by V. Herzau, pp. 197–206. Stuttgart: Ferdinand Enke

HAINLINE, L., TURKEL, J., ABRAMOV, I., LEMERISE, E. and HARRIS, C.M. (1984) Characteristics of saccades in human infants. *Vision Res.*, **24**, 1771–1780

*HAITH, M.M. (1986) Sensory and perceptual processes in early infancy. *J. Pediatr.*, **109**, 158–171

HAYNES, H., WHITE, B.L. and HELD, R. (1965) Visual accommodation in human infants. *Science*, **148**, 528–530

HELD, R. (1968) Dissociation of visual functions by deprivation and rearrangement. *Psychol. Forschung.*, **31**, 338–348

HELD, R. (1984) Binocular vision—behavioral and neuronal development. In *Neonate Cognition: Beyond the Blooming Buzzing Confusion*, edited by J. Mehler and R. Fox, pp 37–44. Hillsdale, NJ: Erlbaum

HELD, R., BIRCH, E. and GWIAZDA, J. (1980). Stereoacuity of human infants. *Proc. Natl Acad. Sci. USA*, **77**, 5572–5574

HOWLAND, H.C. and SAYLES, N. (1984) Photorefractive measurements of astigmatism in infants and young children. *Invest. Ophthalmol. Vis. Sci.*, **25**, 93–102

JACOBSON, S.G., MOHINDRA, I. and HELD, R. (1981a) Development of visual acuity in infants with congenital cataracts. *Brit. J. Ophthalmol.*, **65**, 727–735

JACOBSON, S.G., MOHINDRA, I. and HELD, R. (1981b) Age of onset of amblyopia in infants with esotropia. In *Doc. Ophthalmol. Proc. Series*, **30**, 210–216

JACAOBSON, S.G., MOHINDRA, I. and HELD, R. (1983) Monocular visual form deprivation in human infants. *Doc. Ophthalmol.*, **55**, 199–211

JONES, R. (1983) Horizontal disparity vergence. In *Vergence Eye Movements: Basic and Clinical Aspects*, edited by C. M. Schor and K. J. Ciuffreda, pp. 297–316. Boston: Butterworths

JULESZ, B., KROPFL, W. and PETRIG, B. (1980) Large evoked potentials to dynamic random-dot correlograms and stereograms permit quick determination of stereopsis. *Proc. Natl Acad. Sci. USA*, **77**, 2348–2351

KARMEL, B.Z. and MAISEL, E.B. (1975) A neuronal activity model for infant visual attention. In *Infant Perception: From Sensation to Cognition*, edited by L. B. Cohen and P.Salapatek, *Basic Visual Processes*, Vol. 1. New York: Academic Press

KASE, M., NAGATA, R., YOSHIDA, A. and HANADA, I. (1984) Pupillary light reflex in amblyopia. *Invest. Ophthalmol. Vis. Sci.*, **25**, 467–471

KUPERSMITH, M.J. and NELSON, J.I. (1986) Preserved visual evoked potential in infancy cortical blindness. Relationship to blindsight. *Neuro-opthalmology*, **6**, 85–94

LANG, J. (1971) Congenital convergent strabismus. *Int. Ophthalmol. Clins*, **11**, 88–92

MAURER, D. (1975) Infant visual perception: Methods of study. In *Infant Perception: From Sensation to Cognition*, edited by L. B. Cohen and P. Salapatek, Vol. 1: *Basic Visual Processes*, pp. 1–76. New York: Academic Press

MAURER, D., LEWIS, T.L. and BRENT, H. P. (1987) The effects of deprivation on human visual development: studies of children treated for cataracts. In *Applied Developmental Psychology*, edited by F. J. Morrison, C. E. Lord and D. P. Keating, Vol. 3. New York: Academic Press

MOHINDRA, I., JACOBSON, S.G. and HELD, R. (1983) Binocular visual form deprivation in human infants. *Doc. Ophthalmol.*, **55**, 237–249

MOHINDRA, I., JACOBSON, S.G., THOMAS, J. and HELD, R. (1979) Development of amblyopia in infants. *Trans. Opthalmol. Soc. UK*, **99**, 344–346

MORRONE, M.C. and BURR, D.C. (1986) Evidence for the existence and development of visual inhibition in humans. *Nature*, **321**, 235–237

MORSE, A.R. and TRIEF, E. (1985) Diagnosis and evaluation of visual dysfunction in premature infants with low birth weight. *J. Vis. Impair. Blindness*, June, 248–251

MOSKOWITZ, A. and SOKOL, S. (1983) Developmental changes in the human visual system as reflected by the latency of the pattern reversal VEP. *Electroen. Clin. Neurophysiol.*, **56**, 1–15

NAEGELE, J.R. and HELD, R. (1982) The postnatal development of monocular optokinetic nystagmus in infants. *Vision Res.*, **22**, 341–346

NELSON, J.I. and FROST, B.J. (1978) Orientation-selective inhibition from beyond the classic visual receptive field. *Brain Res.*, **139**, 359–365

PETRIG, B., JULESZ, B., KROPFL. W., BAUMGARTNER, G. and ANLIKER, M. (1981) Development of stereopsis and cortical binocularity in human infants: electrophysiological evidence. *Science*, **213**, 1402–1405

RAMACHANDRAN, V.S., CLARKE, P.G.H. and WHITTERIDGE, D. (1977) Cells selective to binocular disparity in the cortex of newborn lambs. *Nature*, **268**, 333–335

REINECKE, R.D. and SIMONS, K. (1974) A new stereoscopic test for amblyopia screening. *Am. J. Ophthalmol.*, **78**, 714–721

RODIECK, R.W. (1979) Visual pathways. *Annu. Rev. Neurosci.*, **2**, 193–225

SCHNEIDER, G.E. (1967) Contrasting visumotor functions of tectum and cortex in the golden hamster. *Psychol. Forschung.*, **31**, 52–62

SCOTT, J.P. (ed.) (1978) *Critical Periods*. Benchmark Papers in Animal Behavior, Vol. 12. See pp. 344–367. Stroudsburg, PA: Dowden, Hutchinson & Ross (Academic Press, distributors)

SHEA, S.L., DOUSSARD-ROOSEVELT, J.A. and ASLIN, R.N. (1985) Pupillary measures of binocular luminance summation in infants and stereoblind adults. *Invest. Ophthmal. Vis. Sci.*, **26**, 1064–1070

SHEA, S.L., FOX, R., ASLIN, R.N. and DUMAIS, S.T. (1980) Assessment of stereopsis in human infants. *Invest. Ophthalmol. Vis. Sci.*, **19**, 1400–1404

SHIMOJO, S., BAUER, J. Jr, O'CONNELL, K. M. and HELD, R. (1986) Pre-stereoptic binocular vision in infants. *Vision Res.*, **26**, 501–510

SIMONS, K. (1981) Stereoacuity norms in young children. *Arch. Ophthalmol.*, **99**, 439–445

SIRETEANU, R. and FRONIUS, M. (1986) Verzerrte Raumwahrnehmung bei Amblyopen. *Z. praktische Augenheilk.*, **7**, 243–246

SLATER, A.M. and FINDLAY, J.M. (1972) The measurement of fixation position in the newborn baby. *J. Exp. Child Psychol.*, **14**, 349–364

SLATER, A.M. and FINDLAY, J.M. (1975) Binocular fixation in the newborn baby. *J. Exp. Child Psychol.*, **20**, 248–273

TAYLOR, D., VAEGAN, MORRIS, J.A., RODGERS, J.E. and WARLAND, J. (1979) Amblyopia in bilateral infantile and juvenile cataract. Relationship to timing of treatment. *Trans. Opthalmol. Soc. UK*, **99**, 170–175

TELLER, D.Y. (1982) Scotopic vision, color vision, and stereopsis in infants. *Curr. Eye Res.*, **2**, 199–210

*TELLER, D.Y. and MOVSHON, J.A. (1986) Visual development. *Vision Res.*, **26**, 1483–1506

TIMNEY, B. (1981) Development of binocular depth perception in kittens. *Invest. Ophthalmol. Vis. Sci.*, **21**, 493–496

TIMNEY, B. (1984) Monocular deprivation and binocular depth perception in kittens. In *Development of Visual Pathways in Mammals*, edited by J. Stone, B. Dreher and D.H. Rapaport, pp. 405–423. New York: Alan Liss

TREVARTHEN, C.B. (1968) Two mechanisms of vision in primates. *Psychol. Forschung*, **31**, 299–337

VAN SLUYTERS, R.C. and MALACH, R. (1984) Recovery from the cortical effects of visual deprivation in the kitten. In *Development of Visual Pathways in Mammals*, edited by J. Stone, B. Dreher and D. H. Rapaport, pp. 393–404. New York: Alan Liss

VON NOORDEN, G.K. (1985) Amblyopia: a multidisciplinary approach. (Proctor Lecture) *Invest. Ophthalmol. Vis. Sci.*, **26**, 1704–1716

WALK, R.D. and GIBSON, E.J. (1961) A comparative and analytical study of visual depth perception. *Psychol. Monographs* **75** (519), pp. 1–44

WESTHEIMER, G. (1986) Physiological optics during the first quarter-century of *Vision Research*. *Vision Res.*, **26**, 1515–1521

WICKELGREN, L.W. (1967) Convergence in the human newborn. *J. Exp. Child Psychol.*, **5**, 74–85

WICKELGREN, L.W. (1969) The ocular response of human newborns to intermittent visual movements. *J. Exp. Child Psychol.*, **8**, 469–482

YUODELIS, C. and HENDRICKSON, A. (1986) A qualitative and quantitative analysis of the human fovea during development. *Vision Res.*, **26**, 847–855

Further reading

ATKINSON, J. and BRADDICK, O. J. (1981) Development of optokinetic nystagmus in infants: an indicator of cortical binocularity. In *Eye Movements: Cognition and Visual Perception*, edited by D. F. Fisher, R. A. Monty and T. W. Senders, pp. 53–64. Hillsdale, NJ: Erlbaum

BRADDICK, O. J. and ATKINSON, J. (1983) Some recent findings on the development of human binocularity: a review. *Behavioural Brain Res.*, **10**, 141–150

JAY, B. (ed.) (1986) Detection and measurement of visual impairment in pre-verbal children. *Doc. Ophthalmol. Proc. Ser.*, **45**, 1–403

MITCHELL, D.E. and TIMNEY, B. (1984) Postnatal development of function in the mammalian visual system. In *American Physiological Society Handbook of Physiology*, Section 1: *The Nervous System*. Vol. III, edited by Ian Darian-Smith, *Sensory Processes*, Part 1, pp. 507–555. Baltimore: Williams & Wilkins

*Those references with an asterisk could also be used as further reading.

12

Examination techniques

Keith Edwards

In the examination of the child patient, most of the basic clinical skills and techniques are, with a few notable exceptions, the same as for adult patients. However, patient management and the application of these clinical techniques has to be flexible and adapted to whatever degree of cooperation is obtainable from the subject. The fact that the arbitrary classification of 'child' encompasses a wide range of ages, abilities and maturity means that the exact aims of the examination and the relative importance of the individual components of the examination will be varied according to the prevailing circumstances.

The way in which tests are applied to children is often far less scientifically exact than for adults, while still providing significant information. The examiner will often need to apply the tests whenever the child will cooperate for long enough and, for this reason, every assessment made should yield a valid result at first attempt (wherever possible) because another opportunity may not readily present itself. Distractions should be avoided and, in some cases, this may mean leaving the rest of the family at home or at least outside the consulting room. It is normal for the parent to be present, although occasionally this is contraindicated. The practitioner should attempt to gain the child's confidence by talking and playing for a short while before trying to apply tests. The tests themselves should be presented as another form of play and an even temper is a prerequisite for the practitioner.

Aims of the examination

While the parent's aim almost invariably will be to gain assurance that the child's visual faculties are unimpaired, the number and relative sophistication of the tests applied to allow this goal to be achieved will change depending on the cooperation of the child (and parent) as well as on the circumstances that precipitated the visit. For example, the child presenting with signs or symptoms of convergent squint will be given an exhaustive battery of examinations which will include a cycloplegic refraction, while the child brought for routine assessment without signs, symptoms or any relevant personal or family history is unlikely to require the same intensity of assessment. For this reason, it is essential that the practitioner dealing with pre-school-age children, in particular, should develop an ability to determine the aims of the visit as the patient, the symptoms and history are assessed in the earliest stages of the consultation. *Table 12.1* shows some of the principal reasons for considering an exhaustive assessment irrespective of age.

Table 12.1 Possible indications for detailed patient assesment

Poor or unequal acuities
Manifest squint or equivocal cover test result
Report of intermittent squint (*see* text for choice of cycloplegic)
Suspect result to initial indirect ocular motor balance assessment (*see* later text for description)
Reduced accommodation and/or convergence
Significant variation in initial retinoscopy reflex or hypermetropia over 2 D by initial retinoscopy
Relevant close family history
Unexplained signs or symptoms

Methods of assessment
Vision and visual acuity

Depending on the age of the child, the level of vision can be measured with varying accuracy.

Alternate occlusion (suitable from a few weeks)

In the very young child, there is often little that can be performed clinically to measure acuity but, by using alternate occlusion, some assessment of the equality of vision between the two eyes can be made. Each eye is occluded in turn, generally by resting one hand on the child's forehead and then dropping the thumb down in the line of the visual axis. If each eye has approximately equal acuity there will be no difference in response as each eye is covered. However when a dominant eye is occluded leaving vision to an amblyopic or ametropic eye, the child will usually show signs of disquiet by trying to move away from the occluding thumb, trying to move the hand of the examiner or by making a vocal objection! As with all tests for young children and babies requiring some degree of fixation, the fixation target should be whatever can maintain the child's interest for long enough. The technique can be refined further by assessing the child's response to a small target such as sugar strands, hundreds and thousands or cotton threads. If each eye has reasonable acuity, then the interest and attempts to pick up these strands should be the same whichever eye is covered. Caution must be exercised in interpretation, however, since a child's attention span is short and a poor response with the second eye may simply signify boredom. Equally, the test overall relies on hand–eye coordination and dexterity which are developing skills appearing at about 9 months (Sheridan, 1975), but with a high degree of variation even in normal babies.

Stycar ball test (suitable from about 6 months)

This test uses polystyrene spheres as an assessment of vision. In the dynamic test, the child is usually seated on the parent's lap while a helper attracts fixation with a toy or light. The examiner then rolls the sphere into the line of vision and determines whether the child fixates the target as it enters the field of vision. By reducing the size of sphere until no response is obtained, or the smallest is seen, an assessment of acuity is made.

In the static test, the sphere is mounted on a wand and introduced into the periphery of the visual field and the examiner determines whether the child fixates the target. The target size is reduced as before.

Matching toy tests (suitable from 2 to 3 years)

These tests rely on the child's ability to recognize toys held up by the examiner, usually at 3 m, and pick up a matching one from a number held in front of him or placed in the lap. To avoid confusion, the number of choices must be kept to three or four.

The main difficulty in this test is that the various toys are usually so dissimilar that a correct choice can be made without good acuity.

Picture test charts (suitable from about 2 years)

Picture charts employ silhouettes of simple objects or toys which the child should be able to recognize before they are able to read letters. Charts such as the Beale Collins and Clement Clarke types have usually suffered the disadvantage that the silhouettes were dissimilar in detail and thus gave an unreliable measure of acuity (Keith, Diamond and Stansfield, 1972). Some versions were reported to give good results (Hyams and Neumann, 1977), but more recently picture-based charts have been designed which conform to the Snellen principle and are available with single letter (Kay, 1983) and line letter presentations (Elliott, 1985).

Ffookes symbols (suitable from about 2 to 3 years)

This test uses simple shapes (squares, circles and triangles) which are presented as either single symbols or lines of symbols and which the child can match from a series of plastic shapes held in front of them.

Snellen-based tests

Sheridan–Gardiner (Stycar 5 and 7 letter tests; suitable from about 2.5 years)

The Stycar letter tests are based on a standard Snellen letter test and utilize letter matching with a key card held by the child or parent. While using letters designed for 6 m, the test is best employed with younger children at 3 m. At this distance, the examiner can still exert control and the use of mirrors, which are confusing to young children, is avoided, although the best acuity measured will be only 3/6 (i.e. 6/12). The examiner presents a letter on the chart and the child points to the equivalent letter on the card; if necessary, the parent can indicate whether the response is correct.

The major disadvantages of the test is that there is no chance that the acuity is affected by confusion (*see* Chapter 15). To avoid overestimating the acuity in this way, it is better to utilize a line of letters wherever practicable and the standard Snellen chart can be employed with a home-made key card in Letraset or other large type. Caution should be employed in the use of a mirror as explained above. A new purpose-designed chart has been suggested by D.M. Calver (personal communication, 1985) which employs a limited range of letters and has standardized spacing between letters on each row, enhancing reliability and repeatability.

E charts and Llandolt rings (suitable from 2 to 3 years

These charts (described in Chapter 8) are useful for children, especially when the child can hold up a symbol in the same orientation. Caution in interpretation is required since right and left directions are frequently confused, more so if a mirror is used, and thus judgements of acuity should be based essentially on vertical orientations only.

Others

There are a multitude of other tests which rely more or less on the Snellen principle. These include the Sjögren hand test which has silhouettes of hands pointing in different directions, the child indicating the direction. The test suffers the same directional confusion as the E charts and Keith, Diamond and Stansfield (1972) found the performance poor with a group of children aged between 3 and 6.5 years.

A new variation on the Stycar letters has been developed at the Visual Development Unit of the University of Cambridge which uses one letter in a cube with one letter above, below and on each side. This has the advantage that the confusion element is retained while the child only has to concentrate on one letter which is always in the centre of the others.

Validity of subjective acuity assessment

There is little doubt that, once a child is able to cooperate with letter tests, the acuity can be assessed with a reasonable degree of accuracy. Indeed, Adelstein and Sculley (1967) showed that the greatest number of referrals for squint occurred at the age of 2–3 years which is when tests such as the Sheridan–Gardiner become viable, and thus amblyopia could be detected. In a study of the other methods, such as Stycar spheres and toy matching which used a control group of adults to monitor accuracy of assessment, Hall, Pugh and Hall (1982) showed that the other tests were unreliable and overestimated acuity considerably. They recommended that acuity assessment in paediatric screening be omitted if letter tests were not applicable.

Modern methods of acuity assessment

Visually evoked cortical responses (applicable from birth)

This technique, which is described in Chapter 3, will give an indication of the smallest pattern which produces a cortical response. While not strictly a measure of visual acuity, it does indicate the resolving capabilities of the ocular and neural systems.

Optokinetic nystagmus (applicable from birth)

When a target or series of targets capable of resolution is moved across the visual field, the eye will track the target in a smooth pursuit movement until it leaves the field or becomes uncomfortable to follow. At this point, there will be a rapid saccadic refixation movement and the process repeats itself again producing a nystagmic effect. Although subject to some development after birth, this phenomenon can provide useful information on the resolving power of the eye at an early age by controlling the size of the target used (usually spots or lines).

Catford drum (applicable from birth)

The Catford drum is a development of the optokinetic technique which utilizes a spot of variable size that moves across a small aperture with a fast and slow recurring movement. However, standardization is poor and Atkinson *et al.* (1981) have suggested that it can overestimate acuity by a factor of four in emmetropes and more in myopes.

Forced choice preferential looking (applicable from birth)

Based on behavioural response, this technique can be applied to very young babies and seems to be the most likely of modern tests to be developed into a consulting room technique. It relies on the phenomenon where, if two targets are presented to a baby, only one of which has any detail, the child will turn its attention to the target containing the detail in preference to the blank one for as long as the detail can be resolved. It is thus a measure of visual acuity within the limits of the child's boredom threshold. As described by Atkinson and Braddick (1982a), the technique is applicable to infants from 1 to 6 months old, but beyond this the child may become bored and too active.

The child is seated on the parent or helper's lap facing a flickering fixation light which generally attracts their attention. An oscilloscope screen is placed on each side of the fixation target and is illuminated so that, for each presentation, one screen displays a grating of variable spatial frequency (coarseness) while the other remains blank but of matched average luminance. The screen displaying the grating is selected at random (usually by computer) and a hidden observer has to indicate which of the two screens is displaying the grating by deciding which screen the child is viewing. This information can be fed into the computer, which will determine the acuity by assessing the percentage of times that the observer made a correct decision for any spatial frequency. The technique can also be applied to contrast sensitivity by varying grating contrast. It has been suggested that the technique can be used for measurements of monocular as well as binocular acuity (Atkinson, Braddick and Pimm Smith, 1982), but requires more control as the infant is less calm while wearing a patch.

Table 12.2 Visual acuity in infants by different techniques

Age (months)	Tumbling E	Pendular eye movements	Optokinetic nystamus	Preferential looking	Visual evoked potential
1			6/90	6/120	6/90
2			6/45	6/90	6/60
3			6/45	6/60	6/18
4			6/45	6/60	6/15
5			6/18	6/45	6/12
6		6/120			6/6
12	6/42	6/60	6/12		
24	6/14	6/30	6/90		
36	6/14	6/15	6/60		
48	6/12				
60	6/10				

Adapted from *Paediatric Optometry* by Jerome Rosner (1982) with permission.

Alley running

Preferential looking can be extended to older children using an 'alley running' technique where the child runs to whichever target shows the grating pattern and gains a reward, or can be applied to older non-verbal or neurologically impaired children by getting them to point to the target with the pattern (Jenkin *et al.*, 1985).

A more recent development is the Teller card system (McDonald *et al.*, 1985), which is too new as yet to have been thoroughly investigated. While being easier and cheaper to apply in the consulting room, the benefit of 'forced choice' is lost and, with it, potentially, its reliability. (*See Figure 12.1.*)

Interpretation of results

Table 12.2 is reproduced from Rosner (1982) and indicates the relative levels of acuity with age as indicated by various assessment methods. It must be remembered that acuities attained with objective or behavioural methods will tend to give better results than subjective ones because of the role that familiarity, interpretation and personality will have on subjective recognition of and response to letters or targets (*see* Chapter 4).

Subjective tests in younger children have been shown frequently to be inaccurate (Hall, Pugh and Hall, 1982) and those tests regularly used in development screening (i.e. Stycar spheres) are very over-optimistic with Atkinson and Braddick (1982) suggesting that the test is more a measure of attention than acuity. It does, however, indicate a basic integrity of the visual system.

In practice, a measurement of acuity should be attempted by the most refined technique applicable to the child in question. In the very young and in the absence of a practice application of behavioural methods, reliance will have to be placed on the assessment of equality of vision with the assessment of overall visual performance measured in terms of the child's response to his/her own environment. In this respect, the mother's opinion is of paramount importance and, in many cases, the practitioner's assertion that all is well in contradiction of the mother's view to the contrary can frequently be shown to be misguided.

Refractive error

The measurement of refractive error is of varying importance depending on presenting signs and symptoms. In the absence of reliable acuity assessment or with a suggestion or inconclusive assessment of binocular anomaly, it is the most valid predictive test (Ingram *et al.*, 1979).

Retinoscopy

The skill most essential to the practitioner dealing with children is that of rapid and accurate retinoscopy. The principle of the technique is no different to that with adults (*see* Chapter 6) but is complicated by the difficulties of fixation, accommodation and working distance. In very young children, a trial frame is unworkable and it is best to neutralize each principal meridian with spheres using whatever working distance is practical with that particular child. Having achieved a result, a working distance allowance can be made and the result converted to sphere/cylinder form. When dealing with the slightly older and more cooperative child, distance fixation can be attempted using an interesting target (the coloured duochrome panel is often adequate), but frequent reminders to look at the target rather than the retinoscopy light are necessary to maintain fixation and the need for rapid assessment is therefore obvious. With conventional retinoscopy, if more

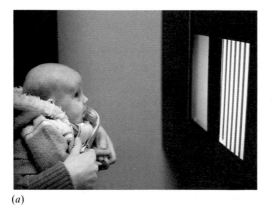

(a)

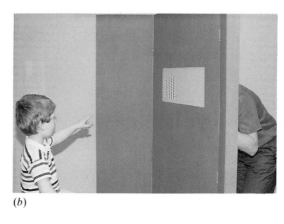

(b)

Figure 12.1 (*a*) Visual acuity assessment using conventional forced choice preferential looking procedures.

(b) Preferential looking technique using Teller cards. (Photographs courtesy of Dr Caroline Thompson)

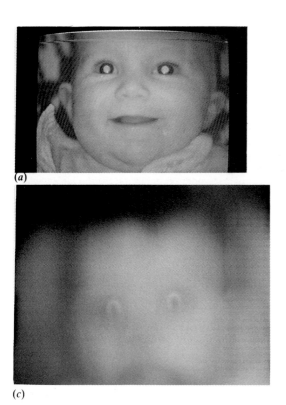

(a)

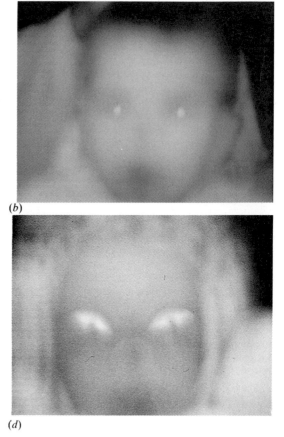

(b)

(c)

(d)

Figure 12.2 (*a*) Isotropic photorefraction: an in-focus picture is first taken to determine pupil size. (*b*) The camera is focused at 150 cm (camera to subject distance 75 cm). A small diffuse blur circle suggests hypermetropia (in this case a small error). (*c*) With the camera focused at 50 cm (and the same camera to subject distance), the blur circles have become enlarged and dif-

fuse. By comparing the images in (*b*) and (*c*) with the known pupil size determined from (*a*), the refractive error can be calculated. (*d*) The appearance of the blur circles in astigmatism where the major and minor axes as well as the refractive error can easily be obtained. (Photographs courtesy of Dr Janette Atkinson)

than a rough estimation of the degree of ametropia present is required, cyclopegia will almost certainly be necessary. The choice of drug will depend on the age of the child and the level of iris pigmentation (*see* Chapter 30).

Near fixation retinoscopy

In an attempt to control accommodation without the use of drugs, a technique has been developed which uses near fixation. The examination room is totally dark with the retinoscopy light then acting as the fixation target. In young babies the fixation of the light is automatic. Retinoscopy is carried out at 55 cm and the result reduced by an empirical 1.25 D to allow for accommodative lag. It has been shown to correlate well with subjective results in adults (Mohindra, 1977), being accurate to 0.50 D on sphere and cylinder power and 5° on axis in people aged under 30 years. In children aged 5–7 years the results were similar to those found by cyclopegic retinoscopy (Mohindra and Molinari, 1979). Moreover, the same investigation found that the correlation with cyclopegic findings was good even when the practitioner had no prior experience of the specific technique. In young babies, the technique can be applied while the subject is being breast fed, thus ensuring an immobile and contented patient.

Autorefractors

Autorefractors have no place in the examination of young children since they are at the same time intimidating, impractical and unlikely to yield accurate results due to poor control of accommodation Any instrument that requires the patient to sit in a head restraint for any period, however short, will not be acceptable. Thus results for both objective automated types (such as the Rx 1—Evans, 1984) and semi-automated types (such as the Topcon RM200—Edwards, 1981, unpublished report) show poor correlation with conventional methods. The only relevance such instrumentation has on the examination of children is where instrument dependence eliminates retinoscopy skills and thus disqualifies the practitioner from any involvement with the young patient.

Isotropic photorefraction

Retinoscopy relies on the reflection of defocused light from the retina to produce a measurement of refractive error. Photorefraction uses a photographic image of a blur circle to facilitate the same measurement. Three photographs are required taken with a standard camera using an on-axis flash source (easily provided by fibreoptics). The child is seated 75 cm from the camera and an in-focus picture taken which provides a record of

pupil size (and can also be used to provide a record of patient information). Two further photographs are required, one focused at 50 cm (0.67 D in front of the pupil) and one at 150 cm (0.67 D behind the pupil plane). If the 150-cm blur is greater than the 50-cm blur then the eye is hypermetropic with respect to the working distance. In myopia the reverse is true and, by measuring the size (and in astigmatism the shape and orientation of the long axis) of the blur circle, the amount of refractive error can be calculated. (*See Figure 12.2.*)

Accurate assessment of the degree of error can be made by computer ray tracing or comparison with adults of known refractive status. With increasing familiarity, an idea of the order of magnitude of the error can be gained just by looking at the photograph. The results indicate good correlation with retinoscopy when conducted under cyclopegia, although not accurate enough to prescribe (Atkinson and Braddick, 1982b). By using the technique without cycloplegia and with variation in the position of the fixation target away from the camera, accommodative function can be checked.

The main advantage of the technique, however, is in screening where the inexpensive equipment, suitability for unqualified staff and speed are particularly useful.

Binocular status

As part of the routine assessment of children it is necessary to determine whether the binocular function is normal. In this respect, it is appropriate to check for manifest deviation, large and/or uncompensated heterophoria and convergence. According to Ingram (1977a), only 50% of squints are cosmetically noticeable. Manifest deviation must be differentiated from the pseudosquinting appearance of epicanthus and can be elicited through direct and indirect tests.

Direct tests

Hirschberg/Krimsky tests

In the normal subject where the two visual axes are joined at the point of fixation, the corneal reflex (first Purkinje image) will be in an equivalent position on each cornea. Where squint is present, there will be a relative displacement of one image and the use of this phenomenon is the basis of the Hirschberg test. In order to determine the amount of the deviation, prisms can be used to align the two reflexes in the same relative position—the Krimsky test.

While there is no doubt about the basic soundness of these two tests, they are both limited in application. An anomalous angle lamda (between the visual and optical axis) may bias the result. More important is the relatively insensitive nature of the test where a small displacement of only 1 mm in relative reflex position is equivalent to approximately 20 prism dioptres (Δ) of squint (Jones and Eskridge, 1971). Therefore, by the time the squint is visible by corneal reflex position, it is probably already visible in the absence of the reflex. The test(s) is therefore only of particular value in cases of apparent squint in the presence of epicanthus. (It is important to remember that children with epicanthus may have squint as well.)

Cover test

The cover test is the only reliable way to determine the ocular motor status in young children, but it is undoubtedly difficult to apply in babies. Wherever possible, the smallest target visible to the eye with the poorer acuity should be used to promote the maximal effect of accommodation on the ocular motor system but, in very young babies, any object that will maintain sufficient attention must be used. If appropriate, a particularly close fixation distance can be applied to maximize the accommodative stress where an accommodative squint is suspected. Near fixation picture charts or bright reflection holograms can be used to attract attention and, in infants, a light may prove the most appropriate target. More cooperation will be achieved in younger patients if the thumb is used as an occluder instead of the more normal type. It is useful to be able to estimate angles of squint/heterophoria so that an assessment can be made without prisms and in the shortest possible time. Where there is no manifest deviation, the size of any heterophoria together with the speed and quality of recovery movement are of interest in determining the likelihood of there being any embarassment to the development of normal binocular vision.

Ocular motility

In addition to the basic status of the ocular motor system, it is important to assess extraocular muscle function. The ability to obtain cooperation in pursuit movements is variable, as is the length of time for which the child will cooperate. In some cases, the addition of an auditory stimulus (squeaky toy) will assist and, although this may produce refixation away from the primary position instead of pursuit movements, it will demonstrate a basic integrity of muscle function.

Indirect methods

Prism adaptation tests

Where it is impractical to obtain a direct assessment of the binocular status, it may be possible to deter-

mine the normality of the binocular system by the reaction to a sudden introduction of base-out prism in front of one eye. In the normally binocular subject, the diplopia resulting from this action will precipitate a fusional recovery movement which is both smooth and immediate. Any failure to make such a movement or a jerky response to the diplopia is an indication that the binocularity is either absent or under stress.

Stereopsis

Stereoscopic acuity is sensitive both to diminished binocularity through squint and decompensated heterophoria as well as blurred retinal imagery. It is therefore possible to gain information about the normality of binocularity/refractive error by an assessment of stereopsis; the test, however, is nonspecific to which is the cause and it is therefore best used as a screening test determining those who require more in-depth assessment. Various tests are available, most of which require some dissociation by filters worn before the eyes. While an absolute measurement of stereopsis is not required, young children will only cooperate with fairly gross tests. Some researchers have advocated the inclusion of stereopsis tests in routine child vision screening (Reinecke and Simmons, 1974), but others have found them impossible to apply in a manner that produces relevant results (Ingram *et al.*, 1986b). There will also always be individual variation in the response of different children.

Ophthalmoscopy

Assessment of the fundus is required in the examination of a child patient, although in the very young direct methods will give a view of little beyond the macular area. In older children, frequent reminders to look in a particular direction may assist in views of more peripheral parts. A better solution, especially where a cycloplegic has been instilled, is the use of indirect methods which give a greater field of view and are thus less fixation dependent. While routine developmental checks by physicians and paramedical personnel should ensure that any major anomalies are detected early, it is still important to ensure that the eyes are healthy.

Vision screening in children

The need for vision screening is dependent on the numbers likely to suffer from anomalies of vision and the prognosis for those who are detected and referred for treatment.

Estimates for the numbers affected by visual problems vary, but recent studies have suggested that just over 11% have refractive errors which are myopic, anisometropic or which are hypermetropic by over 3.5 D (Atkinson and Braddick, 1984), while Graham (1974) has estimated that abnormal cover test movements (i.e. squint or large phoria) were present in 7% of the population; more recently Ingram *et al.* (1986b) have suggested that an average of 8% of their population of 2270 children had abnormal vision which included squint and amblyopia. However, the real benefits of referral on the visual anomalies has only recently begun to be investigated and no figures are yet available which are reliable and unbiased. Some recent papers that are currently available do not suggest much success, even with action as early as age 1 year (Ingram *et al.*, 1985), and this opinion is shared by Stewart Brown (1985a).

Nevertheless, until adequate screening gives a reliable indication of the total incidence of visual problems, inadequate resources will continue to be applied to either researching suitable methods of management or providing sufficiently early screening to prevent the development or establishment of anomalies.

In its most basic form, vision screening in children should include assessment of vision, investigation of ocular motor function and ensuring the absence of morbid conditions. The extent and sophistication of screening will be dependent on the age group being screened and the staffing and monetary resources that are available. The age at which screening is applied will relate, not only to the possible age of onset of visual problems, but to the age at which it is realistic to expect reliable results.

Using Hirschberg, small toys, matching tests, picture and E charts, Oliver and Nawratzki (1971) found little cooperation up to the age of 3 years. At 3–4 years, 53% cooperated rising to 96% at 4–6 years. Mohindra (1975) suggested a comprehensive examination technique which is listed in *Table 12.3*.

Table 12.3 Comprehensive examination format

(1) External examination
(2) Near retinoscopy during breast feed
(3) Internal examination by direct and indirect ophthalmoscopy

then

  (i)   Gross external anatomy
  (ii)   Krimsky–Hirschberg tests
  (iii) Pupillary size and reflexes
  (iv) Unilateral and alternating cover test
  (v)   Ocular movements for concomitancy
  (vi) Near point of convergence
  (vii) Fusion through 4 base-out prism
  (viii) Placido disc
  (i1)   Optokinetic nystagmus

After Mohindra, 1975.

While thorough this is impractical as a screening technique. In young children, Ingram *et al.* (1979) suggested screening by cycloplegic refraction and indicated that, while cyclopentolate is less disruptive to visual function in the long term, it is less effective in determining errors (Ingram and Barr, 1979b). While this technique is valid in predicting amblyopia and squint by the degree of ametropia (especially hypermetropia where 48% of children with a refraction of +3.50 D or more in one meridian have amblyopia and 45% have squint) (Ingram *et al.*, 1986a), it also appears that detection and correction does little to prevent the onset of the conditions (Ingram *et al.*, 1985). If refractive error is of such significance then isotropic photorefraction is a suitable technique, since it is inexpensive and quick, screening up to 20 infants per hour (Atkinson and Braddick, 1982b). It is also reliable missing only one small error in 52 infants (Atkinson and Braddick, 1984). Bishop (1978) suggested different routines dependent on age and these are listed in *Table 12.4*. More recently, a study of children attending toddler and play groups (Dholakia, 1987) has suggested that the most useful information gained related to base-

Table 12.4 Variation of Examination routine with age

At age 1 year
  Near cover test
  Gross convergence and accommodation
  Pupil reflexes
  Ocular movement by pursuit or refixation
  Fusion through 10 base-out prism
  Vision with hundreds and thousands (*see* text for
    limitations)

At age 1–2 years
  As above but with the following additions:
    Attempt at distance cover test
    Fusion through 15–20 base-out prism
    Vision easy with hundreds and thousands
    Reaction to Titmus fly test

At age 2–3 years
  As above with the following additions:
    Cover test, convergence and accommodation more
      accurate due to more consistent fixation
    Fusion through 20 base-out prism either eye
    Vision with matching symbols at 3 m

At age 3–4 years
  As above including:
    Matching symbols at 6 m
    More reliable retinoscopy and ophthalmoscopy
    More detailed stereopsis

At age 4–5 years
  As above including:
    Matching symbols at 6 m

After Bishop, 1978

out prism tests, monocular distance vision and near point of convergence at age 3 years. These tests predicted 66% of cases that would be detected by retinoscopy and cover test. At age 4, the use of prism tests and monocular vision predicted 83% of cases. At age 5, monocular distance vision alone predicted over 76% of the total detected by the more sophisticated methods.

Interpretation of findings, management and prognosis

Before both screening and comprehensive examination results can be interepreted, some knowledge of the normal ranges for each parameter is required.

Visual acuity

The use of sophisticated objective and behavioural methods yields reliable results on visual efficiency and the results have already been given in *Table 12.2*. Subjective tests in older children will tend to give a more pessimistic assessment and it is common to find acuities of less than 6/6 at 6 years old or more. A normal variation between individuals must be accepted. Nevertheless, gross variations from the normal indicates cause for concern and the need for detailed assessment to determine the cause. It is regrettable that, by a narrow view of what constitutes normal vision, the benefits of screening and treatment can be undervalued. For example, Ingram *et al.* (1986) suggest that, because final acuity is not 6/6, detection and occlusion is ineffectual for amblyopia. This is despite an average improvement in the sample of nearly two lines and improvement in the best case of five lines following treatment.

Differences detected between eyes in normal infants using behavioural methods have been attributed to a different speed of development of the two eyes or neural systems (Atkinson, Braddick and Pimm Smith, 1982). A similar but bilateral phenomenon was reported by Hoyt, Jastrzebski and Marg (1983) where eight children (six of whom were premature or small-for-dates) showed no visual responsiveness at 5–11 weeks, but were normal at 26–44 weeks. Seven also showed delayed motor development and thus a theory of widespread maturational delay was suggested.

Refractive error

Historically, it has always been believed that the young infant was habitually hypermetropic and there was a tendency to become more emmetropic with age up to the age of 5 years when a small residual error remained. Recent research has changed this rather simplified view. While average data for the first year of life show a mean refractive

error of between 0.60 D and 2.62 D (Goldschmidt, 1969; Gonzales, 1965—cited by Rosner, 1982), Ingram and Barr (1979a) only found this trend when the initial refractive error was myopic or hypermetropic by less than 2.50 D. Above this level, the final error remained hypermetropic to a significant degree. Myopia is common in premature infants (16%) and is higher still among those with retinopathy of prematurity (50%) (Nissenhorn *et al.*, 1983). The higher incidence of myopia with prematurity is confirmed by Gordon and Donzies (1985). In a study of over 1000 infants aged 6–9 months, Atkinson and Braddick (1984) using photorefraction found that 5% of their sample were hypermetropic by more than 3.5 D and 4.5% were mildly myopic; 0.5% showed myopia of more than 3 D and 1.3% were anisometropic.

The most significant change in current thinking on refractive errors concerns astigmatism. Woodruff (1971) suggested that the incidence of astigmatism was low in children and increased over the first 4 years of life. Mohindra *et al.* (1979), however, suggested that the degree of astigmatism was greatest in the first 6 months of life and declined in incidence by the third year. This decrease in incidence was also found by Ingram and Barr (1979a). Gwiazda *et al.* (1984) found large amounts of against-the-rule astigmatism before the age of 2 which was reduced or eliminated by the age of 4. It was suggested that axis transition occurred at the age of 4–5 years and, thereafter, with-the-rule astigmatism predominated up to the age of 9 years (the limit of the study group). The authors also found total astigmatism was corneal in origin and that myopic astigmatism produced meridional amblyopia. Howland and Sayle (1984) corroborated the findings showing an incidence of 1 D or more of astigmatism in 70% of 1 year olds. This was reduced to 1% at 4 years. The ratio of against-the-rule/with-the rule/oblique was 15:9:1.

From this data some prescribing habits can be gleaned. With hypermetropia of 2–2.75 D in the less hypermetropic eye, Ingram (1977b) found a significant correlation with squint and later results linked this degree of ametropia to amblyopia and squint (Ingram *et al.*, 1986a). Anisometropia was not associated with squint unless there was spherical hypermetropia of more than 2 D, but hypermetropic anisometropia of 1 D (spherical or cylindrical) could be directly linked to amblyopia. As a result, apart from prescribing for accommodative squint, it can be argued that a correction should be considered where there is more than 2.00 D of hypermetropia in the less affected eye as a prophylactic measure against squint. Similarly, anisometropic corrections should be considered where they accompany 2 D hypermetropia or are at least of a difference of 1 D.

Astigmatic corrections of 1–2 D may be normal within the first year of life provided that they are reducing. Greater degrees of astigmatism and incidence beyond the first year are less likely to resolve and could cause amblyopia.

Myopia of less than 3 D is unlikely to be a problem to normal ocular or general development as the child's visual environment is within arm's reach during the critical period of development and this degree of myopia only needs correcting when it starts to hinder the child's life, normally at school age.

However, above this level a correction will be necessary to prevent amblyopia, although the incidence of cases is likely to be small.

Corrections for refractive errors outside those considered are more difficult to justify. There are little or no published data to support the view that low-powered corrections assist asthenopic symptoms, although undoubtedly they can appear to help on occasions. To what extent this is a placebo effect is debatable. Where the ocular motor balance is normal, even moderate hypermetropic refractive errors can be dealt with by the child's ample accommodation and, even where a high positive correction is found under cycloplegia, there is little good reason to prescribe the full correction (after a tonus allowance) unless there is an adverse effect on or reduction in binocular function.

In a recent paper, Stewart Brown (1985b) has suggested that there is a great deal of prescribing of spectacles when acuity is good with little evidence to indicate the reason or benefits. She suggests that, with screening and supply costs being high, solid evidence is required to justify the provision.

Summary

While the practitioner wishing to develop an interest in paediatric optometry needs to acquire a different approach to patient examination and management, the rewards are many. Providing the practitioner maximizes communication, especially with the parent who is often underinformed due to pressures on professional time, there will be a real opportunity to provide an element of primary health care and information that is not readily available elsewhere in the health care services. Both in screening and comprehensive examination, the information acquired will help prevent or minimize the visual consequences of abnormal development and allow referral to other professional disciplines at the earliest appropriate moment.

To contribute fully in this way, care must be given to retain familiarity with the most recent methods of assessment and the current literature.

Acknowledgements

The author would like to thank Richard Llewellyn, David Calver, Richard Broughton and Carole Collins who read the manuscript of this chapter and made many useful comments.

References

ADELSTEIN, A.M. and SCULLY, J. (1967) Epidemiological aspects of squint. *Br. Med. J.*, **3**, 334–338

ATKINSON, J. and BRADDICK, O. (1982a) Assessment of visual acuity in infancy and early childhood. Symposium on early infancy development. *Acta Ophthalmol. Suppl.* 157, 18–26

ATKINSON, J. and BRADDICK, O. (1982b) Use of isotropic photorefraction for vision screening in infants. Symposium on early visual development. *Acta Ophthalmol. Suppl.* 157, 36–45

ATKINSON, J. and BRADDICK, O. (1984) Screening for refractive errors in 6–9 month old infants by photorefraction. *Br. J. Ophthalmol.* **68**, 105–112

ATKINSON, J., BRADDICK, O. and PIMM SMITH, E. (1982) Preferential looking for monocular and binocular acuity testing of infants. *Br. J. Ophthalmol.*, **66**, 264–268

ATKINSON, J., BRADDICK, O., PIMM SMITH, E., AYLING, L. and SAWYER, R. (1981) Does the Catford drum give an accurate assessment of acuity? *Br. J. Ophthalmol.*, **65**, 652–656

BISHOP, A. (1978) Examination of pre-school children. *Ophthal. Opt.*, **18**, 720

DHOLAKIA, S. (1987) The application of a comprehensive visual screening programme to children aged 3 to 5 years—can a modified procedure be devised for screening of by ancillary staff? *Ophthal. Physiol. Opt.*, in press

ELLIOTT, R. (1985) A new linear picture vision test. *Br. Orthop. J.*, **42**, 54–57

EVANS, E. (1984) Refraction in children using the Rx 1 autho-refractor. *Br. Orthop. J.*, **41**, 46-52

GRAHAM, P.A. (1974) Epidemiology of strabismus. *Br. J. Ophthalmol.*, **58**, 224–231

GOLDSCHMIDT, E. (1969) Refraction in the newborn *Acta Ophthalmol.*, **45**, 570

GONZALES, T.J. (1965) Conseraciones en torno a la refraccion del racien nacido. *Arch. Soc. Oftal. Hisp.-Am.*, **25**, 666

GORDON, R.A. and DONZIS, P.B. (1985) Refractive development of the human eye. *Am. Med. Assoc. Arch. Ophthalmol.*, **103**, 785–789

GWIAZDA, J., SCHEIMAN, M., MOHINDRA, I. and HELD, R. (1984) Astigmastism in children: changes in axis and amount from birth to six years. *Invest. Ophthalmol. Vis. Sci.*, **25**, 88–92

HALL, S.M., PUGH, A.G. and HALL, D.M.B. (1982) Vision screening in the under-5s. *Br. Med. J.*, **285**, 1096–1098

HOWLAND, H.C. and SAYLE, N. (1984) Photorefractive measurement of astigmatism in infants and young children. *Invest. Ophthalmol. Vis. Sci.*, **25**, 93–102

HOYT, C.S., JASTRZEBSKI, G.B. and MARG, E. (1983) Delayed visual maturation in infancy. *Br. J. Ophthalmol.*, **67**, 127–130

HYAMS, S.W. and NEUMANN, E. (1977) Picture cube for vision screening of preschool children. *Br. J. Opthalmol.*, **56**, 572–573

INGRAM, R.M. (1977a) The problem of screening children for visual defects. *Br. J. Opthalmol.*, **61**, 4–7

INGRAM, R.M. (1977b) Refraction as a basis for screening children for squint and amblyopia. *Br. J. Opthalmol.*, **61**, 8–15

INGRAM, R.M. and BARR, A. (1979a) Changes in refraction between the ages of 1–3$\frac{1}{2}$. *Br. J. Ophthalmol.*, **63**, 339–342

INGRAM, R.M. and BARR, A. (1979b) Refraction of year old children after cycloplegia with 1% cyclopentolate: a comparison with findings after atropinisation. *Br. J. Ophthalmol.*, **63**, 348–352

INGRAM, R.M., TRAYNAR, M.J., WALKER, C. and WILSON, J.M. (1979) Screening for refractive errors at age 1 year—a pilot study. *Br. J. Ophthalmol.*, **63**, 243–250

INGRAM, R.M., WALKER, C., WILSON, J.M., ARNOLD, P.E., LUCAS, J. and DALLY, S. (1985) A first attempt to prevent amblyopia and squint by spectacle correction of abnormal refractions from age 1 year. *Br. J. Ophthalmol.*, **69**, 851–853

INGRAM, R.M., WALKER, C., WILSON, J.M., ARNOLD, P.E., LUCAS, J. and DALLY, S. (1986a) Prediction of amblyopia and squint by means of refraction at age 1 year. *Br. J. Opthalmol.*, **70**, 12–15

INGRAM, R.M., WALKER, C., WILSON, J.M., ARNOLD, P.E., LUCAS, J. and DALLY, S. (1986b) Screening for visual defects in preschool children. *Br. J. Ophthalmol.*, **70**, 16–21

JENKIN, P.L., SIMON, J.W., KANDEL, G.L. and FORSTER, T. (1985) A simple grating visual acuity test of impaired children. *Am. J. Ophthalmol.*, **99**, 652–658

JONES, R. and ESKRIDGE, J.B. (1971) Re-evaluation of the Hirschberg Test. *Am. J. Optom. Arch. Am. Acad. Optom.*, **47**, 105–114

KAY, H. (1983) New method for assessing visual acuity with pictures. *Br. J. Ophthalmol.*, **67**, 131–133

KEITH, C.G., DIAMOND, Z. and STANSFIELD, A. (1972) Visual acuity testing in young children. *Br. J. Ophthalmol.*, **56**, 827–832

McDONALD, M.A., DOBSON, V., SEBRIS, S.L., BAITCH, L., VARNER, D. and TELLER, D.Y. (1985) The acuity card procedure: a rapid test of infant acuity. *Invest. Ophthalmol. Vis. Sci.*, **26**, 1158–1162

MOHINDRA, I. (1975) A technique for infant vision examination. *Am. J. Optom. Physiol. Opt.*, **52**, 867–870

MOHINDRA, I. (1977) Comparison of 'near retinoscopy' and subjective refraction in adults. *Am. J. Optom. Physiol. Opt.*, **54**, 319–322

MOHINDRA, I. and MOLINARI, J.F. (1979) Near retinoscopy and cycloplegic retinoscopy in early primary grade school children. *Am. J. Optom. Physiol. Opt.*, **56**, 34–38

MOHINDRA, I., JACOBSON, S.G., THOMAS, J. and HELD, R. (1979) Development of amblyopia in infants. *Trans. Ophthalmol. Soc. UK*, **99**, 344–346

NISSENHORN, I., YASSUR, Y., MASKOWSKI, D., SHERF, I. and BEN-SIRA, I. (1983) Myopia in premature babies with and without retinoscopy of prematurity. *Br. J. Ophthalmol.*, **67**, 170–173

OLIVER, M. and NAWRATZKI, I. (1971) Screening of pre-school children for ocular anomalies I. Screening methods and their practicability at different ages. *Br. J. Ophthalmol.*, **55**, 462–466

REINECKE, R.D. and SIMONS, K. (1974) A new stereoscopic test for amblyopia screening. *Am. J. Ophthalmol.*, **78**, 714–721

ROSNER, J. (1982) What is the patient's refractive status? In *Paediatric Optometry*, p. 133. Boston: Butterworths

SHERIDAN, M. (1975) *Children's Development Progress*, 3rd ed. pp. 30–37. Windsor: NFER Publishing Company

STEWART BROWN, S. (1985a) Visual defects in primary school children: which are the ones that need treating? Paper to a one day seminar 'The Child Patient', Middlesex Hospital, London

STEWART BROWN, S. (1985b) Spectacle prescribing among 10 year-old children. *Br. J. Ophthalmol.*, **69**, 874–880

WOODRUFF, M.E. (1971) Cross sectional studies of corneal and astigmatic characteristics of children between the 24th and 72nd month of life. *Am. J. Optom. Physiol. Opt.*, **48**, 650

Further reading

ROSNER, J. (1982) *Paediatric Optometry*. Boston: Butterworths

Part 4

Binocular visual function

13

Amblyopia: the cortical basis of binocularity and vision loss in strabismus

Jerry Nelson

When the retinal images are of unequal quality for any reason, the maturing visual system can react harshly, developing suppression or amblyopia in the disadvantaged eye. In a visual system disadvantaged by mild strabismus, the eyes can see, but binocular cooperation is missing or abnormal. The cellular basis of these changes lies in the visual cortex. This chapter is concerned with the path of visual signals to the visual cortex, and above all with what can go amiss once ascending pathways arrive there. Amblyopia and loss of binocularity are treated as sensory adaptations, the cortical response to altered visual input. Thus, sensory aspects are emphasized rather than oculomotor control. In a nutshell, amblyopia disconnects the visual cortex while anomalous correspondence perverts its function.

Retinocortical pathways

Conscious visual perception depends most directly on the geniculostriate pathways from the retina to the lateral geniculate nucleus (LGN) and thence to the visual cortex (*Figure 13.1*).

Fibres from retinal ganglion cells exit from the globe, acquire myelination and reach the LGN to synapse there with cells which complete the journey to the cortex of the cerebral hemispheres. These retinal ganglion cells fall into at least three classes, with slightly different functional roles and central destinations. If one class failed, vision would be not only worse, but strangely different. Problems in early infancy can differentially cripple one system. These three subdivisions in the main pathway from eye to brain are further discussed at the end of this chapter. Researchers have returned time and again to the LGN, a thalamic nucleus in the diencephalon

(the area between the higher cerebrum and mesencephalon or midbrain), but as yet no important information processing function has been discovered. The first large component of the evoked potential appears on the human scalp 90 milliseconds (ms) after visual stimulation (*see* Chapter 3). Most of the delay occurs in the eye itself, where fibres are unmyelinated and fine. This is fortunate, because the retina has an inside-out construction, and light must pass through these fibres and all other retinal cells to reach the receptors. Diseases of the optic nerve and tract, therefore, leave little scope for altering retinocortical latency. Nevertheless, latency increases of 16 ms are important indicators of disease (e.g. parkinsonism, multiple sclerosis).

Optic chiasma

At the optic chiasma the decussation or branching pattern of ganglion cell fibres from the two eyes sends information about the same half of the visual field to the same cortical hemisphere. For information from the left side of the visual field to arrive at the right cortex means that fibres conveying visual information from the temporal half of one retina and the nasal half of the other must be sent off together. It is nasal retinal fibres which cross (*see* Chapter 1). A problem with this scheme is the need to clarify which system is covering the vertical midline, where displacement of objects in depth sends off the neural responses to separate cortical hemispheres. Anomalies in depth perception tested here (e.g. midline 'notches' in the horopter) may be a reflection of this wiring plan.

The retina-to-cortex relay performed in the LGN is carried out in separate layers for each eye; there is no opportunity here to compare the two eyes' viewpoints of the same visual hemifield. Comparison of signals from the two eyes first occurs in the

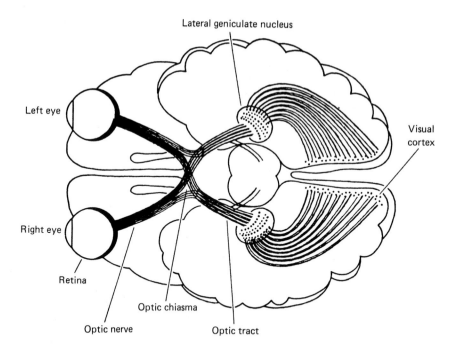

Lateral geniculate nucleus

Left eye

Visual
cortex

Right eye

Retina

Optic chiasma

Optic nerve   Optic tract

Figure 13.1. The retinogeniculate pathway to visual
cortex. Partial decussation at the optic chiasma
ultimately brings information from the nasal and
temporal retinas of different eyes together in one cortical
hemisphere. (From Regan Beverley and Cynader, 1979;
copyright © 1979, Scientific American Inc., all rights
reserved)

striate visual cortex (area 17 or V1; *see* Chapter 1,
for correspondence of areas defined functionally in
animals and structurally in man), where information
relayed from two eyes by the LGN converges upon
one cell. This cell *can* compare the retinal images.
Differences or disparities detected by such cells are
the basis of stereoscopic depth perception (*see*
Chapter 14).

The visual cortex

The importance of the visual cortex for determining
spatial localization is decisive. Amigo (1982) urged
that the word 'retinal' be dropped from terms such
as 'retinal correspondence' and 'anomalous retinal
correspondence' because the cortex determines
both. In a similar vein, primary or anatomical
aniseikonia (not induced by optical factors) is *not*
due to differences in the 'grain' of retinal receptor
elements, but to where the fibre pathways originating there enter the cortical topography. Retinal
elements lack intrinsic spatial values; the cortex
determines the spatial values both within and between the two retinas.

Cortical factors deserve more emphasis in the
analysis of visual performance. The dramatic deterioration in acuity away from the fovea is due in

part to decrease in retinal receptor density and to
increased convergence (pooling) of receptors onto
single ganglion cells. While this *does* produce larger
receptive fields which are less well suited to high
resolution tasks, an equally important factor in
acuity is the amount of cortical machinery available
to process afferent information. The cortical magnification factor (millimetres of cortex serving 1° of
retina; Rovamo and Virsu, 1979; Virsu and
Rovamo, 1979) quantifies the amount of machinery
available at any eccentricity.

Extrageniculostriate paths

Behind the diencephalon (home of the LGN) is the
midbrain or mesencephalon and extrageniculostriate pathways. The mesenchephalon is formed by
the two cerebral peduncles, wherein run many nerve
tracts from the cerebrum above to the brainstem and
spinal cord below. Tectum and tegmentum are the
chief divisions of the mesencephalon. The *superior
colliculus* is a tectal nucleus concerned with generating visual field motion information for driving
alerting responses and many visual reflexes. These
responses include turning of the eye, head and, in
the cat, ear pinnas. Not surprisingly, the superior
colliculus is a multimodal sensory area which has

auditory and somaesthetic (body-sense) information as well as visual responsiveness. In the pretectal area lies the oculomotor nucleus, i.e. the nucleus of the third cranial (oculomotor) nerve. The parasympathetic *Edinger–Westphal nucleus*, controlling pupil diameter, is a part of this nucleus. Here also lies the 'nucleus' of the optic tract (NOT), consisting in the cat of cell clusters scattered along and beside the brachium of the superior colliculus. Directionally selective cells in the NOT detect visual field motion; their output ultimately drives the diagnostically important optokinetic nystagmus reflex (they are not themselves motor neurones).

The receptive field

The receptive field of any sensory neurone is defined as the area where presentation of a stimulus will produce a response. The response may be inhibitory or excitatory. The visual receptive field is a 'field' because the neurone under test is ultimately connected to a patch of retina, permitting the influence by stimulation over some patch of visual field. In cortical areas concerned with high-acuity performance, receptive fields subtend a fraction of a degree; in areas concerned with movement of the whole visual field and with global aspects of perception, one neurone's receptive field may cover everything to one side of the nose.

The receptive field helps to summarize the function of a neurone; a neurone with 'binocular receptive fields' has a role to play in binocular vision. Finding the *structures* which produce this function is an important goal of neurophysiology.

The classic description of a retinal ganglion cell receptive field was provided by Kuffler (1953), who described a concentric disc-and-ring pattern: an *ON-centre* (disc) and antagonistic (inhibitory) *OFF-surround* (ring), and its complement. This pattern has proved to have broad generality across animal species and visual system levels.

Concentric receptive field organization enhances spatial localization: an ON-centre ganglion cell will quickly fall silent as the spot moves onto its OFF-surround, enhancing acuity. If the strength and summation of centre and surround response mechanisms are adjusted for equality, then the cell will make *no response* to field-wide changes in illumination. This is an important first step in isolating local objects (edges) from unimportant changes in global illumination. This system requires the eye to be properly aimed and focused in order to operate. Deprived of proper stimulation, pattern-sensitive elements throughout the visual system from ganglion cells onward may be damaged. When this occurs in amblyopia, it is pattern perception which suffers, as exemplified by acuity loss, while (not surprisingly) colour blindness and loss of light sense are rare (Wald and Burian, 1944).

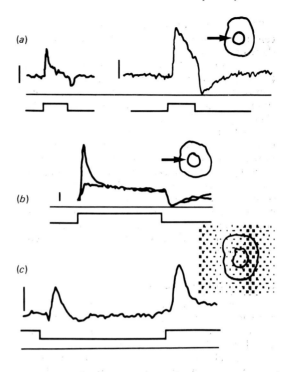

Figure 13.2. Response (discharge rate) of retinal ganglion cells as a function of time. In (a) and (b), a small bright spot (arrow), well-centred on the ON-centre of the receptive field (inset), gives an excitatory response at light onset (lower trace: stimulus timing; upward deflection = stimulus ON) (*a*) X and Y cells compared for identical spots (0.4° across, 4.5 cd/m², half-second ON) at identical background luminance levels of approximately 1.5 cd/m². Under comparable conditions, Y cells (left) are more transient than X (right; *see* text Chapter 1, *Table 1.1*). (*b*) Above a threshold intensity of stimulus plus background, transiency increases for all cells. Thus, transiency can not be a defining characteristic of Y cells. Here, a small, centred stimulus spot is increased 100-fold in luminous intensity. If response shape were then to remain constant for small further increases in stimulus luminous flux, it would be likely that the response came only from the receptive field centre without contamination by surround response mechanisms (stimulus on 1.25 s). (*c*) When stimulation falls across both centre and surround, both make an excitatory contribution, one at stimulus OFF-set and the other at ON-set. This is an OFF-centre Y cell stimulated by the appearance/disappearance of a sinusoidal grating at 0.45 Hz. The response at both contrast onset and offset contributes to the identical responses seen with pattern reversal and *re*-reversal in visual evoked potential recordings. If for some stimulus position the surround response *balanced* the centre in both shape and amplitude, the response could disappear entirely. Such generation and combination of opposite components occurs only with X-type ganglion cells; with Y cells, there is never a null moment. All vertical calibration bars, 25 spikes/s. (Modified from Enroth-Cugell and Jakiela, 1980, B. G. Cleland, *PhD Thesis*, Northwestern University, 1967, and Enroth-Cugell and Robson, 1966.)

The responses of retinal ganglion cells with concentrically organized receptive fields (insets) are shown in *Figure 13.2*.

Inspection of ON and OFF responses shows that temporal transience is built-in to the visual system in a most pervasive way: excitation can occur at both stimulus ON-set and OFF-set (*see Figure 13.2*). Clinically, therefore, it is important to use temporal modulation (flicker) when trying to reach a weak neural population during diagnosis or therapy. This provides a cellular justification for the long-standing clinical practices of flickering the background during afterimage testing (Evans, 1928), or of rhythmically covering and uncovering the deviating eye to break its suppression. At the cortex, stimulus motion becomes even more important than flicker, and at all levels patterned stimulation is more effective than a diffuse flash.

Binocularity in the striate cortex

Binocularity arises in striate cortex by equipping one cell with two receptive fields. In cortical receptive fields, excitatory and inhibitory areas are powerful and elongated, rather than circular as among retinal ganglion cells. Object edges need not move far in position or orientation to greatly excite or inhibit a cell with such a receptive field. The cell acquires selectivity or tuning in its response, and can serve (as would be hoped for neurones in the primary cortical areas) as the basis for encoding patterns in the visual scene rather than merely detecting the presence of spots of light and colour (*Figure 13.3*).

It logically follows from such stimulus selectivity that the pair of receptive fields belonging to one neurone must be closely matched, lest all stimuli adequate for one field find themselves lying squarely across inhibitory regions in the other. When a binocular stimulus is unsuitable for one eye, then no matter how good the stimulus is in the other eye, *there will be no excitatory output* from cells in the binocular visual system. This is the sort of incorrect stimulus provided in strabismus.

Binocular receptive field matching occurs to such an amazing degree (Maske, Yamane and Bishop, 1984) that visual experience is thought necessary to do it (e.g. Nelson, 1978). Genetics alone could not direct so many neural fibres to such precise terminations. The other side of this coin is explored in Chapter 14: small differences permitted to arise between binocular receptive field pairs equip neurones possessing them to detect retinal image disparities and thus stereoscopic depth.

Figure 13.3 shows that the receptive field of a cortical cell is not circular and consequently the cell's response is selective for stimulus orientation. A simple cell in the striate cortex of a cat was stimulated by a small bar (1 x 0.28°) swept rightward along paths passing above, through and below the receptive field centre. The many response profiles

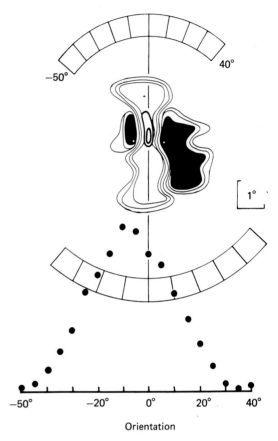

Figure 13.3. Receptive field of cortical simple cell, and the cell's orientation tuning curve. (From Nelson, 1981 courtesy of the Publisher, *Documenta Ophthalmologica*)

thus obtained were statistically processed to produce a contour map of the receptive field. The map's main features are the single, elongated excitatory discharge centre and the two flanking inhibitory sidebands. The two *heavy outlines* in the discharge centre are regions where excitation rose to three and then five times mean levels. *White dots* in black areas mark points of total inhibition.

The orientation tuning curve (bottom) was obtained with a bar long enough to cover the entire receptive field (6 x 0.28°). The average number of action potentials ('spikes') per sweep is plotted as a function of bar orientation (peak: 26 spikes/sweep). Placing a ruler across the receptive field map in the various orientations given by the semicircular reference arcs shows that orientation selectivity is closely related to receptive field topography in simple cells. Optimal response occurs when the bar ruler is aligned with the elongated excitatory centre at about −10°, and falls to zero as soon as the bar encroaches upon the inhibitory sidebands.

If this cortical neurone were binocular, there would be a receptive field in a 'corresponding area' in the other eye, well matched in topography to this one.

Amblyopia

Amblyopia may be defined as visual acuity worse than 6/9 which is not due to refraction errors, ophthalmoscopically detectable anomalies of the fundus or pathology of the visual pathway. Loss of visual function typically affects only one eye, and is most marked in central vision. A significant difference in acuity between eyes, neither worse than 6/9, may therefore also be a sign of amblyopia. Amblyopia is often accompanied by eccentric fixation, strabismus or other motility disorders and by loss of binocular sensory function: regardless of the acuity each exhibits alone, the eyes do not cooperate. For these reasons, visual acuity measurements, motility tests and the cover test for phoria are recommended for all patients suspected of binocular vision anomalies.

'Amaurosis' is a term meaning near or total blindness, and is usually applied to visual loss from organic causes; milder loss would be termed an 'organic amblyopia'. The practitioner is most frequently called upon to treat functional amblyopia arising from strabismus, anisometropia and visual deprivation. The strabismus itself may be primary or secondary to organic problems, such as cerebral palsy, brain damage, Down's or Duane's syndrome. Anisometropia means there is unequal refractive power in each eye; usually, one retinal image is blurred and the other normal. Because the deviating eye falls into disuse, it is easy to view all strabismic amblyopia as a form of amblyopia ex anopsia (literally, blunt sight from not working). More recently, this term has been reserved for amblyopias due to visual deprivation (lack of patterned stimulation), as might occur, for example, in congenital cataract.

The definition of amblyopia attributed by Revell (1971) to Albrecht von Graefe puts the matter most succinctly: 'Amblyopia is the condition in which the observer sees nothing and the patient very little'. This implies that one must look beyond the retina to the visual cortex for the cause of acuity loss.

Monocular occlusion

Inputs from both eyes converge on single neurones to create a basis for binocular vision. About 80% of the cells in the striate and extrastriate cortex of both the adult cat (Wiesel and Hubel, 1963) and monkey (Zeki, 1978) can be excited by both eyes, and are termed 'binocular neurones'. This cortical binocularity is easily lost.

Occlusion of one eye in a developing organism leads to a visual cortex populated by cells driven by the other. An eye without access to cortical machinery is blind. The classic demonstration of deprivation amblyopia was provided by Wiesel and Hubel (1963), who sutured a kitten's eyelid shut. This stimulation deprivation is comparable to that from wearing a translucent contact lens. Earlier research often brought about cellular degeneration, because total light deprivation was used (reviewed by Riesen, 1961, 1982). The change in cortical response induced by a reduced patterned visual input is rapid and profound only during an early 'critical period'. Properly timed treatment can also produce improvement which is rapid and profound; otherwise, the functional loss will be permanent.

Ocular dominance

Because excitatory drive from the two eyes is often unequal, neurones are said to display ocular dominance. Neurones in category or class 1 are excited exclusively by the eye contralateral to the sampled hemisphere, while neurones in the middle class are balanced and binocular (Hubel and Wiesel, 1962). The construction of an ocular dominance histogram is illustrated in *Figure 13.4*. Note that most cells fall into the middle, binocular groups (bottom of the figure).

Ocular dominance is easily assessed with a microelectrode study of the cortex. If the middle (binocular) class of neurones is absent, binocular vision is absent (e.g. no stereopsis: Crawford *et al.*, 1983, 1984). With middle and, for example, left-eye classes absent, the left eye is visually impaired. Cellular 'ocular dominance' describes the primary visual machinery, while ocular dominance in the sense of preferring one eye for sighting a gun (*see* Chapter 15) includes higher-order and more subtle differences between the eyes.

Basic research into binocularity has emphasized excitation at the expense of interocular inhibition. There is evidence that the deprived eye retains cortical connections, but only inhibitory ones (Singer, 1977). Further, most studies have looked only for *monocular* excitation. Today it is known that there are binocularly gated neurones which respond only to simultaneous stimulation of both eyes. Such cells would be missed (classified as visually unresponsive) with monocular tests. Some paths from the eye to the brain may remain even in amblyopia, and can be awakened by extraordinary measures, such as the use of certain drugs (*see later*). A disadvantaged eye does, however, lose cortical access and shifts in ocular dominance provide a rough quantification of this loss. Non-invasive electrophysiological and psychophysical tests for binocularity loss in man are considered in the latter part of this chapter.

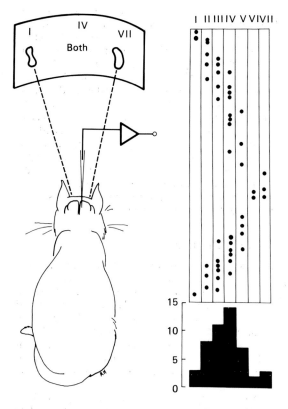

Figure 13.4. The measurement of ocular dominance. The cat is viewing a tangent screen while action potentials are recorded from individual cells in the striate cortex of the right hemisphere. The eyes have diverged under paralysis and anaesthesia, so that receptive fields for the two eyes are well separated on the tangent screen (left). A neurone responsive only to stimulation of the contralateral (left) eye is said to have ocular dominance class I. Binocular neurones (classes III, IV and V) respond well to either eye stimulated alone. During a long electrode penetration, successively encountered neurones (dots, columns on right, plotted vertically in the order in which cells were recorded) often show an orderly progression through ocular dominance categories (hypothetical data; compare Hubel and Wiesel, 1965, Figs. 7 and 8). This regularity was early evidence for the existence of occular dominance columns. A frequency histogram of the ocular dominance distribution of these neurones (lower right; modified from Hubel and Wiesel, 1962) shows a preponderance of binocular neurones in normal cortex. (From Nelson, 1981, courtesy of the Publisher, *Documenta Ophthalmologica*)

The ocular dominance histogram calls attention to the simple but profound idea that there are three visual systems in the sense that it is possible to have populations of cells serving one eye, the other eye or both. The most effective means of destroying cortical binocularity, while leaving vigorous left- and right-eye neural populations, is alternating monocu-

lar occlusion. When binocularity fails in this way, stereopsis fails, even though acuity is normal for each eye alone (Blake and Hirsch, 1975). Surgically induced strabismus also abolishes binocularity in the cat (Hubel and Wiesel, 1965) and monkey (Baker, Grigg and von Noorden, 1974), but *may* leave a monocular neural population for each eye.

Any circumstance in which the eyes receive different stimuli may result in amblyopia. Examples include anisometropia (Eggers and Blakemore, 1978), neutral density attenuation before one eye (Blakemore, 1976), excessive orientation differences between the images (Shinkman, Isley and Rogers, 1983) and astigmatism (Cynader and Mitchell, 1977). Ocular dominance histograms resulting from various forms of deprivation are illustrated in *Figure 13.5*.

A loss of binocularity without amblyopia occurs when the eyes receive equal but separate visual inputs. Manipulations which reduce the quality of visual stimulation for one eye during periods of binocular viewing will impair that eye's access to cortical centres. Amblyopia as well as binocularity loss then ensues (two of the three neural populations are affected).

Competition for ocular dominance

The effectiveness of monocular occlusion as a cause of amblyopia and loss of binocularity is due to *competition* between the eyes for cortical access. While the amblyopic eye decreases in function, the dominant eye gains efficiency. For example, brief occlusion of one eye in man augments evoked potential amplitude from the other (Tyler and Kaitz, 1977). Because ocular dominance shifts arise from competitive mechanisms, penalizing the good eye will tend to reverse ocular dominance, while perfectly good stimulation for *both* eyes following initial deprivation brings little recovery (monkey: Blakemore, Vital-Durand and Garey, 1981; Crawford *et al.*, 1984). This is the cellular explanation for the effectiveness of alternate occlusion therapy.

The first clue to the occurrence of competition came from observations that severe visual loss from monocular occlusion in the kitten could be lessened by occlusion of *both* eyes (Wiesel and Hubel, 1965). Visual input is then indeed less, but it is more balanced. In the end, neither eye completely lacked cortical access.

Monocular areas exist within the disadvantaged eye's visual field; examples are the disadvantaged area paired with the other eye's blind spot, and the 'monocular crescents' in the peripheral visual field. Animal experiments suggest that areas free of competition will be free of amblyopia. This prediction has yet to be confirmed and exploited in visual testing in man.

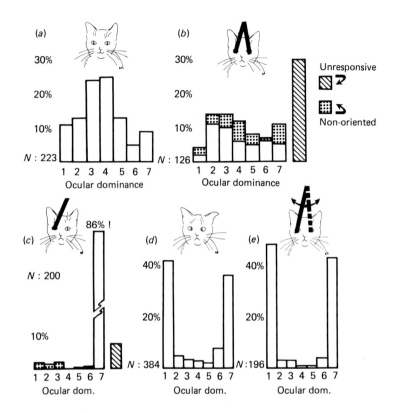

Figure 13.5. Ocular dominance histograms illustrating normal binocularity and its destruction in the cat. (*a*) Normal: most cells are binocular (categories 3, 4 and 5) and more cells fall in category 4 (balanced excitation from the two eyes) than any other. In monkey, binocularity is not so pronounced in area 17, and more stereoscopic processing, especially for motion in depth, is carried on in cortical centres one or two steps higher. (Modified from Hubel and Wiesel, 1962; 223 cells in adult cats.) (*b*) Binocular occlusion prevents cells from developing full adult properties (cross-hatching, visually unresponsive cells; dots, cells without orientation selectivity), but the equality of treatment of the two eyes prevents severe binocularity loss. (Modified from Wiesel and Hubel, 1965; 126 cells in 4 kittens.) (*c*) Loss of binocularity with monocular deprivation. Most cells are excitable only by stimulation of one eye (ocular dominance class 1 or 7), namely the formerly uncovered one. Here, the good eye happened to be ipsilateral to the hemisphere from which recordings were made, so the cells are class 7. This is the animal model of deprivation amblyopia. (Modified from Wiesel and Hubel, 1963; 200 cells from 5 animals deprived for most or all of the critical period.) (*d*) Loss of binocularity from artifical strabismus. Each eye is served by its own population of cells; there is neither amblyopia nor binocular cooperation. Stereoscopic depth will fail, and oculomotor control may be impaired. (Modified from Hubel and Wiesel, 1965; 384 cells from 4 extotropic animals.) (*e*) Alternating occlusion is the most effective means of destroying binocularity. (Modified from Hubel and Wiesel, 1965; 196 cells from two kittens)

Ocular dominance stripes (columns)

In the visual cortex, stripe-like regions 0.5 mm wide are predominantly innervated by fibres from one eye. These stripes alternate with stripes dominated by the other eye (*Figure 13.6*), and are termed 'ocular dominance columns'. More generally, macroscopic groupings of cells differing radically in their function, but indistinguishable in their structure, are termed 'functional architecture'. By ordering cells across the cortical sheet according to the functions they must perform, functional architecture is thought to simplify visual information processing by simplifying the fibres needed for interconnecting related cells (Nelson, 1985). Ocular dominance columns have been demonstrated in man (e.g. Hitchcock and Hickey, 1980).

Monocular deprivation leads to expansion of the ocular dominance columns belonging to the dominant eye at the expense of amblyopic-eye column width in the cat (Shatz and Stryker, 1978), monkey (Hubel, Wiesel and LeVay, 1977; LeVay, Wiesel and Hubel, 1980) and man (Horton and Hedley-

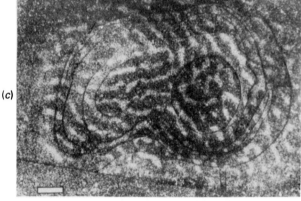

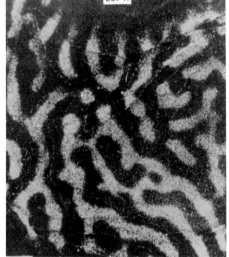

Figure 13.6 Ocular dominance columns in cortical layer IV of the monkey. (*a*) Normal, 6 weeks old. (*b*) Injected at 18 months of age following monocular deprivation begun at 2 weeks. Area 17/18 border at top; width of a left-right column pair is normal (about 750 μ.m) Monkey in (*c*) injected at 6 months of age following monocular deprivation begun at 3 weeks. The column pattern is more irregular further from the 17/18 border. Concentric 'contour lines' in (*b*) and (*c*) are an artefact of the photomontage. All calibration bars, 1 mm. (From LeVay, Wiesel and Hubel, 1980, courtesy of the Publisher, *J. Comp. Neurol.*; (*c*) originally appeared in Hubel, Wiesel and LeVay, 1977, *Philos. Trans. R Soc. Lond.*; photographs courtesy of Simon LeVay)

Whyte, 1984; reviews by Hubel, 1978; Swindale, 1982). In *Figure 13.6*, light areas show where radioactive proline has been transported transsynaptically to cortical layer IV (the input layer) from an injection in one eye. The light bands are the ocular dominance stripes ('columns') belonging to the injected eye and the dark bands are the fibre arrival zones for the other eye. The normal monkey already shows the adult pattern at 6 weeks (*Figure 13.6a*). Following occlusion, injection of the dominant eye produces wide light bands (*Figure 13.6b*), while injection of the deprived eye leads to narrow light bands (*Figure 13.6c*).

These animal observations cast doubt on the possibility of complete functional recovery by showing that structural changes buttress functional losses in deprivation amblyopia. Perhaps because of this, ocular dominance changes from reverse occlusion patching therapy are not as permanent and probably proceed by different cellular mechanisms than the onset of the original amblyopia (Mitchell, Murphy and Kaye, 1984).

Amblyopia therapy is a battle to win tissue back into the service of the deprived eye. Penalization (reverse occlusion) in the monkey can reverse column width expansion, but only infant monkeys (6 weeks old) have been tested (Blakemore and Vital-Durand, 1981).

Optimal occlusion therapy

Further research will define optimal occlusion regimens, at least in animals. It does appear that, if some binocular visual experience is combined with occlusion, the formerly strong (now occluded) eye does not lose ground during recovery of the weak eye. With this minimal visual stimulation, the formerly strong eye (and its pathways) do not reconquer the cortex once both eyes are opened. The formerly weak eye's recovery is permanent. This is shown in *Figure 13.7* where the treatment sequence is shown along the top.

Other plasticities

Morphogenesis (structural development) of the eye itself is dependent on visual feedback. The macaque monkey eye keeps growing until it is 1mm too long if patterned visual input is absent (Wiesel and Raviola, 1979). This is a possible cellular basis for the clinical observation that increasing departures from emmetropia are observed in the deviating eye of a strabismic amblyope after the age of two and a half (Keiner, 1968). It can be surmised the eye was growing into the plane of focus and passed it, either because the images available to the deviating eye

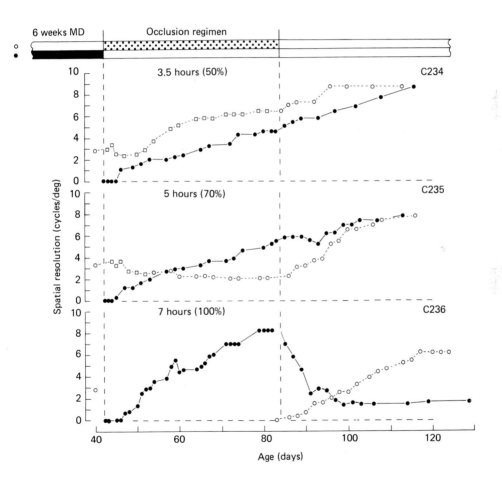

Figure 13.7 Changes in visual acuity with patching. The black bar represents 6 weeks monocular patching, producing severe visual loss in the deprived eye (solid black dots) at the time (left margin, 42 days old) when three different patching regimens for the strong eye were instituted for 6 weeks (stippled bar). Thereafter, both eyes were kept open to see if recovery would last. The three regimens were (top to bottom) 3.5, 5 and 7 patched hours/day out of 7 hours/day total visual experience. If there is no binocular experience (bottom panel), recovery is rapid during patching but collapses thereafter. Normal visual acuity under these conditions is between 6.4 and 8.6 cycles/deg. The open symbols are acuities for the good eye; it is technically possible to obtain these measurements with either one eye (circles) or both eyes (squares) open. (Monocularly deprived cats; from Mitchell *et al.*, 1986 courtesy of the publisher, Pergamon Press)

were often unsharp, or because neural responses from the cortex were already lacking. In human identical twins with eyeball lengths identical to within 0.2 mm, loss of vision in one eye (unilateral, congenital cataract) caused that eye to become 2 mm longer (Johnson *et al.*, 1982). This again emphasizes the need to establish binocularity before the age of two.

Changes in a variety of single unit properties (e.g. orientation selectivity, motion sensitivity) are reviewed by Movshon and Van Sluyters (1981) and by Blakemore (1978).

Critical period

The loss of neurones with access to both eyes and, worse still, the unavailability of any neurones responsive to one eye, are dramatic changes in cortical function and functional architecture triggered merely by changes in visual input. These changes can occur only in young animals. Of greater consequence to the health professions is that these changes can be corrected rapidly only in young patients. A change which endures beyond the critical period becomes permanent. Therapy and monitoring of the state of cortical binocularity may be stopped at this point. If it has not been started, therapy may be futile until some means is discovered of restoring plasticity in a mature cortex.

The critical period in animals

The period of cortical plasticity, or susceptibility to altered visual input, is termed the 'critical period' a concept borrowed from ethology (Erzurumlu and Killackey, 1982). Of concern is how this period is delimited by animal experiments, and what methods may be used to define it in man.

In kittens, occlusion ceases to trigger dramatic cortical changes by the age of 3 months or less (Hubel and Wiesel, 1970). The limit of the critical period may be more sharply defined by using reverse occlusion. With later times of reverse occlusion, it becomes harder to switch ocular dominance. Reverse occlusion pinpoints a sharp drop in the kittens' cortical plasticity between weeks 4 and 8 after birth (Blakemore and Van Sluyters, 1974; *Figure 13.8*). The critical period for loss of binocularity is the same, whether induced by monocular deprivation or strabismus (Levitt and Van Sluyters, 1982).

Recovery beyond the critical period

Assuming that there is a critical period in man, it is important to know what changes, if any, can be expected beyond its limits.

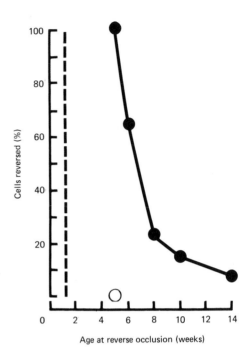

Figure 13.8. Reverse-occlusion defines 10–14 weeks as the end of the critical period in cat. The percentage of cells dominated by the most recently exposed eye is shown for five kittens (filled circles), all of which had one eye occluded from 9 days (dashed line) until reverse occlusion at ages of 5, 6, 8, 10 and 14 weeks. Each cat was tested 9 weeks after reversal. Open circle: control animal not reverse sutured shows complete (unreversed) dominance by normal eye at 5 weeks. (Modified from Blakemore and Van Sluyters, 1974)

In the cat, the critical period begins to shut down at 6 weeks, but the door may not finally close until beyond 4 months (Cynader, Timney and Mitchell, 1980). Cortical plasticity changes can occur in adult animals (Cynader, Berman and Hein, 1976; Yinon, 1978; Pasternak, Movshon and Merigan, 1981), but do not become large or rapid except with draconian measures such as extreme eye rotation, or enucleation of the formerly good eye (Kratz, Spear and Smith, 1976; Geisert *et al.*, 1982). While there is no doubt that therapy should be undertaken early to be most effective, enucleation findings raise hopes that 'hidden' connections from the eye to the brain are present even in the adult, and less drastic means may be found to activate them.

The new look in plasticity and visual training

Oculomotor proprioception and a variety of arousal manipulations are now known to play a role in cortical plasticity (Imbert and Fregnac, 1983; Singer, 1983, 1985). In this respect, animal research has only caught up to orthoptics, where the necessity of a child's attention and motivation has long been emphasized. Bangerter's multisensory training methods (eye and hand, ear or touch coordination) stimulate a large number of cortical areas, arouse the patient, and merit reconsideration.

Visual training programmes have appeared which are soundly based on knowledge of cortical function (Banks *et al.*, 1978), and work in animal tests (Martin *et al.*, 1979). Clinical trials have been disappointing because of poor choice of visual tests. Training which raises sensitivity to low contrast, low spatial frequency stimuli should not be evaluated by high contrast, high spatial frequency Snellen testing. In other clinical trials, arousal and motivation of the patients seemed as important as visual stimulation. Neurophysiological research confirms that both arousal and proper stimulation are necessary for cortical change and effective therapy. The search for more effective programmes should not be abandoned.

The critical period for binocularity loss in man

Clinicians have long been aware that early onset strabismus is more likely to lead to anomalous correspondence, and early treatment provides the most effective cure. Despite this, a clear notion of a critical period did not emerge. Today, the critical period in man has been defined by correlating loss of binocularity with the amount of exposure to altered visual input, typically occurring between well-defined dates of strabismus onset and surgical correction.

Binocularity loss can be assessed with visual after effects. Prolonged inspection of unidirectional motion (a waterfall or scenery outside a moving train window) adapts neurones tuned to such motion. A stationary test stimulus subsequently appears to move in the opposite direction. Suppose that such inspection was monocular and the test stimulus then presented to the other eye. Only neurones serving both eyes will show adaptation. Interocular transfer of after effects taps cortical binocularity at the cellular level.

Another after effect, the tilt after effect, was used in the initial studies of Banks, Aslin and Letson (1975) and Hohmann and Creutzfeldt (1975). Both groups were able to show reduced interocular transfer (reduced binocularity) with earlier strabismus onset, with peak sensitivity to disruption reached at 2 years of age (*Figure 13.9*). The apparent *onset* of plasticity is an artefact of the analysis method (further details in Aslin and Banks, 1978), but can be determined from infant acuity tests (*see* Chapter 11).

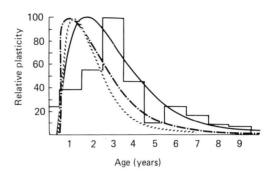

Figure 13.9. Critical period in man. Risk of binocularity loss is greatest at about 2 years of age, as assessed by failure of the tilt after effect to transfer interocularly. (−) Congenital esotropia (modified from Banks, Aslin and Letson, 1975); other lines, late onset esotropia; (−·−) 24 children selected from 300 cases for deviations greater than 20 Δ and good data for age of onset and age of successful surgical correction (Banks, Aslin and Letson, 1975); (...) 12 children (Hohmann and Creutzfeldt, 1975, as replotted by Aslin and Banks, 1978). The histogram shows incidence of anomalous binocular correspondence diagnosis as a function of age; 94 children assessed with Hering after image test (Aust, 1971). The critical period for anomalous correspondence appears to be later than for binocularity loss, only because many parents bring their children to the clinic at the age of three

Clinical correlates

The 1- to 2-year-old range for peak sensitivity is confirmed clinically by data obtained from occlusion therapy. The amount of occlusion necessary to produce a switch in the fixating eye is at a minimum between 14 and 18 months; occlusion is almost futile in this respect after about 5.5 years of age (Assaf, 1982). Acuity becomes immune to the development of unilateral cataract at 8–10 years of age (Vaegan and Taylor, 1980; *Figure 13.10*). With sensitive research methods, plasticity may be detected up to about 8 years of age, but treatment should be undertaken long before this.

Cortical plasticity and orthoptics

Treatment must come early or it will be futile. Hawkeswood (1971) said that there is little or nothing to be achieved in treating adults with abnormal retinal correspondence. The other side of the coin is that the disease must come early, or the sensory (mal)adaptation will be limited. Parks (1971) believed that neither anomalous correspondence nor eccentric fixation develops in children older than about 7–10 years, a guess close to the current estimates of the outer limits of the critical period in man.

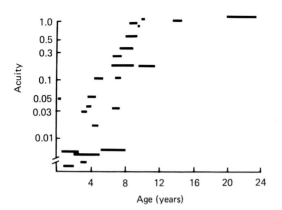

Figure 13.10. Critical period in a clinical setting: increasing immunity to acuity loss with increasing age of cataract onset. Horizontal bars: times of cataract onset (typically traumatic) and removal. Acuities of 1.0, 0.5, 0.1 etc. in the decimal system are 20/20, 20/40, 20/200 etc. in English feet notation. Twenty-three patients: two subjects with the lowest acuity had light perception only. (Modified from Vaegan and Taylor, 1980)

Surgery and/or orthoptic training must be performed early. Orthoptics then has a chance to achieve in days what years of training sometimes fails to do in the school-age child. But what can be done quickly can be undone quickly. Sensory status must be routinely monitored and held at the desired end-point until the patient's visual system emerges safely from the critical period. The main challenge of today is the creation of a new 'infant orthoptics'. Meeting this challenge will require new visual stimuli for diagnosis, training and infant assessment.

Drug-based orthoptics?

In the distant future, basic research holds the promise of re-opening the critical period for intensive visual retraining using drugs. After therapy, the patient would shut his eyes until the drug wore off and the functional changes were permanent.

Something must be making plasticity come and go in young animals, but it is not clear what this is. There is evidence that the critical period is maintained at least in part by noradrenaline (and noradrenaline is itself antagonized by 6-hydroxy-dopamine; reviews by Kasamatsu, 1982; Pettigrew, 1982; Kasamatsu *et al.*, 1984). The results are controversial (Sillito, 1986; Kasamatsu, 1987), and a simple mechanism has not been found for the drug action. This suggests that the factors controlling plasticity are several in number and are not understood at present.

There is reason to be optimistic that cortical circuits are capable of being revived. The classic view of amblyopia as a type of suppression is supported by the re-emergence of receptive fields for a formerly occluded eye when inhibition-blocking drugs are administered (Duffy *et al.*, 1976; Burchfiel and Duffy, 1981), although not all cells respond (Sillito, Kemp and Blakemore, 1981).

Basic research is advancing rapidly enough at the cellular level to warrant formulation of more radical therapies. Additional, unexplored routes to therapy lie in direct stimulation of the weak eye by electrical or magnetic phosphenes, easily induced in man (Gebhard, 1953; Seidel, Knoll and Eichmeier, 1968; Carpenter, 1973), or by temporary retrobulbar blockade of the dominant eye coupled with vigorous visual training of the amblyopic eye. However, structural changes *do* occur and may be irreversible. Such changes include cortical ocular dominance column narrowing and, in the cat, Y-cell loss in the lateral geniculate nucleus. Problems do not end with the restoration of responsiveness. The receptive fields which emerge for both eyes may be stimulus unselective or unmatched and therefore useless for binocular vision.

W, X and Y visual subsystems

Most retinal ganglion cells fall into one of three morphological categories, each having different functional specializations and different pathways to central visual centres. The functional and structural differences are great enough to warrant treating the classic retinocortical pathway as three visual subsystems running in parallel, and designated Y (α), X (β) and W (γ) (*Figure 13.11*).

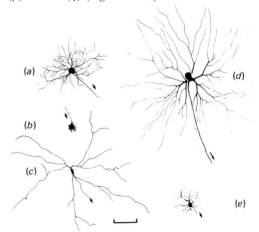

Figure 13.11 (*a,b,c*) α, β and γ ganglion cells at 1.2 mm eccentricity in cat retina. α, β and γ morphological groups parallel Y, X and W functional types. The γ cell's dendritic arbor has been coarsened for illustration; it has a spidery, filamentous appearance. (*d, e*) α (Y) and β (X) cells at about 10 mm retinal eccentricity (roughly 48°) are bigger, but γ cell size is relatively constant across the retina. (Modified from Boycott and Wässle, 1974)

Selective participation of W, X or Y systems is a new theme in the study of many visual problems. In amblyopia, the X system may be selectively impaired. Visual deprivation during a critical period of cortical plasticity can cause functional loss. The X system's specialization for fine detail appears to carry a special vulnerability to degraded visual input. The W X Y groups also merit consideration for understanding the *normal* visual system, where different visual functions draw on different W, X and Y attributes. This seems to apply particularly for visual extremes, e.g. perceiving the direction of the fastest-moving objects or discerning form in fog at low contrast. Research in coming years is likely to show that performance limits are set by one system alone. Such progress is evident in optokinetic nystagmus where, at subcortical levels, cells involved in detecting image motion for this oculomotor reflex appear to be drawn exclusively from the W system.

Characteristics of the W, X and Y subsystems

One way to classify most cat retinal ganglion cell bodies is simply as large, medium, or small (α, β and γ cells, *see Figure 13.11*). A large cell body (soma) has a large axon diameter. Such an axon would be expected to conduct more rapidly and, indeed, cells in the large-soma system are rapid conductors. They capitalize on this boon for signalling *change* by additionally possessing a transient response characteristic: excitatory response is intense at the moment of stimulus change, with relatively less sustained response during periods of constant stimulation (*see Figure 13.2*). Cells in the Y system are also more non-linear in the way they sum their various responses to stimulation within their receptive fields. For example, instead of cancelling, stimuli in the complementary centre and surround regions may both *add* to the response, so that there is excitation at both stimulus ON set and OFF set (*see Figure 13.2*). Such a cell is signalling stimulus transitions regardless of whether they are increases or decreases in light. This system is a major contributor to the visual system's response to flickering lights, as used clinically (e.g. major amblyoscope, after-image test).

Turning from temporal to spatial properties, a large cell body also has a large dendritic field for input. At any given eccentricity, therefore, the receptive fields of Y cells are larger than the fields of X cells, and indeed variation in optimal stimulus size or spatial frequency is due to characteristic α, β and γ cell size differences. *Both* X and Y systems exhibit smaller ganglion cells and higher densities in the central retina, although Y cells are everywhere larger and less numerous than X cells. While the Y system gives high temporal resolution, the X peripheral system has advantages as a high spatial resolution system, advantages amplified by the system's central connections to the striate cortex. By dominating the striate cortex, the X system enjoys information processing by an area with more cortical machinery devoted to central vision than any other, and earns its place as the system most responsible for high-acuity vision at the point of fixation. Normal Snellen acuity represents an X system achievement.

Spatial vision is not entirely concerned with the recognition of detail. The strong, linear surround mechanisms of X cells are a great asset in precise spatial coding: a small stimulus cannot stray off the receptive field centre without incurring enormous losses in the response level it elicits. They do, however, limit sensitivity to stimuli with high velocities and low spatial frequencies. Response to an object big enough or fast enough to stimulate both centre and surround at once will be partially self-cancelling in the X system, but will excite the Y system. Another Y system characteristic is its greater immunity to binocularity losses associated with cortical plasticity. Animal experiments have given results that suggest flicker, motion and motion-in-depth sensitivities, especially in the non-foveal visual field, are more likely to survive in a stereoblind observer lacking conventional cortical binocularity. These functions should be explicitly tested in affected patients.

The different spatiotemporal specializations of the X and Y visual subsystems make grating stimuli a popular means of dissociating the X and Y contributions to psychophysical functions in man. Coarse, low-contrast sine wave gratings are devoid of high spatial frequency content, and may be rapidly drifted or flickered in various ways to favour a Y-dominated response. High spatial frequency gratings presented with little or no temporal modulation favour an X-dominated response. At high contrasts, cells in all systems will respond, but at threshold-level contrasts, one system may drop out, leaving the other to determine visual performance (e.g. Nelson *et al.*, 1984a). Visual function, and particularly the hypothesis that selective X or Y loss may play a role in amblyopia, is increasingly being explored with grating stimuli varied in these ways.

All photopic vision depends on cones, the density of which decreases with distance from the fovea, just as acuity decreases with eccentricity. But when the visual system is seen as differently optimized subsystems operating in parallel, it becomes clear that peripheral vision is not only quantitatively scaled down from central vision, it is qualitatively different (Merchant, 1965; Bouma, 1970; Nelson, 1975b). Much of the difference has to do with loss of fine, local positional information, possibly because Y-cell responses do not encode exact stimulus position within their large receptive fields. Psychophysical findings in this area are reminiscent of the confusion errors found in amblyopia and suggest that an amblyopic visual system is a system thrown back on Y-system responses. In sum, peripheral visual perception is Y-dominated vision.

Some aspects of higher-order colour vision appear to be exclusively X-mediated. Lateral geniculate nucleus and cortical cells with double-opponent colour sensitivity (e.g. where the centre responds ON to red but OFF to green, the surround being the opposite) probably all draw their input from the X stream. Impaired colour discrimination ability of central origin (beyond area 17) will probably prove to be a disorder of this portion of the X system. X-stream cortical neurones capable of detecting colour contrast in the absence of luminance differences have mainly monocular inputs. Many binocular deficiencies arise in normal observers when stimuli are constructed of isoluminant chromatic contours. It is important that, where colour is used as part of a clinical test, there be luminance as well as colour differences if the images are to be combined binocularly.

The W system is heterogeneous. There are cells responding constantly to luminance levels (more luminance, more response), involved in pupillary control and setting our sunrise-sensitive diurnal rhythm (suprachiasmatic nuclei, *see* Chapter 1). Other cells are responsive to contrast edges anywhere on their receptive fields; the sharper the edge the greater is the response. This yields little good position information for pattern recognition, but might drive accommodation because, if so, it is a push–pull system; other W cells are suppressed by standing contrast. There are cells which, by W cell standards, are fast, transient and Y-like, and others which are more sustained. The common characteristics of these cells are thin, slowly conducting axons, sparsely branching dendrites and a sluggish response characteristic.

The W system has widespread connections to older, subcortical centres (the accessory optic system, the nucleus of the optic tract and the superior colliculus) and is itself probably an older subsystem concerned with more fundamental visual tasks. It will probably be shown to play an important role in accommodation, vergence and pursuit eye movements, and especially pupillary control and optokinetic nystagmus. When large areas of the visual field must be covered (albeit loosely), when a great variety of visual processing must be done (but not in a hurry) and when the visual task is important for orienting and servostabilizing the rest of the visual system (but without much conscious awareness), it is probably the W system that subconsciously undertakes the task, while the X and Y systems flash across perceptual consciousness.

Selective YX involvement in amblyopia

X-cell impairment

In unilateral squints, the deviating eye is not pointed at the object of regard. Objects along the line of sight will often be blurred due to inappropriate accommodation, depriving the X system of satisfactory stimulation. Loss of high spatial frequency sensitivity among X cells in the lateral geniculate nucleus (Lehmkuhle *et al.*, 1979) is a generally accepted outcome in a variety of deprivation conditions. Such changes may underlie acuity loss in human amblyopia.

Y-cell loss

Monocular deprivation causes cell body shrinkage and a loss of visual function in Y cells in the cat's lateral geniculate nucleus (Sherman, Hoffman and Stone, 1972). The cells are so unresponsive that early investigators missed them entirely and, based on the remaining X cells, thought there had been no effect upon the LGN. Later investigation showed subtle visual acuity loss even in the surviving X population. A comprehensive hypothesis for the effect has been offered by Sur, Weller and Sherman (1984), based on competitive development between the two systems maturing at different times. It is hypothesized that, with deprivation, the late-arriving Y system finds itself unable to compete for entry into the LGN. It withers, leaving the LGN dominated by the X-fibres which arrived there first. This would be an instance of competition between parallel XY visual subsystems rather than eyes. Such competition may not occur in the monkey's LGN, where X and Y pathways are more segregated by layers than in the cat.

Another instance of Y-selective loss is found in Siamese cats which possess a form of albinism and have fewer Y-type ganglion cells and hence poor flicker–fusion frequencies. Future research may link impoverished innervation of Y-dominated, motion-processing cortical centres with the strabismus and oculomotor control problems often observed in animal and human albinos.

Summary of W, X and Y subsystems

The X system is now strongly linked with what clinicians have traditionally meant by 'good vision', meaning high acuity in the central visual field. Visual neuroscience has yet to link this system with 'locking' the eyes onto the target during fixation. The Y system's role in conscious perception has been underestimated. The domain of this system includes, not only motion and motion in depth, but also global grouping and figure-ground segmentation operations poised at the threshold of pattern recognition. Neuroscience has begun to link this system with the initiation of eye movements. Results from animal experiments, based perhaps too heavily on the cat rather than the monkey, suggest Y-system damage in amblyopia, while the results of studies on human amblyopes suggest a visual system carrying on with Y-system resources despite X-system damage. The W system is unspectacular but vital, contributing heavily, in decreasing order of certainty, to the following classic optometric visual functions: optokinetic nystagmus, pupillary control, accommodation, vergence and tracking. The challenge for neuroscience is to show how W, X and Y pathways, defined in the retina, stream through groups of cortical areas differentially responsible for motion versus pattern/colour-related perceptual processing.

Tests of binocularity loss in man

Monocular and binocular responses

When dealing with amblyopia and binocular vision three visual systems should be kept in mind. These are: the cortical cells serving only the left eye, those serving only the right eye and those serving both (*see* Ocular dominance). Visual performance determined by monocular cell populations does not establish what has occurred in the binocular visual system where correspondence can be set to anomalous values and functions such as stereoacuity may falter or fail.

Summary of binocularity losses in strabismus and anisometropia

There are four possible degrees of disturbance:

(1) The input from one eye, excitatory and inhibitory, may fail to influence the cortex.
(2) Excitatory input from one eye may be missing in the cortex; inhibitory input may survive. This is the current picture of deprivation amblyopia in animals. Presumably the same cortical changes occur in clinical cases of stimulus deprivation, such as in severe anisometropia and possibly in unilateral strabismus. Unfortunately, columnar width changes also occur (*see Figure 13.6*), depriving the observer of tissue to process what few signals do get through from the amblyopic eye.
(3) Excitatory *binocularity* may be lost; each eye is well served by a population of neurones, but the two populations are separate. Stereopsis will fail. There may be no cells to provide fine

control of vergence eye movements (fixation lock), even though monocular acuity may be normal (no amblyopia). Alternating strabismus is a natural cause of such a condition.
(4) Binocularly excitable neurones may be present but 'pathological', such as in anomalous correspondence. A small, constant angle (comitant) squint is a natural cause.

The binocular status can be evaluated using test patterns which powerfully stimulate binocular neurones. Sometimes it can also be advantageous to stimulate only monocular neural populations because their properties remain stable in the face of binocular sensory adaptations occurring elsewhere. Examples are a monocular after-image or Maddox rod streak, assumed to provide an 'objective' indication of where the eye is pointing. The basis of this assumption is that if monocular, unfusible stimuli do not stimulate binocular cortical neurones, they will not elicit anomalous correspondence. This assumption is usually true, but there are limits. *Paradoxical fixation* (e.g. monocular eccentric fixation on temporal retina in an observer who is esotropic during binocular viewing; von Noorden, 1970) is another example of separate adaptations occurring in monocular and binocular cell populations.

Research methods for accessing only monocular or, more importantly, only binocular cell populations are detailed below.

Binocularity and different strengths of after effect transfer

Failure of interocular transfer of a figural after effect in strabismic observers was first observed by a clinician (Brock, 1950), but the observation was forgotten until advances in cortical neurophysiology revealed its significance (Wolfe and Held, 1983). An after effect (illusory shift) in perceived spatial frequency can be demonstrated with *Figure 13.12*.

During monocular adaptation, one monocular cell population and the conventional cell population are exposed and cause an after effect. A 30–40% drop in after effect strength when the previously covered eye is tested reflects the dilution of the effect by the previously unstimulated monocular population. Binocular testing following monocular exposure shows further dilution of the effect (60% total drop in magnitude). The additional neural population responsible for this dilution is presumably a population of obligatorily binocular neurones, which only become activated at this point. Such neurones respond to binocular stimulation only, and can not be excited through either eye alone. As they were never adapted, the obligatorily binocular neurones respond vigorously and detract from the after effect. To summarize, monocular cell populations are blind in one eye, conventional binocular neurones are logical OR gates responding to one eye or the other,

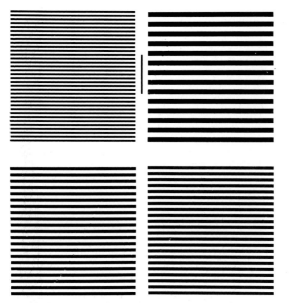

Figure 13.12. Demonstration of spatial frequency after effect. Cover the bottom portion of the figure and look at the top for 30 seconds, letting the eyes rove along the vertical fixation bar between the striped squares, to avoid after-images. Briefly uncover and momentarily transfer gaze to the bottom portion of the figure. Look at the top gratings for at least 10 more seconds before taking another glance at the bottom gratings. Most observers will report the bottom left grating appears coarser than the right, despite their physical equality. If the top is inspected with one eye and the bottom tested with the other, the distortion can only be 'transferred' by cortical neurones which respond to either eye (a binocularly excitable neurone). Interocular transfer of after effects like this one has been used as a probe for cortical binocularity in man

while a minority of binocular neurones are AND gates responding only if one *and* the other eye are stimulated with matched stimuli.

Binocular cell populations can be accessed more directly by inducing an after effect with stripes only visible stereoscopically (cyclopean contours; Wolfe and Held, 1982). Tilt after effects of 2° occur with binocular viewing, but disappear if either eye is shut, because monocularly innervated neurones never experienced the adapting contours.

When different eyes are used, different cell populations are accessed.

Psychophysical tests of binocularity

Without binocular cortical neurones, image disparity detection and stereoscopic depth perception fail. Non-invasive tests of the following functions provide a measure of the state of cortical binocularity.

Binocular summation

In addition to after effect transfer tests, binocular summation offers a straightforward test of binocularity failure. If each eye were served by a separate neural population, processing would proceed independently and two eyes would not be much better than one. As expected, stereoblind observers fail to show benefit from binocular stimulation in a variety of threshold tasks, such as low-contrast grating detection, temporal modulation (flicker) detection, reaction time and the suprathreshold task of putting together dichoptically presented dot patterns to perceive meaningful forms (three-digit numbers). Basic research has confirmed the lack of summation in animals known to lack binocular cortical neurones (cat: Grünau, 1979; monkey: Crawford *et al.*, 1983).

Unfortunately, complications make the above effect small. Summation of the independent left- and right-eye channels can improve binocular threshold performance in the observer who has only monocular capabilities. In the same way that many sweeps can be averaged to retrieve an evoked potential, the brain can average the two samples provided by the two eyes to improve detection (probability summation). Only in the binocular observer will binocular stimulation activate exclusively binocular neurones, and even ordinary (monocularly excitable) binocular neurones will provide an extra response burst with binocular stimulation. But the lack of this binocular machinery does not unduly hamper the stereoblind observer. Instead of *losing* binocular cells, they are converted into monocular cells and thereby augment the (monocular) probability summation mechanisms.

After effect transfer

Interocular transfer of tilt after effects (and other pattern after effects) are effective tests for the loss of binocularity, as described above. Transfer of contrast *threshold elevation after effects*, on the other hand, survive binocularity loss, and are therefore less diagnostically useful.

Other binocularity tests are *utrocular* discrimination (observers with only monocular cell populations may be superior at detecting which eye was stimulated) and interocular masking. The continued occurrence of masking effects suggests the presence of interocular inhibition in stereoblindness.

Evoked potential tests of binocularity

The visual evoked potential (VEP) may provide a rapid, objective test of binocularity, making available comparison to both psychophysics and neurophysiology.

Summation

The obvious test of binocularity is summation, a stronger response resulting from the stimulation of two eyes than from one. Binocularity loss from strabismis amblyopia or any other cause can result in a failure of summation of evoked potential amplitude. Anomalous binocular correspondence can sustain summation, but if the anomalous correspondence reverts to suppression when neutral density filters, vertical prisms or spherical lenses are interposed, then summation will again fail (Campos and Chiesi, 1983).

Many problems make summation a difficult approach. First, the expected effects are small and in practice there is always variability in evoked potential amplitudes (Perry, Childers and McCoy, 1968). Vaegan, Shoerey and Kelsey (1979) obtained summation in an amblyope, so that binocular summation of evoked responses is not a foolproof sign of normal binocularity. Sometimes only one VEP component summates causing confusing changes in the shape of the VEP waveform. The search for a component which reliably summates in normals, and fails to summate or shows inhibition or binocularity loss, has led to the discovery of strong effects and exploration of novel stimuli, but has not yet led to the adoption of a reliable routine (Apkarian, Nakayama and Tyler, 1981).

Interocular contour suppression and latency

The monocular VEP amplitude is decreased when a steady pattern is presented to the other eye (Spekreijse, van der Tweel and Regan, 1972; reviewed by Harter, 1977). A contoured field will cause greater suppression than a diffuse field, and identically oriented contours cause the greatest suppression (Harter, Conder and Towle, 1980). The orientation specificity of the effect, most evident in the early 110 ms component, suggests a cortical origin. The interocular contour suppression effects are a reliable but neglected indicator of binocularity. Like interocular masking, it may be specific to inhibitory interactions.

VEP amplitude does shift in response to short-term occlusion of normal adults (Tyler and Kaitz, 1977), but given the instability of any VEP amplitude measure, latency changes may be a more reliable means of monitoring progress in occlusion therapy (Barnard and Arden, 1979). Future research *in clinical patients* is needed to identify the best means of tapping binocular cortical status with VEP techniques.

Random-dot stereograms: screening with global stereopsis

Early treatment requires early detection and diagnosis. Random-dot stereograms provide a broad-spectrum screening test for binocular disorders because of their high demands for oculomotor precision and central processing. To see them, an observer must possess cortical binocularity, high acuity, disparity detection ability and global processing capability.

A random-dot stereogram which can be stereoscopically fused without special equipment is shown in *Figure 13.13*. The left eye/right eye pattern alternates every centimetre or so, so that a centimetre of diplopia (or 3 cm, or 5 cm) serves to get left and right half-images dichoptically combined. Relaxing convergence will work as well as overconvergence.

Figure 13.13. Chris Tyler's 'autostereogram', a random-dot stereogram (Julesz pattern) which can be seen with free viewing. Place the illustration 50 cm away and hold a finger 7 cm above it. With stable fixation of the finger, a stereoscopic percept will gradually solidify in the plane of the finger, which can then be removed. The first attempt can be time consuming, until one learns to dissociate accommodation and convergence. (From Tyler, 1983)

Matching noise and globality

The carefully repeated half-images and precisely controlled displacements of random-dot stereograms would seem to make disparity detection easy. Instead, the repeating checks of a random-dot stereogram match one another and create ambiguities. A black square in one half-image can be paired with a variety of black squares at a variety of horizontal displacements in the other half-image. In neurophysiological terms, binocular depth-detecting neurones of a variety of disparity tunings will be active; this activity is called matching noise. There is no way to ascertain the correct disparity based on a local, point-by-point analysis of the image without additional processing.

Although matching noise activates random disparity channels at scattered visual field locations, only the correct disparity tuning is *consistently* active across a run of positions.

Stereoscopic globality refers to the visual system's ability to respond to a disparity match which is consistent across an extended portion of the visual field, and to suppress response to isolated, local matches. These random responses, termed 'matching noise', are numerous in random-dot stereograms because of their repeating nature (Julesz, 1971; Nelson, 1975a). The first response at many false disparities, and the additional processing required to get rid of it, are unique to random-dot stereograms and place burdens on cortical machinery not present with conventional stereograms. Once attained, however, the stereoscopic response is strong, because random-dot stimuli are contour rich.

Stereopsis with random-dot stereograms, or global stereopsis, is slow, in part because matching noise must first be suppressed, although an observer's performance improves with practice (reviewed in Nelson, 1985). Because the disparity cue is faint in comparison to matching noise, these stimuli are uniquely poor at eliciting sensory fusion (Fender and Julesz, 1967). Although more research is needed, the stimulus to motor fusion is probably also weak, so that small fixation disparities or tropias constitute greater impediments to stereopsis with random-dot stereograms than with conventional line stimuli.

Because of its additional cortical processing demands, random-dot stereopsis may involve more and higher visual centres than other common visual performance tests. Perhaps for this reason, screening with random-dot stereograms picks up patients with right hemisphere strokes as well as oculomotor inaccuracies. There is evidence that global stereopsis is lateralized to the right cortical hemisphere, particularly the posterior portion (Ross, 1983).

To summarize, random-dot stereograms are good for detecting binocular disorders, leaving differential diagnosis to later examination. Cerebral stroke as well as amblyopia can be detected.

Asymmetrical optokinetic nystagmus and binocularity

The optokinetic nystagmus (OKN) reflex stabilizes the retinal image by turning the eyes. In lower animals, the reflex is stimulated only by nasalward movement of the visual field, so that OKN stabilizes the retinal image during head turning but does not interfere with forward locomotion through the environment. This asymmetrical nystagmus with monocular testing is also found in amblyopia (Nicolai, 1959) and in very young kittens and human infants. Temporalward OKN is present in normal, older individuals, but depends on *cortical* binocular-

ity and drops out with stereoblindness (van Hof-van Duin and Mohn, 1982). The lower nuclei responsible for the nasalward reflex never evolved to respond to temporalward movement, but instead obtain the needed information from the cortex (Schoppmann, 1981; Marcotte and Updyke, 1982). Because the cortex itself must possess binocularity to provide this input, the OKN reflex has been exploited to assess the onset (Chapter 11) and status of binocularity in infants (*see* Chapter 12).

Anatomy

The neural pathways are illustrated in *Figure 13.14*. Visual drive for optokinetic nystagmus originates in the pretectal nucleus of the optic tract (NOT), whose direct innervation comes only from the contralateral eye, probably via very slow W fibres. NOT neurones all have the same directional selectivity: nasalward in the visual field (solid arrows) and temporalward on the retina (outline arrows). To achieve temporalward optokinetic movement of the

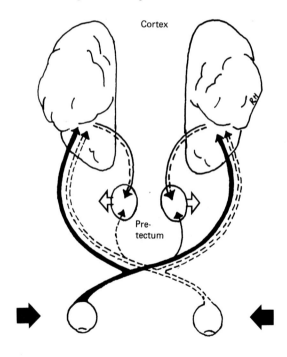

Figure 13.14. Visual pathways involved in optokinetic nystagmus (OKN). Nasalward movement in the visual field (solid arrows) stimulates direction-selective neurones in the contralateral nucleus of the optic tract in the pretectum (outline arrows). Temporalward monocular OKN requires participation of the ipsilateral NOT, which can only be reached via corticofugal pathways. The NOT loses binocularity if the cortex does, rendering monocular temporalward OKN a useful probe of binocularity loss. (Modified from Braddick and Atkinson, 1982)

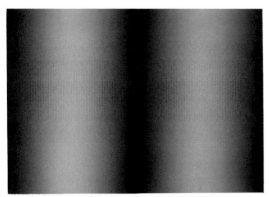

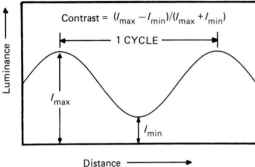

Figure 13.15. Example of a sinusoidal grating and the definition of its contrast. About two cycles of the grating are shown, with the luminance profile of one cycle drawn below. (From Levi and Harwerth, 1982, © The American Academy of Optometry, 1982)

eyes requires activity in an ipsilateral NOT, which must be stimulated indirectly from an external source, insofar as none of its own neurones responds to that direction of stimulus movement. It is the cortex which excites the ipsilateral NOT in such cases.

The W-system role in optometric abnormalities

Temporalward *saccades* and pursuit movements are also weak and variable in strabismic amblyopia (Schor, 1975). Direct and consensual pupillary light reflexes are initiated slowly when driven by the amblyopic eye (Kase *et al.*, 1984), but then proceed normally. Future research may show that a variety of oculomotor and optometric functions have two components, one driven by older, slower subcortical centres via W-fibres from the retina, and the other dependent on faster, binocular, supplementary pathways from the visual cortex. The cortical contribution may fail in strabismus. The suspected diversity of W-system roles is appropriate to the known diversity of W-cell morphology and function.

Investigation of amblyopia

Gratings: spatial and temporal frequency concepts

Discovering the mechanisms of amblyopia requires a more thorough visual assessment than just the measurement of Snellen acuity. Snellen acuity assesses primarily one visual subsystem (the X system) in one place on the retina (the fovea) as served chiefly by one projection area in the cortex (area 17). More comprehensive visual assessment techniques often make use of gratings, which can be linked to everyday images through Fourier transformation (*see* Chapter 2).

Gratings have achieved prominence in vision research for several reasons. If the response to a few gratings is known, performance with any stimulus may be predicted using Fourier transformation. The stimuli are easily varied to test a full range of spatial and temporal sensitivities. The stimuli are quantifiable and mathematically tractable. Gratings can emphasize contributions from higher visual centres (those possessing at least concentric opponent receptive fields), because they can be modulated to produce pattern changes with no change in average luminance. The exchange of black and white areas, termed 'pattern reversal', is a particularly common example of such temporal modulation; others are pattern appearance/disappearance or movement ('drifting gratings'). Gratings provide a means of partially separating X and Y visual system contributions to visual performance. Separate cortical populations may be stimulated with, for example, orientation change. Gratings may be used to provide a well-specified stimulus for the visual field as a whole, and may provide a common ground for comparing clinical and normal, human and animal visual systems.

Gratings and the transfer function concept

Initially, gratings were produced by stretching fine wires across a glass plate, forming a miniature grate which gave the pattern its name. Today it is appreciated that sine wave gratings, readily produced on TV monitors, are more useful. A plot of luminance as a photocell is moved across the blurry grating stripes would show the gradual rise and fall of a sine wave function (*Figure 13.15*). A photocell scanning along any grating stripe sees no luminance variation to act as a pattern stimulus. A sine wave grating is illustrated in *Figure 13.15*. These patterns are unidimensional and are thus said to have orientation purity. This immediately gives us an incisive stimulus for the visual cortex, where most neurones' responsiveness is highly selective for stimulus orientation.

Measurement of contrast sensitivity

The measurement of performance with low and middle spatial frequencies is a necessary complement to measurements of acuity. Coarse stripes are easily seen, and acuity imposes no limits. To bring such stripes to the threshold of visibility for visual testing, they can be reduced in *contrast*. The amount of contrast required to detect the presence of stripes can be measured for a selection of stripes from coarse to fine. These measurements define a contrast sensitivity function (CSF). A graph of the CSF describes sensitivity to patterns (Y axis, the thresholds) as a function of their spatial frequency. The X axis is 'frequency', so that the CSF shows the full spectrum of the visual system's response (*see* Chapter 2). For general applicability, contrast sensitivity should be measured for two series of gratings presented at right angles to each other.

Contrast *sensitivity* functions are a special case of modulation transfer function (MTF) in that they describe an input (grating)/output (perception) function, but only for threshold contrasts. Fortunately, where sensitivities for threshold contrasts are good, perceived vividness of suprathreshold contrasts is likely to be strong as well. Snellen acuity is the final point on the contrast sensitivity function, namely the finest detail (highest spatial frequency) which can be seen when contrast is maximum. A typical contrast sensitivity function is shown in *Figure 13.16 (see also* Chapter 2, *Figure 2.7*). Sensitivity is the reciprocal of threshold; normal observers, able to detect stripes at less than 1% contrast, have peak sensitivities of over 100. The spatial frequency (X axis) of fingers held up at arms' length is of the order of 0.5 cycles/deg; of the lines of text on a double-spaced page at the same distance, 3 cycles/deg. At the acuity limit (*arrow*), stripes become too fine to resolve even at maximum contrast; at the low end, after images and lateral neural interactions have been suggested to explain the mild loss in sensitivity.

Temporal frequencies become important when gratings are turned on and off or reversed. Real motion (grafting drift) also has a temporal frequency, corresponding to the number of white bars crossing a reference point per second. When spatial frequency is zero, temporal modulation produces a uniform field whose luminance fluctuates. Critical flicker fusion frequency is the maximum temporal rate perceivable when luminance fluctuation is maximum (full intensity on, or off). Like Snellen acuity, it represents an extreme case, the tail end of another modulation transfer function called the DeLange curve.

The spatial, temporal and orientation purity of a grating make it a good probe for specific neural populations, whether approached neurophysiologically in animals or as psychophysical channels in man. It is a popular stimulus in modern amblyopia research.

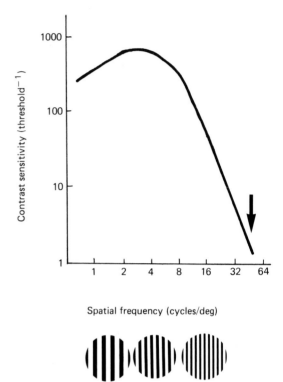

Figure 13.16. Typical contrast sensitivity function

Application to amblyopia

Amblyopia has an incidence of 1–3% in the population. Epidemiological information is lacking (Hillis, Flynn and Hawkins, 1983) due to inadequate screening methods and unresolved diagnostic criteria. Random-dot stereograms (*see above*) and new infant assessment techniques promise improved screening capability. Tests of the following functions may be used to investigate amblyopia.

Contrast sensitivity function

Contrast sensitivity testing of amblyopia often shows a high frequency loss, justifying the historical importance of Snellen testing, and suggesting X-system involvement. Contrast threshold testing, however, is preferable because it has higher diagnostic value than Snellen testing. Still better tests could be developed. First, there are additional abnormalities of spatial localization ('crowding') which are not well detected in tests with grating patterns and, second, suprathreshold performance is important in daily life but is not described by a *threshold* measure.

Two types of threshold contrast sensitivity loss were identified by Hess and Howell (1977) in strabismic amblyopes, one prominent for higher spatial

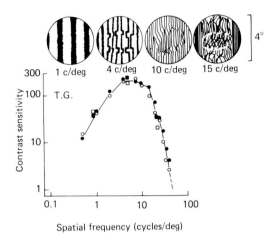

Figure 13.17. Grating distortions (phase errors) are experienced by amblyopes even when contrast sensitivity thresholds are normal. Open symbols: normal eye; filled symbols, amblyopic eye; circles, vertical; squares, horizontal. Light intensity = 30 cd/m². (From Hess, Campbell and Greenhalgh, 1978, courtesy of the Publisher)

frequencies and the other (more common and more severe) showing losses across all spatial frequencies. Loss confined to high frequencies was later demonstrated in anisometropic amblyopia (Bradley and Freeman, 1981). Small display screens and high luminance bring out amblyopic losses by lessening participation of the peripheral visual field, where amblyopes are most likely to have normal function.

Visual reaction times to the presentation of a spot of light are lengthened in amblyopia. Neither eccentricity of fixation nor poorer acuity can explain this observation (Hamasaki and Flynn, 1981). Slowed reaction times persist even at high contrast levels (Loshin and Levi, 1983) and this makes it possible to use reaction times to obtain a contrast sensitivity function based on grating appearance. Results typically show a greater loss at higher spatial frequency (Harwerth and Levi, 1978). While acuity loss is synonymous with X loss, loss of *speed* suggests loss of Y-system cells, whose large-diameter fibres have the most rapid conduction times.

Suprathreshold contrast sensitivity is normal in strabismic amblyopia and nearly so for anisometropes. As the contrast is increased above threshold, the stimulus quickly becomes as vivid to the amblyopic eye as to its fellow in a matching task, something which cannot occur when there has been organic damage to the optic nerve. If sensitivity to above-threshold contrast is normal, amblyopic impairment must have another basis.

Spatial crowding

The Snellen acuity of an amblyopic eye is worse for conventional eye charts than isolated optotypes (crowding effect). Gratings do not appear regular to amblyopes, who describe jagged discontinuities and other spatial distortions (Hess, Campbell and Greenhalgh, 1978; *Figure 13.17*) which are hard to quantify, but easy to detect with non-grating tasks. Such tasks include identifying the location of one dot in an array (Hess and Jenkins, 1980), or vernier alignment (Levi and Klein, 1983). Deficits are more severe in strabismic than in anisometropic amblyopia. With gratings, the jagged discontinuities occur at the border between central and peripheral portions of the visual field although it is not known if this coincides with the border between a central area of suppression and/or anomalous correspondence and a peripheral area of binocularity.

The grating distortions seen by amblyopes are illustrated in *Figure 13.17*. Note that even a complete contrast sensitivity function can fail to detect this visual loss, which takes the form of phase errors. Jumbling of spatial localization is a defining attribute of amblyopia.

Ganglion cell loss in retina tested with pattern electroretinogram

By using grating and checkerboard stimuli, a strong stimulus can be given to pattern-sensitive neural elements without disturbing average luminance of the stimulus field. In the retina, the responding neurones will be predominantly ganglion cells. For their concentric, ON–OFF receptive fields, changes in where luminance flux falls are important, even if the average amount of illumination is constant. An electroretinogram to a pattern-reversal stimulus should be dominated by ganglion cells.

With special averaging techniques, such an electro-diagnostic potential can be recorded, and is termed a 'pattern electroretinogram' (PERG). There is evidence that the PERG originates with the ganglion cells. It is reduced by optic nerve section in animals (which leads to ganglion cell death) and by optic nerve disease in man. The PERG offers another tool for non-invasive, layer-by-layer 'functional dissection' of the retina, and has yet to be fully exploited.

Visual evoked potential

A delay in the reaction time to detect a grating by an amblyopic eye is evident in the prolonged latency of the evoked potential (Arden and Barnard, 1980). The evoked potential amplitude in amblyopes shows a shallower climb as stimulus contrast is increased. The change from normal is greatest at high spatial frequencies and cannot be mimicked with defocusing (Levi and Harwerth, 1978).

Evoked potentials elicited by the vernier offset and realignment of lines can provide an electrophysiological estimate of psychophysical vernier acuity (Levi *et al.*, 1983). This test should be applied to amblyopia because it is sensitive to crowding effects.

Position in the visual field

In many kinds of organic amblyopia, visual losses are either across the whole of the visual field or are peripherally weighted. In strabismic amblyopia, suppression is strongest in the central visual field. For example, in alternating strabismus, the deviating eye is most strongly suppressed in the region corresponding to the fixating eye's fovea (Sireteanu, 1982). Forcing the visual system to rely more heavily on the peripheral visual field by greatly dimming field luminance (3 log unit neutral density filter) can therefore equalize performance of good and bad eyes in strabismic but not organic amblyopia. This classic test for distinguishing functional from organic amblyopia may, however, fail to differentiate *anisometropic* amblyopia from organic amblyopia (Hess, Campbell and Zimmern, 1980).

Both size and scatter of receptive fields increase with increasing eccentricity (Hubel and Wiesel, 1974). Neurones in the peripheral visual field with such receptive fields are better able to respond to large disparities and to survive a small-angle squint. Anisometropia penalizes neurones everywhere more uniformly, and so losses are field-wide.

Amblyopia seems to involve a diminished role for the X visual subsystem and an exaggerated role for the Y subsystem. The consequence is poor phase (Braddick, 1981) and spatial localization capabilities, which leaves amblyopic vision in strabismus and peripheral vision in normal sight with much in common (Levi, Klein and Aitsebaomo, 1984).

Conclusions

Amblyopia: the sensory definition

Amblyopia affects many visual functions. Monocular acuity, luminance detection, spatial localization (egocentric and relative) and optokinetic nystagmus may all be adversely affected. With binocular viewing, stereo-depth perception may fail, interocular suppression can appear and correspondence may become anomalous and variable.

Nevertheless, amblyopia is today still diagnosed by elimination. Outwardly there is nothing to see because the patient's problem is in the brain. Brain research suggests that two distinguishing characteristics of vision loss in amblyopia are loss of binocularity and spatial localization errors. Thanks in large

part to the work of David Hubel and Torsten Wiesel, for which they received the 1981 Nobel Prize in Physiology or Medicine, there is today a structural and functional grasp of binocularity loss which is an inspiration to all workers in this interdisciplinary field. Future developments will lead beyond binocularity and crowding (phase-error) effects, because clearly many systems beyond the striate cortex and indeed beyond the cortex itself are involved in amblyopia. Optometric and oculomotor tests in particular deserve new emphasis.

Amblyopia: oculomotor aspects implicate W and X systems

Amblyopia has oculomotor implications even though it is now treated as a sensory problem of cortical origin. In the nucleus of the optic tract, and perhaps throughout the accessory optic system, loss of binocular and high velocity response seems to accompany amblyopia. For OKN, the story is known (binocularity loss in cortex unmasks an old W system in the subcortex). For pupillary control there are strong hints of a similar story, and for a variety of vestibulo-ocular, ocular and oculomotor reflexes, more research is needed. Amblyopia may also bring loss of fine positional feedback from the cortex to oculomotor centres, owing to impairment of the X system and hence final fixational 'lock' would then become unsteady.

The Y system: greater role in pattern vision

The now classic animal model of amblyopia as a loss of binocularity in the ocular dominance columns of the striate cortex must be an oversimplification. For example, rather than manipulate ocular dominance within the striate cortex, one could remove the striate cortex entirely (Lehmkuhle, Kratz and Sherman, 1982). The peristriate areas in the cat receive their own direct Y and W inputs, so that some residual visual function remains for testing. The resultant amblyopia (in the cat) shows a loss of high spatial frequency contrast sensitivity reminiscent of the milder of Hess and Howell's (1977) two forms of amblyopia. However, the behaviourally assessed amblyopia following conventional monocular deprivation is deeper still, and affects all spatial frequencies. The striate cortex (in the cat) is more dispensable for general visual skills than was thought, and monocular deprivation must be harming other visual areas as well.

In the cat, ablation of the striate cortex effectively removes the cortical X system. The mild nature of the animals' general behavioural impairment and the specificity of its spatial frequency loss reminds us that high acuity performance is only a final refinement, a skill used when reading the newspaper. Spatial egocentric orientation (Howard and

Templeton, 1966; Howard, 1982) — finding that newspaper, creating a representation of the room and moving through it to a chair — involve *motion*, the global visual field, and *gross form* detection. These are more nearly specializations of the Y than of the X visual subsystem.

Broader tests

Clinical visual testing and academic visual research have a natural tendency to emphasize high acuity achievements. To remedy this, for example in binocular vision, more emphasis might be placed on coarse stereopsis (motion in depth, depth in the presence of diplopia). A consideration of a broader range of visual skills will force a consideration of a broader range of visual areas.

From new tests a more positive definition of amblyopia can be expected together with better means of population screening, new means of monitoring infant therapy, and of course a better understanding of the disease.

Why are the sensory adaptations so massive?

Fetal and neonatal neural development often shows overgrowth and retraction. The overgrowth and ensuing crowding brings contact between cells which inhibits the overgrowth and may trigger the cells to differentiate and take up their special functions. The neural machinery begins this sequence of events incompletely specified. There are not enough information bits on the genetic code for it to be otherwise. Postnatal development is therefore required to refine and calibrate the visual system to a degree of precision unattainable and undesirable using genetic means alone. Instead of a system prespecified in every detail experience is used to achieve a visual system precisely mated to the visual environment in which it must function. Precision is the prize for inventing experience-dependent brain development, plasticity is the mechanism, and amblyopia is the occasional cost.

Acknowledgements

Preparation of the chapters by JIN was supported in part by NIMH grant 34793, the Naval Air Systems Command, and the Air Force Office of Scientific Research 83–0225. Linda Misa provided invaluable bibliographic help. I thank colleagues for generously sharing their work and comments, and in particular David Rose, Robert O'Shea and Murray Sherman for reading an earlier draft. Denis Levi, Leo Peich and Donald Mitchell kindly provided original plates. Robin Hannay Nelson did the drawings for *Figures 13.4, 13.5* and *13.14*.

References

AMIGO. G. (1982) Diagnosis and treatment of anomalous correspondence. *Austr J. Optom.* **65** 100–104.

APKARIAN. P. A.. NAKAYAMA. K. and TYLER. C. W. (1981). Binocularity in the human visual evoked potential: facilitation, summation and suppression. *EEG Clin. Neurophysiol.*, **51**, 32–48

APKARIAN. P. A.. REITS. D.. SPEKREIJSE. H. and VAN DORP. D. (1983) A decisive electrophysiological test for human albinism. *EEG Clin. Neurophysiol.*, **55**, 513–531

ARDEN. G. B. and BARNARD. W. M. (1980) Effect of occlusion on the visual evoked response in amblyopia. *Trans. Ophthalmol. Soc. UK*, **99**, 419–426.

ASLIN, R. N. and BANKS. M. S. (1978) Early visual experience in humans: Evidence for a critical period in the development of binocular vision. In *Psychology. From Research to Practice*, edited by H. L. Pick, Jr., H. W. Leibowitz, J. E. Singer, A. Steinschneider and H. W. Stevenson, pp.227–239. New York: Plenum Press

ASSAF. A. A. (1982) The sensitive period: transfer of fixation after occlusion for strabismic amblyopia. *Br. J. Ophthalmol.*, **66**, 64–70

AUST. W. (1971) Results of occlusion therapy in concomitant strabismus. In *The First Congress of the International Strabismological Association*, edited by P. Fells, pp.157–166. St Louis: C.V. Mosby

BAKER, F. H.. GRIGG, P. and VON NOORDEN. G. K. (1974) Effects of visual deprivation and strabismus on the response of neurons in the visual cortex of the monkey, including studies on the striate and prestriate cortex in the normal animal. *Brain Res.*, **66**, 185–208.

BANKS, M. S.. ASLIN, R. N. and LETSON, R. D. (1975) Sensitive period for the development of human binocular vision. *Science*, **190**, 675–677.

BANKS, R. V.. CAMPBELL, F. W.. HESS. R. and WATSON. P. G. (1978) A new treatment for amblyopia. *Br. Orthop. J.*, **35**, 1–12

BARNARD. W. M. and ARDEN. G. B. (1979) Changes in the visual evoked response during and after occlusion therapy for amblyopia. *Child: Care, Health Develop.*, **5**, 421–430

BLAKE. R. and HIRSCH, H. V. B. (1975) Deficits in binocular depth perception in cats after alternating monocular deprivation. *Science*, **190**, 1114–1116

BLAKEMORE. C. (1976) The conditions required for the maintenance of binocularity in the kitten's visual cortex. *J. Physiol.*, **261**, 423–444

BLAKEMORE. C. (1978) Maturation and modification in the developing visual system. In *The Handbook of Sensory Physiology*, Vol. VIII, *Perception*, pp.377–436. New York: Springer

BLAKEMORE. C. and VAN SLUYTERS. R. C. (1974) Reversal of the physiological effects of monocular deprivation in kittens: further evidence for a sensitive period. *J. Physiol.*, **237**, 195–216

BLAKEMORE. C. and VITAL-DURAND. F. (1981) Postnatal development of the monkey's visual system. In *The Fetus and Independent Life*. Ciba Foundation Symposium 86, pp.152–171. London: Pitman

BLAKEMORE. C.. VITAL-DURAND. F. and GAREY. L. J. (1981) Recovery from monocular deprivation in the monkey. I.

Reversal of physiological effects in the visual cortex. *Proc. R. Soc. Lond. B; Biol. Sci.*, **213**, 399–423

BOUMA, H. (1970) Interaction effects in parafoveal letter recognition. *Nature*, **226**, 177–178

BOYCOTT, B. B. and WÄSSLE, H. (1974) The morphological types of ganglion cells of the domestic cat's retina. *J. Physiol.*, **240**, 397–419

BRADDICK, O. (1981) Is spatial phase degraded in peripheral vision and visual pathology? *Doc. Ophthalmol. Proc. Ser.*, **30**, 255–262

BRADDICK, O. J. and ATKINSON, J. (1982) The development of binocular function in infancy. *Acta Ophthalmol. Suppl.* **157**, 27–35

BRADLEY, A. and FREEMAN, R. D. (1981) Contrast sensitivity in anisometropic amblyopia. *Invest. Ophthalmol. Vis. Sci.*, **21**, 467–476

BROCK, F. W. (1950) Visual training. Testing for visual acuity. *Optom. Weekly*, **41**, 1699–1702, 1715–1719

BURCHFIEL, J. L and DUFFY, F. H. (1981) Role of intracortical inhibition in deprivation amblyopia: reversal by microintophoretic bicuculline. *Brain Res.*, **206**, 479–484

CAMPOS, E. C. and CHIESI, C. (1983) Binocularity in comitant strabismus: II. Objective evaluation with visual evoked responses. *Doc. Ophthalmol.*, **55**, 277–293

CARPENTER, R. H. S. (1973) Contour-like phosphenes from electrical stimulation of the human eye: some new observations. *J. Physiol.*, **229**, 767–785

CRAWFORD, M. L. J., VON NOORDEN, G. K., MEHARG, L. S., RHODES, J. W., HARWERTH, R. S., SMITH, E. L. III *et al.* (1983) Binocular neurones and binocular function in monkeys and children. *Invest. Ophthalmol. Vis. Sci.*, **24**, 491–495

CRAWFORD, M. L. J., SMITH, E. L. III, HARWERTH, R. S. and VON NOORDEN, G. K. (1984) Stereoblind monkeys have few binocular neurones. *Invest. Ophthalmol. Vis. Sci.*, **25**, 779–781

CYNADER, M., BERMAN, N. and HEIN, A. (1976) Recovery of function in cat visual cortex following prolonged deprivation. *Exp. Brain Res.*, **25**, 139–156

CYNADER, M. and MITCHELL, D. E. (1977) Monocular astigmatism effects on kitten visual cortex development. *Nature*, **270**, 177–178

CYNADER, M., TIMNEY, B. N. and MITCHELL, D. E. (1980) Period of susceptibility of kitten visual cortex to the effects of monocular deprivation extends beyond six months of age. *Brain Res.*, **191**, 545–550

DUFFY, F. H., SNODGRASS, S. R., BURCHFIEL, J. L. and CONWAY, J. L. (1976) Bicuculline reversal of deprivation amblyopia in the cat. *Nature*, **260**, 256–257; **263**, 531

EGGERS, H. M. and BLAKEMORE, C. (1978) Physiological basis of anisometropic amblyopia. *Science*, **201**, 264–267

ENROTH-CUGELL, C. and JAKIELA, H. G. (1980) Suppression of cat retinal ganglion cell responses by moving patterns. *J. Physiol.*, **302**, 49–72

ENROTH-CUGELL, C. and ROBSON, J. G. (1966) The contrast sensitivity of retinal ganglion cells of the cat. *J. Physiol.*, **187**, 517–552

ERZURUMLU, R. S. and KILLACKEY, H. P. (1982) Critical and sensitive periods in neurobiology. *Current Topics in Development*, **17**, 207–240

EVANS, J. N. (1928) A clinical method to determine the rate of elimination of after images (eikonoscopy). *Am. J. Ophthalmol.*, **11**, 194–202

FENDER, D. and JULESZ, B. (1967) Extension of Panum's fusional area in binocularly stabilized vision. *J. Opt. Soc. Am.*, **57**, 819–830

GEBHARD, J. W. (1953) Motokawa's studies on electrical excitation of the human eye. *Psychol. Bull.*, **50**, 73–111

GEISERT, E. E. SPEAR, P. D., ZETLAN, S. R. and LANGSETMO, A. (1982) Recovery of Y-cells in the lateral geniculate nucleus of monocularly deprived cats. *J. Neurosci.*, **2**, 577–588

GRÜNAU, M. VON (1979) Binocular summation and the binocularity of cat visual cortex. *Vision Res.*, **19**, 813–816

HAMASAKI, D. I. and FLYNN, J. T. (1981) Amblyopic eyes have longer reaction times. *Invest. Ophthalmol. Vis. Sci.*, **6**, 846–853

HARTER, M. R. (1977) Binocular interaction: evoked potentials to dichoptic stimulation. In *Visual Evoked Potentials in Man — New Developments*, edited by J. E. Desmedt, pp.208–233. Oxford: Clarendon

HARTER, M. R., CONDER, E. S. and TOWLE, V. L. (1980) Orientation-specific and luminance effects: interocular suppression of visual evoked potentials in man. *Psychophysiology*, **17**, 141–145

HARWERTH, R. S. and LEVI, D. M. (1978) A sensory mechanism for amblyopia: psychophysical studies. *Am. J. Optom. Physiol. Opt.*, **55**, 151–162

HAWKESWOOD, H. (1971) Some cases of convergent squint with abnormal retinal correspondence. *Austr. Orthop. J.*, **11**, 23–24

HESS, R. F., CAMPBELL, F. W. and GREENHALGH, T. (1978) On the nature of the neural abnormality in human amblyopia: neural aberrations and neural sensitivity loss. *Pflügers Arch. ges. Physiol.*, **377**, 201–207

HESS, R. F., CAMPBELL, F. W. and ZIMMERN, R. C. (1980) Differences in the neural basis of human amblyopias: the effect of mean luminance. *Vision Res.*, **20**, 295–306

HESS, R. F. and HOWELL, E. R. (1977) The threshold contrast sensitivity function in strabismic amblyopia: evidence for a two type classification. *Vision Res.*, **17**, 1049–1055

HESS, R. and JENKINS, S. (1980) Amblyopia cannot be explained by considering only detection thresholds. *Perception*, **9**, 569–576

HILLIS A., FLYNN, J. T. and HAWKINS, B. S. (1983) The evolving concept of amblyopia: a challenge to epidemiologists. *Am. J. Epidemiol.*, **118**, 192–205

HITCHCOCK, P. F. and HICKEY, T. L. (1980) Ocular dominance columns: evidence for their presence in humans. *Brain Res.*, **182**, 176–179

HOHMANN, A and CREUTZFELDT, O. D. (1975) Squint and the development of binocularity in humans. *Nature*, **254**, 613–614

HORTON, J. C. and HEDLEY-WHYTE, E. T. (1984) Mapping of cytochrome oxidase patches and ocular dominance columns in human visual cortex. *Philos. Trans. R. Soc. Lond. B*, **304**, 255–272

HOWARD, I. P. (1982) *Human Visual Orientation*. New York: Wiley

HOWARD, I. P. and TEMPLETON, W. B. (1966) *Human Spatial Orientation*. New York: Wiley

HUBEL, D. H. (1978) Effects of deprivation on the visual cortex of cat and monkey. *The Harvey Lectures*, Series 72, pp.1–51. New York: Academic Press

HUBEL, D. H. and WIESEL, T. N. (1962) Receptive fields, binocular interaction and functional architecture in the cat's visual cortex. *J. Physiol.*, **160**, 106–154

HUBEL, D. H. and WIESEL, T. N. (1965) Binocular interaction in striate cortex of kittens reared with artifical squint. *J. Neurophysiol.*, **28**, 1041–1059

HUBEL, D. H. and WIESEL, T. N. (1970) The period of susceptibility to the physiological effects of unilateral eye closure in kittens. *J. Physiol.*, **206**, 419–436

HUBEL, D. H and WIESEL, T. N. (1974) Uniformity of monkey striate cortex: a parallel relationship between field size, scatter, and magnification factor. *J. Comp. Neurol.*, **158**, 295—305

HUBEL, D. H. WIESEL, T. N. and LEVAY. S. (1977) Plasticity of ocular dominance columns in monkey striate cortex. *Philos. Trans. Roy. Soc. Lond. B.*, **278**, 377–409

IMBERT, M. and FREGNAC, Y. (1983) Specification of cortical neurons by visuomotor experience. *Progress in Brain Research, Vol. 58: Molecular and Cellular Interactions Underlying Higher Brain Functions*, edited by J-P. Changeux, J. Glowinski, M. Imbert and F. Bloom, pp. 1427–1436. Amsterdam: Elsevier

JOHNSON, C. A., POST, R. B., CHALUPA, L. M. and LEE, T. J. (1982) Monocular deprivation in humans: a study of identical twins. *Invest. Ophthalmol. Vis. Sci.*, **23**, 135–138

JULESZ, B. (1971) *Foundations of Cyclopean Perception.* Chicago: University of Chicago Press

KASAMATSU, T. (1982) Enhancement of neuronal plasticity by activating the norepinephrine system in the brain: A remedy for amblyopia. *Human Neurobiol.*, **1**, 49–54

KASMATSU, T. (1987) Norepinephrine hypothesis for visual coritcal plasticity: thesis, antithesis and recent development. *Curr. Top. Develop. Biol.*, **21**, 367–389

KASAMATSU, T., ITAKURA, T., JOHNSON, G., HEGGELHUND, P., PETTIGREW, J. D. NAKAI, K. *et al.* (1984) Neuronal plasticity in cat visual cortex: a proposed role for the central noradrenaline system. In *Monoamine Innervation of Cerebral Cortex*, edited by L. Descarries, T. R. Reader and H. H. Jasper, pp. 301–319. *Neurology and Neurobiology*, Vol. 10. New York: Alan Liss

KASE, M., NAGATA, R., YOSHIDA, A. and HANADA, J. (1984) Pupillary light reflex in amblyopia. *Invest. Ophthalmol. Vis. Sci.*, **25**, 467–471

KEINER, E. C. J. F. (1968) The early treatment of strabismus convergens. *Ophthalmologica*, **156**, 20–24

KRATZ, K. E., SPEAR, P. D. and SMITH, D. C. (1976) Postcritical-period reversal of effects of monocular deprivation on striate cortex cells in the cat. *J. Neurophysiol.*, **39**, 501–511

KUFFLER, S. W. (1953) Discharge patterns and functional organization of the mammalian retina. *J. Neurophysiol.*, **16**, 37–68

LEHMUHLE, S. W., KRATZ, K. E., MANGEL, S. C. and SHERMAN, S. M. (1979) Effects of early monocular lid suture on spatial and temporal sensitivity of neurons in dorsal lateral geniculate nucleus of the cat. *J. Neurophysiol.*, **43**, 542–556

LEHMKUHLE, S., KRATZ, K. E. and SHERMAN, S. M. (1982) Spatial and temporal sensitivity of normal and amblyopic cats. *J. Neurophysiol.*, **48**, 372–387

LEVAY, S., WIESEL, T. N. and HUBEL, D. H. (1980) The development of ocular dominance columns in normal and visually deprived monkeys. *J. Comp. Neurol.*, **191**, 1–51

LEVI, D. M. and HARWERTH, R. S. (1978) A sensory mechanism for amblyopia; electrophysiological studies. *Am. J. Optom. Physiol. Opt.*, **55**, 163–171

LEVI, D. M. and HARWERTH, R. S. (1982) Psychophysical mechanisms in humans with amblyopia. *Am. J. Optom. Physiol. Opt.*, **59**, 936–951

LEVI, D. M. and KLEIN, S. A. (1983) Spatial localization in normal and amblyopic vision. *Vision Res.*, **23**, 1005–1017

LEVI D. M., KLEIN, S. A. and AITSEBAOMO, P. (1984) Detection and discrimination of the direction of motion in central and peripheral vision of normal and amblyopic observers. *Vision Res.*, **24**, 789–800

LEVI, D. M., MANNY, R. E., KLEIN, S. A. and STEINMAN, S. B. (1983) Electrophysiological correlates of hyperacuity in the human visual cortex. *Nature*, **306**, 468–470

LEVITT, F. B. and VAN SLUYTERS. R. C. (1982) The sensitive period for strabismus in the kitten. *Develop. Brain Res.*, **3**, 323–327

LOSHIN, D. S. and LEVI, D. M. (1983) Suprathreshold contrast perception in functional amblyopia. *Doc. Ophthalmol.*, **55**, 213–236

MARCOTTE, R. R. and UPDYKE, B. V. (1982) Cortical visual areas of the cat project differentially onto the nuclei of the accessory optic system. *Brain Res.*, **242**, 205–217

MARTIN, K. A. C., RAMACHANDRAN, V. S., RAO, V. M. and WHITTERIDGE, D. (1979) Changes in ocular dominance induced in monocularly deprived lambs by stimulation with rotating gratings. *Nature*, **277**, 391–393

MASKE, R., YAMANE, S. and BISHOP, P. O. (1984) Binocular simple cells for local stereopsis: comparison of receptive field organisations for the two eyes. *Vision Res.*, **24**, 1921–1929

MERCHANT, J. (1965) Sampling theory for the human visual sense. *J. Opt. Soc. Am.*, **55**, 1291–1295

MITCHELL, D. E., MURPHY, K. M., DZIOBA, H. A. and HORNE, J. A. (1986) Optimization of visual recovery from early monocular deprivation in kittens: implications for occlusion therapy in the treatment of amblyopia. *Clin. Vision Sci.*, **1**, 173–177

MITCHELL, D. E., MURPHY, K. M. and KAYE, M. G. (1984) The permanence of the visual recovery that follows reverse occlusion of monocularly deprived kittens. *Invest. Ophthalmol. Vis. Sci.*, **25**, 908–917

MOVSHON, J. A. and VAN SLUYTERS, R. C. (1981) Visual neural development. *Annu. Rev. Psychol.*, **32**, 477–522

NELSON, J. I. (1975a) Globality and stereoscopic fusion in binocular vision. *J. Theor. Biol.*, **49**, 1–88

NELSON, J. I. (1975b) Motion sensitivity in peripheral vision. *Perception*, **3**, 151–152

NELSON, J. I. (1978) Does orientation domain inhibition play a role in visual cortex plasticity? *Exp. Brain Res.*, **32**, 293–298

NELSON, J. I. (1981) A neurophysiological model for anomalous correspondence based on mechanisms of sensory fusion. *Doc. Ophthalmol.*, **51**, 3–100

NELSON, J. I. (1985) The cellular basis of perception. In *Models of the Visual Cortex*, edited by D. Rose and V. Dobson pp. 108–122. New York: Wiley

NELSON, J. I., KUPERSMITH, M. J., SEIPLE, W. H., WEISS, P. A. and CARR, R. E (1984a) Spatiotemporal conditions which elicit or abolish the oblique effect in man: direct measurement with swept evoked potential. *Vision Res.*, **24**, 579–586

NELSON, J. I., SEIPLE, W. H., KUPERSMITH, M. J. and CARR, R. E. (1984b) A rapid evoked potential index of cortical adaptation. *EEG Clin. Neurophysiol.* **59**, 454–464

NICOLAI, H. (1959) Differenzen zwischen optokinetischem Rechts- und Linksnystagmus bei einseitiger (Schiel-) Amblyopie. *Klin. Monatsb. Augenheilkd.*, **134**, 245–250

PARKS, M. M. (1971) Management of eccentric fixation and ARC in esotropia. In *Symposium on Horizontal Ocular Deviations*, edited by D. R. Manley. St Louis: C.V. Mosby

PASTERNAK, T., MOVSHON, J. A. and MERIGAN, W. H. (1981) Creation of direction selectivity in adult strobe-reared cats *Nature*, **292**, 834–836

PERRY, N. W. Jr, CHILDERS, D. G. and McCOY, J. G. (1968) Binocular addition of the visual evoked response at different cortical locations. *Vision Res.*, **8**, 567–573

PETTIGREW, J. D. (1982) Pharmacologic control of cortical plasticity. *Retina*, **2**, 360–372

REGAN, D., BEVERLEY, K. and CYNADER, M. (1979) The visual perception of motion in depth. *Sci. Am.*, **241**, 136–151, 162, 14

REVELL, M. J. (1971) *Strabismus. A History of Orthoptic Techniques*. London: Barrie and Jenkins

RIESEN, A. H. (1961) Stimulation as a requirement for growth and function in behavioral development. In *Functions of Varied Experience*, edited by D. W. Fiske and S. R. Maddi, pp.57–80. Homewood, IL: Dorsey

RIESEN, A. H. (1982) Effects of environments on development in sensory systems. In *Contributions to Sensory Physiology*, Vol. 6, edited by W. D. Neff, pp. 45–77 New York: Academic Press

ROSS, J. E. (1983) Disturbance of stereoscopic vision in patients with unilateral stroke. *Behav. Brain Res.*, **7**, 99–112

ROVAMO, J. and VIRSU, V. (1979) An estimation and application of the human cortical magnification factor. *Exp. Brain Res.*, **37**, 495–510

SCHOPPMANN, A. (1981) Projections from areas 17 and 18 of the visual cortex to the nucleus of the optic tract. *Brain Res.*, **223**, 1–17

SCHOR, C. (1975) A directional impairment of eye movement control in strabismus amblyopia. *Invest. Ophthalmol. Vis. Sci.*, **14**, 692–697

SEIDEL, D., KNOLL, M. and EICHMEIER, J. (1968) Anregung von subjektiven Lichterscheinungen (Phosphenen) beim Menschen durch magnetische Sinusfelder. *Pflügers Arch. Eur. J. Physiol.*, **299**, 11–18

SHATZ, C. J. and STRYKER, M. P. (1978) Ocular dominance in layer IV of the cat's visual cortex and the effects of monocular deprivation. *J. Physiol.*, **281**, 267–286

SHERMAN, S. M., HOFFMANN, K.-P. and STONE, J. (1972) Loss of a specific cell type from the dorsal lateral geniculate nucleus in visually deprived cats. *J. Neurophysiol.*, **35**, 532–541

SHINKMAN, P. G., ISLEY, M. R. and ROGERS, D. C. (1983) Prolonged dark rearing and development of interocular orientation disparity in visual cortex. *J. Neurophysiol.*, **49**, 717–729

SILLITO, A. M. (1986) Conflicts in the pharmacology of visual cortical plasticity. *Trends Neurosci.*, **9**, 301–303

SILLITO, A. M., KEMP, J. A. and BLACKMORE, C. (1981) The role of GABAergic inhibition in the cortical effects of monocular deprivation. *Nature*, **291**, 318–320

SINGER, W. (1977) Effects of monocular deprivation on excitatory and inhibitory pathways in cat striate cortex. *Exp. Brain Res.*, **30**, 25–41

SINGER, W. (1983) Neuronal mechanisms of experience-dependent self-organization of the mammalian visual cortex. *Acta Morphol. Acad. Sci. Hung.*, **31**, 235–260

SINGER, W. (1985) Activity-dependent self-organization of the mammalian visual cortex. In *Models of the Visual Cortex*, edited by D. Rose and V. Dobson, pp. 123–136. New York: Wiley

SIRETEANU, R. (1982) Binocular vision in strabismic humans with alternating fixation. *Vision Res.*, **22**, 889–896

SPEKREIJSE, H., VAN DER TWEEL, L. H. and REGAN, D. (1972) Interocular sustained suppression — correlations with evoked potential amplitude and distribution. *Vision Res.*, **12**, 521–526

SUR, M., WELLER, R. E. and SHERMAN, S. M. (1984) Development of X- and Y-cell retinogeniculate terminations in kittens. *Nature*, **310**, 246–249

SWINDALE, N. V. (1982) The development of columnar systems in mammalian visual cortex. The role of innate and environmental factors. *Trends Neurosci.*, **5**, 235–240

TYLER, C. W. (1983) Sensory processing of binocular disparity. In *Vergence Eye Movements: Basic and Clinical Aspects*, edited by C. M. Schor and K. J. Ciuffreda, pp.199–295. Boston: Butterworths

TYLER, C. W. and KAITZ, M. F. (1977) Binocular interactions in the human visual evoked potential after short-term occlusion and anisometropia. *Invest. Ophthalmol. Vis. Sci.*, **16**, 1070–1073

VAEGAN and TAYLOR, D. (1980) Critical period for deprivation amblyopia in children. *Trans. Ophthalmol. Soc. UK*, **99**, 432–439

VAEGAN, SHOEREY, U. and KELSEY, J. H. (1979) Binocular interactions in the visual evoked potential using a modified synoptophore. In *Evoked Potentials*, edited by C. Barber, Proceedings of an International Evoked Potentials Symposium, Nottingham, England, pp.291–312. Lancaster: MTP Press

VAN HOF-VAN DUIN, J. and MOHN, G. (1982) Stereopsis and optokinetic nystagmus. In *Functional Basis of Ocular Motility Disorders*, edited by G. Lennerstrand, D. S.

Zee and E. L. Keller. Wenner-Gren Symposium Series, Vol. 37, pp.321–324. Oxford: Pergamon

VIRSU, V. and ROVAMO, J. (1979) Visual resolution, contrast sensitivity, and the cortical magnification factor. *Exp. Brain Res.*, **37**, 475–494

VON NOORDEN, G. K. (1970) Etiology and pathogenesis of fixation anomalies in strabismus. II: Paradoxic fixation, occlusion amblyopia, and microstrabismus. *Am. J. Ophthalmol.*, **69**, 223–227

WALD, G. and BURIAN, H. M. (1944) The dissociation of form vision and light perception in strabismic amblyopia. *Am. J. Ophthalmol.*, **27**, 950–963

WIESEL, T. N. and HUBEL, D. H. (1963) Single-cell responses in striate cortex of kittens deprived of vision in one eye. *J. Neurophysiol.*, **26**, 1003–1017

WIESEL, T. N. and HUBEL, D. H. (1965) Comparison of the effects of unilateral and bilateral eye closure on cortical unit responses in kittens. *J. Neurophysiol.*, **28**, 1029–1040

WIESEL, T. N. and RAVIOLA, E. (1979) Increase in axial length of the macaque monkey eye after corneal opacification. *Invest. Ophthalmol. Vis. Sci.*, **18**, 1232–1236

WOLFE, J. M. and HELD, R. (1982) Binocular adaptation that cannot be measured monocularly. *Perception*, **11**, 287–295

WOLFE, J. M. and HELD, R. (1983) Shared characteristics of stereopsis and the purely binocular process. *Vision Res.*, **23**, 217–227

YINON, U. (1978) On the question of neuronal plasticity in the mature visual cortex. *Arch. Italian Biol.*, **116**, 324–329

ZEKI, S. M. (1978) Uniformity and diversity of structure and function in rhesus monkey prestriate visual cortex. *J. Physiol.*, **277**, 273–290

Further reading

BISHOP, P. O. (1984) Processing of visual information within the retinostriate system. In *American Physiological Society Handbook of Physiology*, Sect. 1: *The Nervous System*, Vol. III, edited by Ian Darian-Smith, *Sensory Processes*, Part 1, pp.341–424. Baltimore: Williams & Wilkins

CAMPBELL, F. W. (1983) Why do we measure contrast sensitivity? *Behavioural Brain Res.*, **10**, 87–97

CYNADER, M. S. (1982) Competitive neuronal interactions underlying amblyopia. *Human Neurobiol.*, **1**, 35–39

ELLENBERGER, C. Jr. (1984) Recent advances in the understanding of vision. *Neuro-Ophthalmology*, **4**, 185–206

FAVREAU, O. E. (1981) Evidence for parallel processing in motion perception. *Acta Psychol.*, **48**, 25–34

HARWERTH, R. S. and LEVI, D. M. (1983) Psychophysical studies of the binocular processes of amblyopes. *Am. J. Optom. Physiol. Opt.*, **60**, 454–463

HOFFMANN, K. P. (1983) Control of the Optokinetic reflex by the nucleus of the optic tract in the cat. In *Spatially Oriented Behaviour*, edited by A. Hein and M. Jeannerod, pp.135–153. New York: Springer

HUBEL, D. H. (1978) Effects of deprivation on the visual cortex of cat and monkey. *The Harvey Lectures*, Series 72, pp. 1–51. New York: Academic Press

HUBEL, D. H. (1982) Exploration of the primary visual cortex, 1955–78. *Nature*, **299**, 515–524

HUBEL, D. H. and WIESEL, T. N. (1979) Brain mechanisms of vision. *Sci. Am.*, **241**, 150–162, 14, 18, 250 (Sept.)

KUFFLER, S. W. NICHOLLS, J. G. and MARTIN, A. R. (1984) *From Neuron to Brain. A Cellular Approach to the Function of the Nervous System*, 2nd edn Sunderland. MA: Sinauer Assoc.

LEVI, D. M. (1985) Binocular interactions and their alterations resulting from abnormal visual experience. In *Models of the Visual Cortex*, edited by D. Rose and V. Dobson, pp.200–210. New York: Wiley

LEVINE, M. W. and SHEFNER, J. M. (1981) *Fundamentals of Sensation and Perception*. Reading, MA.: Addison-Wesley

MacLEOD, D. I. A. (1978) Visual sensitivity. *Annu. Rev. Psychol.*, **29**, 613–645

MITCHELL, D. E. and TIMNEY, B. (1984) Postnatal development of function in the mammalian visual system. In *American Physiological Society Handbook of Physiology*, Section 1: *The Nervous System*. Vol. III, edited by Ian Darian-Smith, *Sensory Processes*, Part 1, pp.507–555. Baltimore: Williams & Wilkins

RATCLIFF, G. and ROSS, J. E. (1981) Visual perception and perceptual disorder. *Br. Med. Bull.*, **37**, 181–186

REGAN, D. (1982) Visual information channeling in normal and disordered vision. *Psychol. Rev.*, **89**, 407–444

SANAC, A., VAEGAN and WATSON, P. G. (1980) Restoration of the visually evoked potential to normal after intensive visual stimulation. A case report. *Trans. Ophthalmol. Soc. UK*, **99**, 455–456

SHERMAN, S. M. (1982) Parallel pathways in the cat's geniculocortical system: W-, X-, and Y-cells. In *Changing Concepts of the Nervous System*, edited by A. R. Morrison and P. L. Strick, pp. 337–359. New York: Academic Press

SHERMAN, S. M. (1985) Development of retinal projections to the cat's lateral geniculate nucleus. *Trends Neurosci.*, **8**, 350–355

SHERMAN, S. M. (1985) Functional organization of the W-, X-, and Y-cell pathways in the cat: a review and hypothesis. In *Progress in Psychobiology and Physiological Psychology*, edited by J. M. Sprague and A. N. Epstein, pp.233–314. New York: Academic Press

SINGER, W. (1985) Activity-dependent self-organization of the mammalian visual cortex. In *Models of the Visual Cortex*, edited by D. Rose and V. Dobson, pp.123–136. New York: Wiley

STONE, J. and DREHER, B. (1982) Parallel processing of information in the visual pathways: a general principle of sensory coding? *Trends Neurosci.*, **5**, 441–446

VAN ESSEN, D. C. and MAUNSELL, J. H. R. (1983) Hierarchical organization and functional streams in the visual cortex. *Trends Neurosci.*, **6**, 370–375

WIESEL, T. N. (1982) Postnatal development of the visual cortex and the influence of environment. *Nature*, **299**, 583–591

WOLFE, J. M. and BLAKE, R. (1985) Monocular and binocular processes in human vision. In *Models of the Visual Cortex*, edited by D. Rose and V. Dobson, pp.192–199. New York: Wiley

14

Binocular vision: disparity detection and anomalous correspondence

Jerry Nelson

It has already been described in Chapter 13 how binocularity arises in the converging pathways from the eyes to the brain. During an early critical period of cortical plasticity, imbalances in the quantity, quality and congruity of the eyes' signals can deprive the disadvantaged eye of cortical access. The result is amblyopia, i.e. a loss of visual function. When the retinal images are equally sharp, but there is strabismus (lack of good binocular alignment), each eye retains cortical access, but to separate neural populations. There is vision, but it is not binocular. If the strabismus is small, constant and early, then the binocular visual system can adapt. The result is anomalous correspondence (AC), a shift in perceived visual directions for one eye during binocular viewing. In AC, a non-foveal region of the deviating eye acquires a corresponding visual direction with the fovea of the other. The amount of shift in perceived visual direction is termed the 'angle of anomaly' (subjective angle). When the angle of anomaly matches the angle of the strabismus (objective angle), the AC is said to be harmonious.

Understanding of binocular vision has reached a turning point because of advances in neurophysiology. Since the mid-nineteenth century, a fixed set of points in one retina was thought to correspond to a fixed set of points in the other retina. But direct study of cells responsible for detecting disparity and defining correspondence shows that multiple states of correspondence must be possible. Indeed, shifts in correspondence of 3° in the *normal* observer have been reported in new studies of sensory fusion (Panum's area). Variability in normal correspondence is also seen in the horopter and in the visual system's failure to respond to disparity inputs ('depthless fusion') generated by oculomotor imprecision (e.g. fixation tremor), by laboratory manipulations (e.g. the telestereoscope) and, above all, by strabismus.

These discoveries and rediscoveries mean that the place of anomalous correspondence in binocular vision will change drastically: anomalous correspondence is not an anomaly, it is an exaggeration, a lawful extension of mechanisms operating in normal vision. A closer unification of laboratory and clinical research has become possible; from it will emerge simpler diagnostic methods and more effective treatment.

The new approach requires an understanding of the cellular basis of disparity detection, and how populations of disparity detectors define correspondence. Disparity detecting binocular neurones actually define a *range* of possible correspondences, so that a mechanism is needed for selecting one correspondence at a time from among the many states which are possible. The domain interaction model provides the needed selection mechanism. It is the same sort of model widely suggested for achieving global stereopsis, i.e. the decoding of random-dot stereograms.

Shifts in correspondence occur when the visual system responds to disparity stimulation. Variable angles of anomaly and conflicting outcomes from various tests can be understood by taking a closer look at what the patient is viewing.

This cellular basis for a modern, dynamically alterable kind of correspondence must be linked to clinical experience, notably the observation that the subjective angle of anomaly in strabismus varies over a great range, and that shifts can be continuous in some patients and abrupt in others. Simple changes in the disparity tunings of binocular neurones can be suggested to produce these and other known variations in anomalous correspondence.

Comparison to clinical stages

In the surgical and orthoptic treatment of strabismus, recovery often follows the stages presented below.

Simultaneous binocular vision: neurophysiologically, this implies both eyes have cortical access, but diplopia may be present.

Single vision without diplopia or suppression: sensory fusional mechanisms are operable.

Stereodepth: disparity detectors are operating and sensory fusional mechanisms are not pathological. A pathological exaggeration of variability in correspondence would be incompatible with detection of depth.

Amblyopia, in brief, implies that the neurophysiological basis of binocular vision is lost, while in AC the substrate is present but malfunctioning. To understand these distortions in AC, we must first consider how the binocular vision system functions in normal depth perception.

Stereopsis and fusion

Cues to depth

Stereoscopic depth and binocular disparity

There are many cues to depth, but steroscopic depth is phenomenologically special and can be elicited almost exclusively by the cue of retinal disparity. Retinal disparities are small positional displacements between otherwise well-matched visual images (*see Figure 14.1*).

If a practitioner has presented unmatched images (the 'bird and cage' stimulus or horizontal and vertical Hering after-images), then the visual system

has had no disparity stimulus and the binocular visual system has probably been inhibited.

Disparities are presented in a laboratory or clinical setting by presenting the two eyes with separate images (dichoptic stimulation). Two separate images or 'half-images' with parallax differences between them are a stereogram. A dichoptically presented binocular stimulus is not a stereogram unless the images are similar in form but not identical. They must contain some disparity information. When a patient is said to have full stereopsis, it should be clear that phenomenological depth as well as single vision was experienced.

Depth relation of disparities

There are many disparities in the retinal images, but not all arise from objects' depth differences. Disparities also arise from *tremor* and microsaccades uncoordinated between the eyes, from *magnification differences* caused by spectacles (an aphakic correction is an extreme case) or by simply looking sideways, from *fixation disparity* and from *strabismus*. Such 'extraneous' sources of image mismatches generate disparities far larger than the parallax signals themselves.

Disparity signals unrelated to depth could cause annoying diplopia. A fundamental task in binocular vision is thus the maintenance of single vision in the face of mismatched retinal input. Even in observers *without* strabismus, using sensory fusional mechanisms to maintain single vision may be a more important task than generating stereoscopic depth itself. The unavoidable and constant image shifting our

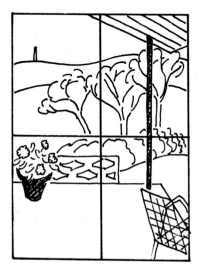 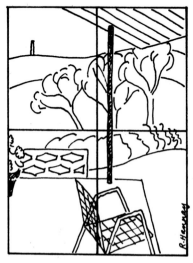

Figure 14.1 Upon stepping up to one and then another window to view a scene from two different vantage points, horizontal shifts in objects' images arise which are proportional to the separation in depth of the objects. Such parallax shifts arise in binocular viewing and are the *retinal disparity* cue for stereoscopic depth perception. Because the eyes are horizontally separated, only horizontal disparities convey depth information

brains must perform is the seed of anomalous correspondence contained in every normal visual system.

Monocular depth information

There are non-stereoscopic cues to both absolute *distance* of an object from the observer, and to *depth*, which refers to the three-dimensional solidity of objects and to the relative distances among them. Monocular, pictorial cues (atmospheric perspective, geometric perspective, texture gradients, relative size, superposition; *see* Hochberg, 1971; Murch, 1973; Levine and Shefner, 1981) do not produce the same vivid phenomenological experience as does retinal disparity, probably because the neural substrate for stereopsis is different from the substrate for these more cognitive cues. The only monocular stimulus capable of evoking the same vivid depth impression as disparity is the kinetic depth effect (KDE). A typical KDE stimulus is the flat shadow cast by a rotating, three-dimensional wire figure (Nelson, 1975b; Stong, 1975; *see also* Epstein, 1967; Braunstein, 1976). Only disparity cues are considered further.

Sensory fusion

Sensory fusion is the achievement of single vision from imperfectly matched retinal images. All disparities (horizontal, vertical, magnification differences) are subject to fusion and the fusion of vertical disparities in particular has secondary effects on the perception of depth from horizontal disparities.

In sensory fusion, the binocular visual system shifts monocularly perceived visual directions to a compromise direction which is the same for both eyes. The new perceived visual direction is an illusion. Sensory fusional shift is sometimes termed 'allelotropia'. Particularly when describing work in strabismus, where both oculomotor and sensory shifts occur, it is important to specify fusion as either sensory or motor. Panum's area is the range of retinal disparities for which single vision may be achieved through sensory fusion.

Fusion and depth

Sensory fusion and perceived depth are two separate responses to disparity. Either can occur alone in normal binocular vision. Nelson (1977) and Hyson, Julesz and Fender (1983) have emphasized the need for sensory fusion without perceived depth, to absorb undesirable differences in the retinal images. The opposite case, perceived depth in the absence of sensory fusion, has been recognized since the earliest experiments in binocular vision (Fröhlich, 1895; Tschermak-Seysenegg and Hoefer, 1903; Heine, 1904; Kaila, 1919); depth can be discriminated in the presence of diplopia — athletes and ballplayers do it all the time.

Because fusion and depth may be independently manifested, it is incorrect to define stereopsis as depth perception caused by the fusion of disparities within Panum's area. The visual system does not have to work at pushing disparate contours into alignment in order to get depth out of the effort.

Rivalry and suppression mechanisms in normal vision

Physiological or normal suppression can alleviate diplopia in everyday visual experience. The suppression which occurs in amblyopia is termed 'pathological suppression'. Pathological suppression of diplopia in strabismus is said to be *facultative* if vision returns with monocular viewing and *obligatory* if it does not. An obligatorily suppressed area is a scotoma.

Retinal rivalry: separate left, right and binocular channels

Grossly dissimilar images presented to the two eyes do not result in a mixed percept. Instead, patches or even the whole image from one eye alternate with input from the other eye. The separateness and alternation of the percepts experienced in such retinal rivalry suggest that separate neural substrates serve each eye and compete with each other (mutual inhibition — Sloan, 1985) for access to a higher neural centre. Modern models of rivalry and binocular summation (Cogan, 1982, 1987; Wolfe and Blake, 1985) express this intuitive view by postulating a monocular channel for the left eye, a monocular channel for the right eye and a binocular channel. The monocular channels each have access to consciousness and inhibit it one another whenever excited: this inhibition is the basis of rivalry. The binocular channel is only activated by well-matched (fusible) binocular stimuli. Such models are a reminder that most patients present three visual systems; when tests are performed with incongruent stimuli, the diagnosis may pertain to those two of the three systems which interest us least.

Despite its simplicity, the cellular basis of retinal rivalry remains elusive (Sloan, 1985). The problem is that binocular neurones are adapted to detecting small disparities and are *silenced* by grossly mismatched stimuli. What is needed, instead, are left and right whole-eye channels which remain active and then compete at a higher, as yet undiscovered, centre.

The clinical philosophy of using a dissociating test to 'penetrate' an anomaly warrants re-examination in light of the concept of three visual systems or channels. 'Penetration' is into one of the monocular systems — being disparity insensitive, this system cannot adapt to a strabismic deviation or show anomalous correspondence and therefore, it should come as no surprise that the diagnosis is normal retinal correspondence. Little is learned about the state of the binocular visual system when one penetrates to a monocular channel.

Other types of image suppression

Other image loss phenomena are the Troxler effect and the fading of images stabilized on the retina against oculomotor tremor. In the Troxler effect (Levelt, 1968), a cipher lying at the end of a line and seen in peripheral vision fades from visibility with prolonged fixation. Does normal suppression of any kind explain amblyopia?

Suppression in amblyopia probably occurs early, certainly as early as the primary visual cortex. Image fading phenomena involve grouping and other figural factors and thus require a higher neural locus. Unlike interactions studied electrophysiologically in binocular neurones, the interactions between the patch of image from one eye and from the other are unspecific: the channel of one eye is shut off as a whole, without regard to what pattern representations are flowing in the channel. The neural sites and mechanisms of suppression effects remain unidentified and, despite their disarming simplicity, no suppression effect provides a good model for either amblyopia or sensory fusion.

Properties of sensory fusion

The hallmark of anomalous correspondence is its variability. Panum's area in *normal* correspondence is interesting because it shows variability in perceived visual direction, an important aspect of correspondence. In fact, perceived depth as well as perceived visual direction can be shown to be variable in normal binocular vision: correspondence variability is universal. It is likely that common mechanisms underlie this variability in both normal and anomalous correspondence.

Panum's area, the range of fusible disparities, is broader horizontally than for vertical disparities. Classic values for Panum's area, still widely quoted today, are 12′ of arc horizontally and 6′ vertically (Ogle, 1964). Panum's area is also broader in the peripheral visual field. Therefore, in the face of oculomotor imbalance the periphery will be more disparity tolerant and less suppression prone than the central visual field.

Large amounts of sensory fusion

Modern research has shown that Panum's area is far larger than previously supposed, extending over 3° horizontally and over 2° in orientation disparity, it is stimulus dependent and it can be divided into two

areas, the limiting disparity for spontaneous fusion and the limiting disparity of extended fusion (*see below*). The larger modern values are due to the use of larger stimuli, less impoverished stimuli with more contour content, more accurate stabilized image measurement techniques and the elimination of monocular 'pointer' or cipher stimuli in the visual field, because of the use of objective eye position measurement techniques. The presence of zero disparity ciphers in the visual field interferes with the fusion of the test disparities. The larger patterns are stronger stimuli for fusion because they are stronger stimuli for the cortical neurones that must perform the fusing.

Hysteresis and stimulus dependency

The existence of two fusion limits is familiar from orthoptic practice with the amblyoscope: after obtaining simultaneous binocular vision at one angle, the amblyoscope arm may be swung to new positions (new disparity input values) without losing single vision. Single vision can be *re*tained at these disparities, even though it could never have been *ob*tained there initially. A difference in output state (fused versus diplopic percept) depending on which way the input is approached is termed 'hysteresis'. The fact that both Panum's area and the expression of correspondence show hysteresis suggests that their basis is similar. In orthoptic training, a change in the angle of correspondence is the goal; in diagnosis, a stable angle is desired. Different stimuli can produce these different results. It is probably safe to say that long contours are effective for obtaining a shifted angle of anomaly in patients with strabismus and eliciting harmonious anomalous correspondence, while random-dot stereograms (RDSs) are not. RDSs are excellent for retaining fusion once obtained. Panum's extended area with random-dot stereograms can reach an average of 3° (Hyson, Julesz and Fender, 1983; four observers; maximum departure in one direction from zero disparity, 5°; confirmed by Piantanida, 1986); the difference between Panum's spontaneous and extended areas can be 2.6°.

Although disparities of 2° or more can be aligned (fused) by the normal binocular visual system, disparity changes may fail to produce perceived depth changes (Erkelens and Collewijn, 1985; *see also below*). It is time to discard the classic value of 12′ arc for 'the' Panum's limit. With Panum's area, a move has been made from the sensation of brightness, colour and acuity to something requiring so much cortical processing that it is no longer a fixed threshold and, indeed, the threshold concept is misleading. The stimulus put in determines the fusional and correspondence shifts produced, i.e. there is information processing, not thresholds.

The horopter

Correspondence is the 'zero' from which stereopsis begins and so the definition of corresponding points is a central problem in binocular vision. Matched or corresponding points may be defined by equality of perceived visual direction, absence of difference in perceived depth or, less commonly, zero motor value for initiation of vergence movements. In the nineteenth and early twentieth centuries, great effort was expended to determine the surface formed by all corresponding points. The surface in depth of zero disparity points, in which the fixation point is ideally embedded, is termed the 'horopter'. Because it is too much work to determine the horopter for the entire visual field, a horizontal cross-section cutting through the fixation point is measured instead. This is the longitudinal horopter. Today, the horopter can be given a neurophysiological interpretation and suggestions can be made for measuring it in ways best able to show binocular function.

Uniformly distributed retinal points produce a circular horopter (Vieth–Müller circle; also termed the 'geometrical horopter'). Earlier in the present century, a horopter research showed that small departures from uniformity always occur: a point 3 mm temporalward from the fovea of one eye is paired with (converges on the same neurone receiving input from) a point more than 3 mm away from the fovea (on the nasal retina) in the other eye. These 'stretches' made in one retina before mapping it onto the other give the horopter a shape (flatter) and a tilt (approaching the perpendicular to the line

of sight, termed the 'objective normal plane') which make it more useful as a frame of reference for depth judgements (*see* Nelson, 1977, 1986). In sum, the Vieth–Müller circle is an idealized horopter not observed in practice.

Horopter types

Correspondence has several aspects, notably perceived visual direction and perceived depth. Different horopters arise from the choice of measurement techniques which emphasize one or another aspect.

Nonius horopter

This horopter, which has been studied the most, is based on the judgment of perceived monocular visual direction: the observer must bring two vertical bars, each seen by one eye alone, into vernier alignment (*Figure 14.2*). This can be done with great accuracy; the technique's drawback is its use of monocular stimulation. Little is learned of binocular function and correspondence may, furthermore, be different when retinal disparity is present and sensory fusion is triggered.

Maximum stereoacuity horopter

With fixation constant, the observer's ability to discriminate a slight depth separation is tested for a series of target distances away from the observer. As with all longitudinal horopters, the test series has to be repeated at increasing eccentricities while the

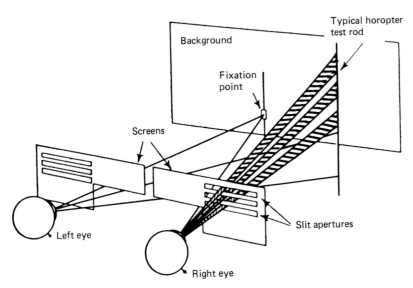

Figure 14.2 The nonius horopter apparatus. Different parts of a single rod are presented dichoptically using baffles; the vernier alignment of the images (line segments) is shifted by varying the actual depth of the rod compared to the fixation point. Today, right and left eye images would be separated by polarization techniques. Only the small fixation point is seen binocularly. (From Ogle, 1964, p. 37, by permission of the Mayo Foundation)

observer holds his fixation. The disadvantage of this method is the large number of measurements needed to establish the point of maximum stereo-acuity. However, this horopter is based on a true test of binocular function.

Fusional horopter

Panum's area is determined and its middle is taken as the horopter. Subjects find the discrimination of fused versus diplopic percepts difficult and the disparate targets are a stimulus to refixate the eyes. However, this horopter tests a true binocular function and one of particular interest in anomalous correspondence, because anomalous correspondence is characterized by exaggerated fusional range (Pasino and Maraini, 1966).

This list is not exhaustive. A horopter could be defined as the surface of disparities eliciting neither convergence nor divergence, thus tapping pathways from retinal disparity detectors in cortex to oculomotor centres. The weight of history behind one horopter (nonius: Ogle, 1964; Tschermak-Seysenegg, 1952) should not be a deterrent to developing new horopters, better suited to modern needs.

The cellular basis of disparity detection

A binocular neurone compares the two eyes' images and detects retinal disparities between them, and links together points on the two retinas and makes these points correspond. Disparity selectivity is one of the most acute spatial skills known at the single-cell level. An arc misalignment of 6' in stimulus position (a movement of 1 mm at arm's length) can bring a cell in cat striate cortex from 90% to 10% of its optimal stimulus response.

The receptive field

In some cortical cells, disparity selectivity can be related to the spatial disposition of excitatory and inhibitory areas in the cells' receptive fields. The receptive field may be defined for the visual system as that place in the visual field where the presentation of a stimulus will change the response of the neurone under test. The response change may be either excitatory or inhibitory. The place producing an excitatory response (increase in the number of action potentials or 'spikes' per second) is termed an 'excitatory discharge region'; there may be several of them in one field. In some types of neurones, excitatory areas may be equated with ON regions (response burst at ON-set of a bright stimulus) and inhibitory areas, with *OFF* regions (burst of excita-

tion at stimulus OFF-set; *see* Chapters 2 and 13, *Figures 13.2* and *13.3*). In receptive fields where inhibitory areas flank the excitatory discharge region(s) they are termed 'inhibitory side-bands'.

The receptive field concept is central: it reaches downward (toward the retina) through the anatomical wiring by which the cell views a small patch of the visual world, and it reaches upward to perception via the neurone's special stimulus encoding abilities.

The existence of strongly inhibitory receptive field areas such as inhibitory sidebands is important for making neural responses highly specific. Besides the disparity cue to stereoscopic depth, specificities (stimulus selectivities) which are common among neurones in the striate and peristriate cortex are length of bars and edges, bar width, orientation, movement direction, velocity, spatial frequency, colour and, of course, position in the visual field. Inhibitory areas also bring the problem that large segments of the binocular population will be silenced when the stimulation is unsuitable.

Table 14.1 Caricature of simple/complex cell differences*

Simple	Complex
Separate *ON/OFF* areas	Mixed
Separated response areas to the light edge/dark edge of a moving bar	Mixed
Small receptive field	Large
No spontaneous discharge	Action potentials emitted in the absence of visual stimulation
Response summates as stimulus length and width are increased, up to full size of the RF	Response saturates when stimulus is still smaller than RF
Sensitive to stimulus position within RF	Phase insensitivity
Linear	Non-linear, saturating, frequency doubling
Sharp orientation tuning	Less sharp
Tend to be stellate cells, tend to be local to cortex	Tend to be pyramidal cells, tend to project out of one cortical area
Tend to receive primary or second-synapse visual input in striate cortex	Tend to occur later in the information processing chain

*Listed in decreasing order of certainty and general acceptance.

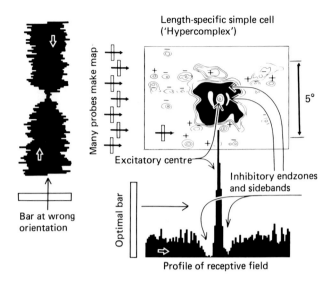

Length-specific simple cell ('Hypercomplex')

Many probes make map

Bar at wrong orientation

Optimal bar

Excitatory centre

Inhibitory endzones and sidebands

5°

Profile of receptive field

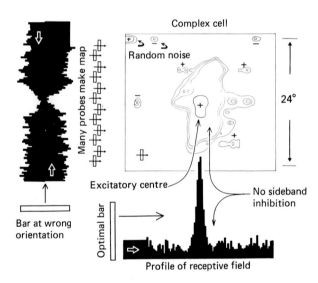

Complex cell

Random noise

Many probes make map

Bar at wrong orientation

Optimal bar

Excitatory centre

No sideband inhibition

24°

Profile of receptive field

Figure 14.3 Topographical maps of simple (top) and complex (bottom) cells recorded in cat striate cortex, and corresponding peristimulus time histogram profiles (PSTHs). Map inset: the stimulus bar and its motion direction (arrow) used to elicit maps and the profiles below them. Profiles on left: when the bar is horizontal and moved up and down (arrows), there is no excitatory response

Simple and complex cells

There are two broad classes of cell in the visual cortex: *simple* and *complex*. Their characteristics are compared in *Table 14.1*. There are several kinds of evidence (e.g. receptive field size and stimulus selectivity differences listed in *Table 14.1*) that suggest many simple cells converge on one complex cell, so that the complex cell can be thought of as performing higher levels of information processing and exporting the results to the next cortical area. *Hypercomplex cells*, however, no longer occupy the next step in this hierarchy. Nowadays, they are viewed as cells (either simple or complex) which

happen also to be length specific owing to the presence of some additional inhibitory areas (*Figure 14.3*).

Actual contour maps of the receptive fields of a simple and a complex cell are shown in *Figure 14.3*. The excitatory discharge regions (white central spot) and inhibitory sidebands (black) are separate in the simple cell, and correspond roughly to ON and OFF areas. These areas are mixed in the larger complex cell receptive field. Unlike the simple cell shown in *Figure 14.3*, inhibitory areas (end zones) here occur above and below the excitatory centre as well as in sidebands, and confer length specificity or hyper-complexity upon the cell. The conventional peristimulus time histograms (PSTHs, black bar graph profiles) below the topographic maps show the response to an optimal moving bar. When the bar is rotated 90°, the profiles (left) show only inhibition for movement up or down (arrows), because visual cortical cells are typically orientation selective.

Lastly, cortical neurones have surprisingly specific response characteristics even in cortical areas lying early in the information processing chain. The selectivities of cortical neurones define the dimensions of perceptual analysis: this is the way the brain takes apart the visual scene and these are the important stimulus dimensions to use in diagnosis and visual training.

Disparity detection by binocular neurones

To be disparity selective, a neurone must deem most disparities inappropriate and not respond to them. Because disparity detectors are inhibited by almost any difference between the retinal images, the dark horse of suppression shadows the achievements of binocular vision.

A system for disparity detection must possess, not only disparity-selective neurones, but neurones covering a *range* of disparity values. This range or scatter sets the limits of disparities which can be successfully detected and discriminated, but it also creates a range of disparities within which correspondence may vary. The belief that correspondence is anatomically determined was widely held in the past, but today it is seen that the determination is loose. One binocular neurone links a pair of retinal points, but a group of disparity detectors makes a range of correspondence links possible. *One cannot have both a modern, cellular basis for binocular vision and only one, unique, anatomically · determined set of corresponding points.*

Types of disparity detectors

The ability to track an object moving in depth over a large range of disparities demands large and broadly tuned receptive fields, whereas fine spatial resolution for working with the hands requires fields which are small and tightly tuned. Different kinds of disparity detectors exist to serve these divergent needs and different kinds of stimuli are optimal for reaching them. It should be no surprise that a patient stereoblind to one stimulus can detect depth with another (Sireteanu, Singer and Fronius, 1983).

Specific depth detectors

The classic disparity detector responds optimally to a specific depth (Joshua and Bishop, 1970). The response as disparity is varied is shown in *Figure 14.4*; this is the neurone's disparity tuning curve. The number of 'spikes' or action potentials is shown

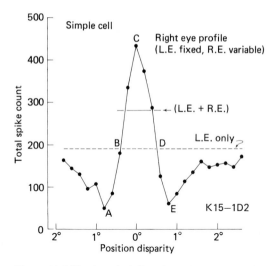

Figure 14.4 Classic retinal disparity tuning curve for a simple cell in cat striate cortex. Dashed line = left eye; solid line = sum of monocular responses. B, D reflects the width of the excitatory discharge centre in the receptive field; A, E reflects the locations of inhibitory sidebands. Noteworthy are the tuning curve's sharpness (important for stereoacuity); the presence of interocular facilitation which makes the binocular response greater than the sum of responses to stimulation of each eye alone (important for summation tests of binocularity); the presence of inhibition rather than merely response cessation when the disparity is inappropriate (important for suppression). (From Nelson, Kato and Bishop, 1977, courtesy of the Publisher, The American Physiological Society)

as a function of position disparity, where zero is the optimal disparity for this cell alone. Special interocular (binocular) facilitation makes the peak response (C) 54% greater than the sum of the monocular responses of left and right eyes. Interocular inhibition from the inhibitory sideband regions of one eye's receptive field (*see Figure 14.3*) reduces response nearly to zero when disparity is not optimal. A 50% reduction in peak response is achieved by 21' and 29' arc disparity (left and right sides of curve).

The disparity tuning curve of *Figure 14.4* is easily related to the perception of depth in free space as shown in *Figure 14.5*. From recordings of a single cortical neurone, receptive fields can be plotted on the tangent screen (T) for both the right (R) and left (L) eyes. The receptive field profile is given more accurately by the PSTHs (peristimulus time histograms). A single moving bar (B) must *simultaneously* stimulate the excitatory peaks shown in the two PSTH profiles to elicit the optimal response. This can only occur if the bar crosses point P in space (when the animal is fixating point F). Other positions in depth cause the bar's image to fall on the inhibitory sidebands in one eye's field at the time it could be exciting the other eye, so that, under binocular viewing conditions, there is no response (*see* points A and E in *Figure 14.4*). When monocular viewing produces more response than binocular viewing, then an early step in binocular suppression has been reached.

Inhibitory specific depth cells

The complementary specific depth cell, the *inhibitory* specific depth cell (Pettigrew, Nikara and Bishop, 1968; Poggio and Talbot, 1981) shows 'occlusion' or sharp response reduction at one particular disparity. This cell is active until the retinal images are in register; it could clamour that vergence was needed until fixation went accurately to completion.

Specific depth cells defining correspondence

Specific depth cells tie together specific retinal points with high acuity. They are, therefore, the most appropriate type of disparity detector for building a cellular definition of correspondence (*see below*).

Near/far detectors

Fine discriminations are possible without sharply selective neurones. In colour vision, the ability to discriminate wavelength differences as small as one nanometre, and perhaps 20 000 hues throughout colour space at equal luminance, arises from three broadly tuned detectors (retinal cones). Depth discrimination could be similar.

Evidence that depth is encoded in three broad bands of 'near', 'in the fixation plane', and 'far' first came from confusion errors made by observers in psychophysical experiments (Richards, 1970, 1971; *Figure 14.6*). Some observers confused large 'near' disparities with zero-depth stimuli, suggesting that a hypothetical 'near' class of detector was absent or defective. The probability that observers lack one class of detector in at least one hemisphere (i.e. when tested in one visual hemifield) is estimated at 0.3 (Richards, 1970).

Neurophysiological research in the cat, sheep and monkey has demonstrated disparity tuning curves appropriate for near and far depth detectors (Bishop, Henry and Smith, 1971; Clarke, Donaldson and Whitteridge, 1976; Maunsell and Van

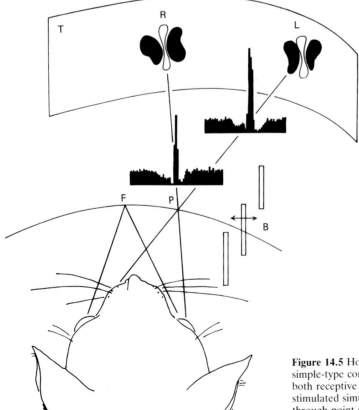

Figure 14.5 How disparity selectivity arises in a simple-type cortical neurone. The excitatory peaks in both receptive fields of the binocular neurone will be stimulated simultaneously only when bar (B) passes through point (P). Solid black = PSTHs. (From Nelson, 1981, courtesy of the Publisher, W. Junk)

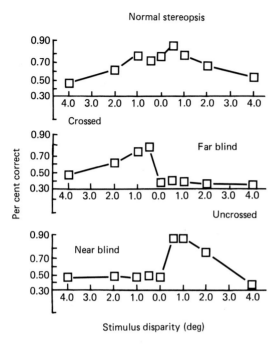

Figure 14.6 Confusion errors between large crossed (or uncrossed) disparities and the fixation plane made by human observers. This form of stereoblindness suggests that large, briefly presented depth intervals are encoded in three broad categories: near, far and in the fixation plane. (Redrawn from Richards, 1971, courtesy of the Publisher, The Optical Society of America)

Essen, 1983; Poggio, 1984). A typical tuning curve is shown in *Figure 14.7*. The sharp transitions in responsiveness occur at zero disparity in the awake, fixating monkey (Poggio, 1984), so that the disparities for which the neurone is responsive are truly nearer or further than the fixation plane (horopter).

The near/far system: coarse stereopsis and vergence initiation

The near/far detector system would be an appropriate substrate for the coarse stereopsis system (Bishop and Henry, 1971). This system can mediate only qualitative judgments of depth, typically for stimuli of very large disparities (up to 7°), brief exposure times or mismatched local contour content (unfusible shape — Ramachandran and Nelson, 1976). The near/far system may also be transient (Y dominated) because the classic near-only and far-only stereoblindness effects can only be observed with short stimulus exposure times (Patterson and Fox, 1984).

The near/far system is also a possible substrate for vergence initiation, which can be triggered by disparities as great as 5–10°, and stimuli as dissimilar between the two eyes as a circle and a cross. But another kind of detector system must take over from near/far neurones to drive vergence into its final lock and sustain it, because the near/far system is not precise enough.

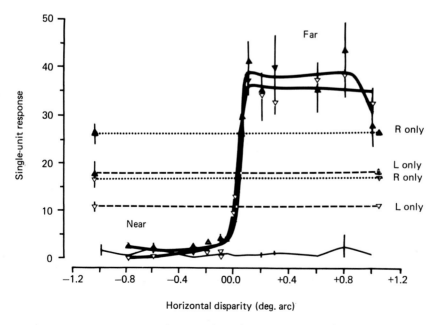

Figure 14.7 Position disparity tuning curve for a 'far' type depth-sensitive cell. This binocular neurone is excited for a broad range of uncrossed disparities (right), but shows an abrupt transition to weak or inhibited responsiveness at the plane of fixation. Lowest curve: spontaneous activity level. Open/closed triangles: two sweep directions. (From Poggio and Poggio, 1984, courtesy of the Publisher, Annual Reviews Inc.)

Motion in depth

While you look at a stone thrown accurately at your head, retinal images are moving in opposite directions. Cells preferring opposite directions of motion could inform you of such impending discomforts and have been observed in the cat (Bishop, Henry and Smith, 1971; Pettigrew, 1973). Even if the motion directions are not opposite, they will have different velocities for any 'near miss' trajectory toward (or away from) the observer. Velocity disparity selectivity has been measured in a variety of areas (monkey: superior temporal sulcus — Zeki, 1974; striate cortex — Poggio and Talbot, 1981; middle temporal visual area — Maunsell and Van Essen, 1983; cat: peristriate cortex — Cynader and Regan, 1978; 17/18 border — Cynader and Regan, 1982; Clare-Bishop area — Toyama and Kozasa, 1982). In clinical patients, the ability to map areas of depth perception with stimuli moving in depth in an observer who is stereoblind to static stimuli throughout the visual field, probably occurs because separate motion-in-depth pathways and separate cortical areas are uniquely probed by the dynamic disparity stimulus and can survive in strabismus when others fail (Sireteanu, Singer and Fronius, 1983; Kitaoji and Toyama, 1987).

Orientation disparity

A straight edge tilted in depth gives rise to retinal images differing in orientation. Tilt may be specified by either this single orientation disparity (cyclodisparity), or by an infinite progression of increasing position disparity values.

Binocular neurones in the cat striate cortex can detect a range of orientation disparities (Blackmore, Fiorentini and Maffei, 1972), but the binocular tuning curves are no better than monocular ones (Nelson, Kato and Bishop, 1977). In the monkey, on the other hand, von der Heydt *et al.* (1982) found 8 out of 170 cells with binocular orientation disparity tunings 10 times as sharp as conventional monocular tuning. Perhaps there are so few 'tilt detectors' because one orientation disparity value so efficiently specifies the tilt of an entire surface. How a powerful cue picked up by a handful of cells can provide heuristic guidance for the computations of entire cortical areas is a problem for both artifical intelligence modellers and neuroscientists.

Detection of vertical disparity

Vertical disparity can be a source of fixation distance and fixation asymmetry information needed to stabilize horopter curvature and tilt. Vertical disparity also triggers the induced effect — a shift in horizontal correspondence. Neurophysiological mechanisms for the detection of vertical disparity exist. Because the binocular visual system is vertical-disparity selective, it is also true that small, unwanted vertical disparities (e.g. hyperphoria) can affect many binocular neurones, typically inhibiting them. Vertical disparity is not a cue to stereoscopic depth, but it is a powerful input to the binocular visual system.

Global stereopsis

Random-dot stereograms (Julesz, 1971) are important screening tests for children (*see* Chapter 11). Their diagnostic usefulness stems from their inability to be faked: no forms can be discerned in the random texture unless stereoscopic depth defines one. However, a certain rivalrous, binocular lustre can appear where disparity is present, so that the observer should be asked, not merely whether he can see the form, but whether the form's depth is in front of or behind the fixation plane. With the Frisby test, head movements must be prevented because of motion parallax cues.

Globality: a more complex kind of disparity detection

Random-dot stereograms (*see Figure 13.13* and *Figure 2.8*) require detection mechanisms different from all others. Their mechanical nature would seem to make local detection of disparity easy, but the precisely repeating nature of the patterns also creates ambiguities termed 'matching noise'. This noise consists of false disparity signals due to accidental pattern pixel matches. Because of matching noise, disparity cannot be detected locally by depth-selective neurones of the sort considered above; instead, the responses of large groups of depth-selective neurones must be pooled (summed), presumably by network interactions in the visual cortex, to decode the stimulus. The pooling operation for deciding on the correct disparity by consensus is termed 'globality'. Besides pooling (strengthening) of the correct retinal disparity response, globality involves the suppression of matching noise.

The domain interaction model of globality

The first neurophysiologically plausible model for globality was suggested by Nelson (1975a), who pointed out that the network interactions required for globality would also produce sensory fusional shifts in normal binocular vision, and variability in anomalous correspondence (Nelson, 1977, 1981). If specific-depth detectors with closely matched disparity tunings, but widely spread spatial positions, were mutually *facilitatory*, response to the globally correct disparity would be strengthened. If mutual *inhibition* spread broadly within the disparity domain and narrowly in all directions across space, matching noise would be eliminated. This is termed a 'domain interaction model' of globality, because the interactions only acquire their usefulness by being ordered along stimulus dimensions or domains. This qualitative model has been followed by more rigorous formulations (reviewed by Poggio and Poggio, 1984; Nelson, 1985). The need for network interactions to create globality is now generally accepted.

Cellular definition of correspondence

The convergence of retinogeniculate inputs from the two eyes onto single binocular cortical cells ties together retinal points (patches) and makes them correspond. But there are multiple correspondences because the neurones involved fall into several disparity detector classes and because, within one class, there must be positional scatter to make a range of disparities detectable.

Variability of normal correspondence

Even normal correspondence must be variable, because of:

(1) Fixation disparity (Ogle, Martens and Dyer, 1967; Schor, 1983), classically said to be less than 30' arc, but really at least twice as great, based on photographic evidence from Stewart (1951).
(2) Fixation tremor. Using the data of St Cyr and Fender (1969), Fender (cited by Bishop, 1981) has shown that the standard deviations for the horizontal and vertical departures of one eye from the position of the other were 4.8' and 8.9' arc, respectively. These disparity fluctuations do not produce fluctuations in perceived depth, even though a disparity of 4' arc is about 12 times above threshold.
(3) Image magnification (Wheatstone, 1838; excerpted in Dember, 1964).
(4) Telestereoscopic stereobase magnification in the laboratory.

In all cases disparity input occurs, but vision remains single and depth does not arise. Therefore, correspondence must have changed.

A formal basis for variability: depthless fusion

The fusion of a physical disparity without perceived depth has been termed 'depthless fusion'. Depthless fusion is, by definition, a shift in correspondence because both depth perception and perceived visual direction have changed. The stimulus characteristic which seems to produce depthless fusion is a dispar-

ity shift which is uniform across the visual field. This is exactly what happens in strabismus and fusion without depth perception is common there.

Correspondence in cellular terms

A rigid definition of corresponding points

The range of detectable disparities defines a range of possible correspondences (functional pairings) between the retinas. For simplicity, only specific depth detectors in striate cortex (area 17 or V1) will be dealt with. How is one state of correspondence chosen from among those possible? A bold start was made by Bishop (Joshua and Bishop, 1970; Bishop, 1973, 1981), who proposed that corresponding points were points covered by the most common single-unit tuning: they asserted that the modal tuning is the zero disparity tuning. This point of view embodies a basic truth about visual system development: the mean fixation position of the eyes and the average visual ecology of the maturing animal will determine the alignment of binocular neurones. But biological systems being what they are, a scatter remains about the modal disparity tuning.

Bishops's correspondence model has been extended to account for the horopter and Panum's fusional area, as shown in *Figure 14.8*. Precisely simultaneous (spatially aligned) stimulation of a binocular neurone's two receptive fields produces the optimal response. The receptive fields may be simplified to a point in the visual field and from the retina through the nodal point of the eye to this receptive field centre point, a so-called receptive field axis may be constructed. The optimal stimulation point (disparity tuning) in three-dimensional space for any given neurone occurs at the intersection of the neurone's receptive field axes. The axes do not all intersect at the same distance from the animal.

Receptive field axis angles are scattered like the bell-shaped curves shown in *Figure 14.8*, but one axis angle or one intersection point is represented by the greatest number of neurones. This angle, lying at the top of the distribution curve, defines corresponding points for this position in the visual field. Corresponding points for a complete cross-section of the visual field defines a horopter. A maximum stereoacuity horopter should match such a neurophysiological horopter because, where there are the most cells, there should be the finest sensory coding. The modal angle (intersecting point) changes somewhat as one moves towards the periphery, so that the distribution of corresponding points is not uniform on nasal versus temporal retina and a Vieth–Müller circle is not generated. Instead, the horopter based on singly recorded binocularly excit-

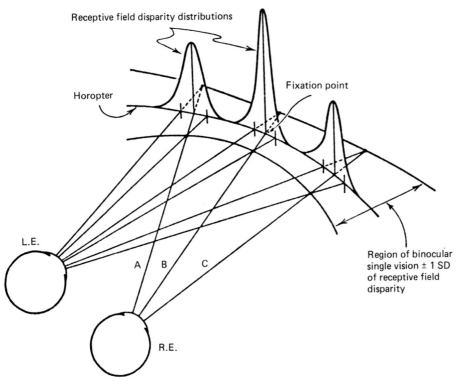

Figure 14.8 Bishop's model for deriving the horopter and Panum's areas from the distribution of optimal disparity tunings in populations of binocular cortical neurones. Bishop defines the retinal disparity to which the most units are tuned as the zero disparity. This definition may be extended to a neurophysiological definition of the horopter and Panum's fusional limits. Although correspondence is now a parameter of a neural population, the parameter is fixed. For anomalous correspondence, correspondence must vary. For an explanation, *see* text. (From Joshua and Bishop, 1970, courtesy of the Publisher, Springer)

able neurones in the cat is somewhat flattened, although not abathic (perfectly flat).

Panum's areas are incorporated into Bishop's model by defining the limits of sensory fusion as the disparity tunings lying plus/minus one standard deviation from the mean tuning (i.e. from the line labelled 'horopter'). These limits are illustrated by the receptive axes shown in *Figure 14.8*. For neurones with receptive axes 'a' and 'b', the disparity tuning (schematized as if arising entirely from the left eye) is uncrossed by one standard deviation of the population scatter and the axes intersect at the further Panum's limit; neurone 'c' exemplifies the near limit. Receptive field scatter is indeed greater in the visual field periphery and so the increase in Panum's area with retinal eccentricity is accounted for.

If increasing disparities were presented, fewer binocular neurones would be available to respond. At the same time, two additional populations of neurones not illustrated (left eye only, right eye only) *will* respond. The activity of these two popula-tions signal stimulation from separate visual directions; diplopia is eventually perceived.

A flexible definition of corresponding points

A fixed definition of corresponding points (plus/ minus one standard deviation of a tuning distribu-tion) does not fit the facts of variability in normal or anomalous correspondence. Further, for sensory fusion, the boundary between single vision and diplopia must vary with the contour content of the stimulus, as a function of past stimulation history (hysteresis effects) and with the context of surround-ing disparities.

A more flexible model of correspondence can still link the state of correspondence to a population of disparity-selective cortical neurones, but the link must be drawn to the activity pattern across the disparity domain, not just to the number of detectors at each tuning. Activity will of course change with stimulation and it will change because disparity detectors are hypothesized to be linked by mutually facilitatory and inhibitory interconnections. These network interactions produce important changes in activity; through them, an active tuning affects many other tunings (disparity domain interactions) and many other visual field positions (spatial domain interactions).

Definition of correspondence: **corresponding points are those paired by the specific-depth detectors which are most active at a given moment. The most active tuning is determined globally.**

This definition extends the Bishop model by asserting that the visual system cannot distinguish between a disparity domain firing pattern produced by a peak in the distribution of *numbers* of units (all of which are equally active) and a similar pattern produced by a peak in the *activity* of fewer units which are vigorously stimulated.

Definition of sensory fusion: **sensory fusion is a local change in the most active disparity tuning.**

Total correspondence shift under field-wide disparity input

With the new definition above and powerful stimulation, correspondence can be driven to new values. The disparity stimulation must be presented across the entire visual field.

Definition of shift in correspondence: **when the dominant tuning changes to a similar value in disparity domains throughout the visual field, retinal correspondence shifts to the new dominant tuning. The disparity which has become corresponding cannot generate perceived depth.**

This extended model has important benefits:

(1) Correspondence can be variable, as it often is in strabismus.
(2) Stimulation is what makes correspondence vary. It is possible to understand why normal correspondence is elicited by the Hering afterimage test whereas the Bagolini striated glasses elicit harmonious anomalous correspondence.
(3) The loss of depth perception in anomalous correspondence becomes clear: a binocular visual system which shifts correspondence to a new zero in response to even minor disparity inputs cannot detect local departures from zero disparity (i.e. objects in depth).

A neurophysiological approach to anomalous correspondence

Anomalous correspondence (AC) requires an intact but abnormal binocular cortical substrate. Abnor-

malities can occur at the single units level (the receptive fields of binocular neurones), the population level (shifted distributions of tunings) or the information processing level (exaggerated domain interactions).

Changes in the neural substrate
Changes at the single cell level

A normal specific depth detector is schematized in *Figure 14.9a*. Binocular neurones like this one (a simple-type cell) are normally plentiful, with well-matched, monocularly excitable receptive fields in each eye. The well-localized receptive field regions (excitatory discharge centre, 30′ arc wide) generate tightly tuned position disparity curves (half-width at half-height 30′ arc). It is known that a group of such detectors taken as a whole will be scattered plus/minus several degress about the group's mean tuning. In deprivation amblyopia (*Figure 14.9b*; *see also* Chapter 13), excitatory signals from one eye fail to enjoy cortical access under binocular viewing conditions. Some neurones recorded in the cortex may even have purely inhibitory receptive fields in the amblyopic eye, symbolized here by the all-black receptive field.

In anomalous correspondence, it can be assumed that cortical plasticity would enable disparity tunings to shift during an early critical period. With a small-angle, comitant squint, the receptive field separation of a binocular cortical neurone would change (*Figure 14.9c*). If the entire population of neurones changed to a new mean tuning, then, in accord with either the Bishop model or Nelson's extension of it, retinal correspondence would shift to an anomalous value. Because this is an abnormal path of development for the sensory cortex (and motor control of the eyes in addition may not be so precise), the amount of variability around the new mean tuning is likely to be broader than normal, as indicated by the broader scatter of the arrows which represent other receptive field pairs. There is experimental evidence that such shifts in position disparity tuning (Shlaer, 1971), orientation disparity (Bruce, Iseley and Shinkman, 1981; Hänny and von der Heydt, 1982) or both together (Dürsteler and von der Heydt, 1983) can occur.

Just as the distribution of tunings is likely to be more scattered in an abnormal population of disparity detectors, so each particular neurone may itself be less selective (*Figure 14.9d*; for evidence from subthreshold interaction in man, *see* Levi and Harwerth, 1982). The loss in selectivity could arise from a broad or multiply peaked excitatory discharge centre, weaker monocular inhibitory regions, or weaker interocular facilitation and suppression (of the kind shown in *Figure 14.4*).

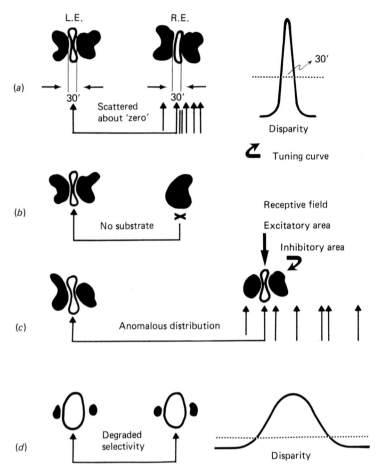

Figure 14.9 Possible receptive field changes in strabismus. (*a*) Normal binocularity. Black areas: inhibitory sidebands. White region: excitatory discharge centre. Curve, right: disparity tuning curve. Arrows: scatter of other disparity detectors' tuning. (*b*) Loss of binocularity (amblyopia). (*c*) Preserved binocularity, but anomalous correspondence. (*d*) Deterioration in binocularity and disparity discrimination. (From Nelson, 1981, courtesy of the Publisher, W. Junk)

Changes at the population level

The most likely changes in the distribution of disparity tunings within a neural population are summarized in *Figure 14.10*. In general, a shift in mean disparity tuning is expected because of cortical plasticity (*Figure 14.10b,c,d* versus *a*); in the Bishop/Nelson model, this tuning shift brings a shift in correspondence. How large the mean shift is (the *angle of anomaly*) is independent of how sharp the peak is (*Figure 14.10b* versus *c*). More broadly scattered disparity tunings will permit a more *variable* angle of anomaly. According to the model, the range of available disparity tunings sets the limit on the angles of anomaly which are possible. In principle, any angle of anomaly may be expressed if the appropriate disparity value is stimulated vigorously enough. With no stimulation or the poor binocular

stimulation available in dissociating clinical tests, the resting state of correspondence is expressed. The resting state is given by the peak of the population tuning curves shown here and in the Bishop model (*see Figure 14.8*).

With normal development before the onset of strabismus, normally tuned binocular neurones will be present and the resting state of correspondence will be normal. With the onset of strabismus, neurones tuned to abnormal disparities will be added to this normal ('zero') peak. This implies the ability to express at least two correspondence states, either alternately or simultaneously. Two *simultaneously* expressed correspondence states would be a form of monocular diplopia, or double vision in one eye evident only under binocular viewing conditions (i.e. binocular triplopia).

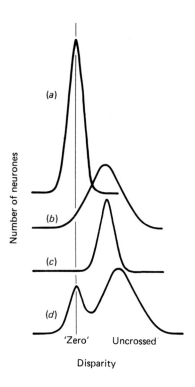

Figure 14.10 Possible distributions of disparity tunings in a population of binocular neurones. The peak determines the resting state of correspondence, but strong disparity stimulation can make other, less well represented tunings temporarily corresponding. (*a*) Normal. (*b*) Correspondence has shifted. The range of available tunings is broader, supporting a broader than normal amount of sensory fusion and/or variation in the state of correspondence. (*c*) No cortical substrate for normal correspondence — a 'deeply rooted' anomaly. (*d*) Bimodal distribution of disparity tunings supporting alternation between normal and anomalous correspondence. (From Nelson, 1981, courtesy of the Publisher, W. Junk)

The depth of anomaly concept

The proportion of neurones at the normal versus the anomalous tuning determines the relative ease of eliciting normal versus anomalous correspondence. The difficulty in eliciting normal correspondence is termed the 'depth of anomaly'. In everyday viewing, or with Bagolini glasses, the anomalous tuning is dominant and the strabismic observer experiences AC, because the anomalous tuning lies at the objective angle and is intensely stimulated.

Strabismic concepts in cellular terms: two types of AC variability

Types of variability in anomalous correspondence

The angle of anomaly in anomalous correspondence changes from minute to minute; yet an adult observer long outside the critical period cannot shift receptive fields in an instant. Because rewiring the cortex is out of the question, the source of this variability must be investigated.

Variability in the angle of anomaly has been known since the earliest studies of strabismus. Schlodtmann (1900) had a subject view a foveal after-image in his deviating eye against a completely homogeneous white field (a sheet of paper held close to the eye) while the strong eye's field was darker, coloured and almost empty, save for a haploscopically presented cipher fixated for the duration of the demonstration. Under these unfavourable conditions for sensory fusion, the after-image was seen in normal correspondence. Upon removal of the white occluder, the deviating eye continued to display normal correspondence for an instant, after which another haploscopically presented cipher for the eye was observed to jump to a position of anomalous correspondence. During all this, the after-image in the deviating eye did not move, proving (although not beyond all doubt) that the eyes had held a stationary position. The brain, not the eyes, had shifted correspondence. Bielschowsky (1900), who obtained data for variability of correspondence from 80 of 100 subjects, reported that one observer localized normally with his eyes closed, but saw the same foveal after-images in anomalous correspondence with eyes open.

In both studies above, greater contour input at the objective disparity (occluder removed, eyes opened) produced the change to anomalous correspondence. Correspondence changes may be either abrupt as in these historical examples, or smooth, as considered next. In either case, visual stimulation is what alters the state of correspondence.

Smoothly varying AC

The angle of anomaly is more likely to change smoothly if the disparity input is smoothly varied, either with instruments, or because the objective angle undergoes smooth variations.

Prisms

The deviating eye may participate in binocular vision while yet being disconnected from oculomotor commands to turn for fixation. Therefore shifting the retinal image with prisms shifts the disparity input instead of triggering disjunctive eye movements. Using after-images to prove eye position remained stable. Rønne and Rindziunski (1953) were able to show continuous shifts in correspondence under these conditions.

Synoptophore

Working with children who fused binocular images at an anomalous angle in the synoptophore, Kretzschmar (1955) gradually shifted the image disparity back to zero. The subjects maintained fusion continuously with no observable eye movements. Similar manoeuvres are used in orthoptic training for reinstatement of normal correspondence. Reports of continuously variable angles of anomaly are rare, however, in part because unfusible (weak) stimuli are commonly used with these instruments.

Motility conditions

In ocular motility conditions where the objective angle smoothly varies, the disparity input to the visual system varies also. By asking someone displaying an A or V pattern to look up or down while wearing striated glasses, it is easy to show that the angle of anomaly co-varies with the objective angle of squint. Ciancia (1962; *see also* Ciancia, 1968) reports maintenance of single vision over a disparity range of 35 Δ. Correspondence variation was reduced with the red glass and almost eliminated by the use of unfusible horizontal/vertical after-images. The reduced range of correspondence shift with dissimilar images may be likened psychophysically to a reduced range of sensory fusion (Panum's area) or neurophysiologically to lowered single-unit reponsiveness (and increased interocular inihibition) when images are poorly matched.

Subjective angle changes also occur in asymmetrical convergence, during orthoptic training and 'spontaneously' (Halldén, 1952). Matching shifts in correspondence are observed in all cases.

Conclusion: exaggerated sensory fusion

The similarity of smoothly varying AC to exaggerated sensory fusion is obvious, and has been championed by Bagolini (1974) and von Noorden (Awaya, von Noorden and Romano, 1970; Helveston, von Noorden and Williams, 1970), who termed it 'point-to-area correspondence'. Halldén (1952) has demonstrated co-variation in objective and subjective angles of anomaly and argued convincingly that only sensory fusional mechanisms could keep the two congruent.

Abruptly switching AC

Anomalous correspondence sometimes shows *discontinuous* changes in angle of anomaly which do

not seem like normal fusion. Switching-type AC almost always shows alternation between normal correspondence (NC) and some anomalous angle. Alternation between NC and AC is most commonly reported for subjects with voluntary control over their deviation, i.e. strabismics who sometimes see with straight eyes. Tschermak (1899) was such a person. Upon fixating without deviation, he reported a switch from AC to NC which he believed occurred across the entire visual field.

In today's domain interaction model, the spread across the visual field of a state of correspondence implies spread of one disparity tuning's dominance, and is attributed to mutual facilitation among like-tuned disparity detectors.

Switching-type AC is more common than the smoothly variable type. Revell (1971) claims that most unilateral squinters who can be induced to fixate with the weak eye will show switching. The effect has been made the basis of a method of orthoptic treatment in which NC is elicited and strengthened (Hugonnier, 1967; Wick, 1974).

Neurophysiological basis

Switching-type AC requires a binocular visual system biased toward the expression of two correspondence states. The bias presumably takes the form of greater numbers of binocular neurones with tunings at each of two different disparity values (*see Figure 14.10d*). The domain interaction model's mutal inhibition makes switching bwetween the two different peaks occur suddenly.

The abruptness of AC/NC changes is indeed dramatic. Starting with stimuli over-converged on the haploscope and proceeding outwards, the images 'suddenly, with a jump, pass each other and appear uncrossed' in the absence of observable eye movements (Rønne and Rindziunski, 1953).

Monocular diplopia

This may be viewed as a temporary balance in the activity level of two populations of binocular neurones, each tuned to and expressing a different mean disparity (correspondence). It is a switching type of AC in which the switching mechanism is momentarily in balance. Competition between states of correspondence makes the appearance of monocular diplopia fleeting, although reports are not as rare as commonly believed (*see* Nelson, 1981).

In sum, switching-type AC depends on the same domain interaction mechanisms postulated to underlie sensory fusion and smoothly variable AC, but behaves differently because the disparity detector substrate is different.

Depth perception in anomalous correspondence

In anomalous correspondence, a point in the peripheral retina of the deviating eye is said to acquire the same visual direction as the fovea of the fixating eye; in harmonious AC, this point is directed onto the object of regard and serves as a pseudofovea.

A fovea is not only an area of high receptor density, but a point with zero motor value for fixation. In strabismus, the pseudofovea typically does not have this property under *monocular* conditions; instead, the real fovea takes over. This is why the *alternate cover test* works: switching from binocular (or dominant eye fixation) to monocular fixation with the non-preferred eye causes an oculomotor shift from pseudofovea-centred to real fovea-centred fixation. The eye's refixation movement can be used to measure the squint. An exception is *obligatory eccentric monocular fixation*, which is sometimes combined with AC. The eccentricity invalidates the cover test and does not reveal the angle of AC either.

Modern research with objective eye response measurement has shown that, with dynamic stimulus presentation, other classes of disparity detectors can be reached and vergence responses can be elicited, so that motor fusion to the pseudofovea occurs (Ciuffreda and Kenyon, 1983). Thus, anomalous correspondence commands rudimentary motor function as well as its own set of spatial values.

Studies demonstrating discrimination of depth (disparities) around an anomalous zero point (i.e. based on an anomalous correspondence) are rare. Even subjects with a small angle, stable strabismus and no suppression had a disparity discrimination function three times worse than normal control subjects (Pasino, Maraini and Santori, 1963). Depth perception loss is characteristic of AC.

There is a tradition in academic vision research of ignoring plasticity in correspondence and denying sensory fusional shifts of contours. Egocentric spatial orientation is supposed to be stable. But the strabismic visual system is not traditional. Unable to turn the eye, the visual system rotates the projection of the visual world, a stunning feat of cortical processing and well worth the price of failed depth perception.

Central/peripheral differences in AC

Centrally, binocularity often shows normal correspondence (no adaptation) or disappears entirely (suppression or amblyopia), whereas peripherally, binocularity is both more resistant to loss and more likely to become anomalous.

Anomalous correspondence in the periphery

In the classic pattern of amblyopic suppression, input from the entire visual field is not suppressed. Particularly for esotropia, suppression will be localized in the deviating eye to the fovea, a peripheral region on which the object fixated by the good eye is imaged, and an oval region overlapping these poles (Harms, 1939; Sireteanu, 1982; Sireteanu, Singer and Fronius, 1983). Anomalous correspondence is common in the remaining, peripheral areas.

On neurophysiological grounds, one would expect there to be less suppression in the periphery than in the fovea because single cell receptive fields are larger and tunings broader there, while the population as a whole has more widely scattered receptive field separations (disparity tunings). These factors support continued responsiveness despite a retinal image shifted by strabismus.

Suppression at the pseudofovea

Suppression in the deviating eye during binocular viewing is often most intense at the pseudofoveal region, the area corresponding to the fovea of the fixating eye. The simplest basis for the central visual field's handicap in developing AC is the enormous *magnification factor* for the foveal projection, particularly in area 17 (striate cortex). With many more millimetres of cortical tissue allocated to one degree of visual field subtense, the arborizing fibres carrying the distant, desired disparity inputs cannot reach their targets. Of course, a neural axon can cross the brain or run the length of the spinal cord, so length alone is not the problem. Instead, there must be a barrier. The barrier to a fibre from the weak eye might be the necessity of entering and exiting an ocular dominance column from its own eye in order to converge on a visuotopically more distant neurone innervated by the other eye. Ocular dominance columns (*see* Chapter 13) are of uniform width and one 'width' is worth several degrees in the periphery, so such barriers would not soon be encountered there. (For magnification factor and module concepts in monkey, *see* Hubel and Wiesel, 1974.) With anomalous correspondence out of the question, there remains competition between a true fovea served by many neurones in a highly magnified cortical projection area and fewer neurones serving a pseudofovea out in the periphery. The outcome is suppression of all channels serving the pseudofovea.

Concluding remarks

Advances in neurophysiology force a fresh look at binocular vision. The neurophysiological substrate is rich and a variety of cue systems play a role in binocular vision's early stages. Retinal correspondence itself may have several bases: different detector classes and different cortical areas may have 'different opinions' about what the state of correspondence should be or whether binocularity should be expressed at all (e.g. binocularity may be absent with static but not dynamic disparities). Above all, neurophysiology teaches us that correspondence is inherently variable. This variability in correspondence offers a new opportunity to unite normal and abnormal binocular vision, and calls for quantitative, graded and neurophysiologically informed clinical testing.

The challenge to future binocular vision researchers will be the understanding of spatial localization: the construction of egocentric maps, allocentric maps and their reconciliation. How the parts of our body are arranged must be known in order to calculate how the environment is disposed around us (egocentric map). Only with an egocentric map of our immediate surroundings and an allocentric map of the world beyond it can locomotion and eye movements be effectively planned. Strabismus disturbs the egocentric map. We do not know 'straight ahead'. Strabismologists studying lower oculomotor control centres may be frustrated in understanding why the eye refuses to be re-educated until the map construction going on in higher command centres is understood.

Today's challenges lie at the input end of the binocular visual system, where disparity is detected. The present task is a unification of clinical, psychophysical and neurophysiological concepts. It must be possible to translate 'stimulus elicits small Panum's area' into 'test is dissociating'. It should be possible to reduce both these psychophysical and clinical concepts to cellular terms. Equating concepts across disciplines, and reducing perception to cellular terms, is a speculative business. But the assertion that if one thing is observed then another will be found is a *testable* speculation, and this is what science is all about.

Acknowledgements

Preparation of the chapters by JIN was supported in part by NIMH grant 34793, the Naval Air Systems Command, and the Air Force Office of Scientific Research 83–0225. Linda Misa provided invaluable bibliographic help. I thank colleagues for generously sharing their work and comments and, in particular, Ruxandra Sireteanu for reading an earlier draft. Robin Hannay Nelson did the drawings for *Figures 14.1* and *14.5*

References

AWAYA, S., VON NOORDEN, G. K. and ROMANO, P. E. (1970) Symposium: Sensory adaptations in strabismus. Anomalous retinal correspondence in different positions of gaze. *Am. Orthopt. J.*, **20**, 28–35

BAGOLINI, B. (1974) Sensory anomalies in strabismus. *Br. J. Ophthalmol.*, **58**, 313–318; 323–331

BIELSCHOWSKY, A. (1900) Untersuchungen über das Sehen der Schielenden. *Albrecht von Graefes Arch. Ophthalmol.*, **50**, 406–509

BISHOP, P. O. (1973) Neurophysiology of binocular single vision and stereopsis. In *Handbook of Sensory Physiology*, edited by R. Jung, vol. VII/3, *Central Processing of Visual Information*, pp. 255–305. New York: Springer

BISHOP, P. O. (1981) Binocular vision. In *Adler's Physiology of the Eye: Clinical Application*, 7th edn, edited by R. A. Moses, pp. 575–649. St Louis: C. V. Mosby

BISHOP, P. O. and HENRY, G. H. (1971) Spatial vision. *Annu. Rev. Psychol.*, **22**, 119–160

BISHOP, P. O., HENRY, G. H. and SMITH, C. J. (1971) Binocular interaction fields of single units in the cat striate cortex. *J. Physiol.*, **216**, 39–68

BLAKEMORE, C., FIORENTINI, A. and MAFFEI, L. (1972) A second neural mechanism of binocular depth discrimination. *J. Physiol.*, **226**, 725–749

BRAUNSTEIN, M. L. (1976) *Depth Perception through Motion.* New York: Academic Press/Harcourt Brace Jovanovich

BRUCE, C. J., ISLEY, M. R. and SHINKMAN, P. G. (1981) Visual experience and development of interocular orientation disparity in visual cortex. *J. Neurophysiol.*, **46**, 215–228

CIANCIA, A. O. (1962) Sensorial relationship in A and V syndromes. *Trans. Ophthalmol. Soc. UK*, **82**, 243–251

CIANCIA, A. O. (1968) Practical implications of the present knowledge about subjective space in anomalous correspondence. In *International Strabismus Symposium*, edited by A. Arruga, pp. 347–350. Basel: Karger

CIUFFREDA, K. J. and KENYON, R. V. (1983) Accommodative vergence and accommodation in normals, amblyopes, and strabismics. In *Vergence Eye Movements: Basic and Clinical Aspects*, edited by C. M. Schor and K. J. Ciuffreda, pp. 101–173. Boston: Butterworths

CLARKE, P. G. H., DONALDSON, I. M. L. and WHITTERIDGE, D. (1976) Binocular visual mechanisms in cortical areas I and II of the sheep. *J. Physiol.*, **256**, 509–526

COGAN, A. I. (1982) Monocular sensitivity during binocular viewing. *Vision Res.*, **22**, 1–16

COGAN, A. I. (1987) Human binocular interaction: Towards a neural model. *Vision Res.*, **27**, 2125–2139

CYNADER, M. and REGAN, D. (1978) Neurones in cat parastriate cortex sensitive to the direction of motion in three-dimensional space. *J. Physiol.*, **274**, 549–569

CYNADER, M. and REGAN, D. (1982) Neurones in cat visual cortex tuned to the direction of motion in depth: effect of positional disparity. *Vision Res.*, **22**, 967–982

DEMBER, W. N. (1964) *Visual Perception: The Nineteenth Century.* New York: Wiley

DÜRSTELER, M. R. and VON DER HEYDT, R. (1983) Plasticity in the binocular correspondence of striate cortical receptive fields in kittens. *J. Physiol.*, **345**, 87–105

EPSTEIN, W. (1967) *Varieties of Perceptual Learning*. New York: McGraw-Hill

ERKELENS, C. J. and COLLEWIJN, H. (1985) Eye movements and stereopsis during dichoptic viewing of moving random-dot stereograms. *Vision Res.*, **25**, 1689–1700

FRÖHLICH, R. (1985) Unter welchen Umständen erscheinen Doppelbilder in ungleichem Abstande vom Beobachter? *Albrecht von Graefes Arch. Ophthalmol.*, **41**, 134–157

HALLDÉN, U. (1952) Fusional phenomena in anomalous correspondence. *Acta Ophthalmol. Suppl.* 37

HÄNNY, P. and VON DER HEYDT, R. (1982) The effect of horizontal-plane environment on the development of binocular receptive fields of cells in cat visual cortex. *J. Physiol.*, **329**, 75–92

HARMS, H. (1939) Ort und Wesen der Bildhemmung bei Schielenden. *Albrecht von Graefes Arch. Ophthalmol.*, **138**, 149–210

HEINE, L. (1904) Zur Frage der binokularen Tiefenwahrnehmung auf Grund von Doppelbildern. *Pflügers Arch. Ges. Physiol.*, **104**, 316–319

HELVESTON, E. M., VON NOORDEN, G. K. and WILLIAMS, F. (1970) Symposium: Sensory adaptations in strabismus. Retinal correspondence in the 'A' or 'V' pattern. *Am. Orthopt. J.*, **20**, 22–27

HOCHBERG, J. (1971) Perception II. Space and movement. In *Woodworth and Schlosberg's Experimental Psychology*, 3rd edn, edited by J. W. Kling and L. A. Riggs. New York: Holt

HUBEL, D. H. and WIESEL, T. N. (1974) Uniformity of monkey striate cortex: a parallel relationship between field size, scatter, and magnification factor. *J. Comp. Neurol.*, **158**, 295–305

HUGONNIER, R. (1967) La correspondance rétinienne anormale dans les strabismes divergents. *Doc. Ophthalmol.*, **23**, 425–447

HYSON, M. T., JULESZ, B. and FENDER, D. H. (1983) Eye movements and neural remapping during fusion of misaligned random-dot stereograms. *J. Opt. Soc. Am.*, **73**, 1665–1673

JOSHUA, D. E. and BISHOP, P. O. (1970) Binocular single vision and depth discrimination. Receptive field disparities for central and peripheral vision and binocular interaction on peripheral single units in cat striate cortex. *Exp. Brain Res.*, **10**, 389–416

JULESZ, B. (1971) *Foundations of Cyclopean Perception*. Chicago: University of Chicago Press

KAILA, E. (1919) Versuch einer empiristischen Erklärung der Tiefenlokalisation von Doppelbildern. *Z. Psychol. Physiol. Sinnesorg.*, **82**, 129–197

KITAOJI, H. and TOYAMA, K. (1987) Preservation of position and motion stereopsis in strabismic subjects. *Invest. Ophthalmol. Vis. Sci.*, **28**, 1260–1267

KRETZSCHMAR, S. (1955) La fausse correspondance rétinienne. *Doc. Ophthalmol.*, **9**, 46–208

LEVELT, W. J. M. (1968) *On Binocular Rivalry*. The Hague: Mouton

LEVI, D. M. and HARWERTH, R. S. (1982) Psychophysical

mechanisms in humans with amblyopia. *Am. J. Optom. Physiol. Opt.*, **59**, 936–951

LEVINE, M. W. and SHEFNER, J. M. (1981) *Fundamentals of Sensation and Perception*. Reading, MA.: Addison-Wesley

MAUNSELL, J. H. R. and VAN ESSEN, D. C. (1983) Functional properties of neurons in middle temporal visual area of the macaque monkey. II. Binocular interactions and sensitivity to binocular disparity. *J. Neurophysiol.*, **49**, 1148–1167

MURCH, G. M. (1973) *Visual and Auditory Perception*. Indianapolis, IN: Bobbs-Merrill

NELSON, J. I. (1975a) Globality and stereoscopic fusion in binocular vision. *J. Theor. Biol.*, **49**, 1–88

NELSON, J. I. (1975b) Reversible depth: the Hornbostel effect. *Optom. Weekly*, **66**, 411–413

NELSON, J. I. (1977) The plasticity of correspondence: aftereffects, illusions and horopter shifts in depth perception. *J. Theor. Biol.*, **66**, 203–266

NELSON, J. I. (1981) A neurophysiological model for anomalous correspondence based on mechanisms of sensory fusion. *Doc. Ophthalmol.*, **51**, 3–100

NELSON, J. I. (1985) The cellular basis of perception. In *Models of the Visual Cortex*, edited by D. Rose and V. Dobson, pp. 108–122. New York: Wiley

NELSON, J. I. (1986) Unsolved problems in the cellular basis of stereopsis. In *Visual Neuroscience*, edited by J. D. Pettigrew, W. R. Levick and K. J. Sanderson, pp. 405–420. Cambridge: Cambridge University Press

NELSON, J. I., KATO, H. and BISHOP, P. O. (1977) Discrimination of orientation and position disparities by binocularly activated neurons in cat striate cortex. *J. Neurophysiol.*, **40**, 260–283

OGLE, K. N. (1964) *Binocular Vision*. New York: Hafner

OGLE, K. N., MARTENS, T. and DYER, J. (1967) *Oculomotor Imbalance in Binocular Vision and Fixation Disparity*. Philadelphia: Lea & Febiger

PASINO, L. and MARAINI, G. (1966) Area of binocular vision in anomalous retinal correspondence. *Br. J. Ophthalmol.*, **50**, 646–650

PASINO, L., MARAINI, G. and SANTORI, M. (1963) Caratteristiche della visione binoculare anomala nell'ambiente. III. Acutezza visiva stereoscopica. *Ann. Ottal.*, **89**, 1005–1011

PATTERSON, R. and FOX, R. (1984) The effect of testing method on stereoanomaly. *Vision Res.*, **24** 403–408

PETTIGREW, J. D. (1973) Binocular neurones which signal change of disparity in area 18 of cat visual cortex. *Nat. New Biol.*, **241**, 123–124

PETTIGREW, J. D., NIKARA, T. and BISHOP, P. O. (1968) Binocular interaction on single units in cat striate cortex: simultaneous stimulation by single moving slit with receptive fields in correspondence. *Exp. Brain Res.*, **6**, 391–410

PIANTANIDA, T. P. (1986) Stereo hysteresis revisited. *Vision Res.*, **26**, 431–437

POGGIO, G. F. (1984) Processing of stereoscopic information in primate visual cortex. In *Dynamic Aspects of Neocortical Function*, edited by G. M. Edelman, W. E. Gall and W. M. Cowan, pp. 613–635. New York: Wiley

POGGIO, G. F. and POGGIO, T. (1984) The analysis of stereopsis. *Annu. Rev. Neurosci.*, **7**, 379–412

POGGIO, G. F. and TALBOT, W. H. (1981) Mechanisms of static and dynamic stereopsis in foveal cortex of the rhesus monkey. *J. Physiol.*, **315**, 469–492

RAMACHANDRAN, V. S. and NELSON, J. I. (1976) Global grouping overrides point-to-point disparities. *Perception*, **5**, 125–128

REVELL, M. J. (1971) Anomalous retinal correspondence — a refractive treatment. *Ophthal. Opt.*, **11**, 110–113

RICHARDS, W. (1970) Stereopsis and stereoblindness. *Exp. Brain Res.*, **10**, 380–388

RICHARDS, W. (1971) Anomalous stereoscopic depth perception. *J. Opt. Soc. Am.*, **61**, 410–414

RØNNE, G. and RINDZIUNSKI, E. (1953) The diagnosis and clinical classification of anomalous correspondence. *Acta Ophthalmol.*, **31**, 321–345

SCHLODTMANN, W. (1900) Studien über anomale Sehrichtungsgemeinschaft bei Schielenden. *Albrecht von Graefes Arch. Ophthalmol.*, **51**, 256–294

SCHOR, C. M. (1983) Fixation disparity and vergence adaptation. In *Vergence Eye Movements: Basic and Clinical Aspects*, edited by C. M. Schor and K. J. Ciuffreda, pp. 465–516. Boston: Butterworths

SHLAER, R. (1971) Shift in binocular disparity causes compensatory change in the cortical structure of kittens. *Science*, **173**, 638–641

SIRETEANU, R. (1982) Binocular vision in strabismic humans with alternating fixation. *Vision Res.*, **22**, 889–896

SIRETEANU, R., SINGER, W. and FRONIUS, M. (1983) Residuelle Binokularitaet im peripheren Gesichtsfeld von Amblyopen und Alternierer: eine psychophysische Untersuchung. *Fortschr. Ophthalmol.*, **80**, 271–274

SLOAN, M. E. (1985) Binocular rivalry: a psychophysics in search of a physiology. In *Models of the Visual Cortex*, edited by D. Rose and V. Dobson, pp. 211–222. New York: Wiley

ST CYR, G. J. and FENDER, D. H. (1969) The interplay of drifts and flicks in binocular fixation. *Vision Res.*, **9**, 245–265

STEWART, C. R. (1951) A photographic investigation of lateral fusional movements of the eyes. *Doctoral Dissertation*, Ohio State University. Ann Arbor, MI: University Microfilms, No. 25 474

STONG, C. L. (1975) Amateur scientist. *Sci. Am.*, **232**, 116–119

TOYAMA, K. and KOZASA, T. (1982) Responses of Clare–Bishop neurones to three dimensional movement of a light stimulus. *Vision Res.*, **22**, 571–574

TSCHERMAK, A. (1899) Uber anomale Sehrichtungsgemeinschaft der Natzhänte bei einem Schielenden. *Albrecht von Graefes Arch. Opthalmol.*, **47**, 508–550

TSCHERMAK-SEYSENEGG, A. VON (1952) *Introduction to Physiological Optics*, 2nd edn. Translated by P. Boeder. Springfield, IL: Thomas

TSCHERMAK-SEYSENEGG, A. VON and HOEFFER, P. (1903) Uber binokulare Tiefenwahrnehmung auf Grund von Doppelbildern. *Pflügers Arch. Ges. Physiol.*, **98**, 299–320

VON DER HEYDT, R., HÄNNY, P., DURSTELER, M.R. and POGGIO, G.F. (1982) Neuronal responses to stereoscopic tilt in the visual cortex of the behaving monkey. *Invest. Opthalmol. Vis. Sci.*, **22**, 12

WHEATSTONE, C. (1838) Contributions to the physiology of vision. I: On some remarkable, and hitherto unobserved, phenomena of binocular vision. *Philos. Trans.*, 371–394

WOLFE, J. M. and BLAKE, R. (1985) Monocular and binocular processes in human vision. In *Models of the Visual Cortex*, edited by D. Rose and V. Dobson, pp. 192–199. New York: Wiley

WICK, B. (1974) Visual therapy for constant exotropia with anomalous retinal correspondence — A case report. *Am. J. Optom. Physiol. Opt.*, **51**, 1005–1008

ZEKI, S. M. (1974) Cells responding to changing image size and disparity in the cortex of the rhesus monkey. *J. Physiol.*, **242**, 827–841

15

Techniques of investigation of binocular vision anomalies

Ronald Mallett

Almost every optometric routine examination will involve an examination of the binocular functions, the only exclusion being where the patient is effectively one-eyed. In many cases a few well chosen screening tests will suffice, but in others the conscientious practitioner will need to proceed to a more detailed investigation if properly to fulfil professional and moral responsibilities to the patient. The ensuing description of some of the techniques available to the modern optometric practitioner is necessarily brief and incomplete and the reader is urged to pursue the subject in greater depth with the aid of the references given.

Symptoms

It must be remembered that although concentrating on the symptoms created by the binocular dysfunction, there may be, in those cases where there is an underlying pathological condition, additional indications of a more general nature which are not always disclosed without questioning. Any such enquiry should be made of the patient, or of the parent if this is dictated by age or poor intelligence. One constant cause of confusion is the presence of uncorrected ametropia as this frequently gives rise to many of the symptoms experienced in binocular dysfunction. The age of the patient is relevant throughout the following discussion.

Visual

The only major disturbance of form vision to be considered in binocular dysfunction is amblyopia which is usually uniocular but is occasionally found to be present in both eyes. A diagnosis of amblyopia can only be considered if the vision remains blurred after the correction of any ametropia which is pres-

ent. If there is a marked variation in visual acuity at different viewing distances, there may be accommodative weakness or it may be of hysterical background — inconsistencies of a distance or temporal basis are common in the latter condition.

An occasional complaint is that there is a transient blurring of vision when transferring gaze from distance to near (or vice versa) or from one line to the next when reading. At a monocular level it is due to an inertia of the accommodation mechanism but a more common cause is binocular where there is a tight relationship between convergence and accommodation with very little interplay between the functions.

Occasionally, a complaint of poor vision binocularly which is improved monocularly, may be caused by uncompensated hyperphoria which is tending to give rise to a *slight* vertical diplopia, the latter being misinterpreted as blur.

Visual field abnormalities are not a source of direct complaint by strabismic or heterophoric patients. Nevertheless a field loss — usually bitemporal hemianopia due to a lesion affecting the chiasma — may so reduce the binocular field that fusion begins to break down with periods of transient diplopia.

Diplopia

Binocular diplopia and confusion are the two sensory components of a single phenomenon, the misalignment of the visual axes by an amount in excess of the dimensions of Panum's fusional areas so that the object of regard (and other objects on the horopter) are no longer forming their images on corresponding receptive fields. Diplopia is a very troublesome symptom and can be a great inconvenience and hazard to the patient. Most sufferers readily admit to it, although the young child may regard it as a natural, albeit abhorrent, aspect of vision — consequently it may be eliminated by closing one eye or adopting an anomalous head posture. When diplopia is present it must be determined, as far as is possible, when it was first noticed and whether it is constant or intermittent. If only intermittent, the viewing distance, direction of gaze, the temporal factors and any associated event (e.g. prolonged close work, illness) must be ascertained. The character of the diplopia, i.e. whether horizontal, vertical or oblique, is important, especially if it varies in different directions of gaze.

Binocular diplopia is an invariable accompaniment to strabismus, both concomitant and incomitant, but would not be expected in an uncomplicated gaze palsy. Heterophoria becoming decompensated and convergence insufficiency patients will experience diplopia, often of an ephemeral nature, if binocular fixation is lost.

Many systemic conditions, such as multiple sclerosis and diabetes, may give rise to transient spells of diplopia and, in myasthenia gravis, diplopia may worsen as the day progresses, as the ability of the corrective fusional reflexes diminish with fatigue.

When a patient with well established harmonious anomalous retinal correspondence (ARC) suffers a change in the objective angle of strabismus, usually through trauma, there may not be any co-variation in the subjective angle. This results in the ARC becoming unharmonious with inevitable diplopia. Most of these patients are adult and the diplopia particularly intractable.

A few patients may complain of normal physiological diplopia, having once been made aware of this phenomenon.

Monocular diplopia

A case of monocular diplopia is occasionally found and, although it may be due to irregularities in the optical components of the eye or to a dissociative cerebral lesion, the only relevant binocular cause is that of abnormal exteroception from a deeply amblyopic eye. In this case, the single retinal image is giving rise to a dual visual localization, one from the fovea (normal and innate) the other from the eccentrically fixating area (abnormal and acquired). This type of monocular diplopia is only seen in cases of developing amblyopia where the visual acuity is very low (generally below 3/60) or during pleoptic treatment of the condition.

Onset

The onset of strabismus is certainly an objective symptom and its character should be evaluated as far as possible, i.e. whether the deviation is convergent, divergent or vertical, whether it is intermittent or constant, if it is present in all directions of gaze or just one in particular, whether the angle is constant or variable (as in uncorrected accommodative squints), if the squint is always confined to the same eye or is alternating, and whether the squint is associated with a particular activity or with fatigue or illness.

Headaches and other asthenopic symptoms

Although it has been stated with some force (Carlow, 1976) that 'ophthalmic causes of headache are unusual and uncommon', it must be evident to all those engaged in optometric and ophthalmological clinical practice that discomfort of this nature is a very frequent complaint. Many headaches have their genesis in extraocular conditions — tension, sinus abnormalities, intracranial pathology etc. — but it cannot be reasonably denied by any experienced practitioner that uncorrected ametropia, uncompensated heterophoria and convergence insufficiency cause a great deal of discomfort.

As far as binocular dysfunction is concerned, frontal and supraorbital headaches tend to be of a dull aching variety, and associated mostly with the lateral heterophorias and convergence insufficiency. Esophoric patients may not experience any discomfort during periods of prolonged critical vision, the headache tending to occur later on; exophoria and convergence insufficiency, however, tend to promote headaches after a relatively short period of visual activity, often cutting short the period the patient is prepared to concentrate. Temporal headaches are not particularly common in heterophoria but esophoria and exophoria are the main culprits.

Occipitoparietal headaches may be promoted by hyperphoria, cyclophoria and esophoria. Uncompensated vertical and torsional imbalances usually give rise to headaches without the trigger of concentrated visual activity and many patients with these conditions endure constant discomfort.

General eye ache and fatigue with a desire to close or rub the eyes 'for a rest', may be attributed to any of the heterophorias.

It is doubtful if binocular dysfunction is the cause of migraine headaches, but uncompensated imbalances may aggravate the condition and increase the frequency or severity of the attacks.

Photophobia and visual localization

Many symptoms attributed to heterophoria — conjunctivitis, neurasthenia, stammering and many others — are probably figments of imagination and were introduced into the early orthoptic literature at a time when enthusiasm was unbounded and the subject not well understood. Some symptoms are, however, worthy of consideration: there is a tendency for some heterophoric patients to be rather light sensitive, especially esophores and hyperphores; it is seldom that this reaches a degree of severity warranting the label photophobia, but it can be unpleasant.

Vertigo or dizziness may occasionally be found associated with cyclophoria or hyperphoria, often with an incomitant background. Indeed a feeling of uncertainty and dizziness may be experienced by any patient with incomitancy, especially if newly acquired. There is, in these cases, a disturbance between visual localization and ocular motor innervation in the field of action of the affected muscle(s). This results in past pointing in paretic conditions and under pointing in spastic cases. Difficulty may result with depth perception, associated with a poor performance in ball games. A feeling of stress or strain when looking in one particular direction, could be associated with incomitant heterophoria or an early pursuit gaze palsy; the latter is sometimes known as version heterophoria — conjugate movement is full but not accomplished without some mild discomfort.

It is possible that spatial localization problems might be confused with a loss of binocular stereopsis which occurs in cases of strabismus; diplopia is eliminated by suppressing the deviating eye rather than developing harmonious anomalous retinal correspondence (harmonious ARC). This aspect of the squinter's symptom is usually only revealed when specific questions about ability at ball games are asked. Loss of central stereopsis has been observed following trauma or disease of the corpus callosum.

Visual fatigue

The heterophoric patient may experience a general loss of efficiency at work as the day progresses due to increasing fatigue of the ocular motor system. While not a presenting complaint, work may be slower and less precise than when fresh and alert in the morning.

When discussing symptoms with the patient, reference should always be made to the working and reading environment and in particular to the ambient illumination. Discomfort caused by heterophoria and related conditions may be aggravated by bad posture, poor health, worry and anxiety.

Aniseikonia is an undoubted problem where the disparity between the retinal image size in the two eyes is considerable, but as a primary symptom producing anomaly its importance may have been overstressed in the past (e.g. *see* Charnwood, 1950). Patients with significant aniseikonia may complain of occipital headaches and have symptoms reflecting the spatial distortion that they experience.

Movement of the visual environment (oscillopsia)

may occur in acquired nystagmus and pathology of the medial longitudinal fasciculus (internuclear palsy) or cerebellum (ocular flutter). An occasional complaint is that of agoraphobia, often said to be associated with divergence excess.

History

The age of onset of signs or symptoms is most important. In the case of a strabismus in the young child, the time when the squint was first noticed is likely to be more accurate, but a review of photographs taken at various ages may help to identify the required age.

Aetiology

Most squints develop slowly, breakdown from a heterophoric state first occurring when the child is tired or unwell. Some caution should be shown if the squint appeared suddenly as related pathology is of greater likelihood. It should be noted that most convergent accommodative squints occur between 2.5 and 4 years of age, a time when active interest is being shown in the environment. Divergent deviations occur rather later, as a rule, usually between the age of 4 and 7 years.

The incidence of strabismus is greater with a long labour, following forceps delivery (possibly due to involvement of the sixth nerve) and if the baby experiences respiratory difficulties. Early squinters often have difficult births in which the head is moulded or scarred (Scobee, 1952). Although it is not likely to provide fruitful information, it is always worth enquiring about any relevant prenatal conditions – illnesses, trauma, medication etc. It is worth noting that the incidence of squint is higher in premature than in full-term infants.

It is useful to gain some information about the close relatives of the patients, in particular any ocular motor anomaly known to be present and any major illnesses experienced.

A brief account of the patient's medical history may provide a clue which will assist accurate diagnosis. Some illnesses may have some role in the causation of some binocular problems — they may merely act as a precipitating factor or act by affecting the ocular motor system directly. Examples are the common occurrence of measles just prior to the onset of convergent strabismus and sinusitis or dental infection preceding convergence insufficiency, and some forms of the influenza virus causing high degrees of exophoria or exotropia.

Many drugs affect the ocular motor system and might be partially responsible for the patient's problem. Tranquillizers and barbiturates tend to depress accommodation and convergence, phenytoin (in high doses) can initiate nystagmus, while others attack the retina or optic nerve and cause toxic amblyopia. The adult patient should be asked (tactfully) about use of tobacco and alcohol — a combination of the two, in particular, is potentially dangerous in producing toxic amblyopia, while alcohol alone, and in excess, induces esophoria at distance, exophoria (or convergence insufficiency) at near with a depletion of the fusional reserves (Charnwood, 1950; Hogan and Linfield, 1983).

In addition to physical illness, note should be made of any psychological trauma suffered by the patient — such upsets have been known to trigger marked deviations in the young, perhaps as a form of attention seeking.

Previous treatment

Care should be taken to ascertain what, if any, refractive corrections have been worn with a note of the centration distance as well as the powers of the lenses, and an attempt made to determine what effect they have had on the binocular status. As with other types of treatment, it should be established whether the patient complied with the advice given in wearing the spectacles.

Details of the exact nature of any orthoptic treatment prescribed should be noted together with an assessment of the enthusiasm (if any) shown for such treatment by the parent as well as the young patient.

Surgery may have been undertaken and a note should be made regarding the age of the patient at the time, the eye being treated and whether it effected a small or a substantial improvement.

Occlusion may have been prescribed for amblyopia (and occasionally for certain other conditions) and it is necessary to determine which eye was occluded, for how long the occlusion was carried out (total or partial), for how long each day and whether every day. The age when occlusion first commenced and the effect on visual acuity are also relevant.

Drugs are not commonly used in the UK for treating ocular motor disorders, but would appear to be more fully used in Europe and the USA. Atropine has been used over a fairly long term to inhibit accommodation and therefore convergence following suggestions by Guibor (1958), but it seems to be little used today as a therapeutic measure. Incorrectly used without the necessary near addition (usually in bifocal form) to provide clear near vision, it would embarrass visual or educational development.

Miotics are more commonly used at the present time, the resulting small pupils usually being noticed by the parent. Occasionally, but especially in Europe, atropine is used in one eye and a miotic (diisopropyl fluorophosphonate or Phospholine Iodide — ecothiopate) in the other and is referred to as penalization.

General observations of the patient

The patient's general posture, behaviour, intelligence, speech and hearing can be assessed during the recording of the symptoms and history, these all being relevant factors to both diagnosis and possible treatment.

The cosmetic appearance of the patient should be evaluated, and this is especially significant if a strabismus is known or thought to be present. This empirical assessment is important since it is often impossible to accurately measure the habitual angle of strabismus, i.e. the deviation normally present in conditions free from dissociating influences, as any attempt to quantify the squint with prisms may trigger fusional movements resulting in an inflated finding which is often referred to as the *total angle*.

Factors affecting cosmetic appearance

Factors which affect the cosmetic appearance of strabismus, or indeed give the impression that a deviation is present when the eyes are, in fact, quite straight, are as follows:

(1) Habitual angle of strabismus.
(2) The presence of a marked angle lambda (λ). This is the angle between the line of sight and the pupillary axis, and is normally between 3° and 5° and positive, with the corneal reflex appearing slightly to the nasal side of the centre of the pupil when the eye fixates a light monocularly. If angle λ is in excess of the normal amount (and still positive) the eyes will look relatively divergent, so masking a convergent squint or worsening a divergent one. If the angle is negative (corneal reflex temporal to pupil centre), an appearance of convergence is created which will exaggerate a convergent deviation, but tends to mask a divergent one. The angles α, γ, κ are often erroneously substituted for angle λ — the last named being the one measured clinically.
(3) Marked epicanthal folds. These are generally nasal and will accentuate the appearance of convergent strabismus while masking a divergent deviation. Temporal epicanthal folds simulate divergent strabismus and will thus improve the appearance of a convergent deviation. Although epicanthal folds are common in the young infant, they usually become less marked with time. Their effect on apparent eye position can be demonstrated to a child's parent by moving the skin with a finger, in the appropriate direction.
(4) Orbital separation in relation to facial width. If this is marked, giving rise to a wide interpupillary distance, it will create an appearance of divergence which will modify the cosmesis of

any strabismus actually present. In fact, the wide separation does make convergence more difficult and many patients with this type of skull configuration are exotropic. A narrow orbital separation will have the opposite cosmetic effect making the eyes look more convergent; there appears to be no relationship between a narrow separation and convergent imbalances, however.

(5) Relative proptosis of the eyes. Eyes which are moderately exophthalmic not only look somewhat divergent but tend to be truly divergent more often than normally situated eyes. This is due to an increase in the secondary abducting action of the oblique muscles (Lyle and Bridgeman, 1959). The effect of enophthalmos is to reduce the abducting action of the oblique muscles to favour convergence, while the recessed position of the eye increases the appearance of any esotropia present.

(6) Facial asymmetry. Although sometimes quite marked, the effect on the ocular motor system is often surprisingly limited. A patient may, in fact, be orthophoric or heterophoric in spite of a marked difference in level of the two orbits (and hence eyes).

Abnormal head posture

The patient may adopt an unusual head posture in order to eliminate or reduce diplopia or to render binocular vision more comfortable.

Horizontal incomitance

In esophoria the chin may be depressed; the eyes will be elevated and divergence made easier. Many esophores are said to find reading more comfortable when lying on the floor, abdomen down, with chin cupped in the hands (Scobee, 1952). Exophoric and convergence insufficiency patients, on the other hand, may keep the chin well up so that convergence is easier, a high percentage of exophoric patients showing increase in their imbalance on looking up.

Some patients with a conjugate gaze palsy will adopt an abnormal posture to make vision more comfortable — many of these patients are elderly, however, and they frequently prefer to maintain their normal posture, this being the lesser of two evils. Those who do make an attempt to adapt will turn the head to the same side as the palsy and away from the affected hemisphere — in many cases, however, the causal lesion will have involved that part of the cerebrum responsible for head movements; this will cause a head turn towards the affected side and frustrate the volitional movement.

Postural adaptation to incomitant anomalies is frequently found when the deviation is congenital or occurs during childhood. Patients who develop their palsy or spasm in adult life often find it difficult to make the necessary head adjustment. When the medial or lateral rectus muscle is involved the patient will turn his head towards the field of action of the affected muscle, i.e. where diplopia is maximal. Those with a lateral rectus palsy may also depress the chin to lessen convergence. Similarly symptoms from a medial rectus palsy may be alleviated by elevation of the chin.

Vertical incomitance

When a vertically acting muscle is involved the resulting head posture can be resolved into three components:

(1) Chin elevation or depression: when an elevator muscle is affected (i.e. superior rectus or inferior oblique) the chin is elevated; with a palsied depressor muscle (inferior rectus or superior oblique), the chin is depressed. This will reduce the vertical diplopia.

(2) Face turn: if the face is turned towards the side where the affected muscle has its greatest vertical action and where the diplopia will be greatest, the diplopia is still further reduced, e.g. to the right for right superior rectus, right inferior rectus, left superior oblique and left inferior oblique palsies. Combining these two components, the effects of a right inferior rectus paresis would be minimized by looking down and to the right. When a significant amount of exotropia is present, the lateral component of the head turn in a vertical rectus palsy may be to the opposite side from that described above (Duke-Elder, 1973).

(3) Head tilt: this component of the compensating head posture is to relieve the torsional diplopia which is much more marked with an oblique than with a vertical rectus muscle palsy. Hence the tilt with an oblique palsy is much greater than when the superior or inferior rectus is involved. According to Adler (1965) the head tilt is always toward the side opposite the affected muscle, i.e. in the normal torsional direction of the affected muscle. Duke-Elder (1973) paints a much more complex picture and the reader is referred to his work for an explanation.

Torticollis

The anomalous head postures described above are sometimes called ocular torticollis. They must be differentiated from orthopaedic torticollis which is caused by contracture of the sternocleidomastoid muscle. The taut muscle is easily felt and the head is incapable of passive or voluntary straightening. The head tilt is very pronounced with the chin elevated and away from the side of the head tilt. It is quite easy to distinguish these very different conditions, but it must be remembered that the orthopaedic torticollis patient is not immune from incomitancy, so ocular motility must be examined with care.

Among the less common varieties of abnormal head posture must be mentioned that adopted by some patients with congenital idiopathic nystagmus who may use such a posture to find a null position where the movement is minimal and, perhaps, better visual acuity can be obtained.

Screening for active pathology

It is obviously necessary that all patients with a binocular dysfunction should be examined most carefully in order that any active pathology can be discovered. It must be said that, of the selection of patients *seen in optometric practice*, very few children display any signs of pathology, but it is of paramount importance that those who do should be detected as quickly as possible and referred for appropriate investigation and treatment. With older patients a very different picture emerges, and a greater incidence of suspicious or obvious pathology is found. Vascular diseases, primary and secondary neoplasms, diabetes and demyelinating diseases can all affect binocular status.

A careful consideration of the symptoms and history followed by careful ophthalmoscopy, a study of the pupillary reflexes and a visual field plot should be undertaken. Children react well to field procedures involving flash stimuli, such as the Friedman–Bedwell visual field analyser, this equipment also permitting the investigation of the macular threshold for white and red. Peripheral fields should be checked with a confrontation test and perimetry performed if indicated. Further guidance may be obtained from a Hess (or similar) screen plot as well as from conventional motility tests.

Refraction

Children should be refracted under cycloplegia to obtain a proper refractive balance and to reveal as much latent error as possible. The choice of cyclopegic is important. At one time, 1% atropine was routinely used, but experience has demonstrated two difficulties. It is seldom properly instilled by the parent so that incomplete cycloplegia results, and it may cause a complete breakdown in binocularity if used in infants with heterophoria or intermittent squint. The uncorrected hypermetropic esophore will be left with blurred retinal imagery for 2–3 weeks. This blur will make fusion difficult and the convergence effort made by the patient to induce some accommodation, so that reasonable vision is possible at near during the recovery period, will

often magnify the esophoria with consequent breakdown into esotropia. It is preferable to use a short-acting cycloplegic, such as cyclopentolate, instilled by the practitioner which will give deep short-lived cycloplegia with minimum risk of binocular breakdown and near vision blurred for just one day. The use of atropine is only permissible with constant squint.

The refractive procedure should always include a measurement of the amplitude of accommodation. In amblyopia it is common to find the amplitude of accommodation to be higher in the normally fixating eye, the amplitude recovering somewhat in the amblyopic eye when the visual acuity improves with treatment (Ciuffreda *et al.*, 1983). If the patient is very young, making subjective determination impossible or unreliable, a reasonable result may be obtained objectively by using an interesting object held just in front of a retinoscope (to allow for the usual lag of approximately 0.50 D).

Investigation of binocular vision anomalies

Certain tests should be undertaken in every case:

(1) Visual acuity measurements.
(2) Cover tests.
(3) Motility tests.

With the information obtained from these, the direction in which to proceed should be obvious. If the patient is heterophoric, compensation and foveal suppression tests will be necessary; if incomitant, further examination of the motility may be required using, for example, a Hess screen. Strabismic patients who are amblyopic must have this anomaly investigated, while the binocular sensory status must be looked at in all cases. It will be clear that there cannot be a standard routine procedure to be followed in every case. A certain degree of flexibility must be used to select the tests which will provide the necessary information. It is important that, whenever possible, the tests should proceed so that the more dissociating tests are left until the end of the examination in order to prevent embarrassment to whatever binocularity that exists. Binocular sensory status should therefore be assessed before such tests as visuscopy which require the removal of a refractive correction that is totally or partially keeping the eyes straight. All tests should be undertaken with the ametropia corrected, whenever this is possible and unless there is a specific need to examine the function with the system in a naked state. It follows that it may prove undesirable to use a number of tests in the same sequence as described in this text.

Measurement of visual acuity

The targets used for visual acuity measurements may be letters, illiterate Es, Landolt Cs or Ffooks symbols. Contour interaction is better with the E and Landolt C which also have a much greater uniformity of value at any given acuity level. Furthermore, it is sometimes necessary to record the acuities by more than one method and it is essential to use the same type of symbol so that accurate comparisons can be made. Ffooks symbols are usually more easily understood by young children and should be employed when necessary. To demonstrate the separation difficulty (or crowding phenomenon) in an eye with strabismic amblyopia, the optimum target separation is equal to the overall size of the targets at any particular acuity level (Flom, Weymouth and Kahneman, 1963). A series of 21 slides embodying Flom's ideas is available, using nine Landolt Cs (at each acuity value) for measurement purposes and surrounded by 17 Es to provide contour interaction. These charts provide a very precise measure of visual acuity but are very time consuming in use. The present author has designed a more conventional E chart with the target separation suggested by Flom and with additional acuity values (6/72, 6/48, 6/7.5) to those available on the standard charts.

It is advisable to make an initial *rapid* check on the visual acuity, employing the minimum occlusion necessary to obtain an approximate result, as a means of determining the best target to use for a cover test — in this way, too much dissociation is avoided and the cover test findings will be more reliable.

Morphoscopic acuity

The morphoscopic (linear or line) visual acuity test is of paramount importance in the diagnosis of amblyopia. Indeed, by definition, the concept of amblyopia is dependent on the inability of an optically corrected and apparently healthy eye to achieve normal visual acuity (6/4–6/6). It is useful to record the near visual acuity, again using the same targets as used for distance, the near value being most conveniently expressed in decimal fashion (6/6 $\equiv$ 1.0, 6/24 $\equiv$ 0.25 etc.). The visual acuity in amblyopia is often better at near than at distance. Patients with hysterical amblyopia often exhibit marked inconsistencies in visual acuity at different testing distances. If the morphoscopic acuity is normal in both eyes, there is no need to undertake the angular and mesopic measurements now described. They should be mandatory, however, whenever amblyopia is present. It should be noted that von Noorden and Leffler (1966) found that the morphoscopic acuity of the strabismic amblyope is adversely affected when the normal fixating eye is receiving visual stimulation.

Angular acuity

Angular (or isolated symbol) acuity is measured by presenting single targets to the patient, the recorded acuity being one in which 4/5 (80%) correct answers are achieved. The angular acuity is usually very much better than the morphoscopic in strabismic amblyopia, a difference of four lines being not uncommon. This difference emphasizes the danger of taking *only* angular acuities, as is often recommended with young children. While being an easier measurement than line acuity such a procedure may overlook a strabismic amblyopia by producing a normal finding so that only the morphoscopic measurement should be used as a basis for determining the presence or absence of amblyopia. This does not apply to non-strabismic types of amblyopia because the morphoscopic and angular acuities are virtually identical under normal clinical testing conditions. Angular acuity measurement therefore assists differential diagnosis of the type of amblyopia.

Mesopic acuity

The same applies to morphoscopic acuity measurement under mesopic conditions. This is most conveniently achieved by placing a neutral density filter (2.0 log units) in front of the amblyopic eye, the sound eye being occluded and, after a short period of adaptation (2–3 minutes), recording the acuity through the filter. If there is little or no drop in visual acuity or, as frequently occurs, an improvement, it is an indication that the amblyopia is due to strabismus. A slight drop in acuity usually indicates ametropic or 'idiopathic' amblyopia, while a dramatic drop is the norm when the amblyopia is organic. This test was introduced by von Noorden and Burian (1959) but they employed a much denser filter (neutral density 3.0 log units). This high density proved to be somewhat impractical and the weaker filter suggested here is clinically very satisfactory. It is interesting that the different behaviour of the visual function of organic and strabismic amblyopes was noted as long ago as 1884 by Bjerrum (cited by von Noorden and Burian, 1959).

An alternative to the neutral density filter is a red one (Wratten 92) and while the results are very similar, it functions rather differently by forcing more central fixation which is helpful if the amblyopia is strabismic, but aggravates toxic amblyopia with a central scotoma for red.

The assessment of contrast sensitivity is of increasing interest in the consideration of amblyopia and both the Arden gratings (Arden, 1978) and VCTS (Ginsburg, 1984) are suitable as clinical tests.

Further tests in amblyopia

When morphoscopic visual acuity measurements reveal the presence of amblyopia, the addition of angular and mesopic recordings will aid differential diagnosis. However, these additional acuity findings may not allow a definitive differential diagnosis and one or more supportive tests must be employed. These include an investigation into monocular fixation of the amblyopic eye, visual fields in suspected toxic amblyopia, and Amsler chart studies in microtropia.

Fixation

Fixation seems to be invariably eccentric in patients whose amblyopia is entirely strabismic. Where the morphoscopic visual acuity is 6/60 or better, there is a fairly linear relationship between the acuity and the degree of eccentricity with 15′ arc of eccentric fixation for every line of morphoscopic acuity below the norm of 6/5 or 6/6. Acuities below 6/60 generally show more marked and variable degrees of eccentricity. Many amblyopias are compound — especially mixed strabismic and anisometropic components — and these show less eccentric fixation than the purely strabismic variety. All non-strabismic amblyopias (idiopathic, hysterical, ametropic, early toxic) show central, although unsteady, fixation with the exception of advanced cases of toxic amblyopia with an absolute central scotoma. Occlusion amblyopia, induced by persistent occlusion of one eye or the continued presence of untreated congenital ptosis or cataract etc. during the sensitive period, usually exhibits fixation and acuity patterns similar to those occurring in strabismic amblyopia. Generally, fixation is nasal in convergent strabismus, temporal in divergent deviations (much less common as these deviations usually develop after the visual system reaches a reasonable degree of maturity) and vertical in hypertropia. Where the fixation is in the opposite direction to that expected it is known as paradoxical eccentric fixation and can occur spontaneously or as a result of a reversal of the motor angle by over-enthusiastic treatment.

Objective assessment of fixation

Fixation is best assessed with a modified direct ophthalmoscope containing a suitable graticule in the optical system. Although many ophthalmoscopes in general use do have a graticule for this purpose, they are not generally very satisfactory as the fixation target is often coarse, there is usually no means of focusing the image of the graticule on the retina, an absence of measuring circles making a quantitative investigation difficult and generally having a green background. It has been shown by Mallett (unpublished data) and later by Mendolsohn (1983) that eccentric fixation increases when fixation is performed at the short wave (green) end of the spectrum and diminishes at the red end, the latter observation being previously made by Brinker and

Katz (1963). The Visuscope (Oculus) is one instrument which fulfils the necessary requirements and presents a useful graticule with a central fixation star surrounded by concentric circles which can be focused on the retina. With the eye not being examined occluded, the patient is asked to look directly at the star; if its image is superimposed on the fovea, fixation is central; if it is to one side of the fovea it is eccentric. The direction is given by the direction of the image of the star (i.e. if the star is to the nasal side of the fovea, then nasal eccentric fixation is present) and the degree can be determined by noting the circle in which the foveal reflex (if present) is seen. The 'steadiness' of fixation should be noted. As previously intimated, the green filter should *not* be inserted into the projection system.

Some fundus cameras permit a permanent photographic record of fixation to be obtained.

Most infants will fix a Visuscope star (the isolated star without the concentric measuring circles should be used) and, in the absence of any reliable method for measuring visual acuity, central fixation could be taken as a reliable indication that no strabismic amblyopia is present, although it does not exclude the possible presence of another variant of the condition.

Subjective assessment of fixation

Three subjective techniques are in fairly common usage: the Haidinger brush and Maxwell spot tests (both entopic phenomena) and the 'transferred' after-image test.

Haidinger brushes are produced only at the macular region, and are most easily seen by rotating a polarizing disc (Polaroid) in conjunction with a blue filter in front of the eye being examined, the patient viewing the centre of an internally illuminated tangent scale. The dark yellow or blue propeller-like brushes rotate, and will appear to be superimposed on the object of regard if fixation is central, but to one side if eccentric. As the background is blue, the degree of eccentric fixation found by this technique tends to be greater than that measured by the unfiltered light of the Visuscope. For an explanation of Haidinger's brushes see Halldén (1957) and Stanworth and Naylor (1950).

The Maxwell spot test is performed by alternating a purple dichroic filter (transmitting blue and red light) with a neutral density filter of equal density (Flom, 1961, advises Roscoe purple No. 28 and ND 1.5 log units) in front of the amblyopic eye, the other eye being covered. The patient will see a reddish spot subtending some 3° with a 0.5° central disc superimposed over the fixation point if eccentric fixation is absent. A tangent scale is used as with the Haidinger brush test. Spencer (1967) has investigated the Maxwell spot phenomenon in great detail.

Both Maxwell spot and Haidinger brush tests require a visually perceptive patient and are not suitable for young children.

Brock and Givnor (1952) have described a useful technique which utilizes the foveal localization of the sound eye as a reference for localization from the amblyopic eye. A vertical after-image is formed in line with the fovea of the non-amblyopic eye by exposing it to a vertical strip of light or a vertical flash stimulus (Mallett, 1975b) — the slit aperture in the plate should be narrow in order to create a fine negative after-image (Murphy, 1968) which will still be seen when the sound eye is covered and the patient asked to look at the centre of a tangent scale. The localized after-image will be 'referred' to the fovea of the amblyopic eye and will appear in line with the centre of the scale if fixation is central but to one side if eccentric. The test works well and the only contraindication is the presence of well established ARC — in these cases the after-image will not be separated from the fixation point by the degree of the eccentricity but by an amount corresponding to the angle of anomaly plus or minus the eccentric angle.

Techniques which rely upon finger pointing or corneal reflex position are too crude to warrant discussion here.

Eccentric fixation and localization in amblyopia

In the normal eye the principal visual direction is intimately related to the fovea, an innate association which is only disrupted in exceptional circumstances. The integrity of foveal localization is, indeed, retained in most cases of strabismic amblyopia in spite of the existence of eccentric fixation, a phenomenon previously known as eccentric viewing but now generally termed 'eccentric fixation with normal foveal localization'. A patient with amblyopia of this order would fix a Visuscope star eccentrically but still localize subjectively from the fovea. The patient thus feels that he is looking to one side of the fixation star. Rarely the amblyopia is so profound that the eccentric area usurps the origin of the principal visual direction and the patient will not only fix eccentrically but also refer his sense of direction to that area and not the fovea. This was once simply termed 'eccentric fixation' but is now qualified as being with anomalous foveal localization. In such a case, the Visuscope star would be imaged eccentrically and appear to be 'straight ahead'. Haidinger brush and Maxwell spot tests can also be used to determine the localization of an amblyopic eye but, as with the Visuscope, a very perceptive patient is required, and it is frequently impossible to obtain a definitive answer. Visual acuity may be used as the arbiter of localization, better than 6/60 generally indicating normal foveal

localization, and worse than 6/60 abnormal localization. The problem has been discussed in detail by von Noorden (1970a). The significance of normal and abnormal foveal localization is apparent during treatment of amblyopia by occlusion when those with normal localization may be expected to achieve better visual acuity and more central fixation, while the few with abnormal localization might even experience a reduction in visual acuity as the eccentric pattern is reinforced.

Visual fields in amblyopia

A visual field plot is most important in patients with suspected toxic or hysterical amblyopia. Toxic amblyopes would be expected to show central scotomata for colour, especially red, and a raised macular threshold for white and red on a Friedman field analyser. Hysterical amblyopes often show a star-shaped isopter or a spiral field when examined on a Bjerrum screen or perimeter.

Amsler's chart test

This technique was described by Lang (1970) and utilizes a standard Amsler chart viewed by the amblyopic eye. It is important that this test be used in microtropic patients only, as the findings described do not relate to larger angles of squint. Lang describes three possible appearances in primary microtropia:

(1) A large central blur in anisometropic amblyopia. This is not invariably present in the opinion of the present author (*Figure 15.1*).

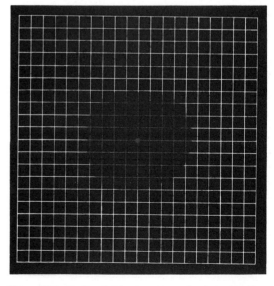

Figure 15.1 Amsler chart appearance of anisometropic amblyopia in microtropia

(2) A small, rather dense, central scotoma in organic amblyopia. Duke-Elder (1973) refers to this as congenital amblyopia — it is also sometimes called idiopathic at the present time (*Figure 15.2*).

(3) A paracentral scotoma, just missing the central fixation point, to the temporal side of the chart whenever nasal eccentric fixation is present. This curious scotoma (*Figure 15.3*) appears to originate from a defect in the nasal retina (or the

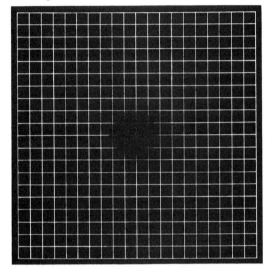

Figure 15.2 Amsler chart appearance of organic amblyopia in microtropia

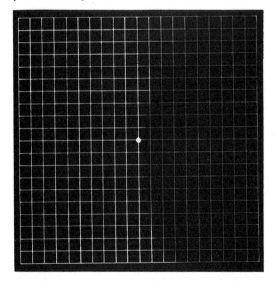

Figure 15.3 Amsler chart appearance of strabismic amblyopia in microtropia. The scotoma shown would be present in a patient with right esotropia with nasal eccentric fixation

cortex or pathways serving it) and extends just as far as the retinal area used for fixing eccentrically. When fixation is temporal in convergent strabismus (this event is rare), the scotoma appears in the nasal field. Mallett and Rundle (unpublished data) have shown that the light threshold in the scotomatous area is normal.

Lang (1971) also describes a binocular version of this test using a reduced Amsler chart in a synoptophore before the amblyopic eye and a skeleton outline (i.e. with no grid pattern) before the sound eye — the tubes are moved to obtain fusion. The chief difference in the clinical appearances is with strabismic amblyopia where the paracentral scotoma now embraces the fixation point.

Table 15.1 summarizes the important differences between the amblyopias.

Measurement of the deviation — the cover test

The cover test is the most important orthoptic procedure available to the practitioner. It should be performed routinely at 6 metres and the near working/reading/playing distance with the ametropia corrected and, in most cases, uncorrected. It is often useful to repeat the near cover test with the eyes elevated or depressed to reveal the V, A, X and Y patterns — an excellent review of these is given by Burian and von Noorden (1974) — and in other parts of the motor field to disclose or evaluate incomitancies. An increasing esophoria or esotropia on dextroversion would, for example, indicate the presence of a right lateral rectus paresis. The face should be well illuminated and the method of uniocular covering employed initially to determine the presence or otherwise of a strabismus. The fixation target should be an isolated symbol of a dimension that can be resolved by the eye with the lower visual acuity; this ideal has to be relaxed when examining young children by using a more interesting object. It is best first to cover the known or suspected dominant eye so that the strabismus is immediately revealed in its habitual form. Its angle is then estimated as precisely as possible before being neutralized with prisms (prism bar) before the deviating eye. An alternate cover test follows to break down the strabismus to the total (maximal) angle or to reveal the full extent of any heterophoria present, prisms again being used to neutralize the deviation.

When examining strabismic patients, the neutralization with prisms of the habitual angle should be undertaken with great care and with maximum speed to avoid prism adaptation; very often the estimate of the angle is more precise than the measured angle owing to compensation effects. Some patients do not transfer fixation to the squinting eye very readily and this is often due to the angle

Table 15.1

Type of amblyopia	Morphoscopic visual acuity	Angular visual acuity	Mesopic visual acuity*	Fixation	Visual fields	Amsler charts	Other
Strabismic, including visual deprivation or occlusion amblyopia	Reduced Usually unilateral	> MVA	⩾ MVA	Eccentric and unsteady	Normal	Lang's one-sided scotoma in microtropia	—
Organic, idiopathic or congenital	Reduced Usually between 6/9 and 6/18 Sometimes bilateral	= MVA	Slightly < MVA	Central Often unsteady	Sometimes small central scotoma	Sometimes a small central scotoma	Fovea looks dull Poor or absent foveal reflex
Ametropic	Reduced Bilateral if ametropia is high in both eyes, especially if hyper-metropic	= MVA	Slightly < MVA	Central Often unsteady	Normal	Faint but large central blur in microtropia	High degree of ametropia present
Hysterical	Reduced and variable Inconsistent at different distances	?	?	Central	Star or spiral field	Normal	Possibly signs of mental instability or personality abnormalities
Toxic	Reduced Bilateral	Usually M = AVA	< MVA	Early-central Late-eccentric	Central scotoma especially for red	Central scotoma especially on red chart	Possibly systemic signs and symptoms Raised macula threshold
Nutritional	Reduced Bilateral	Usually M = AVA	< MVA	Early-central Late-eccentric	Central scotoma especially for red	Central scotoma especially on red chart	General signs of malnutrition Raised macula threshold

* ND = 2.0.
MVA = morphoscopic visual acuity.
AVA = angular visual acuity.
MpVA = mesopic visual acuity.

being of the order of 15° of convergence (Swan syndrome) when the target is therefore imaged on the blind optic nerve head, making the initial attempts to fix dependent on searching movements.

In heterophoria, the quality of the recovery movement is always worth noting. If it is fast and smooth it suggests compensation while a jerky sluggish recovery may be indicative of uncompensated heterophoria.

In all cases, a different angle dependent upon the eye used for fixation may result from incomitancy (the sound eye fixating giving the primary angle and the affected eye the secondary angle) or from a lack of correct refractive balance — if one eye has to accommodate more than the other when fixating, it will generally be responsible for a more convergent or less divergent result.

Subjective cover test

The subjective cover test was introduced by Duane as a sensitive test for detecting and quantifying heterophoria. A cover is passed from one eye to the other, always in the same direction to avoid confusion, and the patient asked to report on the apparent movement or 'jump' of the test target. In exophoria, the target 'jumps' in the same direction as the cover, and the prism which stops this movement is an accurate measure of the heterophoria. The reverse applies to esophoria. The subjective cover test also allows the qualitative evaluation of retinal correspondence in strabismus (Mallett, 1965) and it has sometimes, rather inappropriately, been known as the 'phi' test or phenomenon, when used in this way. Patients with harmonious ARC should merely see a stationary test object when the cover is transferred from one eye to the other. When the strabismus is associated with suppression and latent normal correspondence, a jump will be observed (against the cover in esotropia) which is negated by the same prism which stops the movement objectively. The test is quite sensitive and, with it, around 50% of strabismic patients seen in optometric practice will show harmonious ARC.

The microtropias

Although the objective cover test is the only technique available for differentiating strabismic from heterophoric patients, there is one particular variety of microtropia which might seem to give ambiguous findings: this is the type described by Helveston and von Noorden (1967) in which the objective angle of strabismus is equal to the degree of eccentric fixation in the amblyopic eye — this means that the fixation object is imaged on the eccentrically fixating area even during binocular vision, so there will be no shift when vision is then confined to the squinting

eye. It is important to examine the fixation and the visual acuity by different measurement techniques (as previously described) in suspected cases, in order to arrive at a correct diagnosis. Two other types of 'microtropia' have been described, that most commonly found being the one described by Lang (1970), a small ($< 10 \Delta$) strabismus, usually convergent, with amblyopia and well established harmonious ARC — it may be primary or secondary, and resulting from the treatment of a larger deviation. The deviation described by Parks (1975), and now called the monofixation syndrome, is not a true strabismus at all. Although a definite shift is found when the fixating eye is covered, these patients have normal retinal correspondence with peripheral fusion — they escape central diplopia by developing a large foveal suppression area in the amblyopic eye; they may be said to have a gross fixation disparity, but this is quite unlike the disparity which is found in uncompensated heterophoria or which can be induced in all normal binocular patients. Here foveal as well as peripheral fusion exists and the fixation error is only 5–10' of arc and far too small to be seen by the cover test. Usually a marked degree of heterophoria is found superimposed on the manifest fixation disparity and this has given rise to the quite mistaken impression that these cases have both a strabismus and heterophoria, an absolute contradiction in terminology.

Dissociated vertical divergence

This anomaly has many synonyms including alternating hyperphoria, occlusion hyperphoria and alternating sursumvergence. The most common form demonstrates binocular fixation but whichever eye is covered deviates upwards, often by an unequal amount. These patients often display the deviation through a neutral density filter and sometimes elevation begins when the practitioner's cover is still some 20 cm or so away prior to total occlusion. Exophoria is often present. Although this type of dissociated vertical divergence seldom causes symptoms, it does seem to be responsible for the more easy decompensation of any related heterophoria. Bielschowsky's phenomenon (*see* Duke-Elder, 1973) can be demonstrated in many cases.

A variant of dissociated vertical divergence is sometimes associated with strabismus with cyclotropia, and pendular rotatory nystagmus (Anderson, 1954; Crone, 1954).

Diagnostic occlusion and other tests

Diagnostic or prolonged occlusion was first introduced by Marlow in an effort to expose the full degree of heterophoria, and involves covering each eye in turn, for some 7–10 days. It greatly distorts the true heterophoric picture and large degrees of cyclophoria and dissociated vertical divergence are commonly found. Currently, the test is used for headache patients who may have symptomatic aniseikonia, all other possibilities having been previously investigated and, where necessary, corrected. If the symptoms disappear with occlusion it is reasonable to suggest that aniseikonia might be the culprit (*see* Charnwood, 1950).

Although the cover test is the definitive method for detecting and measuring ocular motor anomalies, it is difficult to use in some young infants who cannot maintain adequate fixation for the requisite time. To gain some idea of the magnitude of a squint in such cases, Hirschberg's test may be used. The child looks at a pen torch held at some 40 cm from his face, and the position of the corneal reflexes is observed. Although angle λ may interfere with the interpretation, as a guide a reflex on the pupillary margin denotes a deviation of some 15°, midway across the iris 25° and at the limbus 45° — crude, but better than no estimate at all.

The Krimsky test is an alternative to Hirschberg's test, prisms (base-out in esotropia) being placed before the fixating eye to induce a conjugate eye movement to the opposite side — the prism which places the squinting eye in a symmetrical position in its palpebral aperture is a rough indication of the strabismic angle.

Measurement of angle λ

As angle λ will influence the appearance of the squint its measurement is considered here. Conventionally, it is measured using a degree scale in a synoptophore, the patient looking from one number to the next until the corneal reflex appears centrally situated within the pupil — the reflex is large, however, and synoptophores not often available in general practice. A better method is to use a pen torch with a naked bulb held just under the practitioner's eye at the end of a millimeter rule held at 50 cm from the patient's face (the eye not being examined should be closed). The patient fixates the lighted bulb and the position of the corneal reflex is noted; if not central, the patient looks at a pen or pencil tip moved along the rule, until the reflex is symmetrically situated within the pupil. A linear displacement of 4 cm at a distance of 50 cm would indicate an angle λ of 8 Δ (or 5°).

Motility investigation

Motility test

This is performed binocularly with the ametropia corrected if possible to avoid instability of the

deviation. The face is well illuminated, the head stationary and erect, and a pen torch or Traquair, or similar, wand used as a fixation target. The patient should report the appearance of any diplopia and unease or discomfort which arises. The practitioner will move the target to the extreme limits of the fixation field in the horizontal and four oblique positions, moving the target in an arc to maintain a constant distance from the patient, to detect any lag or overaction of one eye (i.e. incomitancy). Vertical movement of the target, as well as the previously executed horizontal movement, will show the existence of a gaze palsy of the pursuit system if *both* eyes fail to follow the target to a normal degree. It must be remembered that elevation tends to diminish with advancing years, so a restricted upward movement is not at all uncommon in older patients (Chamberlain, 1971) changing from the normal 40° in young people to 30° at 45–54 years, 22° at 65–74 years and 16° at 75–84 years. Raising the lids when examining the lower motor field should be avoided as it can introduce artefacts into the motility picture. It is preferable instead to raise the patient and view from below head level.

Subjective motility

A subjective motility test can be performed with the patient wearing red and green filters (preferably over any spectacles) while viewing a barlite or pen torch. In the field of action of the paretic muscle(s), the separation of the diplopic images will be maximal, the more distal image belonging to the affected eye. The barlite gives additional information on cyclodeviations because an obliquity of the strip of light seen by the affected eye will be present when one of the vertically acting muscles is involved. The obliquity of the linear light source in such cases will be parallel to the normal torsional direction of the affected muscle. For a full description of the test *see* Lyle and Wybar (1967).

It is sometimes useful to combine the cover and motility tests, especially if there is no restriction of movement in any direction, but the patient complains of distress or discomfort. If, for example, this occurs to his right, it may be due to a right lateral rectus or left medial rectus muscle palsy, or to an early gaze palsy to the right. If a cover test is carried out at approximately 33 cm with the eyes directed to the target in front and 20° to both left and right, differential diagnosis is usually easy. An increasing esophoria in looking from left to right would suggest a lateral rectus palsy, while an increasing exophoria would implicate the medial rectus. If all three measurements prove to be approximately equal, then early gaze palsy is likely. This early or mild gaze palsy was once called a version heterophoria — movements are full but not easy in one particular direction; in the example given a label of laevoversion heterophoria would have been given (note dextroversion heterophoria, anaphoria and kataphoria in which there is difficulty looking to the left, downwards and upwards, respectively). In this early or mild gaze palsy movements are full but not easy in one particular direction. More advanced or obvious gaze palsies exhibit a bilateral restriction of movement to one side, or up or down, and the eyes may deviate to the opposite (affected) direction.

The absence of any manifest restriction of vertical or horizontal gaze does not necessarily imply that the cortical motor areas are intact. A gaze paresis caused by a slowly developing lesion (e.g. astrocytoma) might be concealed by the sound cerebral hemisphere taking over the function of the damaged side, a conjugate deviation only occurring under narcosis, anaesthesia or during sleep. Rapidly developing lesions (e.g. some vascular catastrophies) will normally give rise to an obvious motility problem as will *any* anomaly (of slow or rapid development) affecting the system below cortical level.

Voluntary and postural gaze

Voluntary gaze initiated from the frontal motor areas can be checked by asking the patient to look up, down, left and right. As this procedure is normally followed during ophthalmoscopy, it is not usually necessary to carry out a specific test for this function.

The integrity of the postural reflex is checked by depressing and elevating the patient's chin and turning his head from side to side while facing a blank screen — if the eyes make the appropriate compensatory movement (doll's head phenomenon), the vestibular system would appear to be functioning normally.

The Maddox groove in incomitancy

The Maddox groove, or indeed any suitable dissociation test can be used to isolate a palsied muscle as long as only one muscle is affected. Scobee (1952) has suggested a useful three-step procedure for vertical muscle palsies following measurements at both distance and near with each eye fixating in turn:

(1) It should be determined whether the imbalance is greater with the right or left eye fixating — the fixating eye presenting the larger imbalance is the eye with the affected muscle.
(2) If the imbalance is greater at distance than at near the affected muscle is a vertical rectus; if at near then an oblique muscle is implicated.
(3) It should be noted whether the affected eye is hyperphoric (or tropic) or is deviated downwards. If the former then a depressor muscle is paretic, if the latter, an elevator muscle. This

component is dependent on the fact that the oblique musles have their greatest vertical action during convergence; the vertical recti on the other hand are more effective in this respect when the visual axes are parallel (or divergent).

Example:

Maddox groove   FRE   FLE
used at: 6 m   8 Δ R, Hyper 5 Δ R, Hyper
          33 cm 4 Δ R, Hyper 1 Δ R, Hyper

(i) Paretic muscle is in right eye.
(ii) Deviation is greater at distance, therefore superior rectus or inferior rectus is involved.
(iii) Right eye is elevated, so a depressor muscle is the culprit, i.e. the right inferior rectus.

Field of fixation

The normal monocular field of fixation varies considerably from one individual to the next, but approximate figures are: upwards 35–40°, downwards 54°, nasally 45° and temporally 42°. The binocular field of fixation is more restricted owing to intrusion of facial contours.

The monocular field may be measured by passing a card with a line of small print along a perimeter arc at 30° intervals, blurring of the print indicating the end-point as its image falls to one side of the fovea. Another method, more refined but less practical, is to imprint an after-image on or in-line with the fovea, asking the patient to report when it is no longer coincident with a black spot on a white card moved around a perimeter arc. In both methods the eye not being examined is covered.

A perimeter is also used for the binocular field. With both eyes open, the patient follows a Traquair spot around the arc until diplopia occurs. A dissociated measurement in which the patient wears red and green filters and views a pen torch moving along the perimeter arc is less useful. Very often the dissociated method induces diplopia over the whole motor field. Some practitioners (e.g. Scobee, 1952) have used fixation fields as a basis for their motility diagnosis.

Hess, Lees and similar tests

These are employed to plot the progress or regression of an incomitancy or to identify the presence of those secondary sequelae which are apparent when an incomitancy has been present for some time. All tests of this nature measure the deviation in nine different directions of gaze and with each eye fixating in turn.

The internally illuminated Hess screen, a modern variant of the original model, employs anaglyphic dissociation with the patient viewing nine points of red light in turn, seen through a red filter with one eye (the fixating eye) and with the other (deviating eye) viewing a green slit projected from a Foster torch. Localization is from both foveas (except where there is deeply ingrained harmonious ARC), so the displacement of a motor field represents the actual deviation of the eye being plotted, i.e. if the motor field is displaced nasally then that eye is convergent.

The Lancaster screen is similar but the Hess pattern is replaced by a simple grid and two torches are used, one red and the other green, to be held by the practitioner and patient, respectively. As with the Hess screen test, the red and green filters before the patient are reversed to obtain a plot for the second eye.

The Lees screen employs the same pattern as the Hess. The patient faces a blank screen directly ahead and views the Hess configuration placed at 90° to the blank screen via a bisecting mirror which acts as a dissociating septum. The patient and the illuminated pattern are moved through 90° to plot the motor field of the second eye.

The reader is referred to Lyle and Wybar (1967) for further details.

Interpretation and secondary sequelae

A patient with a new incomitancy (*Figures 15.4* and *15.5*) will show:

(1) Possible displacement of the motor fields, the primary deviation (sound eye fixating) being less than the secondary deviation (affected eye fixating) in paretic conditions.

(2) The fields will be of unequal size, the smaller field being that of the eye with the affected muscle.

(3) The smaller field will demonstrate the paresis, i.e. there will be *less* than the three squares (3 × 5 = 15°) of movement in the field of action of the affected muscle. All counting of squares must be from the centre of the plot and not from the centre of the chart.

(4) A marked overaction of the contralateral synergist to the palsied muscle.

The passage of time will generally modify the appearance of the motor fields, there being a general tendency for the fields to become more nearly equal in size, a phenomenon sometimes known as 'spread of comitance', an unfortunate term, as the ocular motor situation will by now have deteriorated with the establishment of secondary sequelae. These are:

(1) Contracture of the ipsilateral antagonist (*Figure 15.6*) shown by an enlargement of the motor field of the affected eye on looking to the sound side. This normally occurs when the patient elects to use the sound eye for fixating in normal

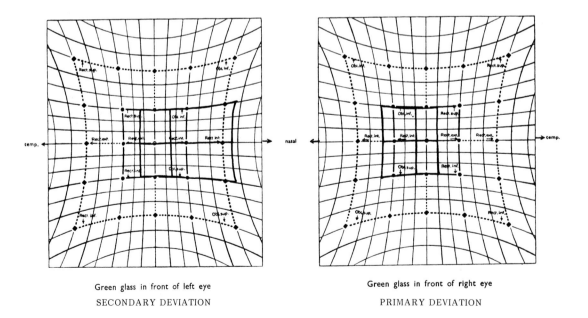

Green glass in front of left eye

SECONDARY DEVIATION

Green glass in front of right eye

PRIMARY DEVIATION

Figure 15.4 Hess screen plot. Recent paresis of right lateral rectus muscle, showing paresis and overaction of contralateral synergist (left medial rectus). Primary angle < secondary angle

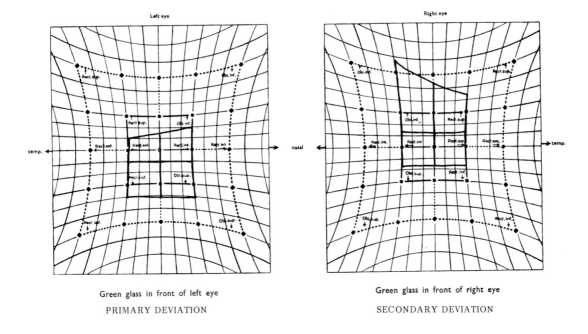

Green glass in front of left eye
PRIMARY DEVIATION

Green glass in front of right eye
SECONDARY DEVIATION

Figure 15.5 Hess screen plot: recent left superior rectus paresis showing paresis, overaction of contralateral synergist (right inferior oblique) and left hypotropia with primary angle < secondary angle. There may be a left ptosis

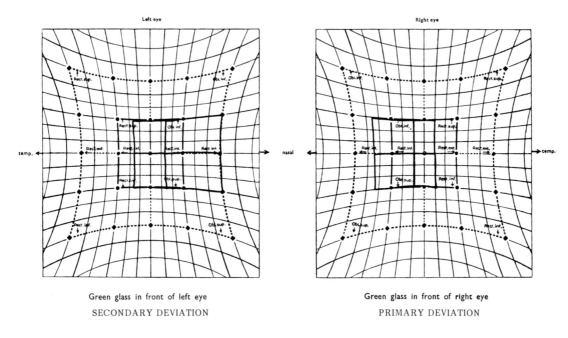

Green glass in front of left eye
SECONDARY DEVIATION

Green glass in front of right eye
PRIMARY DEVIATION

Figure 15.6 Hess screen plot: old paresis of right lateral rectus muscle showing paresis, reduced overaction of contralateral synergist and contracture of ipsilateral ant-agonist (right medial rectus). Patient normally fixates with left eye

everyday vision (Adler, 1965). The contracture is due to the replacement of elastic tissue in the belly of the muscle by fibrous tissue.

(2) Underaction of the contralateral antagonist (*Figure 15.7*) is shown by a reduction in the motor field in the sound eye and away from the direction in which the palsied muscle has its maximal action. If a patient chooses to fixate with the affected eye in normal vision so causing a constant overaction of the contralateral synergist, this type of sequela is likely to develop (Adler, 1965; Mallett, 1969).

In some cases both sequelae develop simultaneously (*Figure 15.8*). The presence then of one or both of these secondary components suggests that the palsy is not of recent onset, although it is possible that the underlying cause is still active.

Concomitant deviations demonstrate equal but displaced motor fields (*Figure 15.9*). Dissociated vertical divergence will exhibit an upward displacement of both motor fields usually by an unequal degree (*Figure 15.10*). Patients with concomitant strabismus and deeply ingrained harmonious ARC will show what is an apparently orthophoric plot (*Figure 15.11*).

Information gleaned from a Hess (or similar) screen together with a knowledge of the symptoms, history, head posture etc. should enable a diagnosis to be established which will determine the future care of the patient.

The reader is advised to consult the standard works for information concerning the ocular motor anomalies resulting from neurological and peripheral pathology and abnormal structure (e.g. Duke-Elder, 1973; Leigh and Zee, 1983).

Bielschowsky's head tilt test

This is normally used to differentiate a recent or long-standing superior rectus palsy in one eye from a palsy of the superior oblique of the other eye, and is dependent upon the utricular reflex. A patient with a right superior oblique palsy will normally have an habitual head tilt towards his left shoulder; if the head is tilted to the right, the otoliths are activated and innervation is sent to the right superior oblique and right superior rectus. The contraction of these two muscles normally would give only intorsion, as their vertical actions would neutralize one another. If the superior oblique is paretic, however, the superior rectus will be unopposed and elevation of the eye occurs. If, however, it is the superior rectus which is palsied and the head is tilted towards the shoulder on the same side, there will be *no* elevation of the eye as the superior oblique is intact and provides an adequate amount of torsion, being a much superior intorter (Adler, 1965).

A three-step procedure for investigating vertical muscle palsy which includes the head tilt test, has

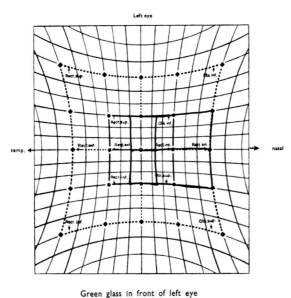

Green glass in front of left eye

SECONDARY DEVIATION

Figure 15.7 Hess screen plot: old paresis of right lateral rectus muscle showing paresis, overaction of contralateral synergist and underaction of contralateral an-

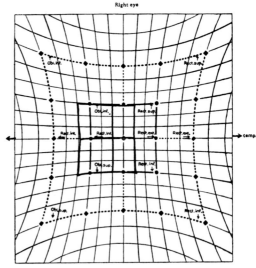

Green glass in front of right eye

PRIMARY DEVIATION

tagonist (left lateral rectus). Patient normally fixates with right eye (the affected eye)

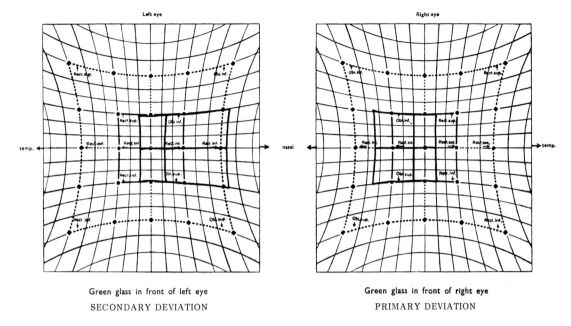

Figure 15.8 Hess screen plot: old paresis of right lateral rectus muscle showing paresis, reduced overaction of contralateral synergist, both contracture of ipsilateral antagonist and underaction of contralateral antagonist

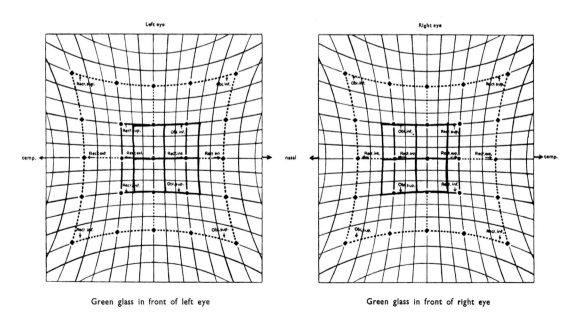

Figure 15.9 Concomitant esophoria, or esotropia (5° = 8 Δ) with normal retinal correspondence

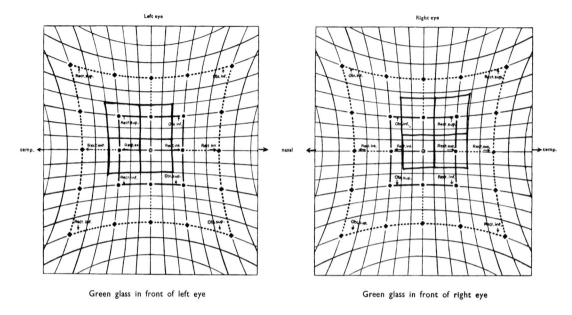

Figure 15.10 Dissociated vertical divergence with exophoria. The vertical movement is greater in the right eye than in the left

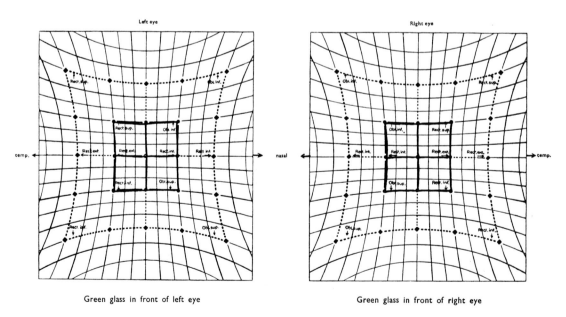

Figure 15.11 Orthophoria or strabismus with well established harmonious ARC

been introduced by Parks (1975):

(1) The hypertropic eye is determined. This eliminates four of the eight vertically acting muscles.
(2) It is determined whether the vertical deviation increases in the right or left eye. This eliminates one of the two possible affected muscles in each eye.
(3) Bielschowsky's head tilt test will isolate which of the two muscles from the preceding step is at fault.

Egocentric localization

Past pointing occurs in the field of action of a palsied muscle; similarly, under pointing occurs in spastic anomalies. It can be detected by placing a pencil in the appropriate part of the field while the patient with the sound eye occluded is asked to put the tip of his forefinger in line with it. The pointing hand must not be visible to the patient, so a horizontal card must be interposed between them. False localization tends to lessen with the passage of time. The various explanations for the phenomenon have been discussed by von Noorden, Awaya and Romano (1971).

Investigation of sensory status in concomitant strabismus

Patients with strabismus usually enjoy single vision due to adaptation phenomena, either suppression or harmonious anomalous retinal correspondence. Others may experience diplopia because the deviation is recent and adaptive mechanisms have not had time to develop, or owing to a breakdown in an objective angle of long standing with very firmly established harmonious ARC. In these latter cases, there is no co-variation and the angle of anomaly remains constant, so giving rise to unharmonious ARC, for example:

Objective angle	10 Δ esotropia
Subjective angle	0
Angle of anomaly	10 Δ
Diagnosis: Harmonious ARC	(single vision)

Objective angle increases to	16 Δ esotropia
Subjective angle	6 Δ esotropia
Angle of anomaly	10 Δ
Diagnosis: Unharmonious ARC	(diplopia)

The increase in angle is usually due to trauma to the head, but may be due to viral or other systemic infection. A similar breakdown in angle occurs when patients with harmonious ARC are examined on dissociating instruments such as the synoptophore, and this explains the confusing diagnosis of unharmonious ARC on such instruments, without the expected complaint of diplopia by the patient.

It is best to consider the diplopic and non-diplopic patients separately.

Diplopic cases

The basis of the investigation to be followed is simply to determine whether the patient has latent normal retinal correspondence without suppression or unharmonious ARC.

The type of diplopia is first ascertained. The conventional method of covering or filtering one eye is not recommended as it may initiate changes in the objective angle. Instead, a non-dissociating marker device should be employed and the Bagolini lens is the best in this respect. The Bagolini lens consists of a plastic film with numerous very fine parallel striations on one surface which is sandwiched between a pair of thin cover glasses; a small light viewed through the lens is seen normally but with a thin streak of light which will be at a right angle to the axis of the striations. There is very little interference with the visual scene and, for all practical purposes, it may be assumed that the lens will not introduce any element of dissociation. The Bagolini lens is placed before one eye and on fixating a spotlight binocularly, the patient will experience diplopia and will find one of the diplopic images to be marked with the streak. If the lens is before the right eye and the right light is so marked then the diplopia is uncrossed, indicating crossed visual axes and esotropia, and vice versa. The Bagolini lens is then removed and appropriate prisms (e.g. base-out in uncrossed diplopia) are then placed before the deviating eye until haplopia is obtained. A uniocular cover test is then carried out. If the prism which eliminates the diplopia also neutralizes the manifest deviation, then the patient has normal retinal correspondence. However, a residual strabismus indicates unharmonious ARC. If the correspondence is abnormal then an after-image test (bifoveal stimulation) can be used as a confirmatory test if desired (*see below*).

Non-diplopic cases

These patients will have either suppression or harmonious ARC, with possible assistance from optic nerve heads if the deviation is around 15° of convergence (Swan blind spot syndrome).

ARC

Generally, patients with an early onset to their deviation, consistent angles and retinal images of similar clarity will have well developed harmonious ARC, while larger unstable angles with marked uncorrected anisometropia are associated with suppression.

Harmonious ARC can exist in many degrees of severity, from a fluid lightly ingrained condition functioning purely to eliminate diplopia and without motor fusion or stereopsis, to the firmly established anomaly with motor fusion and good stereopsis. There can be no co-variation in these intensely ingrained cases and in many respects they enjoy, and suffer, the visual environment in much the same way as binocular subjects with normal retinal correspondence.

Suppression

Suppression can also exist in many degrees of severity. It affects the major part of the deviating eye and only a nasal quadrant of the retina escapes. This is due to the intrusion of the nose into space, restricting the overlapping fields of vision of the two eyes; this causes the temporal fields to be monocular and incapable of experiencing diplopia.

Assessment

The requirement in all of these cases is to establish whether the patient has harmonious ARC or normal retinal correspondence with suppression and then to determine its depth or intensity. Differentiating tests are of two types.

The first type compares the visual localization of the fixating eye with that part of the retina of the squinting eye which receives a similar image (the zero point measure of Jampolsky (1964)). These tests are generally more sensitive in revealing harmonious ARC than those of the second type, which compare the localization of images received on the two foveas; if they are in the same visual direction, correspondence is normal; if not, ARC is deemed to be present.

Experience with the tests described indicates that sensitivity in detecting harmonious ARC is very variable and seems to be dependent on the degree to which the instrumentation disturbs the visual environment. Non-dissociating tests, such as the Bagolini lens, and the modified fixation disparity routine are very sensitive and show that some 80% of all strabismic patients seen in optometric practice have harmonious ARC. They are easily understood by the patient and eminently suitable for use in a routine optometric examination. Disruptive and dissociating tests, on the other hand, are much less sensitive (Burian, 1951; Bagolini and Capobianco, 1965; Mallett, 1970a, 1973). A few practitioners (e.g. Flom and Kerr, 1967) believe that the incidence of ARC is constant whatever test is used, but their conclusions are based on results obtained from a group of tests which excluded those of maximal and minimal sensitivity.

Bagolini lenses

Bagolini lenses are available in two forms identified only by their number (2 or 4), the no. 4 lens giving a slightly brighter streak being generally used. If the squint is unilateral, a single striated lens is placed in front of the deviating eye with the striations horizontal to give a vertical streak. Two such lenses are used at 45° and 135° in patients with alternating deviations. If the single streak, or one of the pair in alternating squints, is not seen, suppression is present. If each Bagolini lens produces a subjectively visible streak, then harmonious ARC is present. The area around the light, subtending approximately 1°, is often not seen (*see Figure 15.12b*), indicating a very small suppression area in the periphery of the squinting eye at the zero point measure of Jampolsky. Perfect alignment of streak and spotlight is often not present, and this represents a slight imperfection in the new sensory relationship and is due to the alliance of receptive fields of unequal dimensions and properties and *not* to unharmonious ARC. Quantification of the ARC is carried out by introducing neutral density filters, in 0.3 log unit steps, in front of the squinting eye until suppression of the streak occurs or, much less often, diplopia. Occasionally, the filter which induces a diplopic end-point is spurious as the objective angle will have been increased by the neutral density filter producing, in effect, unharmonious ARC. A cover test with the filter *in situ* will establish the validity of the diplopic end-point.

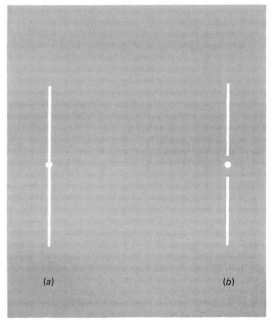

Figure 15.12 Bagolini streaks: (*a*) with no suppression at the 'zero point measure'; (*b*) with suppression (usually 1°) at the 'zero point measure'

Modified fixation disparity test (Figure 15.13)

A modified fixation disparity test (MFDT) procedure gives almost identical results as the Bagolini lens but without the distraction of spurious streaks which sometimes make the latter test a little troublesome (Mallett, 1983). The patient views the distance disparity test at a distance of 1.5 metres, or the enlarged fixation disparity test on the author's near vision unit at 25 cm through Polaroid filters. It is not possible to use conventional distances as the retinal image would fall into the 1° suppression area at the zero point measure and invalidate the test. If both coloured polarized strips are seen then harmonious ARC is present, although the strip seen by the squinting eye is usually somewhat fainter than that imaged in the fixating eye. As with the Bagolini lens, perfect alignment is not always present and no attempt should be made to use prisms to achieve this. The absence of one of the coloured strips indicates suppression which will extend over the whole retina, with the exception of a nasal segment which is not represented in the central overlapping fields (Swan, 1965; Mallett, 1969; Pratt-Johnson and Tillson, 1984). If harmonious ARC is found to be present, a neutral density filter bar is used before the squinting eye progressively to distort the visual environment and to weaken the anomalous association. The end-point is total suppression of the polarized strip seen by the deviating eye. As with the Bagolini lenses, a low density filter would indicate that the harmonious ARC is not firmly established and a certain amount of co-variation, i.e. a change in the angle of anomaly with any coincident change in the objective angle, would be expected. Generally the deeper the filter the more entrenched and immutable will be the ARC. If the MFDT reveals suppression it can be investigated as described below.

After-image tests

Various after-image tests have been suggested which are useful in optometric practice, needing only a small low-powered photographic flash unit, a few opaque plates with vertical slits and fixation marks, and a tangent scale (Mallett, 1975b). At one time a vertical stimulus was presented to one eye and a horizontal one to the other, but it is more precise to utilize vernier alignment. Three of the four tests described here utilize the investigation of fovea—fovea relationship while the remaining test employs polarizing filters and examines the fovea—zero point measure localization. A vertical after-image formed above the fovea of the fixating eye and below the fovea (or eccentric area if strabismic amblyopia is present) of the squinting eye will demonstrate localization from the two stimulated areas by the patient reporting alignment of the two

negative after-images seen against a light surface. There may be a displacement in the presence of eccentric fixation, but it will be substantially smaller than the objective angle unless a microtropia of the von Noorden variety is being examined. Harmonious ARC is indicated by a lateral separation of the two after-images; if the separation is being measured on a tangent scale it will be found to be equal to the objective angle of squint at the fixation distance employed, plus or minus the degree of any eccentric fixation which is present. If the eyes are now closed to form a positive after-image, a much less sensitive environment is created and only the deepest cases will persist in anomalous localization — the incidence of ARC with the eyes open using after-images is about 20%, but only 1% with the eyes closed.

A more sensitive test than those described can be carried out by creating a vertical after-image only in the deviating eye. With both eyes open, the patient views a tangent scale with the zero fixation point acting as a reference for the fovea of the fixating eye.

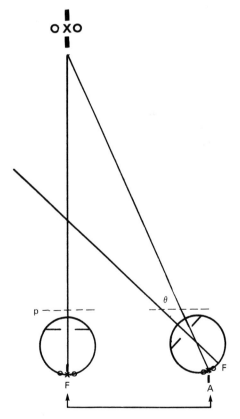

Figure 15.13 Modified fixation disparity test for ARC and suppression: P, Polaroid filters; θ, objective angle of strabismus; F, foveas; A, zero point measure of Jampolsky

The most sensitive of the after-image tests, however, is undoubtedly that using polarizing filters. A plate over the flash gun has a vertical slit with a central fixation mark and is polarized so that the top part of the aperture is visible to one eye and the bottom half to the other eye, appropriate analysers being worn by the patient. A single flash stimulus will form an after-image in line with the fovea of the fixating eye but in line with the zero point measure in the squinting eye. The after-image pattern is, then, the reverse of that seen when both foveas are separately stimulated, and appear to be in alignment when harmonious ARC is present and separated by an amount equivalent to the objective angle in normal retinal correspondence. This technique has a high degree of sensitivity, some 50% or more of squinters exhibiting ARC. It also has the advantage of avoiding eccentric fixation problems in amblyopia as monocular stimulation of the squinting eye is avoided. In some ways this polarized test is similar to the Bagolini test and the MFDT although a little less sensitive. Other after-image tests have been described by Halldén (1952).

Haploscopic methods

The most popular haploscope has always been the synoptophore, an instrument that will measure almost any binocular function, but lacking a certain refinement because of its dissociating properties and the rather unnatural environment presented to the patient. Thus a comparison of objective and subjective angles, normally measured with 'square and circle' slides, will disclose the presence of ARC in about 20% of all squinters examined, but will usually indicate that most of these are of an unharmonious nature. More information on the practical aspects of using the synoptophore can be obtained from Gibson (1955) and Lyle and Wybar (1967).

The single mirror haploscope (Earnshaw *et al.*, 1957) is a rotatable mirror bisecting two grey screens placed at 90° to each other and provides an alternative to the synoptophore. One eye views the screen directly ahead while the other eye observes its own screen through the mirror.

Several attempts have been made to remove some of the disturbing dissociating and proximal convergence properties of the synoptophore and they generally utilize a more natural visual scene than ordinary synoptophore procedures. This is sometimes referred to as examination in 'free space'. The Stanworth modification is one such instrument: the silvered mirrors are replaced by thin glass plates (originally very weak prisms to prevent double reflections) and the position of the collimating lenses changed so that a clear view of the opposite wall at 3 or 6 metres is obtained. Black slides with clear apertures are used and are seen superimposed on the wall which should ideally be patterned to provide a fusionable stimulus. This instrument has proved most useful for examining the sensory status of small angled deviations (Stanworth, 1958; Mallett, 1970a).

Aulhorn and Kreuzer (1968) have described an ingenious haploscope utilizing two rotating sectored discs, one before each eye, and twin projectors with similar synchronized discs to enable rapid (100 Hz) alternate vision which is well above the critical frequency of fusion. It is doubtful if the apparatus is completely free from dissociating effects as von Noorden (1970b) found an appreciably higher incidence of unharmonious ARC than with the Bagolini test.

Twin projectors with polarized filters over the objectives together with a metallic screen (to prevent depolarization) have been used by Pigassou (1968). The visual scene is free from major artefacts but manipulation of the targets in the projectors is difficult.

Evaluation of suppression in strabismus

The Stanworth, Aulhorn and Pigassou instrumentation can all be used to determine the subjective angle and investigate suppression in squinting patients. Many of the techniques previously used to delineate suppression areas have fallen into disuse as there is now a general recognition that the small (approximately 1°) suppression area at the zero point measure in harmonious ARC is of no clinical consequence other than the interference it may give to certain clinical tests, of no therapeutic significance, and the realization that squinters who suppress rather then develop ARC involve the major part of the deviating eye, leaving just a small crescent of nasal retina unaffected. This general suppression is usually more intense in the area between the fovea and the zero point measure, and many of the more dissociating tests previously employed tended to uncover this elliptical or D-shaped region (Jampolsky, 1968) but left the surrounding and more extensive suppression undetected — an instrument artefact.

If the mapping of suppression areas is nonproductive, a more general view of the intensity of the suppression must be undertaken. This can be achieved with neutral density filters to embarrass the dominance of the fixating eye (Mallett, 1965). The patient views a target set in a field with sufficient fusionable stimuli to allow a natural environment. A neutral density filter bar is used before the fixating eye, introducing filters of increasing density in 0.3 log unit intervals until diplopia intervenes indicating a state of equidominance, or the squinting eye itself achieves dominance and takes up fixation. The deeper the filter to achieve this, the more intense the suppression.

Fusional amplitudes in strabismus

That many strabismic patients do have an appreciable amplitude of fusion is obvious to all those who have attempted to neutralize the deviation with prisms and have been perplexed by obviously inflated findings. In many cases, the patient has a well established harmonious ARC and it is not difficult to undertand why they make fusional movements to maintain images of the object of regard on the anomalously corresponding receptive fields. Others, however, have very poorly established ARC or even suppression, yet still manage to compensate for prisms or exaggerated synoptophore tube movements. Sometimes, especially with the synoptophore, the patient retains subjective fusion and single vision of the target, but there is no coexisting eye movement — co-variation. In others single vision and motor compensation for the prism occur simultaneously. It is difficult to believe that true fusional movements can occur when one eye is suppressed and the problem remains unresolved at the present time. The importance of these observations has led to the introduction of various tests for prism adaptation in strabismus (PAT of Jampolsky for example) and the whole topic has been discussed in depth by Bagolini (1985). Fusional amplitudes should only be measured objectively using prisms or a haploscope, careful observation of the patient's eyes being mandatory to find the end-point where motor fusion is relinquished. It must be noted that much of the exuberance shown by the vergence system in strabismic patients is confined to the same direction as the deviation, e.g. high amplitude of convergence in esotropia but only a limited amplitude of divergence.

Depth perception

Whenever possible the stereoacuity of any patient with a binocular anomaly should be determined as part of the investigation of sensory function. A number of tests are available.

Vectographs

The Titmus vectograph test is best known for its 'fly', but the spot test is much more useful and provides a selection of disparities with a lower threshold of 40″ of arc at 40 cm. The 800″ and 400″ arc spots may not provide reliable information in some cases as the lateral displacement seen in patients who suppress may be incorrectly interpreted as depth.

A similar, but in some ways improved, vectograph test is the Randot test. Like the Titmus test it employs polarized targets, four of them being Julesz (random-dot) patterns. The spot tests have a lower threshold of 20″ arc at 40 cm. The Julesz patterns are useful for examining global stereopsis.

Another test which employs Julesz patterns is the TNO test, but anaglyphic separation of the right and left information can cause poor stereoacuities to be recorded. Unequal accommodative efforts are demanded from the two eyes and, as this is normally not possible, one image must always be more blurred than in the companion eye. Furthermore, any test which passes red and green information simultaneously to a single visual cell in the cortex will inevitably be disruptive.

Real depth tests

The Frisby test provides 'real depth' by presenting random-dot patterns on three plastic plates of different thickness, part of the pattern being on one side of the plate, the remainder on the reverse aspect. The greatest distance is found where the sensation of depth is just perceptible with the thinnest plate. Reference to a table will then give the corresponding stereoacuity. Although a little cumbersome in use, the Frisby test is reliable as long as the plates are viewed against (and not too close to) a blank surface while the head is held stationary to avoid parallax clues.

Other tests include the Mallett polarized test which must be used in near darkness, the Lang test which, although not presenting very low stereo thresholds, is delightfully easy to use and for young children to understand, and the rather time consuming Howard–Dolman type of test employing two or three rods for more precise measurements. A study of stereo thresholds has been undertaken by Heron *et al.* (1985).

Strabismic patients with well established harmonious ARC often show stereoacuities better than 100″ arc, and occasionally as refined as 40″ arc. Heterophoric patients normally perform rather better and achieve 20–60″ arc with most tests. The Howard–Dolman apparatus usually suggests much better stereoacuities for both heterophoric and strabismic patients with harmonious ARC.

The further investigation of heterophoria

The most reliable tests for detecting and measuring the degree of heterophoria have already been described — the objective and subjective cover tests. They are alone in approaching the ideal of complete dissociation and have the distinct advantage of simplicity and versatility because they are usable at all fixation distances and directions of gaze.

Many other tests for heterophoria exist and may be grouped as below.

Distortion tests

The Maddox groove is the best known example of this type. It should be green rather than red and used in conjunction with a cover, the latter exposing the eye to a streak for just a moment or so in order that the patient may indicate its position. In other words the streak acts as a marker, leaving the cover to dissociate. Prisms are used to align the streak with the fixation light, or as a bracketing procedure. On occasion, marked esophoria is found at distance which cannot be confirmed with the cover test.

Diplopia tests

The doubling prism of von Graefe is popular in some countries especially for measuring horizontal imbalances. A 6 Δ lens with the base–apex line vertical, induces vertical diplopia and prisms base-in or -out as required are employed to align the diplopic letters or light. Many variants include the Thorington and modified Thorington tests. A desire for symmetry of the diplopic images is a possible source of inaccuracy, but the use of a cover is of assistance.

Tests with independent objects

The synoptophore, various phoriagraphs and the Hess screen are generally too inconvenient and time consuming to use as dissociation tests.

Independent objects seen by selective screening

The Maddox Wing and Mills test are good examples. Although very popular, these somewhat clumsy devices employ a fixed working distance and, in the case of the former, inadequate accommodative stimuli with the contours of the back plate visible to both eyes and hence an embarrassment to complete dissociation. The Mills test employs smaller characters and a larger back plate to overcome these problems. Both tests should be used in conjunction with a cover.

Cyclophoria

Although it is conventional to check routinely for the presence of horizontal and vertical imbalances, a special test for cyclophoria is rarely performed. It is

worth considering when symptoms suggest its possible presence and it may be detected by using two vertical Maddox grooves, one before each eye, with a prism (base–apex line vertical) to separate the streaks. If the two horizontal streaks do not appear parallel to the patient the appropriate groove is rotated until they do. It is more realistic to look for uncompensated cyclophoria as described below because this can easily be carried out routinely if desired.

All of the heterophoria tests described above, and many others, have been discussed by Scobee (1952), Gibson (1955) and Duke-Elder (1973).

Near point of convergence

As with heterophoria, this should be investigated with the ametropia corrected. Several measurements are possible.

Push-up test

The usual test consists of bringing a bold vertical line on a card towards the patient's face until diplopia is experienced or until one eye is seen by the practitioner to deviate. The card is then withdrawn to the recovery position. The normal measurement is some 8–10 cm with a recovery position of 10–15 cm. A patient with long arms who reads at a distance of 45–50 cm might be considered normal with a near point rather more remote than this. This test activates both 'voluntary' and 'reflex' convergence systems.

Jump convergence

The innervation during the jump convergence test is almost entirely of a voluntary nature. The patient looks at an object at 6 metres and observes a near object in physiological diplopia. Fixation is transferred to the near object which is then seen singly with the distant object in diplopia. If this can be successfully achieved, the near object is brought closer to the face and the test repeated, further repeats being made as necessary to record the closest possible distance to which the eyes will converge. Pickwell and Hampshire (1981) consider this test to be one of the most informative for convergence.

Reflex convergence

It is not possible to isolate completely the 'reflex' or occipital convergence system, but Capobianco (1952) described a technique which depends on partial dissociation with a deep red filter placed before one eye. The patient views a small light (preferably a vertical bar of light) which is brought towards the patient until diplopia occurs. This test should be the first convergence test to be used as it is important that no active effort, i.e. voluntary (frontal) convergence, is used to maintain single vision. A considerable difference between this near point and the normal near point (described above) points to a tiring convergence system. The supposition is that during normal close work innervation to convergence should be largely occipital with only rare support from the frontal motor areas of the cortex.

Fixation disparity

Although patients with troublesome convergence normally exhibit a fixation disparity (FD) at near, this is not an invariable finding where the anomaly is induced by severe fatigue. If the convergence is suspect, but there is no FD, the test should be slowly brought closer to the patient until a disparity is noticed. This should not normally be more remote than one half of the patient's reading or working distance.

Compensation tests

It must be emphasized that the degree of heterophoria measured by a dissociation test is small guide to compensation. Although it is reasonable to suppose that smaller deviations will be easier for the fusional reflexes to control than larger ones, there are too many exceptions to this premise for it to be of any significant value.

Tests for compensation can be placed into one of the following categories:

(1) Measurement of the fusional vergence amplitudes opposing the heterophoria and other forced vergence tests leading to graphical analysis or 'middle third' procedures.
(2) Gradient tests.
(3) Partial dissociation tests, e.g. Turville Infinity Balance (TIB), Turville distance balance (TDB).
(4) Tests which embarrass binocular vision by reducing the width of the binocular field — Bishop Harman diaphragm test and the Mitchell stability test.
(5) Dynamic retinoscopy.
(6) Fixation disparity tests.
(7) Recovery from dissociation by cover test (previously described).

Analysis of fusion

Attempts to utilize fusional amplitude measurements have a long and chequered history. It is customary to measure the reserve which opposes the heterophoria, e.g. the positive fusional reserve in exophoria and the right supravergence in left hyperphoria. If the reserve is two or three times the numerical value of the heterophoria, it is assumed (quite wrongly) that there is no lack of compensation. Graphical and middle third techniques demand the measurement of opposing fusional reserves, but the first measurement is always likely to influence the second unless an appreciable interval is allowed. Whether to rely upon blur, break or recovery measurements, is a matter for individual preference, a point well emphasized by reviewing the numerous methods advocated (Borish, 1975). A number of objections to these techniques have been listed by Mallett (1966). The first is that equating the heterophoria with the fusional amplitude is unsatisfactory as the finding will vary with the dissociation technique employed. The second is that the measurement of the fusional amplitudes to blur, break and recovery will vary with:

(1) The instrumentation employed. For example, variable prism stereoscopes generally give higher amplitudes than the synoptophore because of the larger fusion field presented to the patient. Proximal convergence effects also affect the accuracy of the synoptophore.
(2) The targets being viewed as a stimulus will also influence results. Large targets and those with an inbuilt sense of depth will give larger amplitudes than targets which only stimulate foveal fusion without peripheral involvement or which lack binocular disparity.
(3) The speed with which the stimulus to fusional movements is presented will affect the measurement — rapid changes in prism power will effect a smaller amplitude than slowly increased strength of prism. Jump prisms, likewise, give smaller amplitudes than the gradual transition of power created by the rotary prism.
(4) Patient effort and fatigue is a very variable factor which can have a considerable influence on the measurements.
(5) Interpretation of blur is a further uncertain variable which will hinder accuracy.

Morgan (1960) has published a statistical survey of 800 non-presbyopic patients and found the following normal ranges:

At 6 metres *Positive fusional vergences*
(measured with base-out prism)

Blur	7–11 Δ
Break	15–23 Δ
Recovery	8–12 Δ

Negative fusional vergences
(measured with base-in prism)
Break   5–9 Δ
Recovery   3–5 Δ

At 40 cm   *Positive fusional vergences*
Blur   14–20 Δ
Break   18–24 Δ
Recovery   7–15 Δ

Negative fusional vergences
Blur   11–15 Δ
Break   19–23 Δ
Recovery   10–16 Δ

Right and left supra- and infravergences are usually of the order of 3 Δ in each direction.

For a very pragmatic approach to fusional reserve techniques the reader is advised to consult Morgan (1960).

Gradient tests

These attempt to measure the amount of accommodative convergence induced by a known amount of accommodation — the AC/A ratio.

The easiest method is to determine the change in near heterophoria (OMB) when the accommodative stimulus is changed by 1 D and 2 D lenses.

For example: OMB at 33 cm   6 Δ Exophoria
                            10 Δ Exophoria
                               through 1 D
                               lenses
                            14 Δ Exophoria
                               through 2 D
                               lenses

The change is 4 Δ for every 1 D change in accommodation and the AC/A ratio would be expressed as 4 Δ/1 D. An alternative method which is sometimes referred to as the prism lens (PL) ratio, is to find first the sphere and then the prism to eliminate a fixation disparity at near. If no fixation disparity is found, it can be induced with spheres and then prisms, taking care always to effect the slip in the *same* direction, e.g. convex spheres and base-out prisms to give a divergent disparity.

The value of the AC/A or PL ratio is that it indicates whether the degree of heterophoria can be adequately reduced with appropriate plus or minus spheres — a normal or a high ratio (4 Δ/1 D or more) would encourage such management, whereas a low finding (2 Δ/1 D)) would be a contraindication.

It is regrettable that the functions being assessed are not fully understood which may be confused by attaching an unduly important role to accommodation in the convergence/accommodation relation-

ship, an alliance in which development, latent and reaction times, the onset of presbyopia with intact convergence and the very considerable difference in accuracy that is required for normal functions, all point to convergence as being dominant. The precision factor is often overlooked; accommodation is frequently lagging by 0.50 D or more in near vision, which represents an error of some 17% on an accommodative demand of 3 D, yet the patient is quite unaware of any blur. Convergence, by contrast, must be very precise and within the limits of Panum's fusional areas at the fovea in order to maintain single vision — this maximum error of, say approximating 5′ arc is of the order of 0.8% for a fixation distance of 33 cm, and even this misalignment is the exception rather than the rule as the majority of people do not exhibit such a fixation disparity.

Partial dissociation tests

The Turville Infinity Balance (Turville, 1946) is typical of this type of compensation test. There is no foveal fusion but paramacular fusion over a small field is allowed. A polarized version was introduced by Wilmut. Turville (1962) later used an angled mirror (TDB) to provide the necessary partial dissociation at 6 metres and similar instrumentation for employment at near (TNB). These devices are crude fixation disparity tests, but completely negate one of the essential requirements of this type of technique by deliberately embarrassing binocularity. With the simple strip septum, an acceptable, if not ideal, prism for uncompensated hyperphoria can be deduced, but it has little application for lateral imbalances.

An improved technique was introduced by Banks (1954) employing a narrow (21 mm) septum thus allowing a degree of foveal fusion. This gives a reliable correction of hyperphoria and good environment for the detection of foveal suppression at 6 metres.

Variable binocular overlap tests

The first test to measure the smallest vertical strip of fusional detail sufficient to hold the eyes in a normal fixing posture was the Bishop Harman diaphragm test. As the test is no longer manufactured and is little used, the reader is referred to Gibson (1955) and Lyle and Wybar (1967) for details.

The Mitchell stability test (Mitchell, 1953) proved to be a more useful procedure and consisted of a near point rule with a printed card at 33 or 40 cm and a movable septum 30 mm wide (originally 37.5 mm). The septum is moved from the face towards the stability target and in so doing the area of binocular overlap diminishes. When the available fusion field is inadequate to maintain binocular fixation, confusion or separation of the target detail will occur. The width of the binocular overlap (equivalent to the 'ocular poise' of Bishop Harman) can be calculated for the known distance of the target and septum from the spectacle plane, the width of the septum and the interpupillary distance (measured from the *outer* pupil margins) at 33 or 40 cm. If the binocular overlap is 7 mm or less, and the recovery overlap 11 mm or less it is indicative of a compensated heterophoria, while if larger values are obtained, appropriate prisms or spheres are used to achieve the required standard. The technique is fairly accurate but very cumbersome and time consuming.

Dynamic retinoscopy

This technique has engendered much controversial discussion over the years. It is not a popular technique today but it still has its adherents.

The patient fixes a coarse target on a retinoscope at 33 cm while a rack of convex spheres is applied binocularly. Early neutralization of the 'with movement' is supposed to measure the accommodative lag and is sometimes called the low neutral. If the plus power is increased, the negative relative accommodation is invaded, the end-point being denoted by an against movement of the reflex — this is the dynamic or high neutral (DN or HN). The normal DN up to the age of 30 years is 1.50 D; in exophoria and convergence insufficiency a reduced DN is usually found, but a high reading accompanies esophoria or accommodative weakness. Further information on the many procedures advocated can be obtained from Borish (1975; *see* also Chapter 6).

Fixation disparity

Fixation disparity (FD) is a minute error of fixation, the angle being limited by the dimensions of the receptive fields at the foveas. Too small to be seen by the cover test, it usually measures some 5–10′ arc, and may be horizontal, vertical or torsional. It may be present during normal vision whenever the fusional reflexes are incapable of maintaining perfect superimposition of normally corresponding receptive fields. It is therefore an indication that any heterophoria present is causing stress. Any fully efficient binocular system may exhibit FD if binocularity is embarrassed as by blurring one eye, restricting the binocular field, reducing the ambient lighting or dazzling one eye with light. Furthermore the instrumentation employed to detect FD must not introduce any artefacts which will disturb normal binocular vision.

The absence of fixation disparity in normal binocular vision is explained by the work of Joshua and Bishop (1970) who found that the binocular response from optimally superimposed receptive fields is greater by some 45% than the sum of the uniocular responses. Pettigrew, Nikara and Bishop (1968a,b) have found that the binocular facilitation of a striate cell is confined to a receptive field overlap very close to superimposition, a decline in response being evident as soon as the alignment of the two fields becomes less precise. By maintaining perfect superimposition of corresponding receptive fields (i.e. no FD), a maximal cortical response is enjoyed, but this appears to be relinquished when the ocular motor system is subjected to stress such as uncompensated heterophoria.

A competent FD technique merely requires its detection in a perfectly normal environment without any dissociation or other embarrassment to binocularity induced by the instrumentation used. It is *not* necessary to measure the angular extent of the disparity, the detection and then elimination with spheres or prisms being all that is required.

The minimum power of prism or sphere which just eliminates the FD is sometimes called the associated heterophoria, but it really represents the extent of the uncompensated part of the imbalance, and this term is not recommended.

The ideal fixation disparity test must fulfil certain requirements:

(1) There must be a target for bifoveal fixation with surrounding detail to provide both foveal and paramacular fusion. The peripheral field must also provide a fusional stimulus.
(2) Two small monocular markers must be provided, one to be seen by each eye, and their relative alignment must be capable of discernment by the untutored eye of the average patient. The targets should not be easily suppressed.
(3) There must be no dissociation by the instrumentation. A trial frame is superior to the refractor head as it allows a normal head posture and there is no 'tunnel effect' with consequent visual field restriction.
(4) The ambient light should mimic that used by the patient at work or leisure, i.e. it must be capable of adjustment. In the comparatively uncommon case where the patient spends much of his working time in a dark or poorly illuminated environment (e.g. night driving or photographic dark room work), the test must be capable of being used in similar conditions.
(5) A natural head posture must be maintained, a condition of particular importance in incomitant heterophoria. The test should be usable at any reasonable working distance.

The Mallett–Hamblin distance and near tests (Mallett, 1964, 1983) were designed with these factors in mind, the only disturbance to normal binocularity being the reduction of ambient light by the Polaroid visor through which the targets are viewed — this is easily compensated for simply by increasing (roughly doubling) the available light.

In practice, any heterophoria which does not give rise to FD may be disregarded. The clinical appearances in the different varieties of uncompensated heterophoria are shown in *Figure 15.14*. It will be seen that the FD may be uniocular or binocular and, in the presence of uncompensated cyclophoria, there is an obliquity of one or both of the polarized nonius strips.

If a vertical FD is found it is carefully neutralized by adding prisms in 0.5 Δ intervals; refining to the nearest 0.25 Δ is possible in many cases. If the disparity is uniocular, the prism should be placed before the eye displaying the shift, but divided evenly when bilateral.

Esophoric disparities at distance are neutralized with base-out prisms (1 Δ intervals are used in lateral heterophorias), and prisms or binocular convex additions (0.25 D intervals) when at near — in practice the additional plus power is preferred when dealing with such near vision imbalances.

Exophoria at distance is evaluated with base-in prisms, or a binocular concave addition can be used where the patient has a good amplitude of accommodation. Between changes of sphere, the patient should read a line or two of letters or print to ensure that the accommodation is adequately stimulated. Near exophoria and convergence insufficiency can be investigated in a similar fashion. Where it is suspected that the convergence is influenced by fatigue, not present at the time of the examination, the near disparity test should be undertaken at one half of customary reading or working distance.

Mixed hyperphoria and lateral imbalances require careful investigation as correction of one will often influence the other. It is suggested that the vertical FD be eliminated first and then the lateral disparity with the appropriate vertical prism *in situ*; this usually provides a weaker prism combination than the alternative procedure of correcting the lateral component first. There are exceptions, of course, and it is always worth investigating both possibilities.

Uncompensated cyclophoria is not commonly found. Attempts to neutralize the torsional disparity should include the careful correction of any coexisting hyperphoria and the *binocular* evaluation of any astigmatism at both distance and near.

It must always be remembered that the FD is not itself being measured and that the prism or sphere which removes it is in no way related to the degree of heterophoria present.

The technique provides a rapid, precise, consistent and reliable method of evaluating heterophoria. Fixation disparity curves plotted without foveal fusion in operation are suspect, especially when the

curve type, Y intercept and slope are, as a result, given unwarranted clinical priority over the X intercept (the 'associated heterophoria'; Sheedy, 1980). Some of the incongruities found by the absence of foveal fusion have been noted by Wildsoet and Cameron (1985) although they were unable to confirm the effect on the results of varying ambient lighting, this is readily demonstrated clinically, however.

Detection of foveal suppression

Cases of long-standing uncompensated heterophoria sometimes develop suppression. Symptoms tend to disappear as the suppression develops. Any test to detect such suppression must not introduce retinal rivalry or other artefacts, and must be capable of locating small areas of foveal inhibition, preferably quantitatively, of the order of 5–15' arc. A polarized suppression test is shown in *Figure 15.15*; this has central foveal and paramacular fusion detail to prevent 'floating'.

A Javal FLyz card can be used in a plano prism stereoscope (with 9 Δ base-out prisms before each eye), but *not* in a Brewster–Holmes stereoscope. Certain tests for foveal suppression such as the hand diploscope, are too artificial and crude to be of any real value.

Ocular dominance

The detection of marked ocular dominance is sometimes a useful aid to prescribing.

The fixation disparity test will determine motor dominance if a unilateral slip is present, this belonging to the non-dominant eye; patients displaying a new incomitancy are an exception. If there is a bilateral disparity it may be assumed that a state of equidominance exists, for all clinical purposes. A FD can be induced in a compensated heterophore by placing prisms of equal power before the right and left eyes until one or both nonius strips show lack of alignment with the central fixation cross.

Other indications of the dominant eye include:

(1) The eye with the better visual acuity.
(2) The eye which does not suppress on the polarized test or the Javal FL card described above.
(3) The eye which maintains fixation just inside the near point of convergence.
(4) The eye which is used for sighting a distant object through a hole (25 mm) in a card held with both hands at arms' length.
(3) The eye which maintains fixation just inside the near point of convergence.
(4) The eye which is used for sighting a distant object through a hole (25 mm) in a card held with both hands at arms' length.

Orthophoria or compensated lateral heterophoria

Orthophoria or compensated hyperphoria

Uncompensated exophoria with slip in L.E.

Uncompensated exophoria with slip in both eyes

Uncompensated esophoria with slip in both eyes

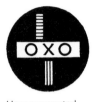

Uncompensated esophoria with slip in L.E.

Uncompensated R. hyperphoria with slip in L.E.

Uncompensated L. hyperphoria with slip in both eyes

R. excyclophoria

Bilateral incyclophoria

Deep central suppression R.E

Deep central suppression L.E

Figure 15.14 Fixation disparity. Clinical appearances using Mallett–Hamblin units. The polarized strips: ▥ seen by right eye; ▤ seen by left eye

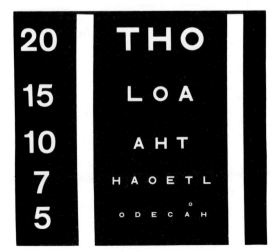

Figure 15.15 Suppression test. The central letters and the vertical stripes provide foveal and paramacular locks, respectively. The remaining letters are polarized so that those on the right are seen by the left eye and vice versa, and subtend 20′, 15′, 10′, 7′, and 5′ arcs at 35 cm. A similar chart can be used at 6 metres for evaluating distance suppression

References

ADLER, F.H. (1965) *Physiology of the Eye, Clinical Application*. Saint Louis: C.V. Mosby Company

ANDERSON, J.R. (1954) Latent nystagmus and alternating hyperphoria. *Br. J. Ophthalmol.*, **38**, 217–231

ARDEN, G.B. (1978) The importance of measuring contrast sensitivity in cases of visual disturbance. *Br. J. Ophthalmol.*, **62**, 198–209

AULHORN, E. and KREUZER, W. (1968) Phase difference haploscopy for investigation of strabismus. *International Strabismus Symposium*, edited by A. Arruga, pp. 245–251. Basel: S. Karger

BAGOLINI, B. (1985) Objective evaluation of sensorial and sensorimotorial states in esotropia: their importance in surgical prognosis. *Br. J. Ophthalmol.*, **69**, 725–728

BAGOLINI, B. and CAPOBIANCO, N.M. (1965) Subjective space in comitant squint. *Am. J. Ophthalmol.*, **59**, 430–442

BANKS, R.F. (1954) A foveal lock for infinity balance. *Br. J. Physiol. Opt.*, **11**, 216–225

BORISH, I.M. (1975) *Clinical Refraction*. Chicago: Professional

BRINKER, W.R. and KATZ, S.L. (1963) A new and practical treatment of eccentric fixation. *Am. J. Ophthalmol.*, **55**, 1033–1035

BROCK, F.W. and GIVNOR, I. (1952) Fixation anomalies in amblyopia. *Arch. Ophthalmol.*, **47**, 775–786

BURIAN, H.M. (1951). Anomalous retinal correspondence: its essence and its significance in diagnosis and treatment. *Am. J. Ophthalmol.*, **34**, 237–253

BURIAN, H.M. and VON NOORDEN, G.K. (1974) *Binocular Vision and Ocular Motility*. Saint Louis: C.V. Mosby Company

CAPOBIANCO, N.M. (1952) The subjective measurement of the near point of convergence and its significance in the diagnosis of convergence insufficiency. *Am. Orthopt. J.*, **2**, 40

CARLOW, T.J. (1976) In *Pathogenesis and Treatment of Headache*, edited by O. Appenzeller. New York: Spectrum Publication Inc, S.P. Books Division

CHAMBERLAIN, W. (1971) Restriction of upward gaze with advancing age. *Am. J. Ophthalmol.*, **71**, 341–346

CHARNWOOD, J. (1950) *An Essay on Binocular Vision*. London: Hatton Press Ltd

CRONE, R.A. (1954) Alternating hyperphoria. *Br. J. Ophthalmol.*, **38**, 591–604

CUIFFREDA, K.J., HOKODA, S.C., HUNG, G.K., SEMMLOW, J.L. and SELENOW, A. (1983) Static aspects of accommodation in human amblyopia. *Am. J. Optom. Physiol. Opt.*, **60**, 436–449

DUKE-ELDER, S.(1973) *System of Ophthalmology*, Vol. VI. London: Henry Kimpton

EARNSHAW, J.R., GOEBBELS, W.F., GRIFFIN, R.G.and MEAKIN, W.J. (1957) A single mirror haploscope. *Optician*, **133**, 289

FLOM, M.C. and KERR, K.E. (1967) Determination of retinal correspondence, multiple testing results and the depth of anomaly concept. *Arch. Ophthalmol.*, **77**, 206–213

FLOM, M.C., WEYMOUTH, F.W. and KAHNEMAN, D. (1963) Visual resolution and contour interaction. *J. Opt. Soc. Am.*, **53**, 1026–1032

GIBSON, H.W. (1955) *Textbook of Orthoptics*. London: Hatton Press Ltd

GINSBURG, A.P. (1980) A new contrast sensitivity test chart. *Am. J. Optom. Physiol. Opt.*, **61**, 403–407

GUIBOR, G.P. (1958) The practical use of atropine in the treatment of strabismus., In *Strabismus Ophthalmic Symposium*, edited by J. H. Allen, Vol. II. pp. 302–311 London: Henry Kimpton

HALLDÉN, U. (1952) Fusional phenomena in anomalous correspondence. *Acta Ophthalmol. Suppl.*, **37**, 5–93

HALLDÉN, U. (1957) An explanation of Haidinger's brushes. *Arch. Ophthalmol.*, **57**, 393–399

HELVESTON, E.M. and VON NOORDEN, S.K. (1967) Microtropia: a newly defined entity. *Arch. Ophthalmol.*, **78**, 272

HERON, G., DHOLAKIA, D., COLLINS, D.E. and McLAUGHLAN, H. (1985) Stereoscopic threshold in children and adults. *Am. J. Optom. Physiol. Opt.*, **62**, 505–515

HOGAN, R.B. AND LINFIELD, P.B. (1983) The effect of moderate doses of ethanol in heterophoria and other aspects of binocular vision. *Ophthal. Physiol. Opt.*, **3**, 21–31

JAMPOLSKY, A. (1964) Ocular deviations. In *International Ophthalmoscopy Clinics*, Vol. 4, No. 3. Boston: Little, Brown and Co.

JAMPOLSKY, A. (1968) Some anomalies of binocular vision. *First International Congress of Orthoptists*. London: H. Kimpton

JOSHUA, D.E. and BISHOP, P.O. (1970) Binocular single vision and depth discrimination. Receptive field disparities for central and peripheral vision and binocular interaction on peripheral single units in cat striate cortex. *Exp. Brain Res.*, **10**, 389–416

LANG, J. (1970) In *Strabismus '69*, pp. 160–164. London: Henry Kimpton

LANG, J. (1971) Binocular Amsler's charts. *Br. J. Ophthalmol.*, **55**, 284–285

LEIGH, R.J. and ZEE, D.S. (1983) *The Neurology of Eye Movements*. Philadelphia: F.A. Davis Company

LYLE, T.K. and BRIDGEMAN, G.J.O. (1959) *Worth and Chavasse's Squint*. London: Baillière, Tindall and Cox

LYLE, T.K. and WYBAR, K.C. (1967) *Practical Orthoptics in the Treatment of Squint*. London: H.H. Lewis and Co. Ltd

MALLETT, R.F.J. (1964) The investigation of heterophoria at near and a new fixation disparity technique. *Optician*, **148**, 547–551, 574–581

MALLETT, R.F.J. (1965) The phi phenomenon and anomalous retinal correspondence. *Optician*, **149**, 535–539

MALLETT, R.F.J. (1966) The investigation of oculomotor balance. *Ophthal. Opt.*, **6**, 586

MALLETT, R.F.J. (1969a) The sequelae of ocular muscle palsy. *Ophthal. Opt.*, **9**, 920–923

MALLETT, R.F.J. (1969) Binocular vision in strabismus *Ophthal. Opt.*, **9**, 812–824

MALLETT, R.F.J. (1970a) Anomalous retinal correspondence — the new outlook. *Ophthal. Opt.*, **10**, 606–624

MALLETT, R.F.J. (1970b) The Stanworth synoptiscope in the investigation and treatment of strabismus. *Ophthal. Opt.*, **10**, 556–573

MALLETT, R.F.J. (1973) Anomalous correspondence. *Br. J. Physiol. Opt.*, **28**, 1–10

MALLETT, R.F.J. (1975a) Neutral density filters in the diagnosis of sensory anomalies. *Ophthal. Opt.*, **15**, 533–535

MALLETT, R.F.J. (1975b) Using after-images in the investigation and treatment of strabismus. *Ophthal. Opt.*, **15**, 727–729

MALLETT, R.F.J. (1983) A new fixation disparity test and its applications. *Optician*, **186**, 11–15

MENDOLSON, G.A. (1983) The effect of red, white and green light on the degree of eccentric fixation and the morphoscopic and angular visual acuities in patients with strabismic amblyopia. City University, final year research project

MITCHELL, D.W.A. (1953) Investigating binocular difficulties. *Br. J. Physiol. Opt.*, **10**, 1–14

MORGAN, M.W. (1960) Anomalies of the neuromuscular system of the aging patient and their correction. In *Vision of the Aging Patient*. Philadelphia: Chilton Company

MURPHY, D. (1968) An examination of suppression. *Optician*, **156**, 4055, 625–627

PARKS, M.M. (1975) *Ocular Motility and Strabismus*. Maryland: Harper and Row

PETTIGREW, J.D., NIKARA, T. and BISHOP, P.O. (1968a) Responses to moving slits by single units in cat striate cortex. *Exp. Brain Res.*, **6**, 373–390

PETTIGREW, J.D., NIKARA, T. and BISHOP, P.O. (1968b) Binocular interaction on single units in cat striate cortex: simultaneous stimulation by single moving slit with receptive fields in correspondence. *Exp. Brain Res.* **6**, 391–410

PICKWELL, L.D. and HAMPSHIRE, R. (1981) The significance of inadequate convergence. *Ophthal. Physiol. Opt.*, **1**, 13–18

PIGASSOU, R. (1968) Examination of binocular vision in polarized light. *International Strabismus Symposium*. Basel: S. Karger

PRATT-JOHNSON, J.A. and TILLSON, G. (1984) Suppression in strabismus — an update. *Br. J. Ophthalmol.*, **68**, 174–178

SCOBEE, R. (1952) *The Oculorotary Muscles*. London: Henry Kimpton

SHEEDY, J.E. (1980) Fixation disparity and heterophoria. *Am. J. Optom. Physiol. Opt.*, **57**, 632–639

SPENCER, J.A. (1967) An investigation of Maxwell's spot. *Br. J. Physiol. Opt.*, **24**, 103–147

STANWORTH, A. (1958) Modified major amblyoscope. *Br. J. Ophthalmol.*, **42**, 270–287

STANWORTH, A. and NAYLOR, E.J. (1950) Haidinger's brushes and the retinal receptors. *Br. J. Ophthalmol.*, **34**, 282–291

SWAN, K.C. (1965) False projection in comitant strabismus. *Arch. Ophthalmol.*, **73**, 189–197

TURVILLE, A.E. (1946) *An Outline of Infinity Balance*. London: Raphaels Ltd

TURVILLE, A.E. (1962) Clinical techniques with the T.D.B. mirror. *Transactions of the International Ophthalmological Congress*, pp. 434–442. London: Crosby Lockwood and Son

VON NOORDEN, G.K. (1970a) Etiology and pathogenesis of fixation anomalies in strabismus. *Am. J. Ophthalmol.*, **69**, 210–222, 223–227, 228–235, 236–245

VON NOORDEN, G.K. (1970b) The phase-difference haploscope. *Am. Orthopt. J.* 7–11.

VON NOORDEN, G.K. and BURIAN, H.M. (1959) Behaviour of visual acuity with and without neutral density filter. *Arch. Ophthalmol.*, **61**, 533–535

VON NOORDEN, G.K. and LEFFLER, M.B. (1966) Visual acuity in strabismic and amblyopia under monocular and binocular conditions. *Arch. Ophthalmol.*, **76**, 172–177

VON NOORDEN, G.K., AWAYA, S. and ROMANO, P.E. (1971) Past pointing in paralytic strabismus. *Am. J. Ophthalmol.*, **71**, 27–33

WILDERSOET, C.F. and CAMERON, K.D. (1985) The effect of illumination and foveal fusion lock on clinical fixation disparity measurements with the Sheedy disparometer. *Ophthal. Physiol. Opt.*, **5**, 171–178

16

The management of binocular vision anomalies

Ronald Mallett

Having subjected the patient to a suitable battery of tests selected from those described in the previous chapter, it is now necessary to consider the appropriate action to take.

Some patients will need to be referred for medical investigation and possible treatment. These include:

(1) Patients with known or suspected ocular or neurological pathology, whether or nor associated with the binocular anomaly.
(2) Suspected systemic diseases, unless already under investigation, e.g. hypertension.
(3) Patients in probable need of psychiatric assistance.
(4) Any binocular anomaly with properties which cannot be adequately treated by the practitioner and which are considered to require attention. Large angles of strabismus outside the scope of refractive and orthoptic treatment, long-standing decompensating incomitancies which cannot be given comfort with prisms, and deviations which are unlikely to respond because of lack of patient or parental cooperation.

Many strabismic conditions are basically quite unsuitable for orthoptic treatment. These include, Duane's retraction syndrome, strabismus fixus (very rare), the superior oblique tendon sheath syndrome of Brown, Franceschetti-type concomitant esotropia and almost all incomitant deviations. These and other orthoptically intractable conditions are discussed in most contemporary texts on binocular anomalies (Burian and von Noorden, 1974).

Other patients may need attention, but only to their ametropia and perhaps to amblyopia when a microtropia is present. It is non-productive for the patient and practitioner to relentlessly pursue a very small and inconspicuous microtropia with well established harmonic anomalous retinal correspon-

dence (harmonious ARC) and consequently reasonable binocularity. It must be understood that perfection is not always achievable or indeed necessary in this imperfect world. The following criteria should be the *minimum* objective of any therapy:

(1) The patient should be free from all subjective symptoms. Any residual heterophoria should be compensated, or rendered so, with lenses.
(2) Cosmetic appearance should be acceptable to the patient and/or parents.
(3) The visual acuity should be improved to as near normal as possible with current available therapies.
(4) Binocular vision should be of a reasonable standard. If a residual strabismus is present, then a well established harmonious ARC with motor fusion and stereopsis would be acceptable.
(5) Any refractive aid, such as a bifocal addition for near or concave addition to control divergent anomalies, should have been dispensed with at the conclusion of the treatment. Ideally, the correction for ametropia should be dispensed with, but this is by no means always possible if the first few conditions are to be met in full.

There are many differing views on the management of binocular anomalies and opinions are usually strongly coloured by the background of the practitioner concerned — thus the ophthalmologist will often lean towards surgical adjustment whereas the optometric practitioner will rely upon refractive and orthoptic therapy. As several professions are engaged in helping strabismic and heterophoric patients, and each will naturally pursue the type of treatment dictated by his training, it behoves each practitioner to ensure that he has respect for the opinion of those who would advocate alternative procedures, always remembering that each discipline is ideally suited to a limited number of cases and yet may be quite unsuited to others. As this summary is part of an optometric text, only limited attention will be given to non-optometric forms of management.

Orthoptic treatment can be tedious and time consuming, and always requires strong patient and, where applicable, parent motivation. Often, therefore, refractive therapy, sometimes supported by relieving or exercising prisms will be preferable. If there is any significant ametropia necessitating the wearing of spectacles it would always seem desirable to modify the refractive correction, where possible, to remedy the binocular dysfunction and obviate the need for orthoptic exercises. In any event, the practitioner should first look to refractive treatment as an initial line of defence:

(1) To provide the best possible visual acuity and freedom from refraction-induced asthenopia.
(2) By carefully neutralizing anisometropia to form the necessary sensory substrate for the developing of fusion and stereopsis.
(3) To reduce the degree of motor imbalance.

Principles of refractive management

The time-honoured recipe of maximum convex (or minimum concave) power in convergent deviations and maximum concave (or minimum convex) power in divergent anomalies, i.e. a full correction of the ametropia taking into account any latent errors revealed by cycloplegia, is all that is required in many cases, particularly Donders' squints. Where the anomaly is strabismic, an objective uniocular cover test is used to determine the effect of lenses on the deviation, whereas in heterophoria this should, wherever possible, be supported by fixation disparity tests to confirm compensation of any residual imbalance. Anisometropia and astigmatism should be corrected in full if there is to be any attempt to achieve a refined degree of binocularity or if amblyopia is subsequently to be treated. Full prescriptions of this nature, however, may not be well tolerated by older patients and some modification will be desirable, though this will probably ensure a reduced level of sensory improvement. If the anisometropia is marked, correction in the form of contact lenses will overcome the problem of induced vertical prism with spectacle lenses on vertical gaze, thus limiting the resulting hyperphoria or hypertropia which is always a hindrance to good binocular vision and, in addition, frequently minimizes the difference in retinal image size. Contact lenses are especially useful when any amblyopia present is of an anisometropic nature.

If a full refractive correction leaves a residual deviation, or perhaps induces one in the opposite direction, some modification will obviously be necessary. Further convex power cannot be added to a patient with a residual esotropia at distance — especially if cycloplegic findings have been used for the assessment, as this will cause blurring and in any event be counterproductive because attempted fusion will be more difficult. If the deviation is at near, on the other hand, the addition of further convex spheres (binocularly) frequently restores bifoveal fixation (in strabismus) or compensation (in heterophoria). It must be remembered that young children have short arms, so up to +4.00 D lens addition may be prescribed in these cases. For children (Burian, 1956), the lenses are best prescribed as large segment (e.g. executive) bifocals with the segment set high so that it is difficult to escape its use — if the top of the segment is level with the lower margin of the pupil when the eyes are in the primary position this requirement will be satisfied. The greater degree of esotropia or esophoria at near is often known as convergence excess and the effect of the additional convex power is due to the inhibiting effect of the convergence system by reducing the accommodative demand. In some cases — hypoaccommodative deviations — the excessive convergence is due to a low amplitude of accommodation, the vergence system being hyperactive in an effort to promote clear vision at near. Again, a convex addition will provide the necessary assistance and can be assessed with a near vision bichromatic chart and cover or fixation disparity test. In all cases where there is latent hypermetropia which is being corrected, the patient (or the parent) must be warned of the possibility of initial blur until accommodation relaxes. If a full hypermetropic correction induces a divergent imbalance it will obviously need to be reduced.

Patients with primary exotropia, and especially those with divergence excess (the deviation being greater at distance than at near), are frequently emmetropic, or nearly so. As long as the patient is in good health and has a good amplitude of accommodation, it is always worth investigating the action of concave lenses on the imbalance. A cover test is used in strabismus, fixation disparity tests in uncompensated exophoria or convergence insufficiency, always using small targets to activate the accommodation reflex. The minimum concave addition which will restore binocular fixation in strabismus or compensation in heterophoric conditions can be prescribed so long as the power is not excessive. In this respect, the amplitude of accommodation and age of the patient will be most important, children tolerating lenses up to −3.00 D very well in most cases. Older patients will obviously not tolerate any substantial minus power and the technique becomes less useful in patients of 25 years or older. It is even worth prescribing concave lenses in many cases where there is no apparent improvement in the consulting room as their salutary effect is not always immediate and spectacular reductions can often be seen after 3–6 months of constant wear. When divergence excess is being controlled with this technique, it may be that an uncompensated esophoria or esotropia is induced at near and must be relieved by a convex addition prescribed in bifocal form. The use of concave lenses has been recommended by many authors (e.g. Duke-Elder, 1973; Parks, 1975).

It is a general rule that lenses which achieve binocular fixation, or compensation of heterophoria, should be allowed to stabilize sensory binocularity for a *few years* and then should, wherever possible, be reduced in strength and eventually abandoned. This applies especially to concave overcorrection and convex near vision addition the former being necessary as the amplitude of accommodation declines. It is suggested that the reduction should be of the order of 0.50–0.75 D at 6-monthly intervals, but the actual amount will always be dependent upon the stability of binocular vision at the time.

Treatment of amblyopia

General principles

An attempt to improve the visual acuity in amblyopia is always worthwhile as it gives the patient the security of a second 'good eye'. Contrary to much uninformed opinion, there seems to be no reasonable upper limit to the treatment of strabismic amblyopia and several patients of 65 years or more have been successfully helped at the London Refraction Hospital — these elderly patients have lost the central vision in their dominant eye due to maculopathy and have been left to cope with just their amblyopic eye. It is not always possible to restore normal visual acuity but an improvement from, say, 6/60 to 6/12 is obviously advantageous to the patient; it is true that a unilateral maculopathy provides a natural form of occlusion, but improvement in visual acuity of the amblyopic eye is slow and hence psychologically disturbing. The present author's views on the age during which visual improvement is possible are now becoming more widely accepted (e.g. Birnbaum, Koslowe and Sanet, 1977).

Another often expressed and disturbing objection to amblyopia treatment in the older patient is the possibility of inducing diplopia. Using the non-occlusive techniques advocated in this chapter, the author has never precipitated diplopia as a result of treating thousands of amblyopic eyes.

The principal cause of diplopia in amblyopia treatment appears to result from an increased angle of strabismus induced by long periods of occlusion

— any well established harmonious ARC will then appear unharmonious (assuming the angle of anomaly remains constant) with resulting diplopia. It is the change in angle and not any improvement in visual acuity which is responsible. Reduced to basic principles, the result of restoring normal visual acuity is to substitute an alternating deviation for a unilateral one, and any existing suppression or harmonious ARC will continue to protect the patient by maintaining haplopia. It must not be assumed, of course, that diplopia can *never* occur, but it cannot be considered a significant hazard with a properly organized treatment regimen.

The management of amblyopia in the young must be undertaken in the light of recent work investigating the normal development of visual acuity from birth through to maturity. The classic authorities usually quoted a very low visual acuity at birth (as low as 6/720) improving to the adulthood level of 6/6 at about 5–6 years. The modern concept is that the resolution at birth is much higher. Dayton *et al.* (1964) found 6/45 using an optokinetic nystagmus/electro-oculography technique, developing to maturity (6/6) at 5–6 months (Marg *et al.*, 1976, using visual-evoked cortical potential). Other studies, using alternative procedures have confirmed these findings. Dobson and Teller (1978) used preferential viewing to find a similar level of resolution at birth and extrapolation of their data suggests an acuity of 6/6 at 6.5–7.5 months. An excellent review of the development of vision has been given by Reading (1983) (*see also* Chapter 11).

The development of visual acuity seems to be intimately related to the sensitive or critical period in the Rhesus monkey (von Noorden, 1971) and clinical experience suggests that there is no reason to suppose that the human is significantly different in this respect. This hypothesis implies that any strabismus or visual deprivation during the first 6 months of life will lead to a partially irreversible retardation of development and subsequent loss of vision (amblyopia of arrest), whereas any interference with normal development after that age is likely to result in a more readily treatable amblyopia, especially if the embarrassment was of a strabismic nature. Even amblyopia resulting from esotropia introduced during the sensitive period (at 1 and 7 days of life) responded to some extent to occlusion of the fixating eye; deprivation of form vision during the first 3 months of the monkeys' life, however, resulted in permanent visual impairment. These findings reflect the generally high success rate of strabismic amblyopia treatment compared with the very much more modest results obtained from visual stimulus deprivation. It is interesting to see that von Noorden's monkeys with *early* induced esotropia all developed amblyopia; his exotropic monkeys, all of which alternated, were found to achieve normal adult visual acuity and this presumably resulted from the alternate use of each fovea to receive, at some time, the image of the most interesting or important aspect of the visual field. It would therefore appear that the prerequisite for the normal development of visual acuity during the sensitive period is the ability of the eye to image the most potent and attractive object on its fovea. Amblyopia is *not*, therefore, a sensory adaptation to overcome diplopia, although this role is often wrongly attributed to it — as with alternating squinters who have good visual acuity in both eyes, diplopia in unilateral squinters with amblyopia is eliminated by ARC or suppression mechanisms.

When the effect of the refractive correction has been evaluated, the question of treatment of the sensory anomalies should be considered. Most practitioners would deal with the amblyopia as a first step and then proceed to the binocular sensory anomalies before finally developing the appropriate fusional amplitude and consolidating binocularity.

Occlusion techniques

Occlusion is a widely practised technique for treating strabismic amblyopia. It is cheap, simple and effective but is really only suitable for pre-school children and a few selected patients from older age groups. It is obvious that it has a detrimental cosmetic effect which can make adherence to the advised wearing times unlikely, many children finding occlusion psychologically traumatic. It must also be realized that occlusion will interfere with education and, in the older person, be an economic embarrassment as well as subjecting the patient to certain physical risks if the visual acuity of the amblyopic eye is very low. For these reasons occlusion is often *partial* — the vision in the fixating eye being reduced with a translucent material (e.g. Scotch tape, Fablon) or with a fogging lens. A plus spherical lens is often employed but this only blurs distance vision and will actually assist that at near — a cylindrical lens (prescribed with axis oblique) will overcome this problem but tends to create another in that the induced astigmatism in the dominant eye is likely to cause asthenopic symptoms.

Although *constant* occlusion during all waking hours is by far the most effective form of the technique, it is often not attempted due to the economic and educational reasons already mentioned and reduced periods are substituted — *part time* or *intermittent* occlusion. However, some of the shorter times suggested for this purpose are quite inadequate and a minimum period of some 2–3 hours each day is recommended. It is usual to confine occlusion to the fixating eye (*direct* occlusion) but some authorities (e.g. Aust, 1970) recommend patching the amblyopic eye (*indirect* occlusion) for several weeks prior to the pleoptic procedures as a 'softening' process — it is doubtful, though, if this has any significant effect on the course of the treatment. In very young children it is important to *alternate* the occlusion with the maximum patching time being devoted to the fixating eye, say in a ratio of 2:1. This is especially important in the 'sensitive period' and during this time, in particular, it is probably desirable to leave both eyes exposed to visual stimuli for at least part of the day, especially if refractive correction or surgery has restored (as far as can be judged) bifoveal vision, so that development of the binocular cells can proceed in a normal fashion.

Various forms of *segmented* occlusion have been suggested as forcing alternate fixation — the upper part of one lens with the lower part of the other, for example — but are often ineffective in that the child quickly learns to adapt his head posture in order to obtain foveal vision with his dominant eye.

Whatever form of occlusion is adopted it will only succeed if the patient is encouraged to use the amblyopic eye to the full. Patients should therefore be encouraged to read, paint, draw, view television, play video games and indulge in any other visually attractive pursuit applicable to age and intelligence.

From a physiological point of view the one major contraindication to direct occlusion is when the monocular localization is abnormal and now originates from the eccentric rather than the foveal area. Occlusion in these cases would merely strengthen the dominance of the eccentrically fixating area and worsen rather than help the amblyopia.

Effective aids to occlusion

Part time occlusion of the sound eye with a red filter before the amblyopic eye is a useful form of therapy (Brinker and Katz, 1963). A Wratten filter No. 92 was originally recommended but is expensive and fragile — more robust substitutes include Primary Red (Lee filters), Ruby Kodaloid and Celastoid POL 15. The patient is encouraged to read, watch black and white television etc. This technique can be used at any age and 2 or 3 hours each day in the privacy of the patient's home will be acceptable in most cases. This treatment must not be confused with a non-occlusive red filter technique suggested by Humphriss (1937) — a deep red filter is used before the *sound* eye and will accordingly distort the colours of the environment by selective absorption; the patient is encouraged to see everything in its known natural colour. To do this the patient must use the amblyopic eye. The patient should wear the filter when watching colour television and when eating.

Pigassou and Garipuy (1967) have used constant direct occlusion with an 'inverse' prism (i.e. base-in with nasal eccentric fixation) before the amblyopic eye. The prism strength should be slightly in excess of the angular subtense of the eccentric fixation but with a minimum of 6 Δ and a maximum of 20 Δ. This places the fovea in a 'straight ahead' position. The localization will then be to the temporal side when nasal eccentric fixation is present — to touch an object the hand position must be modified so that it coincides with the actual position of the object being viewed, i.e. in the direction 'straight ahead' of the fovea. The efficacy of this procedure has been confirmed by Nawratzki and Oliver (1971).

Amblyopia associated with microtropia can be managed by prescribing a 5 Δ base-in prism before the squinting eye, with suffcent partial occlusion of the fixating eye to reduce its visual acuity (by two lines) below that of its fellow (Rubin, 1965).

Active methods of treatment

After-image treatment

An after-image 'transfer' treatment for strabismic amblyopia has been described by Caloroso (1972). A vertical flash stimulus is presented to the fovea of the sound eye which is then covered. If a letter or other test symbol is then viewed, using the eccentric region of the amblyopic eye, the resulting after-image will appear to be to one side as though localized from the fovea. The patient is instructed to move the eye so that the after-image appears to be in line with the letter which, at this moment, will usually appear clearer and can thus be identified. When isolated, 6/6 letters can be resolved, several targets are presented simultaneously to make evident the 'crowding phenomenon' and the procedure repeated until a maximum morphoscopic visual acuity is attained. This is an effective method for dealing with strabismic amblyopia; a session of 30–40 minutes once or twice weekly is usually quite adequate. The only contraindication is the presence of *firmly* entrenched ARC — the lesser degrees do not interfere and some 80% of all strabismic amblyopes (of suitable age) will be found to be eligible for treatment (Mallett, 1975).

CAM stimulator

The CAM (Cambridge) vision stimulator consists of a series of discs with square wave gratings of varying spatial frequency which are rotated in turn before the amblyopic eye, the patient drawing and tracing on a superimposed transparent slide (Campbell *et al.*, 1978). Variable results of the efficacy of the treatment have been reported in the literature and it is the experience of the present author that anisometropic amblyopia is much more likely to succumb than the strabismic variety — a view confirmed by W. M Ludlam (personal communication).

Intermittent photic stimulation

Intermittent photic stimulation (IPS) in a desk unit (for home or consulting room use) or a synoptophore employs a series of slides with varying detail designed to stimulate different types of receptive field. The red background flashes at a frequency of 4 Hz. The detail must be identified, counted (where applicable) and in the case of the desk unit (*Figure 16.1*) traced (Mallett, 1969, 1985). Used for periods of some 30 minutes, once or twice weekly, it can be an effective technique for dealing with many cases of strabismic amblyopia and has the advantage of requiring minimal supervision.

Pleoptics

Pleoptic therapy, as it is usually understood, is based upon the procedures advanced by Cüppers and Bangerter. In recent times these procedures have suffered neglect due to the very disappointing results often achieved. The technique is really only suitable for patients with deep amblyopia and marked degrees of eccentric fixation, smaller degrees of eccentricity not permitting the precise alignment of the discs from the Euthyscope (Cüppers) or pleoptophore (Bangerter) over the foveal region without additionally masking the eccentric area. If a careful selection of suitable patients is made, these techniques have a definite and valuable place in the orthoptic armoury. It must be said, however, that the equipment is expensive, the techniques time consuming and tedious, and mydriasis of the pupil of the amblyopic eye obligatory. Although it is doubtful if inverse occlusion contributes any useful function in the months before pleoptic treatment, it is probably advisable to use this form of patching between treatment sessions to prevent regression. A suitable patient would need to be cooperative, have a visual acuity of below 6/60 with abnormal localization from the fovea and with at least 2° eccentric fixation. Fortunately, early screening techniques ensure that few patients require this intense form of treatment.

In the Cüppers technique the eyes are properly positioned with an object fixated by the dominant eye through a mirror mounted on a headband. An opaque spot is placed over the fovea, and the surrounding area then 'bleached' with an annulus of light. The centre of the resulting annular after-image, which the patient must see in its negative form, is superimposed on symbols of diminishing size which have to be properly localized and then identified.

The Bangerter method is a passive one — after the retinal bleaching of the annulus around the fovea and inclusive of the eccentric area, the pleoptophore is used to stimulate the fovea with a succession of brief light flashes. Once normal foveal

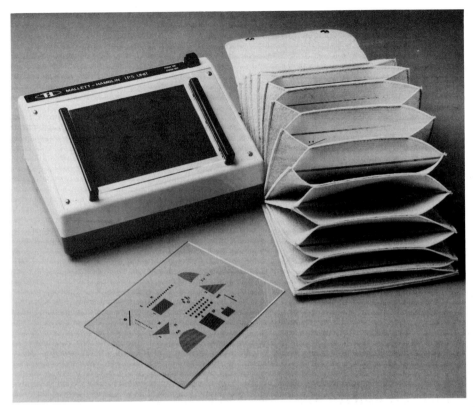

Figure 16.1 The Mallett–Hamblin IPS unit. Each of the eleven slides is designed to stimulate the different types of receptive fields, overcome the 'crowding phenomenon' and promote steady central fixation. The red background flashes at 3–5 Hz. (By kind permission of Keeler Ltd)

localization is restored, the centrophore — a device with a rotating spiral and with the facility to induce Haidinger's brushes — is used to stabilize fixation. Various ancillary instruments (e.g. coordinating localizator) to improve hand–eye localization are also employed by both Bangerter and Cüppers. Although the continental procedure is to hospitalize the patients and pursue treatment on a daily basis, it is often quite adequate (at the London Refraction Hospital) to give a single treatment session each week, with considerable benefit.

A useful overview of pleoptics is given by Aust (1970).

Miscellaneous techniques

Entoptic phenomena (Haidinger's brushes and Maxwell's spot) provide a marker for the fovea of the amblyopic eye and assist in training normal foveal fixation. Pickwell (1984) describes a method for treating amblyopia with physiological diplopia exercises, but there are limitations in that the angle of squint must be small (under 12 Δ) and the patient (and parent) perceptive and cooperative; the starting visual acuity should be 6/24 or better.

Conclusions

Eccentric fixation must not be regarded as being an isolated clinical condition — it is merely one of the clinical signatures of strabismic amblyopia. As treatment progresses, it will be found that every measurable improvement in visual acuity is accompanied by a reduction in the degree of eccentric fixation. If normal visual acuity is restored, fixation will then be central. The time factor is very variable and seems to be more directly related to the enthusiasm and perseverance of the patient than to the age at which treatment is commenced.

Management of non-strabismic amblyopia

It will be necessary to refer certain types of amblyopia such as those with a toxic or nutritional background as well as the more profound hysterical cases as these all need specialized investigation and treatment quite outside the scope of optometric care, hence the need for accurate differential diagnosis in the investigative procedures.

'Congenital' or idiopathic amblyopia sometimes responds to IPS or CAM therapy, but the results of such treatment are generally unsatisfactory. A full refractive correction can only help such patients.

Refractive amblyopia should be managed by the accurate neutralization of all ametropia, and in particular anisometropia. Constant wear of the correction is advocated, especially during childhood, as any improvement in visual acuity is dependent on the formation of clear retinal images. This should obviously be undertaken at the earliest opportunity and recent developments in contact lens practice should encourage the fitting of contact lenses to young patients with marked anisometropia or high degrees of bilateral ametropia. Although occlusion has been recommended for the treatment of anisometropic amblyopia, it is doubtful if this provides any substantial benefit and, where visual improvement does occur, it is difficult to isolate the proven salutary effects of coincident refractive correction. If line stimuli are used with IPS treatment, a modest improvement in vision can sometimes be obtained; the CAM unit, employing a rotating linear grid, is also sometimes helpful but neither technique offers much hope of spectacular improvement. Contrary to the suggestion of McCormick (1978), transfer afterimage treatment has no place in the management of anisometropic amblyopia. Fixation is always central (albeit unsteady) in these cases and it is apparent from the clinical data presented that the anisometropic element was contaminated by strabismic amblyopia and it was the latter component that was treated.

Finally, in this brief review of non-strabismic amblyopia it must always be remembered that amblyopia often exists in mixed form — in particular strabismic and anisometropic variants frequently coexist in unilateral esotropia.

Management of anomalous retinal correspondence

Although anomalous retinal correspondence (ARC) is a frequent accompaniment of strabismus (Mallett, 1970a; Bagolini, 1974), it can frequently be ignored in the mangement of strabismus. Mallett (1970a) has described a classification of ARC which will assist the clinician — a slightly modified scheme is presented here:

(1) Harmonious ARC — this is plastic in nature with co-variation and fulfilment of the function of an antidiplopia mechanism but without conferment of the benefits of any substantial degree of binocularity. The angle of squint is likely to be fluid and often fairly large; there may be uncorrected anisometropia and the onset of the strabismus is unlikely to have been particularly early. This type of ARC is detected only with the more sensitive tests such as the Bagolini striated lens, the modified fixation disparity test, the Stanworth Synoptiscope and the subjective cover test. As this type of ARC is an antidiplopia defensive system, it does not operate in conditions where diplopia is impossible or asymptomatic. The somewhat unusual visual conditions provided by the stereoscope and vectograms used to develop fusional amplitudes seem to fulfil these requirements and attempts to develop the reserves can proceed without interference, the patient utilizing the innate normally corresponding receptive fields under the exercising conditions.

(2) Strabismus of more modest angles, especially those which are relatively stable and where the retinal images are of similar clarity, tends to lead to harmonious ARC of a more profound nature. The age of onset is usually early and because of this a reasonable standard of quasi-binocularity may have developed. It is usually possible to measure fusional amplitudes, the patient employing anomalously corresponding receptive fields, and a useful degree of stereoacuity. The anomalous relationship between the 'retinas' is well established and these patients, together with those in group 3, will develop unharmonious ARC with consequent diplopia if the objective angle is suddenly increased — the most common incident creating this unhappy situation is a blow to the head, though some cases are caused by a recent virus infection. Patients with group 2 ARC will display anomalous correspondence on most tests, the major exception being after-images (positive) with the eyes closed. Using quantitative procedures (Bagolini lenses or MFDT with neutral density filter bars), the abnormal binocularity will generally survive the embarrassment created by filters up to a density of some 1.2 or 1.5 log units or more. These cases often require treatment as they tend to be cosmetically poor and the ARC is sufficiently entrenched to persist in a stereoscope environment. It must, therefore, be weakened or even eliminated before development of the fusional amplitudes can proceed.

(3) The most intense and, in many instances, immutable cases of ARC are found in strabismus of small and stable angles with an early age of onset. The quasi-binocularity is often of a high order although stereoacuity is often low in the von Noorden type of microtropia due to a dense suppression area extending between the fovea (of the squinting eye) and the 'zero point measure'. With this one exception, these squinters enjoy a sufficiently high degree of binocularity to enable them to survive most visual activities without embarrassment. As the deviation is usually cosmetically perfectly acceptable, there

seems to be little point in disturbing the comfortable and effective sensory binocular adaptation which has developed, and the only treatment indicated in most cases is for any amblyopia which may be present.

(4) Unharmonious ARC develops from the harmonious variety (groups 2 and 3) as previously described. The anomalous association is always fairly intense and diplopia invariably present. The chief concern of the clinician will be to eliminate the diplopia.

Before any therapy for harmonious ARC is undertaken it must be understood that restoration of normal retinal correspondence is likely to result in diplopia. There must, therefore, be considerable confidence that the objective deviation can in fact be eliminated by suitable procedures whether these be orthoptic or surgical or a combination of each. This difficulty can often be overcome by merely weakening the intensity of the ARC so that it does not interfere with the development of the fusional amplitude but still acts as an antidiplopia mechanism.

Treatment of harmonious ARC is best undertaken by prismatic techniques, wherever possible. Such techniques depend upon the displacement of the retinal image in the squinting eye so that it stimulates receptive fields which do not correspond (i.e. localize in the same visual direction) with those of the fixating eye. Thus a vertical prism of 6–8 Δ is effective (Mallett, 1979) as is the saturation technique of Bérard (1971) who makes use of the adaptation of base-out prisms in esotropia and saturates the deviation until no further compensation (i.e. fusional movement) can occur — both techniques work but are poor cosmetically in view of the further apparent deviation of the eye behind the prism and, in the latter case, because the prism must often be of very considerable strength to overcome the fusional movements. An improved technique was described by Mallett (1979) who prescribes base-in prisms in esotropia to deflect the image — this actually improves the cosmesis as the eye appears to be more temporal (i.e. less convergent) than before and a much weaker prism is required; this prism is of the order 10–15 Δ base-in, and is prescribed empirically as this power is beyond the divergent fusional capacity of almost all convergent squinters.

Methods of management

If orthoptic procedures are to be undertaken, there is a considerable choice available: bilateral macular massage, kinetic biretinal stimulation, Pemberton's proprioceptive reorientation technique and many

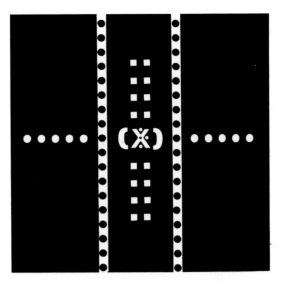

Figure 16.2 The Mallett slide for treating deeply established anomalous retinal correspondence and suppression. The synoptophore tubes are set at the patient's objective angle and the two slides (identical apart from small monocular control marks) are flashed *alternately* at 4 Hz

others (Gibson, 1955; Lyle and Wybar, 1967). These are all slow, demand haploscopic instrumentation and often make little inroad into the sensory anomaly. Perhaps the best way is to use intermittent alternating photopic stimulation in a synoptophore with suitable slides (*Figure 16.2*) set at the objective angle. The targets are flashed at 4 Hz for 30–50 minutes for one or two sessions each week. Free space stimulation with the Stanworth synoptiscope is also possible (Mallett, 1970b; Mallett and Reading, 1971). Lavat's diplopia technique has its advocates and is described by Hugonnier and Clayette-Hugonnier (1969).

Unharmonious ARC

The treatment should be directed towards the elimination of the diplopia. Prisms are sometimes helpful and should be assessed with as little disturbance to the motor anomaly as possible (i.e. using Bagolini lenses to identify the image rather than covering). The vergence system is very labile in many of the patients, however, and prism adaptation is common. Surgical correction to restore the original angle should help, as may hypnosis by a practitioner skilled in eye care and hypnosis, teaching the patient to ignore the unwanted image belonging to the squinting eye. Blurring the image in the squinting eye with a high-powered lens should, theoretically, help but seldom does so in practice.

Management of suppression in strabismus

Suppression in the squinting eye occurs mostly in the larger angles of squint, often unstable in angle and frequently accompanied by anisometropia which has not been corrected in the formative years.

Prismatic treatment is sometimes effective and involves the prescription of prisms which *exactly* neutralize the objective angle. It seems that prism adaptation still occurs in many cases even though the patient is apparently substantially monocular and it may be that the prisms do restore binocularity at a level which the brain rejects and a further deviation develops — a form of horror fusionis, sometimes called evasion squint.

Orthoptic procedures include bilateral stimulation of the maculas using some sort of haploscope or stereoscope, an attempt to induce diplopia using a red glass before one eye when viewing a light (alternate covering is helpful here) and alternating photic stimulation at 4 Hz as described above for treating ARC.

Development of the fusional amplitudes

This is best undertaken as a home exercise involving some three periods, of 15 minutes training each day, the best results being achieved when the patient is fresh, alert and able to concentrate on the task. Care should be taken to exercise the amplitude at the required distance, i.e. with accommodation relaxed for distance imbalances and with a demand of 3 D or so for near anomalies. The lateral fusional amplitudes are easily expanded in most cases, the negative amplitude being developed in convergent deviation and the positive amplitude in the divergent variety. Vertical fusional amplitudes are not easily increased and this form of treatment in hyperphoria is seldom undertaken.

Home instrumentation for fusional amplitude training includes the Brewster–Holmes stereoscope which can be used with any of innumerable stereograms available. Recommended cards are the Bradford series (C and E cards in particular), Wells ONNE cards and, for heterophoric patients, the LRH cards (*Figure 16.3*) which present several targets of varying separation permitting jump vergence training. The patient should fuse targets of increasing separation to develop the negative fusional amplitude and with decreasing separation for the positive fusional amplitude. Generally speaking, large targets (preferably with information demanding a sense of depth perception for correct interpretation) should be employed to begin with and smaller targets substituted as progress is made and any suppression or rivalry diminishes. More expensive instrumentation, but employing very efficient polarized stimuli, is provided by the Bernel vec-

tograms. A cheaper, anaglyphic form of the treatment is less useful as the presentation of a red image to one eye and a green to the other is likely to induce 'retinal' rivalry.

Physiological diplopia techniques are employed by some to influence the motor deviation in strabismus. These techniques are derived from the suggestion by Gillie and Lindsay (1969) that squints are caused by 'aberrant vergence movements' resulting from an inability to cope with normal physiological diplopia. His theory is rather akin to that of an earlier worker van der Hoeve, who in 1922 introduced the term diplopia–phobia. Using a minimum of 'equipment' (e.g. string, light bulbs, pencils, thumbs etc.), the techniques are cheap, simple and popular with some clinicians. The result of this method for treating strabismus is the subject of considerable conflicting opinion at the present time. A full description of the various techniques employed has been given by Pickwell (1984).

Relative vergence can be trained by initially over- or underconverging on a pair of fusible letters placed a metre in front of the patient — a U and an inverted U are suitable for this exercise in which case U ⌒ ∩ or ∩ ⌒ U will be seen. Further separation of the targets demands increased vergence during which an attempt should be made to achieve and maintain clarity. Duplicate pages of large print can be substituted at a later stage (Meakin *et al.*, 1958).

Loose prisms can be lent to patients with precise instructions as to their correct orientation during use. Increasing base-in prism is helpful in exercising the negative fusional amplitude when reading, and is useful for esophoric patients; similarly, base-out prisms can be used for developing the positive fusional amplitudes in exophoria.

In the consulting room any major haploscope (synoptophore, variable prism stereoscope) can be used to develop the fusional amplitudes. Unless this can be done on a daily basis, however, progress will be slow and consequently frustrating for the patient. A prism bar can be used to induce 'jump' vergence as opposed to the rotary prism and similar devices which utilize a smoothly progressive change in fusional stimuli.

In heterophoric patients, the fusional amplitudes should be exercised until the patient does not exhibit any fixation disparity even with an adverse prism of 4 △ — this will be base-out in exophoria and base-in in esophoria.

Whatever method is employed, it is important that the fusional vergences be developed and stabilized with the eyes elevated and depressed as well as in the straight ahead position — this is particularly important in patients with marked V or A syndromes.

Where the relationship between accommodation and convergence appears to be 'tight', it can be

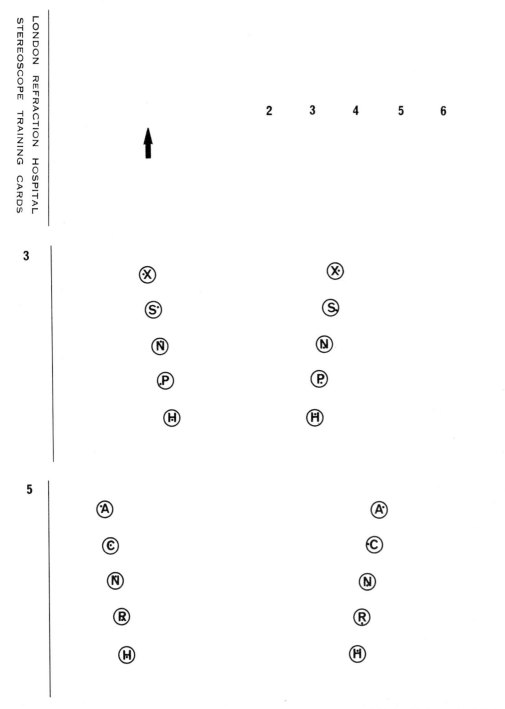

Figure 16.3 Cards 3 and 5 (together with the indicator card) of the London Refraction Hospital series for developing amplitudes of fusion. The six fusion cards cover a range of 48 △ with intervals of 2 △ when used in a Brewster–Holmes stereoscope fitted with 5 D lenses

successfully made more plastic by rapidly interchanging binocular plus and minus spheres (1 D is usually adequate), while the patient attempts to achieve clear vision — this will exercise the negative and positive relative accommodation, respectively. These functions can also be developed by fusing suitable targets in a Brewster–Holmes stereoscope and advancing or withdrawing the card — bringing the card towards the lenses, for example, will stimulate positive relative accommodation which will be helpful in esophoric conditions.

Management of incomitancy

All patients with newly acquired incomitancy should be referred so that the underlying pathology or trauma can be assessed and, if possible, treated. Unfortunately, during the months following the development of incomitancy secondary sequelae will usually develop which often render the ocular motor situation less amenable to treatment later on. Some incomitancies, however, are short lived and recovery is spontaneous and complete.

One method of limiting the contracture of the ipsilateral antagonist to the palsied muscle is to occlude the unaffected eye and prescribe prism before the eye with the paretic muscle — this technique, described by Guibor (1958), is most effective with abducent nerve palsies which require base-out prism. Occlusion is usually abandoned after 1 week and the strength of prism before the affected eye is reduced at the same time as the prism is introduced to the sound eye. The technique is not in common usage, possibly because patients need early attention to benefit from such procedures and this is not always forthcoming.

Elston and Lee (1985) have used injections of botulinum toxin into the ipsilateral antagonist of the palsied muscle with encouraging results. The induced palsy of the contracted muscle gradually diminishes, with a good binocular field and sensory binocular function as a result. This technique appears to be especially valuable, as it does not require immediate instigation, indeed a period of 6 months is allowed to pass by for any spontaneous recovery to take place, before the toxin is used.

Cases of old incomitancy that are asymptomatic are best left alone. Those with symptoms can sometimes be helped with prisms generally prescribed with the patient maintaining any anomalous head posture which is felt to be comfortable. An empirical approach tends to be the rule as any prismatic aid is inevitably a compromise with undercorrection occurring in some parts of the motor field, overcorrection in others. In some cases with a relatively mild anomaly, a fixation disparity unit moved to different parts of the motor field is helpful in assessing the optimum strength of prism. Strips of Fresnel prism are sometimes helpful to provide increasing prismatic power in the field of action of the affected muscle. Patients who experience persistent diplopia, not alleviated by prisms, may require surgery or hypnosis or an occluding correct lens.

Management of gaze anomalies

Many gaze anomalies, if they are not too marked, cause no discomfort and, indeed, the patient is often unaware of their presence because compensation by depression or elevation of the chin in a vertical anomaly or a turn of the head when lateral gaze is affected, is quite common. Generally, difficulty with downward gaze is most disabling and may sometimes be aided by strong base-down prisms before both eyes, although propioceptive and postural adjustments can be disturbing, in particular association between hand and eye. Prisms with the base prescribed in the same direction before each eye are also of value in lateral gaze anomalies. All such prescriptions for prisms must be assessed empirically. With the exception of the physiological restriction of upward gaze occurring as a natural event and associated with ageing, gaze anomalies must be regarded as having a pathological or traumatic basis, so prismatic aids would be considered only when appropriate medical investigations and treatment had been undertaken.

Pharmacological treatment of strabismus

At one time the local use of atropine (a muscarinic receptor blocking agent) was widely advocated for treating the motor aspect of convergent strabismus (e.g. Guibor, 1958). While it did have a beneficial effect in some cases, these were in a minority; perhaps incorrect administration by the parent or failure to combine its use with bifocal lenses to enable clear near vision to be undertaken was responsible. By paralysing accommodation it was assumed that convergence would similarly be inhibited because of synergy of the two functions. Atropine has also been used as a form of amblyopia treatment. The drug is instilled in the eye with the better visual acuity making accommodation in this eye impossible and so forcing the squinting eye to be used for near vision.

Cholinesterase inhibitors have replaced atropine in most strabismus clinics, and appear to function by potentiating neuromuscular transmission and thereby reducing the innervation for accommodation (Chapter 28); this is aided by the small pupils which also allow a considerable depth of focus (and hence depth of field) with a lesser requirement for precise accommodation. The diminished centrally induced innervation for accommodation will, in turn, tend to inhibit convergence. Only the more potent miotics

— Phospholine Iodide (echothiophate) and diiso-propylfluorophosphonate (Dyflos or DFP) — achieve the desired effect. Some practitioners, and especially those in Europe, use a miotic in one eye and atropine in the other.

Various drugs have been considered for systemic administration but almost all have been rejected for their adverse pharmacological or social effects (e.g. alcohol). Galin, Kwitko and Restripo (1971) used diphenylhydantoin (Epanutin) which reduced the angle in convergent strabismus and also reduced the AC/A ratio — a surprising result as the drug induces a mild paresis of accommodation which should, in turn, require *more* convergence to bring about adequate ciliary contraction for clear near vision.

Management of heterophoria

It must be understood that heterophoria will only require attention when suitable tests have shown that there is an uncompensated element present. It can be dealt with in several different ways:

Orthoptic exercises

Orthoptic exercises are aimed at developing the fusional reserve opposing the heterophoria — the negative reserve in esophoria, for example. This technique is normally confined to patients in good health, who are not presbyopic and who have the time and enthusiasm to spend 30–40 minutes each day performing the necessary exercises. There is obviously a lower age limit at which cooperation, perseverance and attention will be too limited. Most practitioners would only treat the lateral and torsional imbalances in this way as the vertical fusional amplitudes are not easily developed — Robertson and Kuhn (1985), however, have found that some hyperphoric imbalances can be compensated by this method.

Exercising prisms

These can be useful in developing the lateral fusional reserves and are especially useful in esophoria — a 4–6 △ base-in prism is usually satisfactory for near imbalances and a weaker prism (2–4 △) for distance. A similar technique, but using base-out prism, is not usually so effective in exophoria. An advantage of prescribing exercising lenses is that they are not demanding of the patient's time or ability to concentrate.

The prism can be temporarily incorporated in the patient's spectacles, or in Fresnel form, or loose prisms can be taped over existing correcting lenses.

Spherical lenses

The prescription of binocularly applied convex lenses in esophoria, concave in exophoria, should have a prominent place in the practitioner's armoury. The indications for this form of management have been reviewed under Principles of refractive management. It is the relative accommodation which is influenced by binocular spherical additions, the position of the visual axes remaining unchanged for a given fixation distance.

Relieving prisms

Relieving prisms will relieve the symptoms of uncompensated heterophoria and constitute a satisfactory form of management for many patients. The often expressed view that they will exacerbate the imbalance because of prism adaptation is quite unfounded in all but the most unusual case. Some patients do, of course, require prisms of increasing strength as time passes, but this is usually related to periods of fatigue or poor health or with certain progressive paretic imbalances. Others can be compensated with weaker prisms at a later date or even abandon them altogether — in this respect the prisms seem to 'rest' the ocular motor system and restore its normal vigour. Prism adaptation, when it occurs, is found when part or all of a *compensated* heterophoria is corrected, a view substantiated by North and Henson (1981).

A review of 140 patients seen in the author's practice, all of whom had been prescribed prisms on the basis of the Mallett fixation disparity tests (Mallett, 1964, 1983) — and hence only the uncompensated component corrected — gave the following information at a minimum of two subsequent examinations over a 5-year period:

(1) Patients requiring unchanged prisms (assumed if there was ± 0.5 △ of vertical prism or ± 1 △ lateral prism) from that prescribed.	98	(70%)
(2) Patients showing an increased requirement (i.e. > 0.5 △ vertically or 1 △ laterally)	16	(11.43%)
(3) Patients showing a reduced (i.e. < 0.5 △ vertically or 1 △ laterally) prism or complete compensation without prism.	26	(18.57%)
Total	140	(100%)

All of the patients had experienced relief from symptoms and the survey demonstrates the efficacy of the treatment and reinforces the belief that *uncompensated* heterophoria can be neutralized with little fear of adaptation occurring. In nine of the 16 patients showing an increase, a deterioration in health had occurred.

Relieving prisms are almost obligatory in uncompensated hyperphoria and are especially useful in all imbalances where the patient is debilitated or elderly and therefore lacks the physical resources, the ocular motor plasticity or, indeed, the enthusiasm needed for orthoptic exercises. It should be noted that although the prescription of base-out prisms in distance esophoria is legitimate and although infrequently necessary, care should be exercised for patients with esophoria which is greater at near (convergence excess) who respond better to additional convex *spheres* for reading and other close visual tasks. Base-out prisms are contraindicated in spastic esophoria as adaptation *does* often occur with a resulting increase in the imbalance.

Prisms are sometimes prescribed for patients with grossly uncompensated heterophoria who, at times, break down into a strabismic state with resulting diplopia. Great care should be exercised in these cases as relief from symptoms tends to be short lived and many such patients go on to deviate constantly. An alternative therapeutic regimen is to be preferred in the majority of these cases.

Management of cyclophoria

Although cyclophoria may be a common condition (especially excyclophoria) particularly in near vision, it seldom promotes symptoms and only a few uncompensated cases are likely to be encountered. In such cases, the correction of any astigmatic error should be based upon a binocular refraction, especially with regard to the cylinder axes. Where necessary, a separate correction should be prescribed with the axes adjusted for close work. Any uncompensated hyperphoria should be corrected and the case reviewed within 2 months. Cyclophoria is frequently secondary to hyperphoria and it may even be appropriate to prescribe for a compensated hyperphoria. If the above procedures are unsuccessful the appropriate cyclofusional reserve should be exercised, incyclovergence for excyclophoria and excyclovergence for incyclophoria. This can be undertaken using fused horizontal lines, preferably with monocular control marks to detect suppression, using a synoptophore or other haploscopic instrumentation. It is easy to develop the cyclofusional reserves although generally unpleasant for the patient, sometimes precipitating vomiting during the exercise period. A pair of fused horizontal Maddox streaks (the cylinder axes of the Maddox groove

being vertical before each eye) can be rotated to develop the reserves.

Cyclophoria which does not respond to the conservative measures suggested above may be responsive to surgery (probably of the oblique muscles) and this should be considered if the symptoms are sufficiently acute.

Management of convergence insufficiency

Some patients with this anomaly have a background of sinusitis, dental infection or debilitation following illness. These or any other conditions thought to be relevant require treatment for the underlying cause rather than optometric assistance. Where recovery from an illness is likely to be prolonged, however, it would be helpful to relieve symptoms with base-in prisms. Before beginning any form of treatment in cases of gross convergence insufficiency, care should be taken to exclude the possibility of convergence paralysis with its attendant pathological undertones.

Three methods are commonly employed for relieving symptoms in convergence insufficiency. The first method involves orthoptic exercises, which are useful in patients in good health, not too elderly and with sufficient motivation and are given where possible. The most common exercise involves bringing a suitable target (some small print with a bold vertical line through the middle is the best target, though a pencil or something similar is often used) towards the face until diplopia occurs — this is repeated during some four or five 10-minute sessions each day. An alternative is to bring the target to a point where single vision is just possible, albeit with great effort, and then to hold at this position while the patient counts (preferably audibly) until a score of 100 is achieved or until diplopia occurs.

Jump convergence exercises are also useful for training voluntary convergence, the patient transferring fixation from a distance to a near object (held just outside his near point of convergence) and vice versa as quickly as possible; the target being fixated must be seen singly at the same time as the second object is seen in diplopia. The objective here is to alternate fixation when the nearer object can be fixated at a normal near point (i.e. closer than 10 cm). Pickwell (1984) places considerable emphasis on this form of treatment.

Development of the positive fusional amplitudes at near is also helpful in some cases. The second method involving concave lens stimulation of the convergence system via the accommodation reflex, is very helpful in young children who cannot be cajoled into putting adequate effort into orthoptic exercises, as well as some older patients with a sufficiently high amplitude of accommodation. The strength of the lenses, which should be worn for all close vision, should be assessed as described in

Chapter 15. This technique is effective in restoring a normal convergence near point in most cases but it should not be used in patients who are debilitated or have a background of fatigue. The third method, using base-in prisms, will relieve the symptoms in almost any patient with convergence insufficiency and the strength should be assessed with a fixation disparity test held at the normal near 'working' distance or at half this distance when a fatigue situation is present. Generally the prescription of prisms is reserved for patients who are debilitated or in poor health, presbyopes and those who are engaged in abnormally long periods of close work (e.g. some students). In presbyopes and younger patients with a low amplitude of accommodation who would benefit from a convex addition at near, this must be assessed before evaluating the necessary prismatic relief. It is frequently the case that prismatic relief can be weakened, or even abandoned, after the period of poor health or visual stress has passed.

Treatment of foveal suppression in heterophoria

Foveal suppression in uncompensated heterophoria is a protective mechanism and its development usually results in an alleviation, or even elimination, of the symptoms associated with the imbalance. Its elimination would be desirable in all younger patients, but in certain older people with long-standing suppression it is probably unwise to disturb a comfortable, albeit imperfect, situation. When the elimination of the suppression is thought to be desirable, careful consideration must be given to the order of therapeutic events. Suppression used to be eliminated before any attempt was made to increase the fusional amplitude which opposes the heterophoria. This procedure, however, often intensifies the symptoms as, at this stage, the heterophoria is still uncompensated.

It is preferable first to correct any ametropia, and then any prisms or adjustment of the spherical component carried out, should this be preferred to giving orthoptic exercises. If the heterophoria is now in a compensated state, it will usually be found that any foveal suppression will gradually disappear without any further treatment.

If orthoptic treatment is thought to be desirable, the appropriate fusional amplitude should be built up to render the heterophoria compensated. This will usually necessitate large fusion targets, e.g. Bradford HOT-DOG or Wells ONNE. It is usual to find that the suppression will spontaneously disappear when compensation is achieved.

If the prescription of prisms or spheres, or the new normality of the fusional amplitudes still allows some foveal suppression to persist, it can be removed by bar reading exercises with a Javal grid

using print of diminishing size as required, by using stereograms in a Brewster–Holmes or plano prisms (9 △ base-out each eye) stereoscope, which employ two paragraphs of print (several cards are normally available with different size of print) with multiple controls which are imaged monocularly when the print is fused. The stereoscope technique requires that accommodation and convergence effort should be in harmony — as the stereograms usually used (Bradford F series, Javal L series) have the fusible print separated by 6 cm, a distance of 33 cm between the card and prism is required for the plano prism stereoscope, while the Brewster–Holmes instrument which has a +5 D (or 5.25 D) lens centred at 8.25–9 cm should be used with the stereogram in the 1 D accommodation demand position, at which point, approximately 1 metre angle of convergence will be in use.

Methods of treatment employing red and green detail and viewed through complementary coloured lenses to provide monocularly seen components have been utilized by some clinicians, but it is difficult to recommend their use as they tend to excite 'retinal' rivalry. The use of tracing exercises on a Pigeon–Cantonnet stereoscope is occasionally useful, but this instrument is now no longer manufactured; the hand diploscope of Remy was once popular but is now obsolete.

After care

No patient should be discharged without a period during which his motor and sensory conditions are carefully monitored to detect any sign of regression or (hopefully) improvement.

If parallelism of the visual axes has been achieved, any residual foveal suppression will normally disappear over a period of time and stereoacuity will generally develop without the need for any specific attention. If fusion at both sensory and motor levels is to be maintained it is important to insist that any necessary refractive correction be worn though its reduction in strength, or eventual elimination, would be a commendable objective. Patients with a residual and cosmetically acceptable strabismus should, whenever possible, be allowed to develop a well entrenched harmonious ARC. If they are to acquire a degree of binocularity (albeit on anomalously corresponding receptive fields), a stable and approximately equal angle of strabismus at all fixation distances is a necessary requirement.

Conclusion

Only a brief outline of the possible therapeutic procedures for managing binocular imbalances has been possible in this chapter. It must always be remembered that the ultimate goal of every treatment regimen is to provide comfortable, efficient and cosmetically acceptable binocularity for the patient — to this end the enthusiasm and dedication of the practitioner is almost as important as the techniques employed.

References

AUST, W. (1970) *The Conservative Management of Squint*. Basel: S. Karger.

BAGOLINI, B. (1974) Sensory anomalies in strabismus. *Br. J. Ophthalmol.*, **58**(3), 313–318

BERARD, P.V. (1971) The use of prisms in the pre- and post-operative treatment of deviation in comitant squint. *The First Congress of the International Strabismological Association*. London: Henry Kimpton

BIRNBAUM, M.H., KOSLOWE, K. and SANET, R. (1977) Success in amblyopia therapy as a function of age: a literature survey. *Am. J. Optom. Physiol. Opt.*, **54**(5), 269–275

BRINKER, W.R. and KATZ, S.L. (1963) A new and practical treatment of eccentric fixation. *Am. J. Ophthalmol.*, **55**, 1033–1035

BURIAN, H.M. (1956) Use of bifocal spectacles in the treatment of accommodative esotropia. *Br. Orthopt. J.*, **13**, 3–6

BURIAN, H.M. and VON NOORDEN, G.K. (1974) *Binocular Vision and Ocular Motility*. St Louis: C. V. Mosby

CALOROSO, E. (1972) After-image transfer: a therapeutic procedure for amblyopia. *Am. J. Optom. Arch. Am. Acad. Optom*, **49**(1), 65–69

CAMPBELL, F.W., HESS, R.F., WATSON P.G. and BANKS, R. (1978) Preliminary results of a physiologically based treatment of amblyopia. *Br. J. Ophthalmol.*, **62**, 748–755

DAYTON, G.O. Jr., JONES, M.H., AIU, P., RAWSON, R.A., STEELE B. and ROSE, M. (1964) Developmental study of co-ordinated eye movements in the human infant. *Arch. Ophthalmol.*, **71**, 865–870

DOBSON, V. and TELLER, D.Y. (1978) Visual acuity in human infants: A review and comparison of behavioral and electrophysiological studies. *Vision Res.*, **18**, 1469–1483

DUKE-ELDER, S. (1973) *System of Ophthalmology*, Vol. VI, London: Henry Kimpton

ELSTON, J.S. and LEE, J.P. (1985) Paralytic strabismus: the role of botulinum toxin. *Br. J. Ophthalmol.*, **69**, 891–896

GALIN, M.A., KWITKO, M. and RESTRIPO, N. (1971) Influence of diphenylhydantoin on accommodation. *The First Congress of the International Strabismological Association*. London: Henry Kimpton

GIBSON, H.W. (1955) *Textbook of Orthoptics*. London: Hatton Press

GILLIE, J.C. and LINDSAY, M.A. (1969) *Orthoptics: A Discussion of Binocular Anomalies*. London: Hatton Press

GUIBOR, G.P. (1958) Some uses of opthalmic prisms. In *Strabismus Ophthalmic Symposium*, Vol. 11, edited by J.H. Allen, pp. 244–260. London: Henry Kimpton

HUGONNIER, R. and CLAYETTE-HUGONNIER, S. (1969) Strabismus, heterophoria, ocular motor paralysis. In *Clinical Ocular Muscle Imbalance*, edited by S. Veronneau-

Troutman, pp. 573–584. St. Louis: C. V. Mosby

HUMPHRISS, D. (1937) Some notes on the treatment of amblyopia. *Dioptric Rev.* **xxxix**

LYLE, T.K. and WYBAR, K.C. (1967) *Practical Orthoptics in the Treatment of Squint*. London: H. K. Lewis and Co.

McCORMICK, B. J. (1978) After-image transfer therapy in non-strabismic amblyopia. *Ophthal. Opt.* **18**, 641–643

MALLETT, R.F.J. (1964) The investigation of heterophoria at near and a new fixation disparity technique. *Optician*, **148**, 547–551, 574–581

MALLETT, R.F.J. (1969) A useful adjunct to the treatment of amblyopia. *Ophthal. Opt.*, **9**, 1033–1034

MALLETT, R.F.J. (1970a) Anomalous retinal correspondence — the new outlook. *Ophthal. Opt.*, **10**, 606–624

MALLETT, R.F.J. (1970b) The Stanworth synoptiscope in the investigation and treatment of strabismus. *Ophthal. Opt.*, **10**, 556–573

MALLETT, R.F.J. (1975) Using after-images in the investigation and treatment of strabismus. *Ophthal. Opt.*, **15**, 727–729

MALLETT, R.F.J. (1979) The use of prisms in the treatment of concomitant strabismus. *Ophthal. Opt.*, **19**, 793–798

MALLETT, R.F.J. (1983) The treatment of congenital idiopathic nystagmus by intermittent photic stimulation. *Ophthal. Physiol. Opt.*, **3**(3), 341–356

MALLETT, R.F.J. (1985) A unit for treating amblyopia and congenital nystagmus by intermittent photic stimulation. *Optom. Today*, **25**(8), 260–264

MALLETT, R.F.J. and READING, R.W. (1971) Variations in the state of retinal correspondence with intermittent stimuli: a case study. *Ophthal. Opt.*, **11**, 847–850

MARG, E., FREEMAN, R.D., PELTZMAN, P., and GOLDSTEIN, P.J. (1976) Visual acuity development in human infants: Evoked potential measurements. *Invest. Ophthalmol.*, **15**, 150–153

MEAKIN, W.J., EARNSHAW, J.R., GOEBELLS, W.F. and GRIFFIN, R.G. (1958) Orthoptic treatment of divergent strabismus. *Optician*, **13**, 323–330

NAWRATZKI, I. and OLIVER, M. (1971) Eccentric fixation managed with inverse prism. *Am. J. Ophthalmol.*, **71**(2), 549–552

NORTH, R. and HENSON, D.B. (1981) Adaptation to lens induced heterophorias. *Am. J. Optom. Physiol. Opt.*, **62**(11), 774–780

PARKS, M.M. (1975) *Ocular Motility and Strabismus*. Maryland: Harper and Row

PICKWELL, D. (1984) *Binocular Vision Anomalies*. London: Butterworths

PIGASSOU, R. and GARIPUY, J. (1967) Treatment of eccentric fixation. *J. Ped. Ophthalmol.*, **4**(2), 35–43

READING, R.W. (1983) *Binocular Vision: Foundations and Applications*. London: Butterworths

ROBERTSON, K.M. and KUHN, L. (1985) Effect of visual training on the vertical vergence amplitude. *Am. J. Optom. Physiol. Opt.*, **62**(10), 659–668

RUBIN, W. (1965) Reverse prism and calibrated occlusion. In the treatment of small-angle deviations. *Am. J. Ophthalmol.*, **59**, 271–277

VON NOORDEN, G.K. (1971) Research in strabismus. *Am. Orthopt. J.*, **21**, 15–20

Part 5

Ocular examination

17

Clinical pathology of ocular disease

Alan Bird and Janet Silver

The effect of disease upon ocular tissues depends upon the site of the disease and the nature of the pathological processes. These, in turn, will determine the influence of the disease upon visual function and upon the appearance of ocular structures. An attempt will be made to typify the nature of the precipitating disorder and the tissue responses of the eye to disease.

Eyelid

The major disorders of eyelids relate to inflammation at the margin of the eyelid and abnormal position of the lids due to defects in innervation of the lid muscle or to degenerative change in the lid structure.

Inflammation

Inflammation of the lid edges, blepharitis, is extremely common and is centred around the orifices of various skin appendages at the lid margin. Eyelashes and sebaceous glands emerge in the anterior half of the lid margin while the orifices of the meibomian glands are in the posterior half. Inflammation may affect primarily the lash follicles or the meibomian glands, although in most patients both systems appear to be involved.

Anterior blepharitis implies inflammation around the lid follicles and is associated with seborrhoea which is seen in its most severe form in acne rosacea. Secondary staphylococcal infection is common. In mild disease, the lid margins are red, there is inflammation around the hair follicles and scales may be seen around the origin of the lashes. Secondary staphylococcal infection may cause ulceration of the lid margin. Obstruction of the sebaceous gland orifices may give rise to accumulation of secretion

and secondary infection within the gland, causing styes. Treatment is aimed at reducing staphylococcal population of the lid edge by local antibiotics and the nature of sebaceous gland secretion may be modified by systemic use of tetracycline. Blepharitis associated with seborrhoea is likely to recur because it reflects a constitutional anomaly of sebaceous gland secretion.

Posterior blepharitis is due to inflammation of the meibomian gland (meibomianitis). Meibomian secretions appear to accumulate within the gland, causing inflammation within the tarsal plate and abnormal contour of the posterior margin of the lid. Mechanical emptying of the glands by lid massage is often all that is needed to control the condition. Acute swelling of the meibomian gland may be accompanied by inflammation; this is known as a chalazion. Once a chalazion has formed, it is usually necessary to incise the posterior margin of the granuloma and remove the contents surgically.

Blepharitis may be complicated by secondary inflammation of the conjunctiva and marginal cornea. This is thought to be related to an immune system response to the bacteria within the lid. Treatment is aimed at reducing the bacterial population by local antibiotics, and the immune response by local steroids.

Involutionary positional defects

The attachment of the lids to surrounding structures appears to become loose causing the lid to become abnormally long; positional defects appear to affect the lower lid more commonly than the upper lid. *Entropion* implies that the edge of the lid turns inward, the lower portion of the tarsal plate moving forwards within the lid. This is caused by abnormal lengthening of the lid and, in particular, dehiscence of the attachments of the lower border of the tarsal plate to the retractor muscle. Entropion causes irritation of the eye largely due to the lashes rubbing against the inferior conjunctiva and cornea. The condition can be treated surgically by tightening the lid and by re-establishing the connection of the lower border of the tarsal plate to retractor muscles.

Ectropion implies that the border of the lid falls forwards, thus exposing the palpebral conjunctiva. This is caused by abnormal lengthening of the lid and can be corrected by tightening of the lid surgically.

Ptosis of the upper lid may occur with age due to dehiscence at the aponeurotic attachment of the upper tarsal plate to the levator. If this is severe enough to obstruct the vision, surgical reattachment of the lid to levator will correct the abnormality.

Blepharochalasis implies redundancy of skin of the upper and lower lids due to lengthening of skin, and is usually associated with prolapse of orbital fat through dehiscence in the orbital septum. Excision of a portion of skin may be required if the abnormality is sufficient to obstruct vision or cause significant cosmetic defect.

Conjunctiva

Conjunctivitis is most commonly infective in origin, or immune system mediated as a result of atopy or chronic exposure to allergens.

Many infective agents have been identified as causing conjunctivitis, the most common being *Chlamydia* and viruses; bacterial conjunctivitis is rare in uncompromised eyes. Trachoma is the commonest cause of blindness in the world; it occurs in communities in which infection is hyperendemic.

Trachoma

Infection appears to occur in early life, the organism being transmitted by eye-seeking flies. Acute conjunctivitis occurs in early childhood and this is followed by chronic disease which results in scarring of the conjunctiva and secondary lid deformity. Secondary staphylococcal infection is common and is a major contributor to ocular damage. Secondary scarring of the cornea occurs in long-standing disease. In its mild form, this may be seen as a pannus of blood vessels in the superior stroma, while in severe disease secondary staphylococcal infections of the cornea cause permanent scarring or corneal perforation.

The infective agent is sensitive to tetracycline. Treatment has been aimed at clearing whole communities of the organism by mass treatment with tetracycline. A major impact on blindness may be achieved by reducing secondary bacterial infection

with the use of antibiotics. Recently it has become evident that regular washing reduces substantially secondary staphylococcal infection and has highlighted the importance of secondary infection as a major cause of blindness in this condition.

Chlamydial infection has also been recognized recently as a cause of acute conjunctivitis in Western communities. It appears to be sexually transmitted and the genitourinary tract may act as a reservoir of the infective agent. Treatment is directed at relief of the conjunctivitis but most also include systemic treatment by tetracycline. Control of the infection includes treatment of sexual partners of the infected individual.

Children born to an infected mother may have ophthalmia neonatorum. The importance of this infection relates to the potential scarring effect on the eyes and requires urgent treatment.

Viral conjunctivitis

Many viruses have been recognized as causing conjunctivitis, the most important being adenoviruses. Adenovirus 8 has been recognized as causing epidemics of keratoconjunctivitis while other types cause isolated conjunctivitis following pharyngitis.

Adenovirus infection of the cornea causes acute inflammation associated with pain, redness of the eye, conjunctival oedema and conjunctival haemorrhage. Punctate keratitis may follow causing extreme photophobia and blurring of vision.

No specific agent has been recognized for treating this inflammation which may continue for up to one year. Symptoms may be relieved by the use of weak local steroids, particularly if they affect the cornea, although withdrawal of the steroids is often accompanied by recrudescence of symptoms.

Allergic conjunctivitis

Atopy is characterized by asthma, eczema and hayfever. These patients are subject to chronic or episodic allergic conjunctivitis which is typified by soreness and redness of the eye, and patients may have giant follicles beneath the bulbar conjunctiva. In some patients, the inflammation appears to be seasonal (vernal conjunctivitis), although many have chronic inflammation throughout the year. Secondary corneal changes may be severe and permanent with consequent visual loss. Patients may be helped by avoiding allergens, although this is clearly impractical if the allergy is to pollens. Steroids have been used for many years in attempts to control the inflammation. Recently, cromoglycate has proved more effective in helping many sufferers.

Giant papillary conjunctivitis is also seen in contact lens wearers and in patients who are regularly instilling ophthalmic preparations. This is thought to be immune mediated, representing an immune response to preservatives in drops, or to chronic irritation. Withdrawal of preservatives from medications or ceasing medications and contact lens wear may be the only method by which the condition can be controlled.

Cornea

General considerations

The cornea is transparent and avascular and its anterior surface serves as the major refracting surface of the eye. The cornea is composed of a central stroma with a single layer of endothelial cells on its inner surface, and a 5- or 6-cell thick epithelium on its anterior surface. Between the epithelium and the stroma is Bowman's membrane which represents the basement membrane of the epithelial cells. On the posterior surface of the stroma is Descemet's membrane which is composed of densely packed fibres. The stroma is relatively dehydrated and its regular fibre arrangement accounts for its transparency. The detergescence is maintained by the endothelium which pumps water out of the stroma. Failure of the endothelial cell layer causes the cornea to become oedematous which results in swelling. The epithelium is not keratinized and is covered by a continuous tear film. The tear film has a surface layer of oil secreted by meibomian glands and the deeper part of the tear film is composed of a mucus/water complex secreted by the goblet cells and lacrimal gland. The stability of the tear film is dependent upon the microvillous anterior epithelial surface. Abnormality of the tear film causes secondary changes in the epithelium.

The cornea is avascular and derives its nutrition from the limbal vessels around its perimeter, from the aqueous and from the tear film. Its avascularity is a reflection of metabolic influences in the stroma; if these are altered by inflammation, invasion of the stroma by blood vessels from the limbus is a common response. The anterior surface of the cornea is well supplied by nerve fibres such that any disturbance to the epithelium causes pain.

The clarity of the cornea is dependent upon the regular arrangement and spacing of its fibres. Any disturbance of their distribution causes loss of transparency. This is a constant consequence of oedema as the extracellular space expands. Similar loss of clarity results from inflammation due to the excess of water, protein and cellular infiltration. Scars appear white because the collagen fibre distribution becomes irregular.

Keratitis

Inflammation of the cornea may occur in response to infection by bacteria, fungi and viruses. Bacterial keratitis is rare in healthy eyes occurring when there is pre-existing disease of the cornea. It represents one of the major blinding disorders of the world in association with protein or vitamin A deficiency (tropical corneal ulcer). In Western communities, it is seen progressively more commonly in contact lens wearers, particularly in those wearing soft lenses. It is also a complication of corneal denervation following inflammation or as a result of a lesion affecting the trigeminal nerve; in such patients there appears to be an abnormal cellular response in the corneal stroma and there is also a defective tear film and epithelium, the epithelium having lost its normal microvillous surface. Fungal infections are rare, usually affecting agricultural workers. They are nevertheless of importance since vision is likely to be lost unless appropriate treatment is given. Amoebic keratitis appears to be a progressively more common problem.

Viral keratitis

The most important virus infecting the cornea is herpes simplex virus which appears to proliferate in the corneal epithelium causing necrosis and a typical dendritic ulcer. This is demonstrated as a branching opacity in the corneal epithelium which may be seen most clearly after staining by fluorescein or rose bengal. The initial infection may heal spontaneously although it will give rise to anterior stromal opacity. The size of the lesion and scarring can be limited by removal of infected epithelium or with antiviral agents. Recurrent infection is common and with each infection there is progressively more inflammation within the stroma resulting in disciform keratitis which implies full thickness infiltration of the stroma and subsequent scarring. In severe disease the inflammation may affect the anterior chamber causing signs of uveitis. The virus is thought to reside in the trigeminal (gasserian) ganglion and infects the cornea by transport of virus via the axons of the trigeminal nerve by axoplasmic transport.

Similar disease is seen with herpes zoster virus in association with shingles affecting the territory of the first division of the trigeminal nerve. The mode of infection is thought to be identical to that of herpes simplex.

Non-infective corneal ulceration

In a variety of disorders, ulceration and thinning of the peripheral cornea occurs in which there is little evidence of direct infection of the cornea. Such lesions are seen in patients with severe rheumatoid arthritis and may also occur rarely as a Mooren's ulcer. In these disorders, it is believed that inflammation at the limbus causes accumulation of inflammatory cells which secrete proteolytic enzymes

— these in turn induce stromal thinning. The thinning of corneal stroma and opacification of the margins of the lesion, can be appreciated by biomicroscopy together with thickening of the limbal conjunctiva and episclera. Similar loss of peripheral corneal thickness is a consequence of blepharitis, particularly in patients with acne rosacea. Treatment consists of careful use of local and systemic antibiotics, and local corticosteriods.

Corneal degeneration

Keratoconus is an uncommon disorder of the cornea whereby the corneal curvature is increased and the apical cornea is thinned. It occurs in a variety of conditions, such as atopy, but in many patients it appears to be an isolated defect. The deformation of the cornea is progressive and can be appreciated by biomicroscopy. The change in the refracting surface of the cornea is readily appreciated by retinoscopy and the change in the anterior reflecting surface by placido's disc or keratoscopy. The loss of vision due to refractive change may be corrected by a contact lens but in severe disease the only treatment is corneal grafting.

Band keratopathy consists of deposition of calcium in the superficial corneal stroma and occurs in many chronic ocular diseases particularly in patients subject to long-term intraocular inflammation, such as pauciarticular arthropathy in children. Labrador keratopathy consists of deposition of lipid droplets in the anterior part of the cornea and occurs in patients exposed to large quantities of ultraviolet light throughout life. It has been described in desert dwellers as well as people from the arctic regions who are exposed to sun for a large part of their lives.

Inherited corneal dystrophies

A large number of disorders have been described in which there is inherited disease of the cornea and they have been arbitrarily subdivided into those affecting the anterior cornea, central stroma and posterior cornea.

Epithelial dystrophies include Meesman's dystrophy which is slowly progressive and characterized by microcystic changes in the epithelium and Reis–Buckler dystrophy which causes vortex-like patterns in the epithelium — both are dominantly inherited. These, together with fingerprint dystrophy, cause epithelial change with consequent pain and irritation although they do not cause severe visual loss. A common problem with fingerprint dystrophy is recurrent erosion. The epithelial changes are readily identified by biomicroscopy.

Three main forms of stromal corneal dystrophy have been recognized; in each there is deposition of abnormal material in the stroma. Granular and lattice dystrophies are autosomal dominant while macular dystrophy is recessive. They all cause a distinctive pattern of opacification of the corneal stroma with consequent blurring of vision, although this is usually only severe in macular dystrophy. Lattice dystrophy and macular dystrophy may cause secondary changes in the epithelium with consequent pain. In granular dystrophy, histopathology shows rod extracellular deposits of amino acids. Macular dystrophy is thought to be a localized mucopolysaccharidosis. There is intracellular accumulation of glycosaminoglycans within the fibroblasts, probably due to a defect in activity of enzymes responsible for degradation of keratin sulphate. Deposits of polymerized light chains are found in lattice dystrophy causing amyloid accumulation.

The most important endothelial corneal dystrophy is Fuchs' dystrophy in which progressive change of the corneal endothelium can be seen. Oedema of the corneal stroma and epithelium will result in blurring of vision and pain. The endothelial changes are readily observed in the specular reflex from the posterior corneal surface. The only effective treatment is corneal grafting. Posterior polymorphous dystrophy is dominantly inherited and causes the appearance of polymorphous opacities in the deep stromal layers. This rarely gives rise to significant visual disability, although corneal oedema and epithelial changes may occur in later life.

The pupil

The pupil is the central gap in the iris diaphragm. It is surrounded by a sphincter which causes the pupil to constrict; the dilator muscle is in the midstroma.

The dilator muscle is supplied by sympathetic innervation derived from the superior ciliary ganglion, while the constrictor muscle is innervated by the parasympathetic system originating in the third cranial nerve, fibres passing forward in the base of the skull to the ciliary ganglion where there is a final synapse. Pupillary size is determined largely by changes in ambient light and also with variation in tone within the autonomic nervous system. Light causes pupillary constriction, light shone in one eye causing equal constriction of the pupil in both eyes. Abnormalities of pupil shape, size and reactivity can be due to mechanical interference with pupil activity, and abnormalities in the afferent and the efferent arc of the light reflex.

Irregular pupil

The pupil may become irregular if there is adhesion of the pupil to the lens or vitreous such as may occur following inflammation or surgery; these irregularities are known as posterior synechiae. Anterior synechiae, in which the iris is adherent to the cornea, may also occur following accidental or iatrogenic perforating trauma to the cornea.

Proliferation of fibrovascular tissue on the surface of the iris occurs in neovascular glaucoma in response to posterior segment ischaemia. The fibrovascular tissue growing on the anterior surface contracts, with eversion of the posterior pigmented layer onto the anterior surface around the pupil, and causes irregularity of the pupil margin.

Segmental atrophy of the iris may occur due to vasculitis (typically with herpes zoster infection) and it may be seen after severe attacks of acute closed-angle glaucoma. Rare inherited conditions may also cause segmental changes in the iris such as iridoschisis, iridocorneal endothelial syndrome (ICE) and in anterior chamber cleavage syndromes.

Irregularity of the pupil is a rare result of abnormal innervation. It is seen characteristically in neurosyphilis in which the site of the neurological lesion is not known; the pupil is typically small and irregular in paretic syphilis and is large and irregular in tabes dorsalis. In the Holmes–Adie pupil, it is thought that abnormal innervation is a result of inflammation affecting the cilary ganglion. This causes segmental denervation of the sphincter muscle while the dilator muscle innervation is preserved. Such patients have large pupils during the acute phase. Small segments of sphincter may be seen to react to light while the response to accommodation appears to be relatively well preserved. With time there is re-innervation of the sphincter such that the pupil becomes smaller and indeed it may become smaller than the contralateral normal eye. The condition is benign, although it may be associated with minor changes elsewhere in the autonomic nervous system — in particular tendon reflexes are reduced.

Defects of the afferent reflex arc

Widespread disease of the retina or optic nerve in one eye will cause a reduction of pupillomotor drive when that eye is illuminated. The reduced constriction is equal in the two eyes. If the contralateral normal eye is then illuminated, the pupils will constrict further. This represents the basis of the swinging flash light test in which the eyes are illuminated alternately. Transferring the light from a diseased eye to the normal eye causes pupillary constriction, while moving the light in the reverse direction is accompanied by pupillary dilatation. The test is important because a diagnosis of unilateral optic nerve disease is indefensible in the absence of a relative afferent pupillary defect.

Efferent reflex arc defects

Loss of dilator innervation occurs with any neurological lesion affecting the sympathetic nervous system. This may occur with disease in the neck and characteristically causes oculosympathetic paresis in which there is reduction of pupil size (miosis), and mild ptosis and movement of the lower lid due to denervation of the retractor muscles. Dilatation of the pupil (mydriasis) is seen with any lesion of the parasympathetic nervous system and in particular in association with third nerve paresis. Involvement of the pupil is a particularly useful sign in third nerve palsy since it appears that a third nerve lesion due to infarction usually spares the pupillomotor fibres, while compression of the nerve almost invariably causes pupillary dilatation. Thus pupil involvement is useful in distinguishing between various causes of third nerve lesions.

Lens

In early life the lens is virtually transparent having a lamellar structure of fibres, a cellular epithelium on its anterior surface and surrounded by capsule. Little is understood of lens metabolism; the metabolic activity is low, nutrition being derived from the aqueous. With age, new fibres are formed on the surface of the lens so that the lens becomes larger. The increased rigidity results in reduction of focusing ability and presbyopia. There is also progressive degradation of protein within the fibres which alters optical properties of the lens, and gives rise to cataract. Certain specific metabolic abnormalities may hasten this process.

The lens is suspended between the anterior and posterior chambers by the zonular fibres which originate in the cilliary body and are inserted into the lens capsule.

Cataract

By far the most common cause of cataract is age and the lens opacities may take various forms. As the lens becomes larger and the refractive index of the nucleus increases, there is a tendency for myopia to develop. Progressive opacification of the nucleus is common (nuclear cataract) and is often accompanied by accumulation of brown pigment. These give rise to the familiar symptoms of blurring, dazzle and lack of sensitivity to blue light. Alternatively, opacities may appear between the lamellae (cortical cataract) which gives rise to the additional symptom of polyopia. If the cataract progresses, it may become mature which implies total opacification of the lens that now appears as a white opacity in the pupil and reduces vision to light perception. Changes in the capsule at this stage may allow egress of protein out of the lens which causes the lens to shrink and the cortex to become liquefied (hypermature cataract). The protein that escapes may be ingested by macrophages which can be seen in the slitlamp beam circulating in the aqueous and which may obstruct the trabecular meshwork causing the lens-induced glaucoma. Rarely, inflammation may be generated by such protein causing lens-induced uveitis.

Certain factors have been recognized which are associated with high incidence of 'senile' cataract, such as diabetes, but the aetiology of cataract apart from these conditions is unknown. It has been recognized that cataract is more common in some communities than others; some believe that high life experience of ultraviolet light or recurrent gastroenteritis may increase the prevalence of lens opacities. A specific acute onset cataract occurs with diabetic coma which may be reversed by rapid correction of the metabolic defect.

No medical treatment has been shown to influence the progress of lens opacities. Cataract extraction involves removal of the lens from the eye. Intracapsular extraction implies that the whole lens has been removed from the eye while in extracapsular extraction the posterior capsule is left intact. The hypermetropia consequent upon lens removal may be managed by spectacles, contact lens or by the insertion of a lens in the anterior or posterior chamber (pseudophakia).

Congenital cataract may be genetically determined and has been recognized as a consequence of maternal rubella during the first trimester of pregnancy. If the lens opacities are bilateral and sufficient to interfere significantly with visual function, dense amblyopia can be expected unless the condition is treated quickly. It is the aim of therapy to remove both cataracts and have the eyes corrected optically by the age of 2–3 months.

Cataract is also common as a consequence of certain ocular disorders. Posterior subcapsular lens opacities may be due to any condition which causes widespread retinal damage, such as retinitis pigmentosa or retinal detachment, in the presence of chronic intraocular inflammation, or with both local and systemic corticosteroid administration. Posterior subcapsular as well as nuclear lens opacities occur with great frequency following any intraocular operation such as vitrectomy or drainage surgery for glaucoma. Certain rare inherited multisystem disorders also induce lens opacities.

The presence of early cataract may be detected by slitlamp biomicroscopy or by observing the red reflex during ophthalmoscopy or retinoscopy.

Subluxation or dislocation of the lens occurs in a variety of general disorders, such as homocystinuria and Marfan's syndrome, and is common in patients with coloboma. The visual problems depend upon the position of the lens. If the lens is completely dislocated the patient is effectively aphakic and requires appropriate hypermetropic correction. If partially dislocated, two refracting systems exist, one through the edge of the lens and the other through the aphakic portion of the pupil. Such patients may suffer from pupil block glaucoma. Dislocation of the lens may also result from trauma which causes rupture of the zonule.

Glaucoma

Glaucoma signifies an increase in intraocular pressure causing damage to the optic nerve head with consequent loss of visual nerve function. Two major subcategories of glaucoma are recognized: acute closed-angle glaucoma and chronic open-angle glaucoma.

Acute closed-angle glaucoma

Aqueous humour which is produced by the ciliary body is secreted into the posterior chamber and then flows through the pupil in the anterior chamber and subsequently leaves the eye via the trabecular meshwork at the drainage angle of the anterior chamber. In acute closed-angle glaucoma, there is increased resistance to flow of aqueous through the pupil due to the contact between the posterior surface of the iris and the lens; this mechanism has given the name pupil block to this form of glaucoma. The increased resistance to flow causes enlargement of the posterior chamber with consequent forward movement of the iris which makes contact with the trabecular meshwork, thus preventing aqueous outflow via the normal channel. Characteristically, this form of glaucoma occurs in hypermetropic eyes with shallow anterior chambers and an anteriorly placed lens. Pupil block may also occur if vitreous prolapses into the posterior chamber as may occur with a subluxated lens or after intracapsular cataract extraction. Adhesion of the iris to the lens occurring in anterior segment inflammation will also have a similar effect.

The pressure of the eye becomes extremely high in acute closed-angle glaucoma reaching levels of 70 mmHg. The high pressure induces dilatation of the pupil due to ischaemia of the iris sphincter and oedema of the cornea. A patient experiences severe pain, the eye becomes red and vision blurred. In some patients the attack may resolve spontaneously and a history may be obtained of previous episodes of high pressure. Such patients may complain of recurrent frontal headache and visual blurring; the corneal oedema often gives rise to the distinctive symptoms of coloured haloes seen around focal lights. Acute closed-angle glaucoma may be precipitated by mydriasis or pupil block occurring during the recovery from pupillary dilatation.

Treatment is aimed initially at reducing the intraocular pressure with acetazolamide and hyperosmotic agents given systemically and constriction of the pupil using miotic drops. Miosis is readily achieved once the intraocular pressure is lowered unless there is total infarction of the iris sphincter. Definitive treatment is achieved by creating a hole in the iris, allowing aqueous to flow freely from the posterior chamber to the anterior chamber. An iridotomy can be achieved either surgically or by use of a laser.

Patients suffering acute closed-angle glaucoma in one eye are recognized as being at risk of suffering similar problems in the contralateral eye, so that it is universal practice to create an iridectomy in the unaffected eye unless it has been shown that the two eyes are anatomically different.

Following the treatment of an acute attack, vision is usually good although some damage to the optic nerve head is commonly observed. In a small number of patients with sustained high pressure, anterior subcapsular lens opacities may be seen — glauconflekon.

In some patients, permanent adhesion of the iris to the trabecular meshwork may result from the acute attack. If a significant proportion of the drainage angle is permanently compromised, there may be sustained ocular hypertension once the acute attack has been successfully treated. In such patients medical treatment for glaucoma or drainage surgery may be indicated.

Chronic closed-angle glaucoma

In a small number of patients progressive closure of the angle by peripheral anterior synechiae may occur in the absence of overt closed-angle attacks. These patients present in a similar fashion to chronic open-angle glaucoma, although the distinction between the disorders can be made by gonioscopy. If sufficient of the drainage angle is available for aqueous drainage, creating an iridotomy may be sufficient to prevent further peripheral anterior synechiae forming. On the other hand, if a large percentage of the angle function is permanently lost, drainage surgery may be necessary.

Chronic open-angle glaucoma

In chronic open-angle glaucoma, it is believed that structural changes in the trabecular meshwork result in an increase in resistance to aqueous outflow from the eye. This causes the ocular pressure to be higher than normal, although the rise in pressure is often quite small. Such an increase in intraocular pressure over months or years induces progressive damage to the nerve head with initial loss of ganglion cell axons

entering the nerve at its superior and inferior poles. The loss of ganglion cell axons at these specific sites causes an enlargement of the cup at the nerve head in a vertical direction. The mechanism of damage to the nerve head is not clear. It is believed by some that the rise in ocular pressure compromises blood supply to the nerve head and that cellular damage is due to ischaemia. Alternatively, it is possible that the rise in ocular pressure causes compression of the individual axons against the fibrous structure of the nerve head, namely the scleral ring or the bars within the lamina cribrosa. Denervation of the retina causes loss of visual field with characteristic arcuate scotomata usually involving vision 15° from fixation. With progression of disease, the scotomata enlarge and in advanced glaucoma the patient may have good acuity although the central field will be extremely small and there may be some sparing of temporal peripheral field.

Symptoms

Patients rarely have any symptoms related to the raised pressure. The loss of vision is extremely slow and patients may be unaware of functional deficit before the disease is advanced. With time the patient becomes aware of the scotomata and poor vision at night is common due to denervation of rod-rich retina.

The diagnosis can usually be made on the basis of raised intraocular pressure and the presence of the cupping of the optic nerve with consequent field loss. However, it is clear that many patients can have sustained ocular hypertension over many years without any damage to the nerve head. It is also the case that patients with cupping of the nerve head characteristic of glaucoma may show no evidence of ocular hypertension. There is diurnal variation in ocular pressure and, if a patient is suspected of having glaucoma but the pressures are normal, it is common practice to measure the ocular pressure at various times of day; a patient may have normal pressures in the afternoon but markedly raised pressures in the early morning. The situation is complicated further by the presence of patients whose ocular pressure is constantly within normal limits and yet who have progressive loss of ganglion cell axons as manifest by increasing field loss and increasing optic nerve cupping: this is commonly known as low tension glaucoma. It is believed that these patients have some abnormality of the nerve head whereby even normal ocular pressures can cause progressive damage. Whether this can be related to a deficit in blood supply or abnormal anatomy of the nerve head is not clear. Diagnosis is further confounded by the apparent similarity of disc changes between these patients and patients who have suffered ischaemic optic neuropathy. The latter have field loss and cupping as a result of a single ischaemic incident, and progressive field loss does not occur.

Management

The aims in the treatment of chronic simple glaucoma is to lower ocular pressure either by reduction of ciliary secretion or by decreasing the resistance to outflow via the trabecular meshwork. Both these can be achieved by medical therapy, although it is evident that in some patients medical therapy is inadequate to stabilize visual function. Decreased resistance to outflow may be achieved by laser photocoagulation to the trabecular meshwork — laser trabeculopasty. Should these methods fail, outflow can be reduced by constructing new outflow channels by surgery.

It is evident that the more advanced the glaucoma, the more difficult it is to achieve stable vision.

Congenital glaucoma

This disorder is due to congenital malformation of the drainage angle causing obstruction to aqueous outflow. The condition may be evident at birth or develop during the first few years of life. The high pressure causes the globe to become enlarged which is associated with increased corneal diameter. Ruptures in Descemet's membrane may occur with enlargement of the cornea presenting as parallel lines on the inner corneal surface. In severe disease, the cornea becomes oedematous and the high pressure inevitably results in disc cupping.

The disorder may come to light if abnormal enlargement of the globe is identified or if the cornea becomes oedematous. The children are often noted to dislike sunlight and this may be the presenting symptom. Therapy is aimed at dividing the abnormal tissue in the drainage angle by goniotomy.

Intraocular inflammation

Intraocular inflammation has been arbitarily divided according to the tissue believed to be the site of disease. In retinitis it is clear that the retina is primarily affected. The term 'uveitis' is used to describe patients in whom the uvea (iris, ciliary body, choroid) is thought to be affected, although the term is used also to describe intraocular inflammation in which the primary site of inflammation is unknown.

Anterior uveitis/iritis

When the inflammation involves the iris, effects of inflammation are seen in the anterior chamber. The changes depend to some extent on the nature of the disease, being different in acute and chronic disease.

Acute anterior uveitis

This results in exudation of cells and protein into the aqueous; the presence of protein causes opacification of the aqueous which can be seen as a flare in the slitlamp beam. Individual cells may also be seen circulating in the anterior chamber. In the rare case where there is massive outpouring of debris from the iris, a layer of pus may occur in the lower part of the anterior chamber (hypopyon). The pupil is often small due to constriction of the sphincter of the iris and the iris may adhere to the posterior lens surface (posterior synechiae).

The most common association with acute anterior uveitis is ankylosing spondylitis (HLA-B27). The nature of the association is uncertain; it is believed that such patients respond in this specific way to non-specific circumstances such as virus infections.

Patients with acute anterior uveitis are aware of pain and photophobia and examination reveals a bright red eye with dilatation of the blood vessels around the limbus. The changes in the anterior chamber such as flare and cells can be detected by slitlamp biomicroscopy and, if there are posterior synechiae, the pupil becomes irregular. The acute attacks of anterior uveitis are severe but respond well to corticosteroids.

Chronic anterior uveitis

This causes changes similar to those seen in acute disease but different in degree. Flare and cells due to egress of protein and cells from the iris vessels are readily seen by biomicroscopy. Inflammatory debris may collect on the posterior surface of the cornea and is seen as white opacities (keratic precipitates). Patients with chronic anterior uveitis are often unaware of pain but may present with blurred vision due to keratic precipitates. In a small percentage of patients the cause of chronic anterior uveitis is identified (e.g. sarcoid), but in the vast majority no basic disorder is found.

The inflammation is normally managed with corticosteroids. If there is risk of formation of posterior synechiae, it is normal to dilate the pupil and prevent a pupil block.

Heterochromic cyclitis

This is a specific syndrome in which there are signs of chronic anterior uveitis, but without formation of posterior synechiae and which may progress for many years without necessarily causing many symptoms. With time the iris loses its stromal pigment giving it a grey colour. The cause of heterochromic cyclitis is not known, although it is associated with microvascular change in the iris and fundus and small focal fundus scars are evident.

Posterior uveitis

This term is used loosely to denote any chronic inflammatory disease affecting the posterior segment in which there is no obvious retinitis. Within this category it is now clear that there are disorders which appear to affect the retinal vessels (*retinal vasculitis*). There are specific conditions in which it is clear that there is true *choroiditis*. Within this group there are entities with well-recognized cause or associations, while in others there is a constant clinical presentation, although the aetiology of the disease is unknown. However, in the majority of cases there are changes of inflammation identified in the vitreous cavity without ophthalmoscopically identifiable choroidal disease and in which the aetiology of the disorder is unknown.

In all patients, changes analogous to those seen in the anterior chamber can be identified in the vitreous. Cells and protein accumulate in the hyaloid cavity and can be identified by biomicroscopy. Collections of debris within the vitreous may be seen inferiorly as discrete white opacities. Changes in the fundus vary from one condition to another and will be summarized individually.

Harada's disease

This causes diffuse infiltration of the choroid by inflammatory cells with focal collections of giant cell and epitheloid cells which may be seen as focal pale areas within the choroid. Inflammation causes secondary changes in the overlying retinal pigment epithelium which, in turn, causes serous detachment of the posterior retina. Optic neuritis is a constant association with active disease and anterior uveitis usually accompanies the disorder. The mechanism of disease is not known although it is believed to be an immune-mediated disorder related somehow to antibody formation to pigmented cells. The disorder may be associated with dysacusis and meningitis in the acute stage, and in chronic disease there is loss of pigment in hair and skin; all of these are believed to be manifestations of the same disordered immune state.

Sympathetic ophthalmitis

This is inflammation in both eyes resulting from perforating injury in one and is virtually identical in its presentation to Harada's disease; it is believed that they share common pathogenesis although the precipitating event is different.

Multifocal choroiditis

This is rarely recognized as a result of infective disease (e.g. *Brucella* sp.), but evidence of old multifocal choroiditis is often detected by the presence of multiple punched-out scars seen throughout the fundus. It has been shown that there is a positive association between these fundus changes and the prevalence of infection with *Histoplasma capsulatum* in certain communities. This has given rise to the concept of the presumed ocular histoplasmosis syndrome which consists of multiple punched-out lesions seen throughout the fundus and the presence of peripapillary retinal pigment epithelial atrophy. Although this syndrome is seen commonly in areas where histoplasma infection is endemic (Ohio, Mississippi valleys), it is also seen in areas where histoplasma infection does not occur. It is assumed that alternative infectious agents may also cause this syndrome, although their identity is unknown. The importance of this syndrome is the threat of disciform degeneration occurring at the site of scars in the posterior pole long after the time of the initial disease.

In some patients it is clear that the choroiditis appears to follow the major choroidal veins giving rise to white lesions at the level of the choroid, associated with signs of low grade chronic inflammation in the vitreous. Whether this represents a single condition or several conditions is not known. The appearance of the fundus has been termed 'birdshot choroidopathy' and is associated with HLA-A29.

Lymphoma

Lymphoma of the choroid presents rarely as multifocal choroidal pale lesions simulating inflammatory disease. Unlike inflammatory disease, the lesions do not respond to anti-inflammatory agents and the disorder is inexorably progressive. Analysis of the tissue has shown that this may be monoclonal or polyclonal.

Retinal vasculitis

This is a term used to denote patients who have signs of intraocular inflammation and in which there appears to be widespread abnormality of the retinal blood vessels. This may be manifest as retinal oedema and the retinal vessels can be demonstrated as the source of the intraretinal fluid by fluorescein angiography. Inflammation of retinal vessels may be accompanied by progressive closure of the peripheral retinal vessels. Symptoms depend on the severity of disease, all patients being aware of floaters due to circulating opacities in the vitreous. If the retinal oedema affects the fovea, visual acuity is reduced. Closure of the peripheral vessels may induce neovascularization on the nerve head or in the retinal periphery with the consequent risk of vitreous haemorrhage; this pattern of disease has been collectively termed 'Eales' syndrome'. Neovascular glaucoma is extremely rare. It is rare for a cause to be found for retinal vasculitis, although it is a characteristic presentation of ocular sarcoid. The appearance of retinal vasculitis can also be caused by large-cell lymphoma of the retina.

The natural history and management of patients with 'posterior uveitis' differs from one condition to another. Management consists of treating those complications which are visually threatening. If there is macular oedema causing loss of central vision, anti-inflammatory agents may cause recovery of vision in some patients. Neovascularization in the presence of closure may be treated by laser photocoagulation to the non-perfused retina. In the case of lymphoma, the disorder is non-responsive to anti-inflammatory agents, but can be effectively managed with ocular irradiation; these diseases may be associated with central nervous system or generalized disease.

Retinitis

Certain infective agents have now been recognized as causing retinitis. The appearance of the lesion depends to some extent on the nature of the infective agent and also upon the host response. *Toxoplasma gondii* has been recognized for many years as a cause of retinitis but more recently evidence has come to light of increasing numbers of patients with viral retinitis occurring in those who are immunologically intact and more importantly in patients who are immunosuppressed, either as a result of treatment or as a result of infection by helper T-cell immune suppressive virus (human immunodeficiency virus — AIDS).

Toxoplasma

Toxoplasma gondii is usually derived from non-domestic cats and the infectivity of the cat appears to be related to the presence of coincident infection of the cat by *Toxocara catis*. The infection is particularly commonly acquired *in utero* during the course of primary toxoplasma infection of the pregnant mother. Such patients may be identified soon after birth as a result of scars in the posterior pole causing visual loss or the effect of cerebral involvement. More commonly such patients come to light as a result of recurrent retinitis occurring in later life. Retinitis may also occur during the course of the primary infection.

Toxoplasma sp. is a protozoal parasite which causes human infection after ingestion. The organism infects various tissues and usually presents with lymphadenitis and pyrexia. The organism enters the cells of the retina and multiplies intracellularly. This causes destruction of the retinal cell and the organisms released from this cell then proceed to infect other cells. The retinal inflammation is due in part to cell death and in part to the response of the immune system to the infecting organism. Certain of the intracellular organisms become cystic and remain dormant within the retinal cell for many months or years and represents the source of recurrent inflammation. During the acute systemic disease, immunoglobulin M (IgM) antibodies can be detected and subsequently disappear. Following the acute attack, IgG antibodies occur and can be detected throughout life. During recurrent retinitis, IgG levels do not change.

The patients become aware of blurred vision due either to loss of retinal function or to opacification of the vitreous. The retinal lesion appears as a pale-white area within the retina and the overlying vitreous contains significant debris. The distinction of a primary infection from recurrent disease may be made on the basis of the absence of a pre-existing fundus scar and the presence of IgM. The lesions, if threatening to vision, are usually treated by corticosteroids to reduce the amount of destruction occurring and specific antimicrobial agents are available to reduce the number of cells which become infected. As the lesion resolves, the swelling subsides leaving a white scar on the retina and choroid, and reactive hyperpigmentation.

Toxocara canis

Epidemiological studies imply that *Toxocara canis* is common, although the characteristic symptoms of the infection are rare. The worm has been recognized as causing retinal granulomata.

Viral retinitis

Viral retinitis is now being recognized more commonly. The viruses most frequently implicated are herpes zoster, herpes simplex and cytomegalovirus. This infection occurs most commonly in patients who have immunosuppression, but it is also seen in patients who appear to be immunologically normal. The area of affected retina appears intensely white with haemorrhages around major blood vessels, the blood vessels becoming closed. In patients who are immunodeficient, the retinitis appears to spread slowly across the fundus over a period of days or weeks. In patients who are immunologically intact, the retinitis appears to spread more quickly, but becomes limited within a short time. Within a few days there is necrosis and patchy clearing of the opaque retina as material sloughs into the vitreous which becomes more turbid. The vitreous debris clears slowly and retinal detachment is a very common late sequel.

Retina

Retinal vascular disease

General considerations

The eye has two distinct sources of blood supply, one in the choroid and the other in the retina, and the two vascular systems have totally different physiological properties. The retinal vessel endothelial cells form a continuous lining to the vascular space and there are well-defined junctional complexes between the cells, so that the retinal capillary wall acts as a metabolic barrier between blood and the extracellular space of the neuroretina. By contrast, the capillary endothelial cells of the choroidal circulation are fenestrated and allow free passage of small molecules into and out of the lumen. The choroid is separated from the neuroretina by the pigment epithelium which has similar properties to the retinal vascular endothelium. Thus the neuroretina is separated metabolically from plasma by these two cell systems. Both the retinal pigment epithelium and the endothelial cells are capable of transporting water and ions out of the neuroretina into the vascular space which serves to maintain homeostasis within the extracellular space of the retina. The two circulations have different regulatory systems. The choroidal arteriolar tone is governed by neural influences as opposed to the retinal circulation which has autoregulation. Both circulations respond to changes in partial pressure of oxygen and carbon dioxide.

Well-characterized ophthalmoscopic phenomena result from disturbed vascular function. Loss of integrity of retinal capillary endothelial cells causes oedema with accumulation of fluid within the extracellular space of the neuroretina. If oedema is localized, the healthy endothelial cells in the surrounding retina pump water out of the retinal extracellular space. This results in localization of the oedema and precipitation of plasma constituents, such as lipids and protein, on the margins of the affected area which are seen as exudates. There is some evidence that the presence of chronic oedema may have a deleterious effect on normal retinal capillaries such that the area of oedema tends to increase in size. Thus retinal oedema may be self-perpetuating of even self-propagating. The presence

of exudates implies that the retinal capillary abnormality is focal rather than diffuse, since in diffuse disease exudates do not occur. The oedema fluid itself gives rise to loss of retinal transparency and cystoid spaces.

Acute retinal arteriolar obstruction causes rapid onset of ischaemia with cellular swelling. This appears as opacification of the inner neuroretina which appears grey in colour. Since, at the fovea, the metabolic needs are satisfied entirely by the choroid, there is no swelling, which gives rise to the characteristic appearance of a 'cherry red spot' in central retinal artery occlusion. The retinal opacification is most prominent in the posterior retina because of its thickness, and tends to fade towards the periphery. The second consequence of ischaemia is obstruction or delay in axoplasmic transport within the ganglion cell axons. It has been shown that protein is constantly being incorporated in the cell body of the ganglion cell in the inner retina and is transported in an orthograde direction along the axon to the lateral geniculate body. There is also a separate transport of axoplasmic material in the reverse direction, from the lateral geniculate body towards the cell body which is known as retrograde transport. Interference of metabolic activity within a segment of the ganglion cell axon causes transport to cease in that segment. This results in accumulation of material at the margins of the affected retina due to continued transport by the viable axon on either side of the diseased area. Thus, if there is infarction of the whole of the retina due to central retinal artery obstruction, material accumulates at the disc due to continued retrograde axoplasmic transport in the axons of the optic nerve. Similarly, infarction of the nerve head in ischaemic optic neuropathy causes accumulation of axoplasmic material in the nerve head due to continued orthograde transport by the retinal ganglion cell axons. If there is a small infarct in the retina, material will accumulate on either side of the infarct. Axoplasmic material appears as an intensely white deposit in the inner retina and is known as a cotton-wool spot.

Obstruction of retinal veins causes increased resistance to retinal blood outflow with consequent reduction of flow within the retinal vascular system and increased transmural pressure. Two distinct responses to this disorder can be identified. If there is sufficient slowing of blood flow, there is a tendency for widespread thrombus formation to occur within the capillary system with closure of the retinal vessels within that territory. Apart from total cessation of flow within the capillaries, there is widespread egress of red blood cells from the deep retinal capillaries which appears ophthalmoscopically as diffuse midretinal haemorrhage. If widespread thrombosis does not occur, permanent interference of endothelial metabolism may occur causing chronic leakage of plasma constituents from the capillaries.

Secondary responses to closure of retinal capillaries have been well recorded. There is good evidence that the non-perfused retina produces a diffusible substance that induces blood vessel growth at a site distant from the site of retinal ischaemia. Proliferation of iris blood vessels gives rise to neovascular glaucoma. New vessels derived from the retina often proliferate anterior to the plane of the retina on the posterior surface of the detached vitreous, arising either at the optic nerve or in the peripheral retina. These give rise to the complication of bleeding into the vitreous cavity and, in certain disorders, the vasoproliferation appears to be inexorably progressive and is accompanied by fibrosis. Contraction of these membranes may result in traction detachment of the retina.

Retinal artery obstruction

The most common cause of retinal artery obstruction is an embolus derived from the heart or the major vessels of the neck. The visual loss and retinal changes correspond with the territory of infarcted retina. Central retinal artery obstruction causes total or near-total blindness while branch artery obstruction causes a scotoma. The area of infarcted retina appears opaque and embolic material may be seen within the retinal artery. Patients may have suffered previous transitory episodes of ischaemia and visual loss, due to emboli which lodge in a blood vessel and then pass into the peripheral circulation. Similar, self-limited, neurological symptoms occur if the emboli enter the cerebral circulation and are known as transient ischaemic attacks.

Retinal vein obstruction

The retinal veins may be obstructed at an arteriovenous crossing causing branch vein obstruction or just behind the lamina cribrosa causing central vein obstruction. Central retinal and branch vein obstruction appear to be more common in diabetics and patients with a high blood pressure than in the general population. Central retinal vein obstruction may also be seen as a consequence of ocular hypertension and glaucoma.

The area of affected retina is thickened, grey and contains haemorrhages. If there is retinal capillary closure, the blood tends to be diffuse and in the midretina, while in the absence of retinal capillary closure, there may be little haemorrhage or the haemorrhages are restricted to the innermost retina. Such nerve fibre bundle haemorrhages tend to conform with the orientation of ganglion cell axons giving the characteristic 'splinter' appearance.

The symptoms will depend upon the extent of dysfunction and this is determined by the intensity, duration and severity of obstructed flow. Central vision is poor if there is macular oedema or if there is closure of blood vessels at the foveola. If the foveola is unaffected, the patient may be unaware of the problem because branch vein obstruction may not affect the fovea and the changes in central vein obstruction may be mild. Patients who fail to notice the initial visual loss may present with the consequences of neovascularization such as neovascular glaucoma or vitreous haemorrhage.

In some cases with macular oedema, the visual prognosis can be modified by laser photocoagulation. The proliferative consequences can be prevented by laser photocoagulation to non-perfused retina.

Diabetic retinopathy

The initial structural change in the retinal vessels of diabetics is loss of pericytes and subsequent loss of endothelial cells. This causes the capillaries to dilate and subsequent formation of microaneurysms. As the disease progresses, there is loss of the capillary bed. The capillary changes are accompanied by functional alteration whereby plasma constituents leak from the capillary lumen into the neuroretina causing oedema, exudates and haemorrhage.

It appears that the quality of diabetic control has some influence upon the development of retinopathy because severe disease is much less common in well-controlled patients than in poorly controlled patients. The retinopathy may become particularly active during pregnancy.

In type 1 (insulin-dependent, juvenile onset) diabetes, the disorder is usually identified during the first two decades of life and retinal disease is unlikely to be significant until 12 years after the onset of disease. By contrast, in type 2 (non-insulin-requiring, adult onset) diabetes the retinopathy may be identified at the time that the diabetes is diagnosed.

In patients with loss of central vision due to diabetic maculopathy, laser photocoagulation can reverse the changes to some extent and treatment appears to be most beneficial in early disease. There is evidence that laser photocoagulation induces increased mitosis of endothelial cells and pericytes, thus causing the capillaries to become repopulated with cells. Retinal vessel closure induces new vessel formation, either in the posterior segment (proliferative retinopathy) or on the surface of the iris causing neovascular glaucoma. The proliferative retinopathy represents a major threat to vision and, unless treated, is inexorably progressive in the vast majority of patients. Both neovascular complications of diabetic retinopathy can be prevented or reversed by destruction of non-perfused retina by laser photocoagulation.

Retinal vaso-occlusive disease

This occurs in a variety of other disorders. In sickle-cell retinopathy there is progressive closure of peripheral vessels; this occurs in both homozygous sickle-cell and sickle-C haemoglobinopathies. The progressive closure of peripheral vessels induces vasoproliferation in the equatorial region which may cause, in turn, vitreous haemorrhage, or traction retinal detachment. Similar vascular changes are seen in Eales' syndrome — *see* Intraocular inflammation.

In premature infants placed in a high oxygen environment, closure of the distal retinal vasculature occurs with subsequent vasoproliferation and contraction of fibrovascular sheets in the retinal periphery (retinopathy of prematurity). In many the condition settles. Cryotherapy or surgery may also improve the visual outcome. An identical condition occurs as a dominantly inherited disease (dominant exudative vitreoretinopathy).

Hypertension

In accelerated hypertension the high blood pressure is due to the presence of circulating pressor agents. In response to the raised blood pressure, retinal arterioles constrict as a manifestation of autoregulation which tends to protect the retinal capillary bed from the effects of high blood pressure. By contrast, the choroidal circulation is relatively unprotected and it is believed that the increased blood pressure is transmitted throughout the choroidal vasculature. Thus, in accelerated hypertension, there are changes resulting from dysfunction both in the retinal and choroidal circulations. Choroidal ischaemia is manifest as focal opacification of the retinal pigment epithelium due to choroidal infarction and serous detachment of the posterior retina. In severe disease, large choroidal infarcts may occur which present as triangular-shaped opacification of the pigment epithelium. The retinal vessels become narrowed and there are frequently haemorrhages and periarterial exudates. Disc swelling is a regular feature of accelerated hypertension.

In essential hypertension there is a sustained rise in blood pressure due to changes in the tone of the autonomic nervous system. Choroidal changes are rarely seen since the arterioles become constricted in response to raised sympathetic tone. In the retina, the arteries become narrow and often show a heightened reflex. The veins are dilated and there may be haemorrhages and exudates, indicating significant capillary disease. Branch vein obstruction and macroaneurysm may occur as secondary phenomena.

Macroaneurysms

These occur on the retinal arteries as non-endothelial line out-punchings from the lumen of the vessel. In some cases this appears to be induced by weakening of the vessel wall as a consequence of an embolus lodging at that site. The aneurysm is readily seen by ophthalmoscopy and may induce oedema or cause haemorrhage. Under certain circumstances the lesion can be treated by laser photocoagulation.

Coats' disease

This disease is a disorder occurring typically in boys, in which large leaking vascular channels (telangiectasias) develop in the retinal periphery of one eye causing exudates, retinal detachment and haemorrhage. The lesions can be treated by photocoagulation or cryotherapy. A similar disorder is seen in adults which is considered to have a different aetiology and which causes less extensive change.

Outer retinal dystrophies

General considerations

The choroidal capillaries which occupy the inner portion of the choroid, the retinal pigment epithelium and the retinal receptors are closely linked functionally. The retinal receptor cells are highly active metabolically and receive their metabolic requirements from the pigment epithelium. In turn, the pigment epithelium receives its nutrition from the choriocapillaris. There is also interdependence between the cell systems in the clearing of metabolic waste material. It has been demonstrated that both rods and cones shed short segments of the distal outer segment daily and these fragments of outer segment are ingested as phagosomes by the retinal pigment epithelium. They are subsequently broken down by lysosomal enzymes within the retinal pigment epithelial cell and the products discharged into Bruch's membrane. These are then believed to diffuse through Bruch's membrane towards the choriocapillaris, entering the bloodstream and thus being cleared from the eye. It is also evident from the study of disease that receptor cell death is followed by the pathological changes in the retinal pigment epithelium and that pigment epithelial cell death induces closure of the choroidal capillaries. The situation is further complicated by secondary cellular responses in the inner retina to outer retinal atrophy. Loss of retinal receptor cells may induce visible secondary changes of the ganglion cell layer consisting of thinning of the retina, narrowing of the retinal blood vessels and optic atrophy. In certain conditions there is also invasion of the neuroretina by pigmented cells derived from the pigment epithelium.

These cellular interrelationships and secondary responses explain the inability to identify the site of primary disease, on the basis of ophthalmoscopy and histopathology in well-established retinal disease.

Because of these limitations, it is impossible to identify individual disorders causing inherited retinal receptor cell death on the basis of fundus appearance. Many conditions affect the midperipheral fundus initially and cause loss of scotopic vision and midperipheral field; a large number of such conditions falls into the category of retinitis pigmentosa. By contrast, macular dystrophies cause death of central cones with loss of visual acuity and colour vision. This division is not absolute because simultaneous loss of central and peripheral receptors characterizes some disorders. Nevertheless, the subdivision is useful and is used here. The term 'tapetoretinal degeneration' is sometimes used to refer to this group of disorders on account of the surface reflex seen in some conditions on ophthalmoscopy.

Retinitis pigmentosa

Retinitis pigmentosa is a term used to refer to a large number of inherited conditions which are variable in their severity, age of onset and speed of progression. Traditionally the disorders were thought to cause initial loss of rods. Recently it has been shown that, in some forms of retinitis pigmentosa, cone function and rod function are lost in early disease in a patchy fashion. In other patients there appears to be loss of rod function throughout the visual field, but relatively good preservation of cone function. In the first case the disease appears to be patchy, affecting both rods and cones whereas, in the second case, the disease appears to be diffuse, affecting rods rather than cones in the early course of the disorder. The inheritance may be autosomal dominant, autosomal recessive or X-linked.

In all patients the initial symptoms are of poor night vision. At a variable time afterwards, the patients notice visual field loss by day and poor vision in bright light. In well-advanced disease, the visual field is reduced to a few degrees around fixation, but visual acuity is characteristically well preserved until the last phases of the disorder. At this stage patients are severely handicapped in terms of mobility although reading may be easy. Visual acuity may be reduced by posterior subcapsular lens opacities, although these are only seen in long-standing disease. Earlier in the disease, macular oedema may also cause loss of visual acuity.

The diagnosis of retinitis pigmentosa is often suggested by a typical history of visual loss and by the presence of affected members within the family, and supported by the demonstration of midzone visual field loss. In early disease the fundus frequently appears to be normal. Thereafter, there is loss of pigment within the pigment epithelium and, in some patients, there are white or grey patches which may represent accumulation of metabolic residue. At this stage, fluorescein angiography may be valuable in identifying the pigment epithelial changes which are revealed as transmission defects allowing better visualization of the choroid. Ten years after disease onset, the pigment epithelial atrophy is more obvious and there is migration of pigmented cells into the neuroretina; by 20–30 years the pigmentation is often marked. Secondary atrophy of the inner neuroretina is accompanied by narrowing of the retinal blood vessels and optic atrophy. In very late disease, atrophy of the choriocapillaris is frequently observed. Electrophysiological testing often shows apparent disproportionate loss of electrical responses of the eye to light. The light-induced rise in ocular potential may be abolished and the electroretinogram potentials extremely small in the presence of apparently early disease. Dark adaptation tests show reduced scotopic sensitivity in all the affected areas and in most there is associated loss of photopic sensitivity.

Retinal disease indistinguishable from retinitis pigmentosa occurs in a variety of disorders affecting other systems. The best known are Usher's syndrome, in which there is congenital and non-progressive hearing loss, and Bardet–Beidl syndrome which is typified by reduced intellect, obesity, polydactyly and hypogenitalia. Congenital rubella and syphilis may also simulate the disorder.

Other generalized retinal receptor dystrophies have been identified with identical symptoms and visual defects, but which can be distinguished from retinitis pigmentosa by the fundus appearance. In choroideremia, which is inherited in an X-linked fashion, atrophy of the choroid is identified much earlier in the course of the disorder. Gyrate atrophy is autosomal recessive and causes well-defined lacunae of choroidal and pigmental atrophy in the midperipheral fundus.

With three exceptions, the basic metabolic abnormality of the various disorders within retinitis pigmentosa is unknown. The three exceptions are abetalipoproteinaemia in which there is a major disorder of lipid absorption and metabolism, gyrate atrophy in which low activity of the enzyme ornithine amino acid transferase gives rise to high blood levels of ornithine, and Refsum's syndrome in which the patient is unable to break down phytanic acid causing it to accumulate in the tissues. In these conditions, treatment is available by which the abnormal metabolism can be modified. In other forms of retinitis pigmentosa no definitive treatment is known.

Macular dystrophies

Macular degenerations cause loss of central vision with preservation of peripheral fields. Typically, patients will be aware of slow loss of visual acuity, the peripheral visual field remaining relatively well preserved. In some conditions, there appears to be more generalized involvement of cone function such that vision in bright light and colour vision become poor. Patients retain good mobility but reading becomes progressively more difficult.

As in generalized retinal disorders, a variety of tissue responses to disease can be identified. In many, loss of receptors and corresponding pigment epithelium is identified early in the course of the disease. Atrophy of the choroid also takes places and appears to be more prominent in some disorders than others. Choroidal atrophy is readily identified by ophthalmoscopy and, in some conditions, it has been thought that the initial pathological process is closure of the central choriocapillaris, although there is little scientific evidence to support this theory. In some disorders, accumulation of pale material at the level of the pigment epithelium and Bruch's membrane is prominent. This appears to be due to accumulation of phagosomal debris which reflects an inability of the pigment epithelium to break down products of phagosomal activity. In some disorders where such accumulation is prominent, there may be invasion of the abnormal deposit by new vessels derived from the choroid — *see* Disciform macular disease. Loss of inner retina causes loss of central ganglion cells axons and atrophy of the temporal quadrant of the optic nerve head.

In contrast to generalized retinal disorders, many single nosological entities can be identified within macular dystrophies. A large proportion of the remaining conditions have been divided broadly into two subcategories: bulls's eye dystrophies and fundus flavimaculatus. The term 'Stargardt's disease' has been used to refer to many of the dystrophies of early onset, but it has been imprecisely used and as such its value has been largely lost.

Bull's eye dystrophy

Within this subcategory are a variety of disorders which may be inherited as an autosomal recessive or autosomal dominant disorder. In the early stages, there is loss of paracentral vision accompanied by ophthalmoscopic changes of the perifoveal retinal pigment epithelium. This is often difficult to identify in early disease but is evident on fluorescein angiography as transmission defects. With progression, the area of involvement slowly becomes larger such that central vision is lost.

Fundus flavimaculatus

In these conditions there is multifocal deposition of pale material in the central 20° of the fundus which is accompanied sooner or later by atrophy of the outer retina at the fovea.

In both bull's eye dystrophy and fundus flavimaculatus the age onset is highly variable. Typically, they become apparent between the ages of 8 and 18 years, but in some disorders patients may not be symptomatic until the sixth decade of life. The conditions can be subdivided on the basis of inheritance. In about 70% of cases, an additional fluorescein angiographic abnormality has been identified. This consists of obstruction of all choroidal fluorescence by even deposition of abnormal material at the level of the retinal pigment epithelium; this has been termed the sign of dark or silent choroid. It implies a generalized abnormality or handling of phagosomal material without there necessarily being any corresponding ophthalmoscopic change.

Best's disease

This dominantly inherited disorder presents typically in the first 15 years of life with a raised white lesion centred at the fovea which is characteristically about 10° in diameter. At this stage visual acuity is often good. During the subsequent 10 years, the yellow material appears to break up and this is often accompanied by invasion of the mass by new vessels derived from the choroid. Thereafter, the lesion may become atrophic or a fibrous scar may form if there is prominent invasion by new vessels. Many patients with Best's disease have less prominent manifestation of the disorder and, in a few, the fundus may appear entirely normal. All patients with the abnormal gene have loss of light-induced rise in ocular potential which indicates diffuse abnormality of retinal pigment epithelial cell function, although there is no clinical consequence of this diffuse abnormality.

X-linked schisis

This condition is thought to be due to a diffuse abnormality of Müller's cells which is a class of glial cell within the neuroretina. Classically, this condition causes splitting of the retina with detachment of the innermost layer of the retina which appears as veils in the hyaloid cavity. About half the patients do not manifest this change but rather have an appearance of cystoid change at the fovea which is associated with variable loss of central vision. The electroretinogram gives a characteristic waveform with a deep a-wave and no b-wave.

Macular disease with serous detachment of the retina

General considerations

In a variety of conditions fluid collects between the neuroretina and the pigment eithelium or between the pigment epithelium and Bruch's membrane. Such an accumulation reflects a metabolic abnormality of the cells in the outer retina with respect to fluid flow. Normally, there is a net outflow of fluid from the centre of the eye towards the choriocapillaris. This is due to the small differences in hydrostatic pressure between the vitreous and extracellular space of the choroid as well as the active transport of ions by the pigment epithelium from the outer retina into Bruch's membrane with consequent movement of water. It has been suggested that a localized reversal of pigment epithelial cell transport may be the cause of fluid collecting between the neuroretina and the epithelium in central serous retinopathy, and may also explain serous detachment of the neurosensory retina in accelerated hypertension and certain forms of choroiditis. Accumulation of fluid between the retinal pigment epithelium and Bruch's membrane causes detachment of the pigment epithelium. In age-related disease, this may be due to increased resistance of water flow through Bruch's membrane.

Serous detachment of the retina may also occur if blood vessels invade the subretinal space occupying a position between the neurosensory retina and Bruch's membrane; fluid appears to exude freely from these blood vessels causing serous detachment of the posterior neuroretina. Growth of new blood vessels from the choroid is the basic pathological process in disciform macular disease which occurs as a consequence of almost any disorder that causes diffuse or multifocal abnormality of Bruch's membrane and the pigment epithelium. By far the most common, and therefore most important, disorder is age-related macular disease. Although neovascularization is a secondary phenomenon, it is frequently the main determinant of visual loss. The importance of this process is illustrated by the fact that in Western society these disorders account for over one-third of registered blindness.

When vessels invade the subretinal space, there is initially serous detachment of the neuroretina, the size of the detachment being determined by the behaviour of the new vessel complex. During the early period of subretinal neovascularization, there is rapid growth of the new vessel complex. Growth tends to be directed towards the fovea, such that extrafoveal lesions almost inevitably become subfoveal if the growth period is long enough. This is relevant to management — *see below*. Following the period of rapid growth, the neovascular complex tends to remain stable in size and this is followed by closure of the capillaries within the new vessel complex. During this final period the retina tends to flatten. Closure may be accompanied by variable fibrosis. If fibrosis is minimal the old lesion may appear as atrophy of the outer retina, pigment epithelium and choriocapillaris. On the other hand, prominent fibrosis will give rise to a hypertrophic subretinal scar. The appearance of the lesion may be altered by the presence of blood derived from the new vessel complex. In a few patients, bleeding may be quite prominent with blood in the subretinal and subepithelial spaces as well as blood within the neuroretina. Secondary changes in the overlying neuroretina may also occur. The retinal capillaries may become functionally abnormal due to prolonged detachment. This is manifest as intraretinal retinal oedema, exudates and haemorrhage in the area around the detached retina. In age-related macular disease, growth of the new vessel complex occurs over a period of as long as one year giving rise to large lesions. By contrast, in the young with multifocal pigment epithelial disease such as choroidal rupture, presumed ocular histoplasmosis syndrome and myopia, the growth period is often brief and, therefore, the lesions are small.

Central serous retinopathy

This condition occurs characteristically in men in middle life and is widely believed to affect tense individuals and to be related to mental stress. During active disease the neurosensory retina is detached from the retinal pigment epithelium. It is believed that the fluid between the neuroretina and pigment epithelium is derived from the pigment epithelium and fluorescein angiography indicates that there is a small population of pigment epithelial cells which are actively transferring water in an inward direction from the choriocapillaris into the subretinal space. Patients with this condition are aware of some reduction of visual acuity which is, at least in part, due to induced hypermetropia. Distortion of vision is common, and is presumably due to the loss of normal contour of the posterior retina. Other symptoms include dyschromatopsia and a prolonged recovery time from retinal bleach; these deficits are presumably due to an abnormality of metabolic exchange between receptors and retinal pigment epithelium across the subretinal space.

The serous detachment of the posterior retina is often evident ophthalmoscopically, although the pigment epithelial lesions are rarely indentifiable. Fluorescein angiography is used to identify the origin of the fluid, from whence the dye is seen to leak into the subretinal space.

In the vast majority of patients, good visual function is retained despite active disease lasting weeks or months and spontaneous resolution occurs in all patients. Resolution of the disease is accompanied by improvement in symptoms, although a small residual deficit may last for weeks, months or may be permanent after such an attack. Recurrent disease can be expected in over one half of the patients and in a small proportion multiple recurrences may cause diffuse pigment epithelial disease with permanant loss of visual function.

No medical treatment has been shown to influence the disorder. Laser photocoagulation applied to the areas of pigment epithelial cell dysfunction is followed by rapid resolution of the serous detachment, although it is most unlikely that this has any influence on the long-term visual outlook, and does not reduce the likelihood of recurrent disease.

Age-related macular degeneration

Alternative terms that have been used are 'senile or involutional macular degeneration'. The changes in senile macular degeneration appear to be a response to abnormal deposition of material at the level of Bruch's membrane due to disordered handling of phagosomal material. With age, material accumulates in the inner part of Bruch's membrane and may be recognized as drusen. Initially, these are seen as well-defined small yellow deposits beneath the neuroretina, and with time the deposits become larger and less well defined. A second change has been identified in which epithelial cells form a reduplicated basement membrane; this is known as basal linear deposit. With age there is also progressive loss of receptor cells. In the elderly, the number of receptors may be reduced to 10% of the number seen in the young. There is consequent reduction of the phagosomal load and drusen become crystalline before resolving completely.

Three distinct consequences of this accumulation have been identified. In some patients there appears to be detachment of the pigment epithelium from Bruch's membrane. It is thought that accumulated debris within Bruch's membrane may contain high lipid in some patients which would render Bruch's membrane hydrophobic. A significant increase in the resistance to water flow in Bruch's membrane would result in accumulation of fluid between the pigment epithelium and Bruch's membrane and consequent detachment of the pigment epithelium. The most important result of these changes is invasion of Bruch's membrane by blood vessels. The final manifestation is extreme loss of receptor cells with consequent atrophy of the pigment epithelium and closure of the choriocapillaris; this is known as geographic atrophy. Pigment epithelial detachments and disciform disease are collectively known as exudative or 'wet' macular disease and account for about 85% of all patients suffering major visual loss in this category of disease. Geographic atrophy or 'dry' macular dystrophy accounts for the remaining 15%. Exudative lesions occur over the age of 55 and become progressively more common until the mid-

to late-70s. Geographic atrophy is more common in patients over 80 years.

Pigment epithelial detachment

Pigment epithelial detachment causes distortion of central vision. Visual acuity is often good, at least in the early stages of the disease, since the neurosensory retina is not detached from the underlying pigment epithelium. Ophthalmoscopically, such lesions appear as well-defined dome-shaped elevations of the posterior retina.

The lesion may remain stable for months or even years. Spontaneous resolution of the pigment epithelial detachment is uncommon and is generally accompanied by loss of central vision. Two particular complications of pigment epithelial detachments are recognized. The subpigment epithelial space may be invaded by blood vessels from the choroid which may grow on the inner surface of Bruch's membrane or the outer surface of the detached pigment epithelium. Their presence may be indicated by haemorrhage or subpigment epithelial exudate or uneven pigmentation of detached tissue. Should the blood vessels remain confined to the subpigment epithelial space, vision may remain stable. On the other hand, if the blood vessel transgresses the pigment epithelium, central vision is affected. Finally, the pigment epithelial detachment may become progressively larger and more deeply detached and a tear may occur around a part of the perimeter of the detachment. This occurs as a sudden event and is accompanied by rapid loss of visual function. The presence of a tear may be implied by haemorrhage or the appearance of a flap of pigment epithelium with a free edge in the subneuroretinal space. With time, the pigment epithelial flap may flatten onto Bruch's membrane or the edge may be reattached to Bruch's membrane giving rise to a smaller pigment epithelial detachment and an area of bare Bruch's membrane. The area of Bruch's membrane may become recovered by pigment epithelium or more commonly is replaced by a fibrous plaque.

At present no treatment is known which alters the visual prognosis in pigment epithelial detachments.

Disciform macular disease

Invasion of the subretinal space by blood vessels causes serous detachment of the neuroretina and distortion of central vision. Once the new vessel system is subfoveal, visual acuity is lost; some recovery of vision may occur as the blood vessels close down and the retina flattens but recovery is limited by tissue damage.

The detachment caused by the disciform lesion is often apparent by ophthalmoscopy. Its presence may also be signalled by the presence of blood and accumulation of exudates in the subretinal space or by changes in the overlying neuroretina such as exudates, oedema or haemorrhage. As the lesion become more mature, the fibrous content of the lesion increases and is seen as white material beneath the neuroretina. If the fibrous tissue is minimal, then the lesion will appear as atrophy of the retina, the pigment epithelium and choriocapillaris.

During the early stages of blood vessel growth, fluorescein angiography shows the lesion clearly and there is profuse leakage of dye into the subretinal space. As the lesion becomes more mature, the blood vessels are less well seen and leakage becomes reduced.

The importance of disciform macular disease is related to the recent demonstration that laser photocoagulation may destroy the subretinal new vessel complex. If such a complex is identified before it reaches the foveola, central vision may be preserved although there will clearly be a dense scotoma at the site of therapy. Unfortunately, only a small percentage of disciform lesions are identified at a stage at which they are amenable to therapy. It is clear that a lesion that is not subfoveolar is likely to become subfoveolar with time and that a majority of disciform lesions are subfoveolar at the time of their diagnosis.

The properties of a treatable lesion have been well characterized. It has been shown that a patient with good acuity and recent history of visual loss is likely to be treatable, while a patient with poor vision and long history is most unlikely to be treatable. As a general guideline, a vision of 6/24 or better and a history of visual loss of less than 1 month implies that a lesion is likely to be amenable to therapy. Such a history associated with progressive distortion of vision identifies a patient who should be assessed urgently with a view to treatment.

Geographic atrophy

In this condition, there is progressive appearance of well-defined areas of atrophy of outer retina, pigment epithelium and choriocapillaris. The progress of geographic atrophy appears to be slow and irregular. Initially, patients notice paracentral scotomata which correspond to the areas of atrophy. No treatment is known by which the course of the disorder can be modified. In particular there is no evidence that vasodilators influence the visual prognosis. It is much more likely that loss of choriocapillaris is a consequence of loss of neighbouring tissue, such as pigment epithelium and receptor cells, rather than being a consequence of primary choroidal ischaemia.

Disciform lesions

Disciform lesions from other causes have similar qualitative attributes to those in age-related disease in terms of their behaviour characteristics and in clinical presentation. In presumed ocular histoplasmosis and in disciform macular disease of the young of unknown origin, it has also been shown that laser photocoagulation improves the visual prognosis.

Other retinal conditions

Preretinal fibrosis

This is a common condition in the older population and appears to be a consequence of vitreous detachment. It is believed that detachment of the vitreous causes small defects in the retinal inner limiting membrane at sites of vitreoretinal adhesion. Accessory glial cells derived from the defect proliferate on the surface of the retina giving rise to an abnormal sheen (cellophane maculopathy). If the fibrous complex contracts, there is distortion of the inner retina and occasionally there is associated limited detachment of the posterior retina. In the vast majority of patients with this condition, acuity remains good but occasionally patients may have distortion or loss of central vision. In the few with poor vision, surgical peeling of the membrane may result in improved function.

Retinal detachment

Retinal detachment due to retinal tear is caused by an accumulation of fluid between the retinal receptors and pigment epithelium. The retinal tears are produced during the vitreous detachment and occur by traction of the detaching vitreous at sites of vitreoretinal adhesion. Potential adhesions can be recognized sometimes prior to detachment at the sites of lattice degeneration and fibrocystic tufts. During the period of retinal traction, the retina tears and is lifted from the underlying pigment epithelium, fluid entering the subretinal space from the hyaloid cavity. In some cases, small segments of retina may become completely detached from the rest of the retina thus relieving traction, and detachment may not occur. Population surveys have shown that peripheral retinal holes may be identified without detachment in 8% of the population above the age of 60 years. Once the detachment is initiated or traction continues as in U-shaped tears, the detachment is generally progressive.

During the period of traction, patients may be aware of flashing lights and, as the retina is broken, there may be accompanying haemorrhage which is recognized by the patient as floaters. Enlargement of the detachment may be recognized as an increasing area of visual field loss and, once the macula is detached, visual acuity is lost. Surgical treatment of detachments results in successful re-application of the retina in about 95% of cases, although the visual recovery may be incomplete due to structural change occurring at the time of retinal detachment.

In a small percentage of patients, cells appear to proliferate on the inner surface of the retina and along structures within the vitreous. These cells are believed to be of pigment epithelial origin. They proliferate and form collagen and fibrocellular membranes which contract. This represents the most common cause of treatment failure and is termed 'preretinal fibrosis'. It appears as white strands in the vitreous and causes folds to occur in the retina. The only effective treatment in such cases is surgical removal of the fibrous material.

Degenerative retinoschisis

This is common and is due to splitting of the peripheral retina. It causes high elevation of the inner retina in the affected area, and corresponding visual loss. Retinal detachment is a rare complication of this otherwise benign condition.

Fundus tumours

Two principal primary malignant ocular tumours are recognized: uveal melanoma and retinoblastoma.

Melanoma

Melanomata may occur in any part of the uvea although they are most common in the choroid and least common in the iris. Choroidal melanomata may arise from naevi and are initially seen as brown, slightly elevated lesions in any part of the fundus. As the lesion grows there may be serous detachment of the neuroretina and, if the tumour grows through Bruch's membrane, there is often rapid growth forming a 'collar-stud' tumour; the term 'solid detachment' is sometimes used to describe this condition. There may be some variation in pigment and tumours may appear pale. The symptoms depend upon the site of the tumour, the visual loss corresponding with the area of retinal detachment. Iris tumours appear as slowly enlarging brown lesions within the iris stroma. Ciliary body lesions may be seen if they displace the iris away from the limbus as a brown mass in the peripheral part of the anterior chamber; they may also cause displacement of the lens with consequent refractive change or cataract. Choroidal tumours have the highest malignancy and iris tumours are considered almost benign.

Melanomata have been traditionally treated by removal of the eye although it is not proven that this improves prognosis for life. There are now attempts to treat these lesions in a more conservative fashion; small tumours may be destroyed by photocoagulation, irradiation or local excision.

Retinoblastoma

Retinoblastoma is a tumour of the retina occurring typically in children and may occur in two circumstances. It may be dominantly inherited in which case both eyes are affected and the tumour usually appears within the first 2 years of life. Alternatively, it may occur sporadically, in which case one eye is usually affected and it presents, on average, 2 years later. The inherited form may be detected as a result of routine examination of a child known to be at risk of developing such a tumour. Sporadic cases may be identified because of visual loss, development of a squint or as a result of the characteristic white reflex seen in the pupil. On examination the tumours are seen as white or pale-yellow masses growing into the eye from the neuro-retina or, more rarely, the retina is detached and the tumour appears to invade the subretinal space. In very advanced disease, the tumour may extend into the orbit causing proptosis or may metastasize.

This tumour can be effectively treated by radiation, light coagulation or cryotherapy provided that the case is identified early enough in the course of the disorder. Patients with hereditable disease are at risk of developing other tumours in later life, particularly osteosarcoma of the femur.

Metastatic lesions

These may be identified in the eye. The secondary deposits usually appear as slightly elevated pale lesions in the choroid and are frequently multiple. The most common sources of such metastases are breast and lung. These tumours are often effectively treated by radiation, although clearly the prognosis for life depends upon metastatic spread elsewhere.

Choroidal haemangioma

This is a benign tumour of the choroid which causes elevation of the retina, distortion of vision if the lesion is in the posterior pole and retinal oedema with consequent loss of visual function in the affected area. In large tumours there may be serous detachment of the retina which may be widespread. The lesion may not appear markedly different from the surrounding retina, although it is clearly seen on ultrasound and fluorescein angiography. The importance of the lesion is its distinction from choroidal melanoma. It can effectively be treated by laser photocoagulation.

Phacomata

This term is used to denote a variety of conditions which are familiar and in which there are tumours or malformations of the retina. In von Hippel–Lindau disease, retinal angiomata occur and may be accompanied by angiomata in the cerebellar hemispheres and abdominal tumours. The retinal tumours appear as well-defined red lesions which grow causing serous retinal detachment or traction retinal detachment. In Sturge–Weber disease, diffuse choroidal haemangioma is associated with a dermal haemangioma corresponding with the first division of the the fifth cranial nerve. The fundus appears intensely red due to the vascularity of the choroid and, in a minority of cases, serous retinal detachment may occur. Such patients are also at risk of suffering glaucoma. Bournville's disease causes astrocytic hamartomata in the retina which appear as pale mulberry-like lesions. These patients are at risk of having abdominal tumours and similar astrocytic malformations in the central nervous system and skin changes. Neurofibromatosis (von Recklinhausen's disease) causes multiple neurofibromata in the skin and associated with the central nervous system, and 'café-au-lait spots' in skin. Such patients may have congenital glaucoma, optic nerve gliomata and choroidal neurofibromata.

Optic nerve disease

General considerations

Disc swelling is seen in a variety of circumstances, such as optic neuritis, ischaemia, accelerated hypertension, ocular hypotony and raised intracranial pressure. In all these conditions, the disc swelling is due to delay in axoplasmic transport at the cribriform plate causing the axons to swell. This causes vasodilatation in the nerve head which, in turn, induces oedema and haemorrhage. That the mechanism of disc swelling is the same whatever the initiating disorder, explains the inability of the clinician to identify the basic disease on the basis of the appearance of the nerve head. Clinically, the swelling is seen initially as blurring of the disc margins, and spontaneous pulsation of the central vein ceases. With progression, the swelling becomes more obvious, haemorrhages are seen on the disc surface and in the inner peripapillary retina, and axoplasmic debris accumulates within the nerve head.

Optic atrophy results from loss of ganglion cell axons with consequent closure or constriction of the papillary blood vessels. Loss of ganglion axons is also apparent in the inner retina. In the young, the axons appear as a fine parallel pattern in the reflex from the inner limiting membrane. They are most easily seen around the nerve head and in the temporal arcuate areas. Mild loss of axons appears as

linear defects in the reflex; complete absence of the axons appears as linear defects in the reflex; complete absence of the axons causes the retinal blood vessels to have sharp borders and the normal linear reflex is lost.

Optic neuritis

Acute optic neuritis

Acute optic neuritis may occur as a manifestation of primary intrinsic demyelination, either as an isolated phenomenon or as part of disseminated sclerosis. The patients experience loss of colour vision and visual acuity and pain which is aggravated by eye movement. Visual field testing typically reveals a central scotoma, and colour vision is invariably abnormal. In unilateral disease, there is a relative afferent pupillary defect. The optic nerve head is usually normal at this stage unless the inflammation is in the anterior nerve in which case it is swollen. The diagnosis can be made on the basis of a typical history, particularly if there is evidence of previous demyelination. It may be confirmed by the demonstration of optic nerve swelling, by imaging techniques such as magnetic resonance imaging or computerized tomography. The most characteristic abnormality is a delay in visual evoked response due to slow transmission of the impulse with the segment of affected nerve. This delay may be permanent even though visual recovery may appear complete. Recovery of function occurs within a few days or may be delayed for several weeks and is so good that the residual deficit is often hard to identify. Although systemic steroids may hasten recovery, the final level of vision does not appear to be altered by treatment. Permanent loss of ganglion cell axons is a constant feature, although this does not become apparent for several weeks, at a time when vision may be good. Defects in the ganglion cell layer, and delay in the visual evoked response may be the only evidence of previous optic neuritis. Loss of function with rise in body temperature and with exercise may also occur; this phenomenon, known as Utthof's symptom, is thought to be due to loss of conductance in compromised neurones as the temperature rises.

Leber's optic neuropathy

This is a specific familial disorder which affects men more often than women and presents with acute visual loss affecting both eyes, although the visual loss is usually not simultaneous. Typically, visual loss occurs between the age of 15 and 30 years, and recovery is usually poor. Prior to visual loss the nerve appears mildly swollen and there is dilatation of the peripapillary radial capillaries. Profound optic atrophy occurs but may only become apparent 9 months after visual loss.

Ischaemic optic neuropathy

The blood supply to the optic nerve head is dual, the posterior portion at the lamina cribrosa being derived from the choroidal circulation while the anterior part is from the retinal circulation. Infarction of the nerve head results from obstruction of the ciliary supply of the optic disc. It is a common feature of giant cell arteritis in which there is generalized inflammation of medium-sized arteries. The vision is usually very poor and total blindness is common. The disc appears markedly swollen on ophthalmoscopy. The diagnosis may be suspected if there is polymyalgia rheumatica, night sweats, loss of appetite and non-ocular ischaemia, and is confirmed by a highly elevated sedimentation rate and the finding of characteristic histopathological changes in a temporal artery biopsy. Treatment consists of high doses of corticosteroids in order to prevent infarction of the contralateral optic nerve or infarction elsewhere. Treatment may be required for many years. In the absence of giant cell arteritis, infarction of the nerve tends to cause altitudinal field loss, often with good acuity. No cause is known, there is no evidence of ischaemia outside the eye and yet involvement of the other eye occurs in about 50% of cases.

Infiltration

Infiltration of the nerve may occur in inflammatory disease, such as sarcoid, or by tumour. The visual loss is usually severe and the optic disc markedly elevated.

Toxic amblyopia

'Toxic amblyopia' is a term used to denote a number of conditions in which there is bilateral symmetrical visual loss due to optic nerve disease. The visual loss is slowly progressive and causes poor colour vision and bilateral centrocaecal visual field loss. It is seen in people with vitamin deficiency, particularly vitamins B_1 and B_{12}. Vitamin B_{12} deficiency occurs in pernicious anaemia, in patients who have had chronic gastric disease or gastrectomy, and is common in vegans, while alcoholics on poor diet often suffer hypovitaminosis-B_1. Similar disease is seen in pipe tobacco smokers; it is believed that certain tobaccoes give rise to high cyanide intake which is not detoxicated adequately causing optic nerve damage. The fundus appears normal in early disease and optic atrophy may not be apparent for many months. An identical condition is also seen in patients of Jamaican origin; the nature of the disorder in Jamaican optic neuropathy is not understood and, in particular, it does not appear to be familial. The optic disc pallor is usually confined to the temporal quadrant, the remainder of the disc retaining its normal colour; there is corresponding loss of ganglion cell axons in the papillomacular bundle.

The severity of visual acuity loss depends on the nature of the condition. In vitamin deficiency, vision may be regained if treatment is initiated early. In tobacco amblyopia, cessation of smoking and administration of large doses of hydroxycobalamin may cause visual recovery. No treatment is known which will alter the course of Jamaican optic neuropathy, although the progress is extremely slow.

Dominant optic atrophy

This is the most common inherited optic atrophy and causes mild reduction of visual acuity in childhood associated with localized atrophy of the temporal quadrant of the disc. During subsequent years there may be further functional loss. It is unusual for acuity to fall below 6/60 and it may remain as good as 6/9. For this reason, familial involvement is not always evident by history alone and, if there is any doubt as to diagnosis, it is essential to examine other family members.

Congenital abnormalities

Congenital abnormalities of the nerve head may take many forms. Colobomata cause the disc to appear enlarged mostly consisting of lamina cribrosa. The lamina may extend to the edge of the disc over a significant proportion of its circumference. This may be associated with colobomata of the uvea. Smaller defects appear as optic disc pits which are small and dark in colour. Serous detachment of the posterior retina is a rare complication of such colobomata.

Apparent swelling of the disc is produced by hamartomata or optic disc drusen. These are sometimes associated with non-progressive visual loss. Pseudopapilloedema is seen in patients with small optic discs in which crowding of the ganglion cell axons gives the impression of disc swelling; such patients are often hypermetropic.

Tropical eye disease

Certain communities of the world have a very high prevalence of blindness due to hyperendemic infective disease or to nutritional defect. The commonest cause of blindness in the world at present is trachoma (*see* Conjunctivitis).

Onchocerciasis

Certain communities in Sub-Saharan Africa and Central America have hyperendemic infection by *Onchocerca volvulus* which is transmitted by the fly *Simulium* sp. The condition has been termed 'river blindness' due to the high infection near fast-flowing rivers. Distribution is determined by the fly which can only develop in this environment. Individuals are infected in very early life and may become infected *in utero*. The immature worm is inserted into the skin by this blood-sucking fly and matures in subcutaneous sites. Adult worms produce microfilariae which spread throughout the body and evoke remarkably little inflammation. An infected individual may have dozens of adult worms within the body which may live for as long as 20 years. Each adult produces up to 1000 microfilariae per day and the microfilariae appear to survive for about 2 years. Inflammation occurs only around dead microfilariae. Dead microfilariae will evoke corneal stromal infiltrations which are seen as fluffy opacities. These resolve over a period of a few days, but with chronic presence of microfilariae, progressive corneal opacification starts at the inferior limbus — sclerosing keratitis. The microfilariae also cause characteristic chorioretinal scarring and optic atrophy. The importance of the disease is a high prevalence of blindness in the affected communities. In Africa as many as 10% of certain communities may be blind, and half the community will be blind before death.

Attempts have been made to control the infection by destroying the vector. This has proved to be effective but expensive. The traditional medical treatment by diethylcarbamazine is accompanied by high risk of permanent damage to the visual system from reactive inflammation. The introduction of a new drug, ivermectin, has brought some hope of mass treatment for this condition.

Leprosy

Leprosy is a chronic inflammatory disorder caused by an acid-fast bacillus, *Mycobacterium leprae*. In certain communities this appears to cause marked inflammation resulting in 'tuberculoid leprosy'. In other communities, the inflammatory response is much less marked — lepromatous leprosy. The organism survives in only those parts of the body which are cold so that the major effect is on skin and the extremities. Ocular damage may result from facial nerve palsy and exposure keratitis or the organism may cause keratitis directly. In cooler climates, the organism appears to survive in the iris and dysfunction of the dilator muscle causes the pupils to become very small. The small pupil associated with minor lens opacities results in severe visual disability.

Nutritional blindness

In undernourished communities, patients suffer ocular damage from low intake of proteins and vitamin A. Vitamin A deficiency results in keratinization of the conjunctiva (Bitot's spot) and of the cornea. Progressive loss of receptors results in night blindness and eventually outer retinal atrophy. Patients with protein deficiency may also suffer catastrophic infection of the cornea (tropical ulcer). The causative organism has not been defined and there may not be a single organism responsible for this inflammation. It may be associated with measles and there is some evidence that herpes simplex virus may play a major aetiological role.

18

Anterior eye examination

Harry Stockwell and Janet Stone

The major instruments used for this purpose are the slitlamp biomicroscope, for observation of fine detail, and the keratometer or ophthalmometer, for measurement of central corneal curvature. More detail of corneal contour as a whole is obtained with a keratoscope. There is a multitude of smaller instruments which may be used for observation and measurement of certain aspects of the anterior eye. These range from the ophthalmoscope and the hand-held pen-slit torch used with a loupe of × 6 to ×10 magnification, to pupillometers and the Wessely keratometer used for diameter measurement. Norn (1983) has given a good description of these minor instruments and techniques.

Slitlamp biomicroscopy
General considerations

A typical slitlamp is shown in *Figure 18.1*. Observation of the normal eye and adnexa, and detection of pathological conditions of the anterior segment, as well as the examination of the quality of contact lens surface, is best carried out by studying the fine details of the structures through a binocular microscope using slit beam illumination as described, for example, by Stockwell (1983a). Ideally, the microscope has a magnification range in the region of × 5 to ×50, a Zoom lens system being the most convenient, although many instruments have a turret of two or three pairs of objectives used with one or two pairs of eyepieces. Müller (1981) and Henson (1983) both give details of the optical systems used in modern slitlamp biomicroscopes and include comprehensive diagrams of the illuminating and viewing systems.

For general examination of lesions and small opacities direct viewing of the slit section is first used. For ease of manipulation, the slit beam is

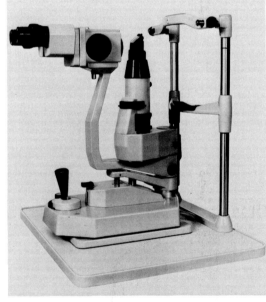

Figure 18.1 The Rodenstock Slit Lamp RO 2000 S which has a microscope permitting magnification of × 6 to × 48. The following accessories are among those which may be attached to it: Goldmann-type applanation tonometer, pachometer, anterior chamber depth gauge, retinal visual acuity meter, camera and flash attachment, television camera, Hruby lens, teaching eyepieces, oculars for length and angle measurement. (Photograph kindly supplied by Rodenstock)

usually directed so that its focus coincides with the focus of the microscope objectives (*Figure 18.2*). This common focus is usually arranged to be mounted in the vertical axis of rotation of the two systems which can be positioned with respect to the observed eye so that the viewing angle (α) between

309

the slit and the microscope can be varied. This arrangement is known as a 'coupled system'. Other things being equal, a long working distance between the slit system, the microscope objectives and the eye is desirable because there will thus be a greater depth of focus when viewing the slit section. This is particularly noticeable in crystalline lens work as both systems are shortened by the power of the observed eye to converge the rays.

Because of the observer's awareness of the nearness of the object, stereopsis is more easily achieved if the microscope eyepieces are convergent rather than parallel. Spectacle wearers should check that the microscope exit pupils suit them. To avoid misinterpretation of irregularities in the structure of the eye, the slit must be sharp, of good contrast, free from aberrations as well as being white and free of harmful radiations. However, it must have sufficient strength in the deep violet to permit useful illumination through a cobalt filter for staining techniques, used mainly in contact lens work, preferably in conjunction with a yellow filter in the observation system. The slit aperture should be adjustable down to 0.1 mm in width and up to 16 mm in length, and convertible to a circular aperture of the same dimensions to facilitate full viewing of a contact lens fit. A very small aperture of about 0.6 mm diameter is useful for examination of vacuoles, or in association with a very fine slit set horizontally to search for cells in the anterior chamber.

Types of illumination

A general view of the lids and external eye by diffuse illumination is made possible by the use of a ground glass 'filter' placed just in front of the 45° mirror which reflects the slit onto the eye. This is particularly helpful when studying everted eyelids in

conjunction with blue filter and fluorescein or when studying limbal vasculature by red-free illumination.

Illumination from the iris or lens, or when examining by sclerotic scatter from the limbus, may require the slit to be moved slightly off its axis of common focus and coincidence, and slightly defocused to the surface of reflection (*see Figure 18.2b*, angle θ). In such cases any surface other than that

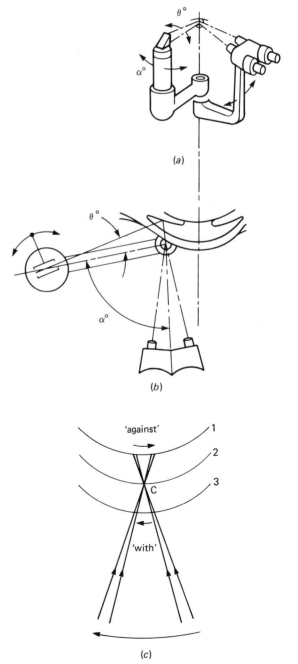

Figure 18.2 Focusing the slit beam and microscope. (*a*) Both microscope and illuminating systems have supporting arms which rotate about a common pivot situated directly below the focus point of each. (*b*) Angle α is the angle between slitlamp and microscope which may be varied from 0° to 180°. However, the slit beam may be offset from this common focus by angle θ, by rotating the tube and/or mirror of the illuminating system. (*c*) Since the common focus of both slit beam and microscope is situated directly above the pivot point around which each supporting arm rotates, this pivot is placed under the eye to be examined. The slit beam supporting arm is then rotated slightly from side to side. If correctly focused, there will be no movement of the focused light patch on the eye (the closed eyelid is preferable)—as shown in (*c*) position 2 at C. If the instrument is too far away from the eye, there will be an 'against' movement—as shown at position 1; and if too close to the eye a 'with' movement—as shown at position 3. (Angle θ should of course be 0° when this is carried out.) (Reproduced by kind permission of *The Ophthalmic Optician*)

under inspection may be used to change the contrast so that the difference in structure may be better observed. It is advantageous if the detent mechanism for returning the slit to its direction of coincident focus is a deadlock and not one of the type located by a spring and ball in a 'vee' notch which prevents small angles of displacement from being achieved. This type of position may be useful in the examination of corneal endothelial cells, their pattern and count. For this the viewing axis is set at about 45° to the vertical slit. The area is located with low magnification and switched to ×40 with a McIntyre reticule, (Micro-surgical Technology, Inc.) (*Figure 18.3*). The slit may then need to be moved very slightly off axis to obtain the optimum specular reflection view. Specular microscope attachments are also available on some more sophisticated slitlamps, thereby allowing both observation and photography of endothelial cells.

The 1986 model Haag/Streit Slit Lamp offers a 'stereo-variator' attachment built into the body of a reversible Galilean drum-type microscope which permits reduction of the stereoscopic viewing angle from 13° to 4.5°. This retains converging eyepieces yet provides binocular viewing of stereoscopic slit sections of the media through to the retina, as well as stereoscopic viewing and photography of endothelial cells. In conjunction with the Eisner (1985) lens which incorporates a red filter to eliminate light of short wavelength and stray rays from corneal stroma, increased magnification of 2.2 times the microscopic magnification is available.

Supplementary attachments

Most slitlamps accept an applanation tonometer for estimation of intraocular pressure (IOP) after Goldmann — for a description *see* Chapter 23.

In some slitlamps a greenish 'red-free' filter is incorporated to enhance contrast when using rose bengal stain and when viewing blood vessels, either of the anterior eye or when the fundus is viewed. Both stain and blood vessels then appear black. In the latter case, either a Hruby lens, which is planoconcave of power −58.6 D (Hruby, 1941), may be employed, with concave surface facing the patient's eye, forming a virtual image of the fundus within the focusing range of the microscope thereby permitting direct observation of the fundus, or alternatively the El Bayadi (1953) positive planoconvex lens (+60 D), which forms an aerial image of the fundus (similar to the indirect ophthalmoscope) may be used. A Polaroid filter is sometimes used to eliminate unwanted reflections from these lenses, neither of which is easy to use without a good patient and much practice. A fundus (or high minus) contact lens is preferable.

Anterior chamber examination is not complete without inspection of the iridic angle — the technique of gonioscopy (Becker, 1972; *see* Chapter 24). This is best performed with a fine slit which can be rotated about its centre of projection to view a section at right angles to the mirror or prism of the gonioscopy lens used. There are several types of lens for this purpose. The patient will be grateful and the examination easier if a light one is chosen. The single mirror type has to be rotated, gently; the two-mirror type gives two sections at one setting and is not much heavier, but the three-mirror variety is difficult to manoeuvre and perhaps initially to interpret. The originals of these were due to Goldmann (1938) and are now made in acrylic material. They should not be confused with the special glass types used for laser work.

Follow-up work on keratoconics and contact lens patients is more comprehensive with corneal thickness measurement (pachometry). The pachometer attachment is arranged so that a part of each of the vertically bisected slit images—one each from the front and back surfaces of the cornea—may be viewed simultaneously. A scale is attached to the image splitter (usually a parallel plate) which provides a direct thickness reading. It is important to use a fine slit and focus precisely with the slit set at the correct angle to the microscope objective. An attachment for anterior chamber depth measurement works on the same principle.

Facilities for the attachment of 'teaching eyepieces' by means of extra observation tubes are most useful. These extend from the microscope body permitting one or two extra observers. A slitlamp may also be used to provide a mount on the microscope body for an aesthesiometer, for recording corneal or ocular surface sensitivity (Norn, 1983). Thus the tip of its nylon monofilament may be observed as it is gently touched onto the eye.

There are several camera attachments for slitlamps. Most are suitable only for external or anterior chamber work. Only two types of principle are really satisfactory:

(1) Those which are pre-set by the manufacturer with respect to the slit focus and are independent of the microscope, and used bearing this fact in mind.
(2) Single lens reflex types, some of which may view through the microscope eyepiece but which must use the camera viewfinder to evaluate the picture taken.

Other types whose focal plane images are not capable of direct visual assessment are not to be recommended. Expert photography is a special study involving special angulation techniques for illumination and reflection.

Attachments to hold contact lenses exist to facilitate inspection of their edges, surfaces and inclusions. Indirect illumination is useful in conjunction

Horizontal section to
show position of microscope
and light beam

Vertical
section seen

Photograph of vertical
section

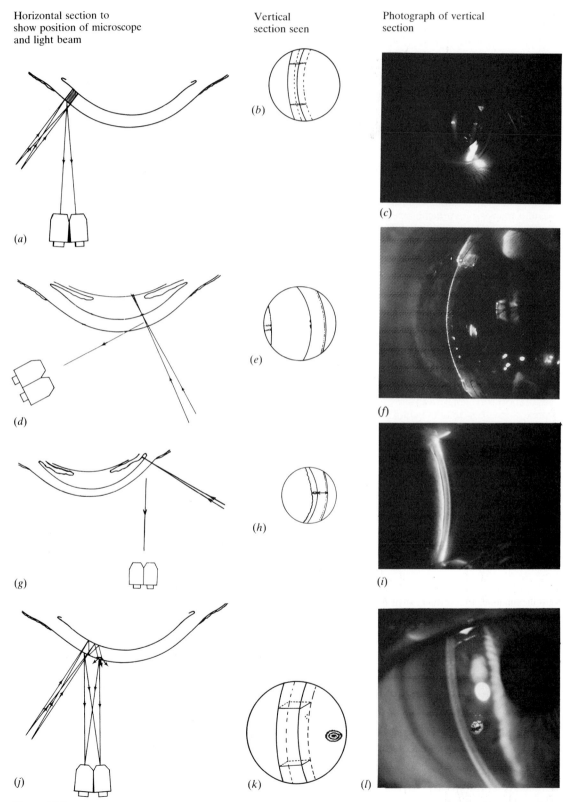

Figure 18.3

Figure 18.3 Traditional techniques of illumination. (*a*) Direct focal illumination: both beam and microscope are focused at the same point. To assist easy viewing the angle between the two may vary from 0° to 180°, commonly being around 30° to 60°, and their relative positions in front of the eye may also be varied to aid observation. The focally illuminated area may be circular or slit-shaped, of any width or length within the capability of the instrument, and additional filters may be used and the light intensity varied. The whole of the anterior eye and adnexa may be examined thus. Only when a ground glass is introduced into the beam path does the illumination become non-focal. This is known as diffuse illumination and is useful with or without other filters for cutting out annoying reflections. (*b,c*) Parallelepiped section: a fairly wide (2 mm) slit is useful in examining the cornea as it allows both epithelial and endothelial surfaces, as well as the substance, to be observed simultaneously. Thus such features as epithelial abrasions, stromal scars and nerve fibres, as well as pigment deposits on the endothelium, may all be seen during one sweep of the cornea. The microscope is usually best in front of the eye and the slit, anything from 20° to 70° to one side or the other. As with all types of illumination, the microscope is first set to give low magnification, which is increased when interesting features are to be studied in detail. (*d*) Narrow section: useful for observation of depth of any notable feature such as a corneal or crystalline lens opacity. For corneal observation (*e,f*) the beam should be focused from in front with the microscope anything up to 90° from it, whereas for studying the crystalline lens, unless the pupil is dilated, the angle between beam and microscope should be very small, between 5° and 10°, needing to be even smaller if the rear surface of the lens and anterior vitreous are to be seen. A particular application of this technique is assessment of anterior chamber angle width, known as the Van Herick technique, whereby a narrow beam is focused on, and perpendicular to, the corneal limbus in such a position that a corneal section and a section of the anterior chamber at the extreme limit of the angle can just be observed through the microscope placed directly in front of the eye (*g*). The angle between slit and microscope is about 60°, and the patient looks at the microscope throughout. Low magnification is used to give good depth of field. The width of the anterior chamber is compared in dimension with the corneal thickness (*h*) and if the ratio is 1:4 or less then a dangerously narrow angle may be suspected (*i*). (*j*) Indirect focal illumination: to a certain extent this method of illumination is used every time observation by direct focal illumination is carried out, because the field of view of the microscope is usually much larger than the area being focally illuminated. Hence any areas of the eye seen beyond the focally illuminated area are being viewed by indirect illumination (*k*). Corneal nerve fibres and endothelial or stromal striae are often most easily detected in this way as are foreign bodies, when they lie just adjacent to the slit beam (*l*). Alternatively the beam is offset and focused to one side of the microscope focus by rotating the mirror as shown in *Figure 18.2b*.

with, for instance, a diffusing card held behind the lens. If the slitlamp be placed to one side at 180° to one of the microscope objectives, the eyepiece can be used to project an image of matter placed at the focus of the microscope. Simple eyepiece graticules, such as millimetre and protractor scales, are useful when observing contact lenses *in situ*, for recording sizes as well as angles of truncation and cylinder axis markings.

Before contemplating certain surgical procedures, it is desirable to ascertain preoperatively the probable integrity of the fundus although the view may be hampered by a cataractous lens. An attachment to the Rodenstock slitlamp employs twin low power coherent laser beams to produce variable spatial frequency interference gratings which can be rotated by means of a Dove (Amici) prism and may be projected through to the fundus. The patient is asked to indicate the axis of the grid. A similar but cheaper attachment, the Lotmar visometer (Lotmar, 1980), which uses projected Moiré interference fringes, is available for the Haag–Streit slitlamp.

The slitlamp is used as a delivery vehicle for ruby lasers in fundus photocoagulation, for argon lasers and others more anteriorly where the absorption spectra are more suited. More recently, YAG (yttrium–aluminium–garnet) lasers have been built into compact slit systems: their effects and side-effects require further study. In such adaptations, the slitlamp requires accessory lenses of very special surface quality and the microscope, of course, requires a special interactive shutter which is opaque to laser emissions.

The various methods of illumination traditionally used in slitlamp work are shown in *Figure 18.3* with photographs to illustrate the types of appearance seen.

Keratometry (and allied techniques)

A curved reflecting surface produces an image whose size is a function of the radius of curvature of that surface, provided that the size and distance of the object and the means of viewing are fixed. The purpose of the keratometer is to measure this radius which is normally that of the cornea, but may be a calibrating ball or the concave or convex surface of a contact lens. The reflected object usually consists of an illuminated pattern of special form called a 'mire', or else two distinct 'mires' whose separation and orientation may be variable. The means of viewing is usually a monocular microscope of long focal length, which may also be used to inspect the edge and surfaces of a contact lens. The distances of both the microscope and the object mires to the image are fixed. This is shown in *Figure 18.4a* in diagrammatic form, along with the mathematical

Horizontal section to
show position of microscope and light beam

Vertical
section seen

Photograph of vertical section

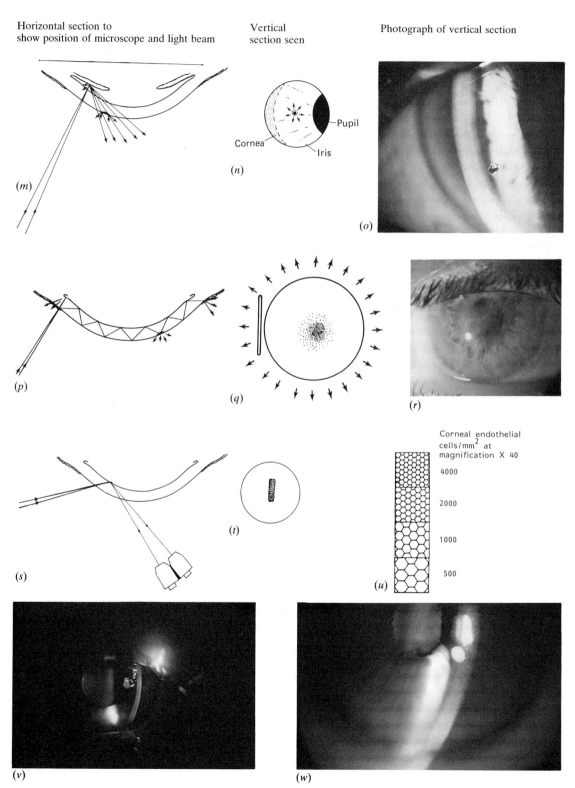

(m)

(n)

Pupil

Cornea

Iris

(o)

(p)

(q)

(r)

Corneal endothelial
cells/mm^2 at
magnification X 40

4000

2000

1000

500

(s)

(t)

(u)

(v)

(w)

Figure 18.3

Figure 18.3 (*cont.*) (*m*) Retro-illumination: when the microscope may be independently focused, so that the focally illuminated area is beyond the focus of the microscope, interesting features in the cornea show up as dark areas against a light background; for example corneal opacities against the light iris background (*n*, *o*) and limbal neovascularization shown up by oblique retro-illumination where the nasal limbus is viewed by the beam directed towards it from the temporal side and focused on the back of the cornea (*p*). Sclerotic or scleral scatter is another form of indirect focal illumination usually carried out without observing through the microscope. A slit beam is focused at the limbus. Light from it is totally internally reflected by the normal cornea before being scattered again by the sclera giving rise to a glow of light around the entire limbus region. Any corneal irregularity or opacity will similarly scatter the light (*q*), showing up as a light area against the darker background of the pupil or iris. Localized areas of corneal oedema, often called central circular clouding when it follows oxygen deprivation following the wear of hard contact lenses, shows up in this way as do corneal dystrophies (*r*). Subtle corneal changes can only be seen in a completely darkened room, and may then only be detected if the observer studies the cornea from several different directions while keeping the illumination fixed. Once any such light scattered from the cornea has been detected, the area involved may be viewed by direct focal illumination through the microscope and then the beam offset to the limbus again, while viewing through the microscope. (*s*) Specular reflection: specular, or regular, reflections of the light source are usually annoying and only occur when the angle of incidence of the beam at one of the eye's surfaces is such that the microscope axis is located along the line of reflection. The brightest reflections are obtained at the front surface of the eye. The back and front surfaces of the crystalline lens and the back surface of the cornea give rise to much dimmer reflections because the refractive index differences at these surfaces are much less. Specular reflection gives a lot of information about the quality of the surface at which the light is being reflected, permitting, for example, the study of conjunctival surface irregularities, the 'orange peel' effect caused by the cellular nature of the front surface of the crystalline lens and the nature of the corneal endothelium (*t*). All that is necessary is to focus the microscope on the surface to be viewed and then move the slit beam so that the incident light will be reflected back directly into the microscope. In this way the observer is viewing an out-of-focus image of the light source often referred to as the 'zone of specular reflection'. In reality the surface is being viewed against the background of the Purkinje image which it forms. Studied at high magnification (× 50 or more) the size and density of corneal endothelial cells can be judged by the use of the McIntyre eyepiece graticule (*u*). Mire traverse: occasionally it is helpful to focus the microscope on the actual Purkinje image of the light source formed by the corneal or crystalline lens surfaces. Much as a keratometer mire image gives an indication of the regularity or otherwise of the front of the cornea, so reflections of the lamp filament can give an indication of surface quality. To locate the Purkinje images (*v*, *w*), the beam should be moved slightly from side to side, and viewing without the microscope, the first, second and third Purkinje images will be seen to give a 'with' movement, although the second is difficult to locate as it is so

close to the first (*v*) and very dim by comparison. The fourth (*w*), because it is a reflection from a concave surface—the back of the crystalline lens—will give an 'against' movement. If the diffuser is put in place, this becomes the light 'source' and the Purkinje images are then small rectangular reflections. The first Purkinje image is really formed at the precorneal tears film and this technique can form a useful way of observing it. (The illustrations (*c*), (*i*), (*l*), (*o*), (*r*), (*v*) and (*w*) are by courtesy of Keith Edwards and (*f*) and (*u*) by courtesy of Carl Zeiss (Oberkochen) Ltd)

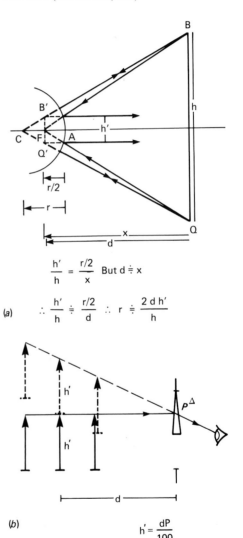

$$\frac{h'}{h} = \frac{r/2}{x} \quad \text{But } d \doteq x$$

(a)

$$\therefore \frac{h'}{h} \doteq \frac{r/2}{d} \quad \therefore r \doteq \frac{2\,d\,h'}{h}$$

(b)

$$h' = \frac{dP}{100}$$

Figure 18.4 Optical principles used in keratometry. (*a*) Derivation of the 'keratometer formula'. (*b*) The doubling principle—the size of an image, *h'* may be measured precisely when its doubled image, seen through a prism, is formed exactly adjacent to it—as shown in the central position here. Where the power of the doubling prism, *P* (in △) and the distance, *d* (in cm), at which it is used are fixed and known, then *h'* (in cm) = *dP*/100. (Reproduced from Sheridan, 1984, by kind permission)

derivation of the 'keratometer formula', $r = 2dh'/h$. This is only strictly correct if the mire images are formed exactly in the focal plane of the cornea acting as a convex mirror and, for this to occur, the keratometer must have collimated mires. However, any error introduced by non-collimated mires is very small and easily allowed for during calibration of the instrument by the manufacturers. The formula also assumes paraxial theory which is an oversimplification with the steeply curved surfaces involved.

Doubling

The reflected mire images are continually moving because the cornea is never still. In order to measure the length of a moving image it is necessary to view both its ends simultaneously. This is achieved by the use of an optical doubling system in the microscope. Thus one end of one of the doubled images is displaced to coincide with the opposite end of the other doubled image (*Figure 18.4b*). Henson (1983), and Bennett and Rabbetts (1984) give details of the various doubling systems employed in keratometers which include parallel glass plates, double image prisms and prism and lens systems. In practice, each end of the image corresponds to a specific reference point on one of the mires and the amount of displacement of the doubled images may be by a fixed amount or by a measurably varied amount. Hence keratometers are often classified into two main types according to whether the doubling is fixed or variable.

Fixed doubling

This necessitates a variable object size, by means of movable mires to achieve the necessary image displacement. The Javal type of instrument employs this mode of doubling.

Variable doubling

This is used to give the required image displacement when the mire pattern is of fixed size as in the instruments of Helmholz, Zeiss, Sutcliffe, Bausch & Lomb, American Optical and Gambs.

Mires

Some of the mire patterns used by different instrument manufacturers are shown in *Figure 18.5*.

The central 3–4 mm of the cornea usually approximates to a spherical or toroidal form, unless it is very irregular, as for example in keratoconus. However, beyond the central region the cornea flattens off and, in cross-section, its form is mathematically very close to that of an ellipse (Kiely, Smith and Carney, 1982). Keratometers are normally designed to measure the curvature of the central region of the cornea only, and as this is most often toroidal a maximum and a minimum curvature need to be recorded. These are known as the principal meridians. Some instruments have mires in mutually perpendicular meridians, making the assumption that once one principal meridian has been located, then the other is at right angles to it. The Bausch & Lomb instrument is of this type, having two separate doubling devices to allow mire image doubling along both principal meridians to be made concurrently. This follows rotation of the mire pattern about the optical axis of the instrument until correct orientation with either of the principal meridians is achieved. Such instruments are known as 'one position' instruments. 'Two position' instruments utilize mires in one meridian only which can be rotated about the optical axis to any desired meridian, usually to the two principal meridians to allow maximum and minimum radii to be recorded. Because corneas are often slightly irregular, the two principal meridians may not be perpendicular to each other, and hence the latter type may permit greater accuracy. Also, for extremely toroidal corneas, refocusing the instrument will be necessary for each meridian, because the mire images fall in slightly different planes. Again the 'two position' type of instrument is easier to use in this respect.

Sources of error

The main sources of error in keratometry are:

(1) Failure to adjust the eyepiece to allow for the user's refractive error.
(2) Accommodation being exerted by the user, resulting in incorrect mire setting.
(3) Focusing the instrument too close to the measured cornea (associated with the use of accommodation).
(4) Failure to centre the mire images in the field of view.
(5) Incorrect fixation by the patient.

Wilms (1968) has been responsible for several devices to reduce errors in keratometry. Those instruments which employ fixed eyepieces and telecentric optical systems remove the probability of the first three sources of error above. A good quality optical system removes the fourth source of error. Such foolproof instruments are very expensive. Correct fixation by the patient is achieved by occluding the other eye and by locating the fixation target so that no accommodation is required by the patient. Use of the keratometer objective is made for this purpose. It is important to ensure that the patient's head remains stationary throughout the procedure. Most instruments provide adequate chin and fore-

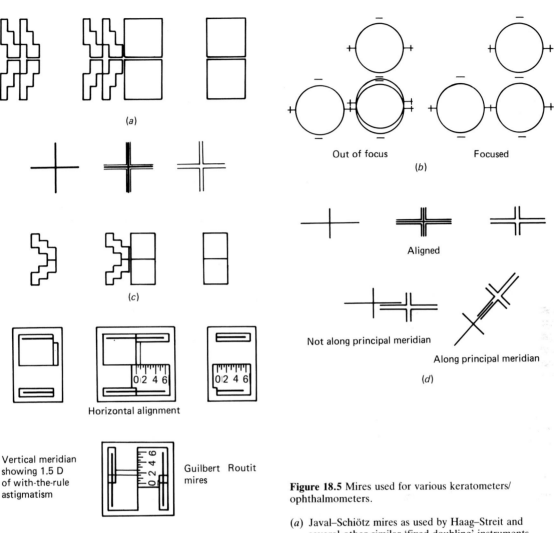

Horizontal alignment

Vertical meridian showing 1.5 D of with-the-rule astigmatism

Guilbert Routit mires

Mires not along principal meridian

(e)

Out of focus   Focused

(b)

Aligned

Not along principal meridian

Along principal meridian

(d)

Figure 18.5 Mires used for various keratometers/ophthalmometers.

(a) Javal–Schiötz mires as used by Haag–Streit and several other similar 'fixed doubling' instruments.
(b) Bausch & Lomb mires, also used in other 'one position' instruments such as the Topcon.
(c) Gambs mires: two different types have been employed one type very similar to the Javal–Schiötz.
(d) Zeiss (Oberkochen) mires.
(e) Guilbert Routit mires

head rests and allow the microscope axis to be aligned with the patient's visual axis using reference markers. A quick, reliable way of aligning the two is to shine a pen torch through the eyepiece, and to adjust the height and direction of the microscope so that a (doubled) light patch falls on the patient's cornea.

To minimize the risk of errors on less expensive instruments, those with adjustable eyepieces should be checked against the highest precision steel balls (others are not likely to be truly spherical) and the

eyepiece wound in until the graticule is just sharp, with accommodation fully relaxed. Then any error between the scale reading and the radius of the steel ball can be noted and allowed for in future measurements. A graph may be plotted of scale reading against correct (steel ball) radius to assist this. To aid accurate focusing the Scheiner disc principle is employed in some instruments. Thus the doubled images are themselves seen double unless accurately focused. The Bausch & Lomb, Rodenstock and Sutcliffe instruments employ split field adaptations of this principle. Greater detail of the optical systems used in various instruments is available from the individual instrument manufacturers whose brochures give a wealth of information. Textbooks on instruments and visual optics, such as those by Henson (1983) and by Bennett and Rabbetts (1984), allow comparative assessment of the instruments to be made.

Measurement of the peripheral cornea

Henson (1983) and Bennett and Rabbetts (1984) also give information on instruments designed to measure peripheral corneal curvature, sometimes called 'topographical keratometry'—for example the Guilbert Routit instrument which had collimated mires and a Michelson doubling system, which is no longer made. Adaptations to conventional instruments to permit their use for peripheral corneal measurement have also been discussed by Stone (1962, 1975). Attachments which move fixation for exploration of corneal topography should be treated with caution unless there is a full understanding of the true corneal areas involved (Wilms and Rabbetts, 1977). The Rodenstock C-MES and CES instruments have reliable topographic attachments (Wilms, 1981) and the latter permits corneal eccentricity values to be derived by means of a programmed pocket calculator. The Zeiss (Jena) 110 instrument also has a topographic attachment.

Measurement of mire images

It should be realized that the position and extent of the measured surface used to form an image of each point on the mire, vary with the aperture of the keratometer objective, the mire position and the radius of curvature of the surface itself. With most keratometers the two mires are reflected by two areas of cornea either side of its apex and separated by between 2 and 4 mm, the areas themselves being between about 0.1 and 0.7 mm in extent, depending on the instrument (Stockwell, 1983b). For instruments having fixed mire separation, the separation of the reflection areas increases as the radius of curvature of the cornea increases, whereas the reverse applies in instruments with variable mire separation. The work of Lehman (1967) and Mandell (1964) has demonstrated this, and their findings have been summarized by Sheridan (1984). The assumption is made that the two areas used for reflection as well as the region of surface between them are all part of a surface of constant curvature. Because this is not so, different keratometers give different measurements for the radius of curvature of the same cornea. Also, the visual axis along which

the instrument axis is directed, does not necessarily intersect the cornea at its apex, in which case pseudo-astigmatic errors may be introduced.

Due to aberrations, the size and plane of the reflected mire images depend on whether the surface is convex or concave. Corrections are built into the keratometer scale to compensate for the aberrations of convex surfaces, but for concave surfaces such as the back surfaces of contact lenses a correction factor must be applied (Emsley, 1963; Bennett, 1966).

Keratometers not only measure the radius of curvature of each principal meridian of the cornea, they convert this into a measure of the refractive power of the cornea in that meridian. To do so entails the assumption that the cornea as a whole can be represented as a single refracting surface separating air from a medium of refractive index somewhat lower than that of the actual cornea, the refractive index being chosen on the assumption that the back surface of the cornea neutralizes approximately one-tenth of the power of the front surface. This assumption has led different manufacturers to use slightly different indices of refraction for the calibration of their keratometers, varying from 1.332 to 1.3375. Although this leads to different power values for a particular radius, the difference in the refractive indices used is too small to lead to any errors in the astigmatic differences so determined between the two principal meridians (Stone and Francis, 1984). Some 'two position' instruments have mires which are graduated in dioptric steps. Then, if the flatter, least powerful, meridian of the cornea is measured first and the mires rotated to the steeper, more powerful, meridian there will be an overlap of the mire images. The amount of overlap of these images indicates the amount of astigmatism of the cornea. The Javal–Schiötz mires consist of one stepped mire and one rectangular mire (*see Figure 18.5a*), each step of coverage by the rectangular mire indicating 1 D of astigmatism. The Guilbert Routit instrument has a dioptric scale on one mire, the amount of overlap of the other mire being read off on the scale of a vernier marker on this second mire.

Extreme variations

If necessary, steeper and flatter radii than the keratometer is normally designed to measure, may be successfully determined by extending the range of the instrument. For measuring steep radii, such as those of keratoconic corneas and very steep contact lens radii, a low positive trial case lens, e.g. +1.25 D may be taped in front of the keratometer objective. Precision steel balls of suitable known steep radii are mounted in front of the instrument. The positive trial lens serves to magnify the mire images reflected by the steel balls so that a reading within the normal radius range of the instrument is recorded for each steel ball measured. A graph is then plotted of steel ball radius against instrument radius reading, which, provided that the same trial case lens is used on subsequent occasions, may then be referred to whenever such steep radii are encountered. In similar fashion, a low minus trial case lens may be taped in front of the objective and flat steel balls used to obtain a graph for the measurement of flat radii, such as those found in cases of cornea plana and for flat contact lens surfaces. It is important that the supplementary trial case lens used is always of the same power and form, and correctly centred on each occasion if differing aberrations which might affect the results are to be avoided.

Contact lens measurement

The measurement of contact lens radii is often simply carried out by placing the lens on a suitable holder with a 45° inclined mirror above it to reflect light from the instrument mires onto the lens surface. A reading is made in the usual way, but correction tables must be referred to when concave surfaces are being measured due to non-paraxial aberrations causing slight differences in image size between convex and concave surfaces. The measurement of soft lenses (Chaston, 1973; Loran, 1984) requires a saline cell, increased light output from the mires and trial case lenses to extend the range of the instrument as described above.

Corneal topography

A general impression of the topography of the cornea may be obtained from the Placido disc: a series of concentric black and white rings on a flat evenly illuminated round disc is held facing the cornea. The image of these rings formed by the cornea is viewed through a lens in the centre of the disc. The form and quality of the image indicate the state of the cornea. In photokeratoscopes, a camera is mounted in place of the viewing lens. To render the image suitable for photography, the ringed surface must be dished and the width and spacing of the rings varied. This then permits a record capable of computer analysis. The Wesley-Jessen System 2000 PEK (Photo Electric Keratoscope) is an example of this technique (Townsley, 1970) enabling a contact lens to be specified from the result obtained.

A variation by Ysoptic has two series of small bright steel cylinders arranged like the rungs of two curved ladders at right angles to each other lying on the surface of an imaginary dome. A camera is mounted at their intersect and directed towards the cornea at the dome centre. The photograph is scanned and the resulting analysis used to program a lens-generating machine.

The Humphrey Auto Keratometer, as its name implies, carries out corneal measurement automatically. It also makes two extra measurements either side of the apex horizontally and uses this information to produce a 'shape factor' for the cornea. It uses sophisticated electronic techniques to make the measurements and has an inbuilt computer. Henson (1983) and Bennett and Rabbetts (1984) give more details of its mode of operation.

Other automatic keratometers are the Canon K1 and Nidek KM 800 using television viewing systems, and the Sun PKS-1000. All provide information about the peripheral cornea, and the Sun instrument, by means of a suitable supplementary system, permits three-dimensional graphics of the cornea to be computer printed (Port, 1987).

For additional information on techniques of examining and measuring the anterior eye, readers should consult the manufacturers' literature and the reading list together with the references where more comprehensive treatments may be found.

References

BECKER, S.C. (1972) (*Clinical Gonioscopy.* St Louis: C.V. Mosby

BENNETT, A.G. (1966) The calibration of keratometers. *Optician*, **151**, 317–322

BENNETT, A.G. and RABBETTS, R.B. (1984) *Clinical Visual Optics.* London: Butterworths

CHASTON, J. (1973) A method of measuring the radius of curvature of a soft contact lens. *Optician*, **165** (4271), 8–12

EL BAYADI, G. (1953) New method of slitlamp micro-ophthalmoscopy. *Br. J. Ophthalmol.*, **37**, 625–628

EISNER, G (1985) Endothelioscopie à large champ simplifiée. *Bull. Mem.* SFO, **96e**, 129–134

EMSLEY, H.H. (1963) The keratometer: measurement of concave surfaces. *Optician*, **146**, 161–168

GOLDMANN, H. (1938) Zur Technik der Spaltlampenmikroskopie. *Ophthalmologica*, **96**, 90

HENSON, D.B. (1983) *Optometric Instrumentation.* London: Butterworths

HRUBY, K. (1941) Ueber eine wesentliche Vereinfachung der Untersuchungstechnik des hinteren Augenabschnittes im Lichtbüschel der Spaltlampe. *Albrecht von Graefe's Arch. Ophthalmol.*, **143**, 224–228

KIELY, P.M., SMITH G. and CARNEY, L.G. (1982) The mean shape of the human cornea. *Optica Acta*, **29**, 1027–1040

LEHMAN, S.P. (1967) Corneal areas utilised in keratometry. *Optician*, **154**, 261–264

LORAN, D.F.C. (1984) The verification of soft contact lenses. In *Contact Lenses*, 2nd edn, edited by J. Stone and A.J. Phillips, Chap. 15. London: Butterworths

LOTMAR, W. (1980) Apparatus for the measurement of retinal visual acuity by Moiré fringes. *Invest. Ophthalmol.*, **19**, 393

MANDELL, R.B. (1964) Corneal areas utilized in keratometry. *Am. J. Optom.*, **41**, 150

MÜLLER, O. (1981) *Ocular Examination with the Slit Lamp: A treatise on the instrument with hints on its practical application*. Oberkochen, West Germany: Zeiss

NORN, M.S. (1983) *External Eye: Methods of Examination*. Copenhagen: Scriptor

PORT, M.J.A. (1987) Keratometry and keratoscopy. *Optician*, **193** (5085), 17–24

SHERIDAN, M. (1984) Keratometry and slit lamp biomicroscopy. In *Contact Lenses*, 2nd edn, edited by J. Stone and A.J. Phillips, Chap. 5. London: Butterworths

STOCKWELL, H.J. (1983a) Considering the slit lamp and biomicroscope. *Optician*, **185** (4796), 16–20

STOCKWELL, H.J. (1983b) Considering ophthalmometers. *Optician*, **186** (4800), 16–19

STONE, J. (1962) The validity of some existing methods of measuring corneal contour compared with suggested new methods. *Br. J. Physiol. Opt.*, **19**, 205–230

STONE, J. (1975) Keratometry. In *Contact Lens Practice*, edited by M. Ruben, Chap. 7. London: Baillière Tindall

STONE, J. and FRANCIS, J.L. (1984) Practical optics of contact lenses and aspects of contact lens design. In *Contact Lenses*, 2nd edn, edited by J. Stone and A.J. Phillips, Chap. 4. London: Butterworths

TOWNSLEY, M.G. (1970) New knowledge of the corneal contour. *Contacto*, **14** (3), 38–43

WILMS, K.H. (1968) Improvements to ophthalmometers. Rodenstock's British Patent 1,227,016 patented 12 July 1968

WILMS, K.H. (1981) Topometry of the cornea and contact lenses with new equipment. *Ophthal. Opt.*, **21** (16), 516–519

WILMS, K.H. and RABBETTS, R.B. (1977) Practical concepts of corneal topometry. *Optician*, **174** (4502), 7–13

Further reading

BEDFORD, M.A. (1971) *A Colour Atlas of Ophthalmological Diagnosis*. London: Wolfe Medical Books

BERLINER, M.W. (1943) *Biomicroscopy of the Eye*, Vol. 1 and 2. New York: Paul B. Hoeber

EISNER, G. (1973) *Biomicroscopy of the Peripheral Fundus*. Berlin: Springer.

EMSLEY, H. H. (1936) *Visual optics*, Chap. IX, London: Hatton Press

GOLDBERG, J.B. (1970) *Biomicroscopy for Contact Lens Practice*. Chicago: Professional Press

MAYER, D.J. (1984) *Clinical Wide-field Specular Microscopy*. London: Baillière Tindall

SPALTON, D.J., HITCHINGS, R.A. and HUNTER, P.A. (1984) *Atlas of Clinical Ophthalmology*. Edinburgh: Churchill Livingstone

STONE, J. (1979) The slit lamp biomicroscope in ophthalmic practice. *Ophthal. Opt.*, **19**, 439–455

TORTOLERO, J., WESLEY, N.K. and BRONSTEIN, L. (1959) *Fluorescein Staining: Characteristics of Corneal Insult*. Chicago: The Plastic Contact Lens Company

19

Fundus examination

Richard Llewellyn

Introduction and historical development

Ophthalmoscopy is performed routinely during the eye examination. At what stage it is undertaken is dependent upon the preference of the practitioner, although a good case can be made for leaving it until near the end when the induced after images will cause no disruption to subjective assessments by the patient.

It is worthwhile reviewing the history of ophthalmoscopy briefly before looking at examples of the optics and use of current instruments. Babbage in 1848 and then von Helmholtz in 1850 devised the first ophthalmoscopes, although it was only with the latter that the real significance of the invention was appreciated.

The early techniques involved the illumination of the internal eye by means of light reflected by a plane piece of glass. The illuminated fundus was then observed by the examiner looking through the glass reflector (*Figure 19.1*). Efficiency was improved by increasing the number of glass plates to reflect more of the incident light towards the subject. Finally, von Helmholtz suggested silvering the reflector and allowing observation by means of a small hole. Reute in 1852 included a concave mirror to further improve the illumination and this system is the basis of all modern direct ophthalmoscopes.

Current instruments allow a range of apertures to be inserted into the illuminating system and the use of filters to modify the spectral characteristics of the light source is common. From the examiner's point of view, the task of examination is simplified by

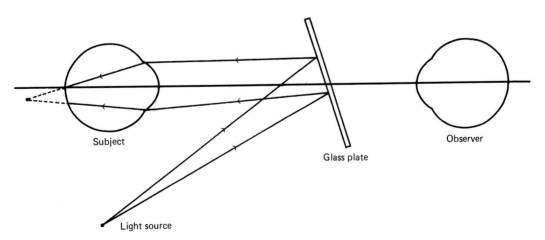

Figure 19.1 The original ophthalmoscope of von Helmholtz, showing the illuminating system, which is still the basis of modern instruments

means of positive and negative spherical lenses that can be positioned behind the mirror to correct for any refractive errors that may be present in the subject or the examiner and to focus to the desired level within the eye. This can provide an estimate of the patient's refractive error but is inaccurate for reasons detailed by Emsley (1952).

The early instruments were non-luminous, requiring an external light source, usually positioned approximately in the plane of the subject. The hand-held ophthalmoscope was then adjusted to reflect light from this source into the eye to be examined. Special lamps were used to provide the necessary illumination, having a blackened envelope, with a small clear portion left for the light to escape.

Modern instruments are self-luminous having a small lamp, usually positioned beneath the mirror and supplied with current either from internal batteries or via a lead to a suitable power supply. An alternative to this is to have a remote projector with the light being carried to the instrument in a fibreoptic light guide (*Figure 19.2*). This reduces the bulk of the hand-held part of the instrument and allows a greater range of sources and filters to be used.

Corneal reflex

One of the main difficulties during ophthalmoscopy is avoiding the reflection of the source from the corneal surface. This forms an image of the source about 3.5 mm behind the front surface of the cornea and can mask the detail of the inner eye. This problem has been largely overcome by the use of small light sources and the careful positioning of the filament image, as far as possible separating the viewing and illuminating paths.

The reflection can be eliminated entirely by means of crossed polaroid filters inserted into the illuminating and viewing systems, an idea proposed by Cardell (1935). However, the advantages of this system are heavily outweighed by the need to quadruple the illumination in order to allow for the light loss induced by the filters.

Direct and indirect ophthalmoscopes

Direct ophthalmoscopy is so called because the image of the subject's fundus is projected directly onto the fundus of the examiner with no intermediate image being formed. *Indirect* ophthalmoscopy employs the technique of forming an intermediate, or aerial, image and it is this which is viewed by the examiner (*Figures 19.3* and *19.4*). Indirect ophthalmoscopes may be *monocular* or *binocular* and take the form of either *hand-held* or

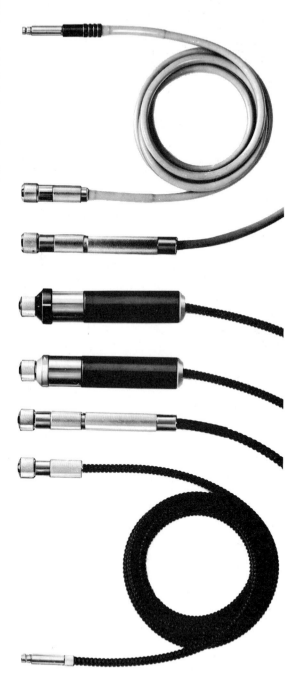

Figure 19.2 A selection of various light guides, used to convey light from the remote projector to the instrument in use. (Reproduced with the permission of Clement Clarke International Ltd and Heine Optotechnik)

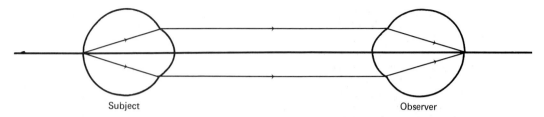

Figure 19.3 The viewing path for direct ophthalmoscopy. The image of the subject's fundus is projected directly onto the fundus of the observer

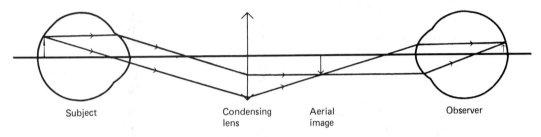

Figure 19.4 The viewing path for indirect ophthalmoscopy. The condensing lens forms an aerial image of the subject's fundus to be viewed by the observer

headband devices, usually employing a separate condensing lens held close to the subject's eye. Major stand instruments are now less common, except as fundus cameras or in the form of slitlamps with auxiliary fundus viewing lenses.

An indirect ophthalmoscope gives an inverted image as shown in the ray diagram, unless a separate lens system is used to correct it. Significant differences exist between the direct and indirect methods in terms of the field of view and the magnification at which the fundus is seen. An approximate comparison is shown in *Table 19.1*, but the absolute values will vary according to the amount and type of the patient's ametropia.

The greater convenience of the instrumentation means that it is generally the direct opthalmoscope that is used routinely in optometric practice. It usually enables the practitioner to undertake detailed examination of the media and fundus without the need for pupil dilatation by utilizing the various apertures and the rheostat provided on the instrument. For viewing the extreme periphery, pupil

dilatation using a recognized mydriatic is advantageous. Bennett and Rabbetts (1984) listed the design criteria of a direct ophthalmoscope as follows:

(1) Adequate illumination.
(2) Controllable illumination.
(3) Control over the area of fundus to be illuminated.
(4) Freedom from harmful radiation.
(5) Freedom from stray light reflected from the edges of the sight hole and lens mounts, known as sight hole flare.
(6) Minimization of the corneal reflex.

Indirect ophthalmoscopy is certainly useful where an overall view is required, for example in determining the relative positions of landmarks or the extent of a detachment. It may also give a clearer view of the fundus in cases where the media are irregular.

Difficult viewing conditions

Problems will be encountered where central opacities in the media obscure the view. It may be that, in trying to see around these opacities, the observer encounters the corneal reflection of the light source. In order to see the fundus adequately under these conditions, it is necessary to dilate the pupil. Similarly, patients who are on miotic therapy, usually for glaucoma, will present with their habitually con-

Table 19.1 Comparison between direct and indirect ophthalmoscopes

Ophthalmoscope	Field of view (°)	Magnification
Direct	8	×15
Indirect	40	× 4

stricted pupil(s). There is a reluctance to use a mydriatic on these patients in optometric practice. In most cases they will be under ophthalmological care where such procedures will be undertaken routinely. It is, however, helpful to ask such patients to delay the instillation of their drops until after the examination. Care must be taken in interpreting refractive results that have been obtained when the pupil is more dilated than usual.

Indirect ophthalmoscopes will always give a better quality image when the pupil is dilated and, indeed, most instruments will only work satisfactorily if this is done. Some, for example the Reichert hand-held indirect ophthalmoscope, are able to operate through an undilated pupil and can perform well within the limits of normal pupil size and media clarity. Indirect ophthalmoscopes of any sort suffer more than direct ophthalmoscopes when small pupils are present.

Record keeping

Before examining the specific techniques of using direct and indirect ophthalmoscopes, it is appropriate to look at the means by which observed details may be recorded. Defects in the media must be identified and their depth and position noted. Close examination of such defects may be better performed with a hand slitlamp and magnifier or with a slitlamp biomicroscope if they are positioned in the anterior part of the eye, but they may well first be noticed during routine ophthalmoscopy.

An initial impression of the depth of a defect will be obtained by noting the lens power in the ophthalmoscope when it is first seen. The higher the plus power necessary to focus the edges sharply, the more anterior is the defect. By noticing the 'with' or 'against' movement of the object relative to lateral movements of the ophthalmoscope, the position in front of, at, or behind the nodal point may be assessed. As shown in *Figure 19.5*, defects in front of this point (e.g. corneal foreign bodies) appear to move in the opposite direction to the ophthalmoscope, defects at this point (e.g. nuclear sclerosis lens changes) appear to remain stationary and defects further back (e.g. vitreous opacities) move in the same direction as the ophthalmoscope. The further away is the point from the defect, the greater will be the movement seen. In this way it is possible to record the site of a lesion by sketching it in on diagrams representing both the front and side views.

Opacities further back within the vitreous may be related in position to the retinal structures over which they lie.

The apparent size of retinal detail will vary according to the power of the refracting surfaces of the eye, the axial length and, of course, their physical structure. For example, the retinal structures in an aphakic eye look very small because of the loss of the magnifying power of the crystalline lens, while the fundus details of a high axial myopic look very large and the field of view is correspondingly small. This magnification or minification can be minimized by viewing the fundus through the patient's own spectacle correction, but it is still difficult to quantify the size of any details that need to be recorded without reference to something to which it can be compared. The retinal detail of a patient with high astigmatism can be similarly enhanced if the fundus is viewed through the patient's spectacles. Obviously such record keeping

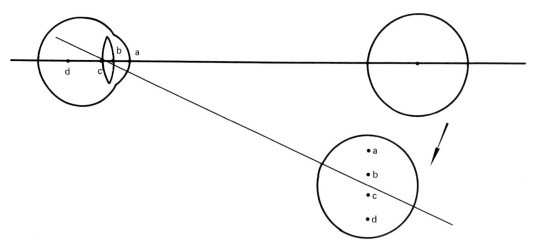

Figure 19.5 The use of parallax to determine depth. The objects a, b, c, d all lie on the midline and appear to move in the directions shown when viewed obliquely

is important for the practitioner's future reference and for anyone else who subsequently examines the patient.

Size of retinal detail

There are two main ways of defining the size of a lesion or abnormality. Reference may be made to other structures within the same eye, for example describing a patch of old choroiditis in terms of its size relative to the disc or, alternatively, smaller objects can be related to the width of an adjacent blood vessel. This, coupled with a sketch showing its position relative to the disc or macula, will enable the observer to pinpoint the object in future.

Distances across the fundus can be described in terms of 'disc diameters' or in angular terms if it is assumed that the disc to macula distance represents approximately 12°.

Cupping of the disc may be defined by specifying the cup/disc ratio; this ratio is the proportion of the total disc diameter occupied by the cupping (*Figure 19.6*).

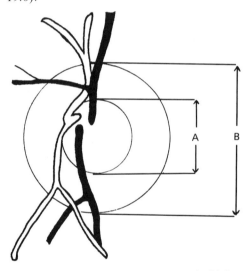

Figure 19.6 The cup : disc ratio is A : B; in this instance it is 1 : 2 or 0.5

Relative widths of the retinal vessels may be recorded by noting the retinal artery/vein ratio. Chester (1977) however points out that, although the alteration of the artery/vein ratio from the normal 2:3 relationship to 1:2 or 1:3 is an expected result of retinal artery narrowing, the same result is produced by engorgement of the veins. He suggests that the artery/vein ratio is not meaningful unless the calibre of the vessels is individually described as well. This argument overlooks usefulness of such data when used for comparisons on subsequent visits.

Some instruments enable graticules, or other measuring devices, to be projected onto the fundus itself. The size of an object can then be described in terms of the amount of the target covered by the object. The distance to a fixed point, such as the disc, can also be measured to aid in subsequent localization. Using this system, some quite fine measurements can be made, for example the direction and distance of the eccentric point used for fixation in a strabismic amblyope can be related to the macula. Some specialized ophthalmoscopes have been specifically designed for this purpose, e.g. the Keeler Projectoscope and the Visuscope.

Even if this facility is not available, the diameter or length of the projected spot or streak of light on the fundus can be used to define size or distance. It must be remembered though that this will vary depending upon the ophthalmoscope used.

Sometimes it is necessary to assess the depth or elevation of structures on the fundus, for example in cases of cupping or holes in the disc tissue, where a knowledge of the depth is required and in papilloedema or retina detachment, where the elevation above the surrounding tissue is required. In dioptric terms, a change in depth of approximately 0.3 mm is accomplished by a change of focus of 1 D and thus an estimate of the actual amount of vertical displacement can be made. In practice, it is usually specified by simply stating the dioptric value necessary to focus from the highest to the lowest, for example 'Central physiological cupping, c : d 0.4, depth 3 D'. As stated earlier the most frequently used instrument for examining the fundus in optometric practice is the direct ophthalmoscope (*Figure 19.7*). This is available in many guises, examples of which are shown in *Figure 19.8*. However, despite the different instruments, the techniques for examination are, on the whole, much the same and individual practitioners will develop their own style with practice.

Clinical use of the ophthalmoscope
Examination of the media

The media, comprising the cornea, anterior chamber, crystalline lens and vitreous, are best viewed initially against the red glow of the fundus reflex. The examiner stands alongside the seated patient who looks straight ahead. A fixation object on the opposite wall or viewed in the chart mirror may prove useful initially. Using a low positive lens in the instrument sight hole (2 or 3 D), the examiner directs the ophthalmoscope light into the patient's eye and views the fundus reflex from a distance of about 25 cm. If the media are clear, an even red reflex will be seen in the pupil area once the eye is being properly illuminated. Any defect in the media will be seen as irregularities or opacities against this

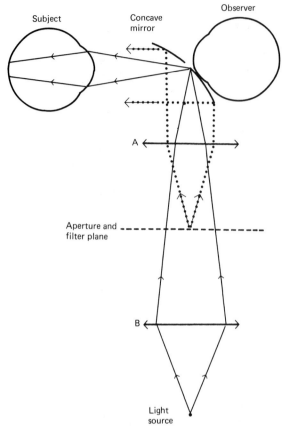

Figure 19.7 Basic illumination system for a modern, direct ophthalmoscope. The positive lens systems at A and B enable a light patch to be projected onto the patient's fundus through the focused apertures, positioned as shown

red background. Non-central areas of the media may be best examined by getting the patient to look up, down, right and left. Any vitreous opacities will be seen as characteristic spots or fibre-like strands swirling or moving as the eye moves and frequently continuing to move, slowly settling once the eye stops. Mucus and other debris on the front corneal surface will also be seen to move, especially with blinking, and it is important to establish the depth of the irregularity being viewed. This is achieved by the parallax method described earlier. The same applies to stationary opacities in the cornea or lens.

Examination of the fundus

Once the media have been examined in this general way, a closer look at the various structures can be undertaken. The lens power is increased in the ophthalmoscope sight hole to about +15 D and the instrument moved forward to within a few centimetres of the eye. This will bring the front corneal surface into focus. Adjusting the distance from the eye and (generally) reducing the lens power make it possible to focus down through the eye until the fundus is reached. In order that as much of the media as possible can be viewed it is again important for the patient to move the eye in all directions. If there is no defect, then, of course, nothing will be seen. If a defect is found a record is made of its size, shape, position and density as explained earlier. Anterior defects may be further investigated using a focal light source and magnification.

When the fundus is reached, a systematic search begins using the disc as a starting point and the fundus is mentally sectored into four through the disc. The colour and any peculiarities of structure, such as cupping, elevation of the margins, visibility of the lamina cribrosa etc., are noted as are the vessels at the disc, both major and minor, and any unusual paths they take.

From the disc, and with the patient's eyes still looking straight ahead, the superior temporal blood vessels are followed as far as possible and the surrounding fundus examined. Any departures from the normal are noted. This is repeated for the superior nasal quadrant vessels and for the inferior temporal and nasal quadrants. The outer limits of each of these sections are examined by getting the patient to look up, down, right and left as far as possible, ensuring that the ophthalmoscope is turned to increase the obliquity of the view. At all times it is imperative to keep the instrument as close to the eye as possible. This maximizes the field of view obtained and very little of even the extreme periphery of the fundus will be missed, providing the pupil is not too small. It is usually difficult to examine the central area and the fovea itself without restricting the aperture of the illuminating system. If this is not done, the reflections from the cornea mask the view of this area, especially as pupil constriction will be at a maximum while this area is being examined.

In the event of an adequate view not being possible because of obstruction of the central media or a small pupil, the use of a mydriatic will greatly increase the ease of examination (*see* Chapter 30).

Apertures and filters

Normally the large aperture is left in the illumination system during the first part of the examination and the macula stop used as described above. In addition to these apertures (*Figure 19.9*), many instruments also have a slit aperture, which may be projected onto any retinal structure in order to help determine whether or not it is higher or lower than the adjacent tissue, as can be found in a cyst, or

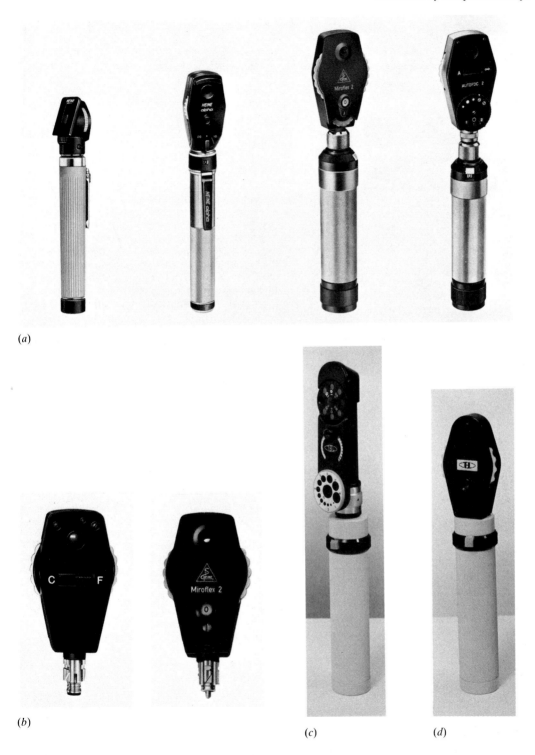

(a)

(b)

(c)

(d)

Figure 19.8 A selection of modern ophthalmoscopes. (a) The Heine range with details of the Miroflex 2 head in (b). (c, d) Two of the range of Hamblin ophthalmo-scopes. (With the permission of Clement Clarke International Ltd, Heine Optotechnik and Hamblin Instruments Ltd)

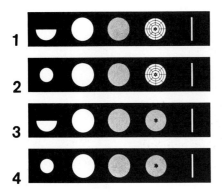

Figure 19.9 A range of typical light apertures. (With permission of Clement Clarke International Ltd and Heine Optotechnik)

retinal detachment (*Figure 19.10*). The slit is positioned such that it falls across the apparent boundary and it can be seen whether a change in level really exists or if it is an artefact—as for example in pseudopapilloedema. Intermediate-sized round apertures are helpful sometimes for examining the peripheral fundus when the patient has a small pupil.

Most instruments also allow the practitioner to insert filters into the illuminating and/or viewing system. The purpose of these filters is to modify the contrast of the structure being observed against the background. For example, the use of a green filter will make red structures appear darker and may be useful in increasing the visibility of retinal circulation defects as well as increasing the visibility of

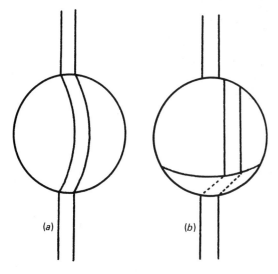

Figure 19.10 The use of a slit aperture to look at a retinal elevation, such as a cyst in (*a*), and a depression, such as a macula hole in (*b*)

haemorrhages and microaneurysms. Ballantyne and Michaelson (1962) provide a useful review of ophthalmoscopy with modified and various spectral sources.

Indirect ophthalmoscopy

Indirect ophthalmoscopy is usually performed through a dilated pupil, the eye being illuminated by a light source mounted on a headband. A positive condensing lens is held by the examiner close to the eye being examined. This lens forms an aerial image between the patient and the observer and it is this image which is viewed (*see Figure 19.4*). The proximity of the image to the examiner means that some degree of accommodation must be employed to view it clearly, or a supplementary viewing lens used. A second examiner can also look at the image if an angled 'teaching mirror' is inserted in the viewing path (*Figure 19.11*).

It is possible to obtain an indirect view of the fundus without specialized equipment by using a retinoscope as a light source and a lens of approximately +15.00 D sphere (DS) with which to form the required aerial image (*Figure 19.12*).

Whatever the equipment, the light source must first be directed towards the eye under observation and the viewing path established. The condensing lens is then inserted into the illuminating beam, immediately adjacent to the eye under examination. Following this, the lens is withdrawn from the eye, ensuring that the illuminating beam is kept central on the patient's pupil and that attention is directed towards the lens itself. At the point when the lens renders the entrance pupils of the eyes of both examiner and patient conjugate, an aerial image of the fundus is seen. The image is inverted, hence to view different parts of the fundus the patient must move his eye up, down, right and left remembering to allow for this inversion, and of course, the examiner can shine the light from oblique directions as well, making the same allowance.

Filters may be inserted into the light path to modify the light reflected from the tissues as described earlier.

The principal difference between the illuminating system of the direct and indirect ophthalmoscope is in the vergence of the emerging light beam. This is because of the greater distance between the examiner and patient when undertaking indirect ophthalmoscopy; the vergence is correspondingly less in this type of instrument.

Other means of viewing the fundus

For the sake of completeness, although rarely used in general optometric practice, the following are included, since they represent alternative means of viewing the media and fundus detail.

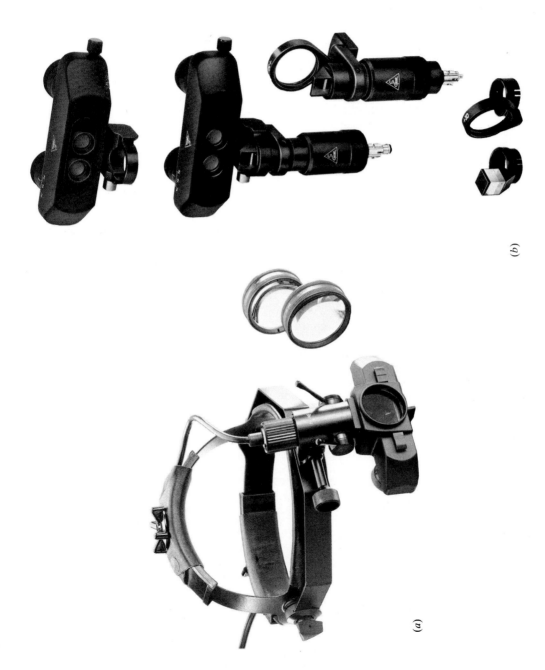

Figure 19.11 (*a*) Heine headband binocular indirect ophthalmoscope; (*b*) Heine headband monocular/binocular indirect ophthalmoscope (with the permission of Clement Clarke International Ltd and Heine Optotechnik).

(*b*)

(*a*)

330

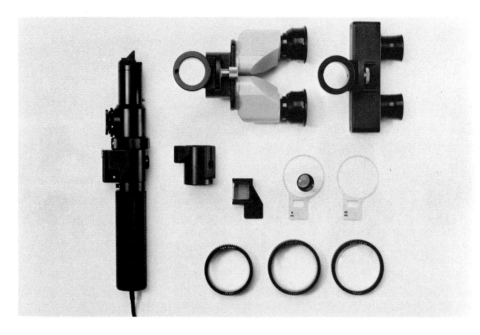

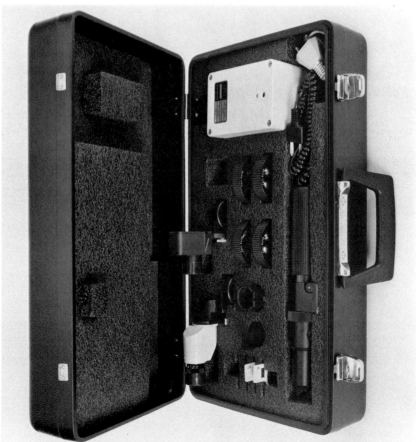

(d)

(c)

Figure 19.11 (contd) (c,d) Zeiss hand-held monocular/binocular indirect ophthalmoscope and condensing lens (with the permission of Carl Zeiss (Oberkochen) Ltd)

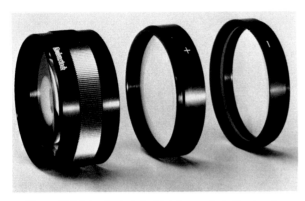

Figure 19.12 Aspherical doublet for use in indirect ophthalmoscopy. (With the permission of Rodenstock Instruments)

In the biomicroscope/slitlamp arrangement usually used for anterior eye examination, there is already established a viewing and illumination system. In order to use this for fundus examination, some means must be found of neutralizing the refractive power of the cornea or of forming an aerial image as in indirect ophthalmoscopy. There are several ways in which this can be achieved:

(1) A Hruby lens is a plano/concave lens of approximately -55 D (*Figure 19.13*). The concave surface is placed close to the eye to be examined and the inner eye illuminated by the slitlamp, through the lens. The lens can be tilted to avoid reflections from the front surface. A binocular view of the fundus can be obtained using the microscope which gives a better impression of depth than a monocular view. The slit width can be varied to

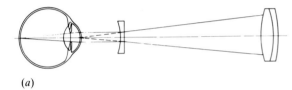

(a)

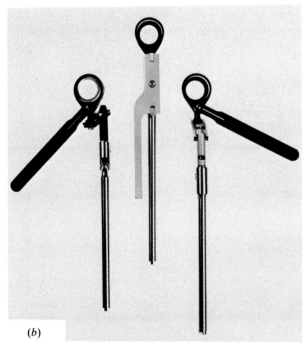

(b)

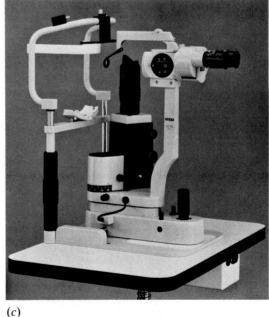

(c)

Figure 19.13 (*a*) The beam paths of a Hruby lens in use (with the permission of Carl Zeiss (Oberkochen) Ltd). (*b*) A selection of Hruby lens for use on slitlamps (with the permission of Clement Clarke International Ltd). (*c*) Hruby lens mounted on a slitlamp (with the permission of Carl Zeiss (Oberkochen) Ltd)

Table 19.2 Slitlamp examination of the fundus: comparison of fields of view

Ocular refraction	Hruby lens (−55 D)		El Bayadi lens (+55 D)	
	Monocular (mm)	Binocular (mm)	Monocular (mm)	Binocular (mm)
−10.00	3.7	0.2	7.4	4.0
Emmetropia	4.1	1.4	6.2	2.7
+5.00	4.3	1.9	5.7	2.2

After Bennett and Rabbetts, 1984.

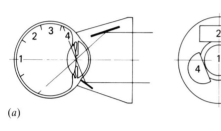

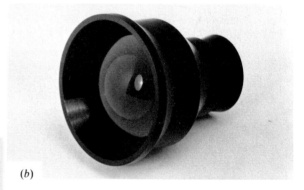

(a)

(b)

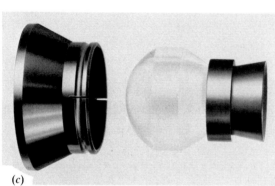

(c)

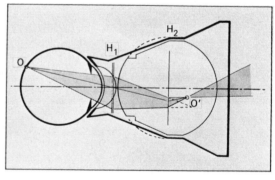

(d)

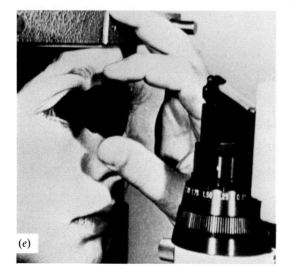

(e)

Figure 19.14 (*a*) Goldmann triple-mirror fundus viewing lens (with the permission of Carl Zeiss (Oberkochen) Ltd). (*b, c, d, e*) Rodenstock panfunduscope fundus viewing lens (with the permission of Rodenstock Instruments). (*f*) Range of Goldmann gonioscope and fundus viewing lenses (with the permission of Clement Clarke International Ltd)

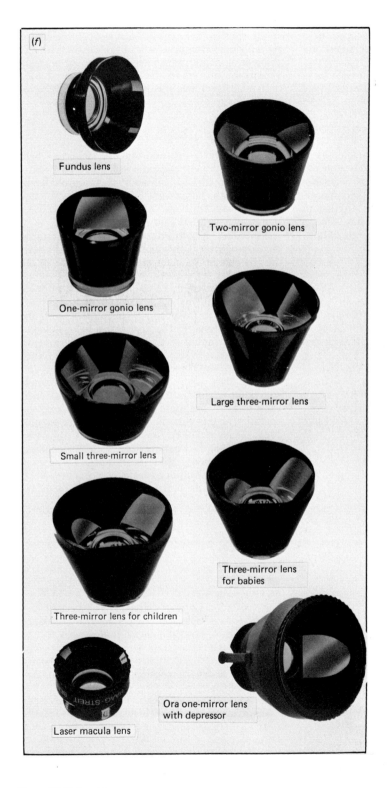

Figure 19.14 (contd)

project either a full circle of light onto the fundus for a general view, or reduced to a narrow beam for looking at elevations and depressions.

(2) A high-powered plus lens may be used instead of the above. This will form a real aerial image which can be viewed by the microscope. The El Bayadi lens used for this purpose is +55 D. Bennett and Rabbets (1984) produced a table comparing these two lenses (*Table 19.2*).

(3) A variety of fundus-viewing contact lenses is available, some examples of which are shown in the figures. The cornea needs to be anaesthetized when such lenses are used. By incorporating mirrors in a similar way to the Goldmann gonioscope lenses, a view of the whole fundus can be obtained right out to the extreme periphery (*Figure 19.14*).

Transillumination

This technique is used to examine the translucency of the tissue layers of the globe (*Figure 19.15*). A transilluminating head is used in contact with the sclera to direct light against the eye.

With a dilated pupil, and by applying the transilluminator head over different parts of the sclera from the limbus to as far back as possible, a large part of the eye can be transilluminated. Care must be taken to avoid too bright a light, as this can mask early changes in the tissues.

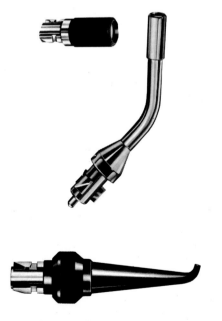

Figure 19.15 Transilluminator heads and lamps. (With the permission of Clement Clarke International Ltd)

The purpose of this exercise is to detect variations in the density of the tissue, such as might be caused by a pigmented new growth of the choroid, when a diminution of the transmitted light would be seen. During this procedure, the inner eye is viewed using a standard ophthalmoscope with its own illumination turned off.

Light sources

All of the above instruments depend upon a light source to illuminate the inner eye. In the early days, candles, gas jets and eventually, incandescent lamps were used, the latter being constantly improved and filaments and envelopes made smaller to produce a more easily focused light patch in the eye.

Nowadays, a halogen gas is introduced into the envelope of the lamp which has the effect of reducing the amount of blackening on the inside of the lamp.

This is achieved by reducing the rate of burn-off of the filament and by ensuring that the particles that do burn off are able to recombine with the filament material. For these reasons, halogen lamps can be run hotter, and therefore brighter, than standard incandescent lamps and will last much longer.

These days many ophthalmoscopes, slitlamps, and fibreoptic projectors use these lamps as their light source. The light source should always be operated at the minimum level necessary to give adequate illumination. Great care should always be exercised when experimenting with high power sources and photographic flash tubes. The energy levels reached by these devices and the spectral characteristics can make them injurious to ocular tissues.

References

BALLANTYNE, A.J. and MICHAELSON, I.C. (1962) *Textbook of the Fundus of the Eye*, Chap. 1, pp. 10–15. Edinburgh: E & S Livingstone Ltd

BENNETT, A.G. and RABBETTS, R.B. (1984) Visual examination of the eye and ophthalmoscopy. *Clinical Visual Optics*, Chap. 16, pp. 323–350. London: Butterworths

CARDELL, J.D.M. (1935) Recent developments in the use of polarized light in ophthalmology with special reference to its use in ophthalmoscopy. *Trans. Ophthalmol. Soc. UK* **55**, 158

CHESTER, E.M. (1977) *The Ocular Fundus in Systemic Disease*. Chicago: Year Book Medical Publishers Inc.

EMSLEY, H.H. (1952) *Visual Optics*, 5th edn, Vol. 1. London: Hatton Press

20

Ophthalmic photography

Colin Hood

Photography has become, in the twentieth century, a simple everyday occurrence—almost every family owns or has access to a camera. The introduction of automation, computerization and miniaturization to these cameras now enables everyone to produce excellent results with further important improvements enhancing these results, for example the improvements in the quality of lenses, film emulsions and flash guns. Because of these advances, people naturally expect that it will be possible to produce excellent results in more specialized areas of photography and cannot understand why, in many cases, these results are not achieved. This situation occurs because photographic equipment is designed to produce excellent results when photographing commonplace everyday types of image. If the same equipment is then used to photograph more specialist subjects, naturally it is found not to be capable of handling this new situation. When this happens, the photographer becomes aware that a limited knowledge of photography has suddenly become a problem. It is the aim of this chapter, therefore, to give the reader an understanding of the basic principles of photography and how these can be used in conjunction with their own photographic equipment to produce good usable images.

Background and terminology

Before looking at the specialist applications of ophthalmic photography, the basic principles of photography should be understood. The first permanent photograph was produced by a Frenchman called Nice'phore Nie'pce in his garden in Gras, France in 1826. This first exposure took approximately 8 hours which gives some idea of just how slow the early film emulsions were, but it did prove that images could be recorded and preserved permanently. Over the next 60 years, many improvements were made to the quality and especially the speed of

emulsions, and also to the design of cameras. Photography, however, was still the domain of the scientist and professional photographer and it was not until 1888 that the major breakthrough came which would bring photography to the amateur. This was the introduction in that year, by George Eastman, of his Kodak 'Everyman's Camera'. This camera totally changed the role and future of photography and brought this new science within everyone's range. Over the ensuing years, and in particular the last 20 years, cameras have made fantastic strides both in size and versatility; the most popular type today has become the 35 mm single lens camera of which there are two main types produced:

(1) Single lens reflex (SLR).
(2) Rangefinder or direct vision cameras.

Single lens reflex cameras

The single lens reflex (SLR) camera allows a single lens to be used both for taking the photograph and for viewing the image. This works by using a hinged mirror which lies behind the lens at an angle of 45°, and produces a reflected image onto the viewing/focusing screen. When the image has been framed and focused, the shutter is then depressed causing the mirror to lift and, as the mirror reaches the horizontal position, it triggers the shutter allowing the photograph to be taken. Once the shutter has closed, the mirror then drops down allowing the next image to be framed and focused. The one main advantage of the SLR camera over rangefinder cameras is that it eliminates the factor of parallax, a phenomenon described below. The other main advantages of the SLR cameras are:

(1) Interchangeability of lenses.
(2) Critical focusing for any subject at any distance which can be imaged by the photographic lens or any other optical system which may be used.

(3) The potential to visually check the depth of field.

These main advantages make this type of camera particularly suitable for medical and scientific types of photography, by allowing them to be attached to equipment such as microscopes, slitlamps etc.

Rangefinder cameras

The main difference between rangefinder and SLR cameras is that the rangefinder has a separate photographing and viewing system. This means that the viewfinder and lens are separated by approximately 25 mm (1 inch) which results in the field of view seen through the viewfinder being slightly different from that being recorded through the lens. The difference is of no importance when working at a reasonable distance from the subject, but becomes very serious when focusing at close quarters. This separation results in the photographic image including more of the bottom of the picture and less of the top than was seen through the viewfinder.

Films and emulsions

Now that a way has been found of producing the image, a convenient method of recording it permanently must be acquired.

There are many substances which are altered by the action of light, i.e. are light sensitive, but the one chemical which provides the sensitivity to record the visual spectrum and a reaction which produces a finely detailed permanent record is a salt of silver; this substance still remains the cornerstone of photographic emulsions. The two main features of films that have to be considered are film speed and grain, as these two areas have a direct bearing on the quality of results that can be produced. The degree of sensitivity of an emulsion to light is referred to as its 'speed' and the more responsive or sensitive an emulsion is to light the *faster* it is said to be; conversely, the less sensitive the *slower* the emulsion. Consequently, the sensitivity of one film to another can be accurately compared and an international speed rating system has been devised; the one most commonly used in Britain is ASA (American Standards Association) and this system applies numbers to different emulsions to denote their speed—the higher the number the greater the film speed.

An example of this system is as follows. If an exposure of 1 s at an aperture of f8 using a film with a speed of 100 ASA is required, then the exposure would have to be altered to 4 s at f8 if a film with a speed of 25 ASA was to be used.

The other main element of films is that of grain. There are many aspects which can affect grain, but

which are far too complex to include in this chapter. However, a rough rule of thumb can be used to explain the problem. The emulsion contrast of a photographic emulsion is the range of grey tones it is capable of forming between dense black and clear emulsion, and this depends upon the size of the grain and its distribution. A film that has grains of a small equal size will produce a high contrast emulsion with a low film speed; therefore, a film constructed with grains of a different size would produce a wide range of greys and would have a faster film speed. The choice of the correct film is therefore a balance between contrast and speed and it is important to chose the correct film for the type of work being undertaken.

Ophthalmic photography

Ophthalmology is probably the one specialization in medicine that relies on photographic images both for diagnosis and for teaching. The main aim of this section is to look at the different types of equipment available and the special functions that can be performed. Ophthalmic photography can be divided into three main categories:

(1) External photography.
(2) Slitlamp photography.
(3) Fundus photography.

External photography

This is the area of ophthalmic photography that is undertaken most frequently by non-qualified personnel who believe that it is just the same as taking conventional photographs. Unfortunately, this is not the case because lighting and magnification play a very vital role in this particular type of work.

Camera

A typical camera set-up is shown in *Figure 20.1* and the reasons that make this camera most suitable for the specialist applications of external photography can be considered. A single lens reflex 35 mm camera should be used as this allows the photographer to actually see what is being photographed which is not the case with rangefinder cameras.

Viewfinder screen

The camera should also have a good viewfinder screen which the user finds satisfactory to their own particular needs, this being very important because most of the photographs will be taken at fairly high magnification when focusing must be precise. There are different types of screen and they can usually be interchanged quite easily.

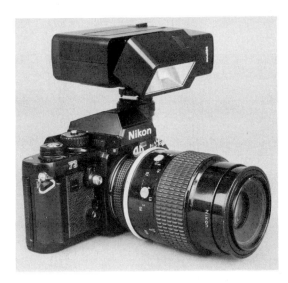

Figure 20.1 Typical camera set-up for external photography. Note the standard magnification marks on the lens. This is to ensure the precise reproducibility of photographs. (Photograph published by kind permission of Nikon UK Ltd)

Lenses

Two of the most commonly used lenses are the Nikon micro-nikkor 55 mm lens and the Nikon 105 mm lens. The first lens allows the photographer to focus from infinity down to 74 mm (3 inches) and the latter permits focusing from infinity down to 240 mm (9.5 inches). This latter lens gives a greater working distance from the patient which is particularly important when working in the clinic or operating room etc. If the use of extension rings is required to increase the magnification, then the camera should be placed on a firm base or tripod and the patient's head placed on a head rest, thus preventing any movement which may blur the result.

Lighting

This is probably the least important element in the system, but there is one very important point to remember which is to avoid using a 'ring' flash. This creates a large reflex on the cornea which can obliterate any pathology being photographed. Any small on-camera flash will produce sufficient illumination to photograph an area large enough to record images up to head and shoulders. It is essential to ensure that the flash is placed as close as possible to the optical axis.

Film

The correct film is also very important and Koda-chrome (Kodak) gives the best colour quality, but

has to be processed by the manufacturer. This makes the turn-round time between the photograph being taken and the results being returned rather long and many photographic departments have transferred to Ektrachrome 64 or 200 (Kodak) or other equivalent films. These films give acceptable colour rendition and resolution.

Camera settings

The final point to be considered concerning external photography is the camera setting. The f/stop refers to the opening of the iris diaphragm, the lower the f/stop (f/3.5) the larger the iris opening, while the higher the f/stop (f/22) the smaller the iris opening. Because the camera lens is less efficient at the periphery, then it is essential to ensure that the iris diaphragm should be stopped down (closed) to at least f/8. The higher the f/stop the greater is the depth of field, i.e. the distance in front and behind the point of focus which is still in focus. Exposure should always be determined by trial and error and never by using the built-in exposure meter of the camera. Once the standard procedures have been decided upon, then a series of photographs should be taken—one for each f/stop. After the film has been processed, the correct exposure should then be assessed and all subsequent photographs should be taken at this setting. Standardization is vitally important to ensure that clinical photographs taken over a period of time are uniform. The clinical value of photographs is greatly reduced if standardization is not strict. Specific distance values, i.e. magnification should be marked onto the lens for specific views such as full face, two eyes, single eye etc. When one of these standard views is required, then the lens should be set to the corresponding setting: focusing is then achieved by moving the camera backwards and forwards.

Slitlamp photography

The photo slitlamp

This instrument combines all the features expected in the traditional slitlamp with the essential requirements for photography. Although there are many makes of photo slitlamp on the market, the best known is probably the Zeiss (West German) version and it was in fact this company that managed to produce the first practical photo slitlamp in 1965. However, the story started back in 1911 when Gullstrand developed the slitlamp illuminator and when, in 1916, this was coupled with Czapski's corneal binocular microscope, the first photo slitlamp appeared. Developments have then occurred over the decades until 1965. The main problem with these early instruments was obtaining sufficient illumination while still retaining all the features of the slitlamp plus the additional photographic ones

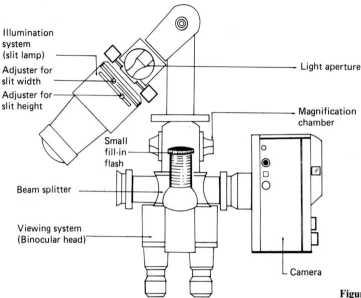

Illumination
system
(slit lamp)

Adjuster for
slit width

Adjuster for
slit height

Light aperture

Magnification
chamber

Small
fill-in
flash

Beam splitter

Viewing system
(Binocular head)

Camera

Figure 20.2 Diagram of (Zeiss) photo slitlamp

(*Figure 20.2*). Photographs are always a flat one-dimensional image unless stereo photography is used, and one of the main problems facing the photographer when recording clinical detail is to show exactly in which plane of focus the condition appears. The photo slitlamp allows an optical light section through the anterior portion of the eye to be imaged, thereby allowing the identification of a precise location of a certain condition. It would be unfair to imply that this instrument is limited to recording the anterior segment only. Without modifications, the photo slitlamp can record well into the vitreous and, by using a panfunduscope lens, it is possible to photograph the retina (*see* Chapter 19). The anterior chamber angle can also be recorded by using gonio photography (*see* Chapter 24 for a discussion of gonioscopy).

The photo slitlamp is a fairly difficult instrument to use because of the many variables. These include the slit height, slit width, and the angle between the light source and the camera, and the magnification can also be varied. All these factors can, therefore, have a combined effect on the final exposure. It is only by practice that the inter-relationship between all the different functions can produce good, useful results. The instrument can be divided into two main parts:

(1) The illumination system (slitlamp).
(2) The viewing system (binocular head).

The illumination system provides an accurate and adjustable light source which is essential for recording detail in almost transparent tissue. The viewing system comprises a mounted binocular head which

gives a three-dimensional image that can be either viewed or recorded. The magnification system is incorporated into the viewing head and provides a magnification range of between approximately × 6 and × 25. It is essential that the light source and the viewing system both focus at the same point (plane of focus), and the slit beam must be in the centre of the field irrespective of the angle between the slitlamp and the viewing system.

Filters

The filters in the slitlamp are used on the same basis as general photographic filters and include the uses discussed below.

Fluorescein excitation

By preferentially filtering specific wavelengths from the light source, fluorescein can be made to fluoresce. A 'cobalt' blue filter has such an effect when placed in the optical path of the illuminating/flash system.

Contrast filters

Contrast filters create their effect by differential absorption between the object of interest and its background. Thus a red-free filter will render blood vessels dark against an unchanged, light scleral or corneal/iris background and therefore make the detection of neovascularization easier. Similarly, a yellow barrier filter in the path of the observation/photographic system with fluorescein observation will heighten the contrast of the fluorescence against the background.

Neutral density

Neutral density filters can be used to reduce ambient illuminance without affecting colour thus allowing more comfort to the patient as well as larger camera apertures which, by reducing depth of field, will help visually to isolate the subject of interest from its background.

Polarization

Polarizing filters, if used at right angles over the illuminating/flash and observation/photographic systems, will eliminate or substantially reduce reflexes from the major ocular reflecting surfaces. There is a corresponding loss of light requiring larger apertures for photographic purposes.

The binocular system incorporates varying magnification and an adjustment for the user to set the correct interpupillary distance and the correct dioptric setting. The photo slitlamp also has additional components, the more important being: camera body, beam, splitter, electronic flash tube, ground glass diffuser, eyepiece graticule.

(1) A 35 mm body is fitted onto the beam splitter and is an integral part of the system.
(2) The beam splitter is a piece of optical equipment which produces two images, one of which is relayed to the observer and the other to the camera. Normally the beam splitter divides the amount of light into two equal parts and this would be referred to as a 50/50 splitter. However, different configurations are available, for example the 70/30 which divides the illumination into 30% to the observer and 70% to the camera, which is very beneficial if the illumination is very low, thereby allowing as much light as possible to pass to the camera.
(3) Electronic flash is essential because it is of such short duration (1/1000 of a second) that any movement which is likely to occur during exposure is eliminated. Because electronic flash also has a colour temperature of approximately 6000 K, this allows the use of daylight colour film.
(4) The ground glass diffuser is placed over the light exit aperture on the light source unit and allows diffuse general photographs to be taken of the external eye and/or records of contact lens fit.
(5) The eyepiece graticule is essential for the production of sharply focused photographs, and because an aerial image is being recorded, it is essential that the eyepiece is correctly set for each individual user's refractive error, which is achieved by focusing the graticule first. When taking the photograph, both the image and the graticule must be in focus and the other advantage of the graticule is in ensuring the correct centring of the image.

There are various ways of fitting cameras onto slitlamps and the easiest one of all is to mount the camera into one of the ocular tubes. This, however, means that the user can only view through one ocular, while the camera records through the other which can lead to the camera recording a slightly different view to that of the photographer—the problem of parallax. Another system which is often used is to mount a camera onto the slitlamp in what is often called the 'piggy back system'. Because a normal 35 mm system is used, the photographer has the use of both oculars and can also focus through the camera system itself. Unfortunately, when focusing through the standard viewing screen, the quality of image is degraded and it is therefore very difficult to focus on the very fine detail. The main problem with both these methods is that photographs have to be taken using the available light provided by the slitlamp's illuminating system, which means that high speed film has to be used; this, in turn, means that the film has a larger grain structure resulting in images with lower resolution.

In the photo slitlamp, the camera is linked to the microscope objectives via the beam splitter as described, and the flash source is coincident with the normal source acting through the instrument's illuminating system.

Fundus photography

This is the most commonly practised area of ophthalmic photography and is performed at most large hospitals. Fundus photography is a vital clinical aid in the documentation and diagnosis of intraocular disease and has been available since the early part of the century. The first retinal photograph was produced by Webster in 1886, when, unfortunately, only the optic nerve was visible as a fairly irregular area with no detail of the retinal blood vessels being seen. However, the great advantages of this type of photography had already been noted and great strides were quickly taken to ensure that retinal photography could be used to provide useful clinical information. In 1961, Novotny and Alvis described their method of producing fluorescein angiograms and this was to transform retinal photography from documentation to diagnosis. Retinal photography requires the purchase of specialized fundus cameras which are fairly expensive (costing from £8000 to £20 000) and, unfortunately, there is no other way of producing high quality fundus photographs (*see Figure 20.3* for typical fundus camera).

The main function of the equipment is to produce sharp edge-to-edge images from an extremely curved surface. The optics, therefore, are extremely specialized and, when the camera is used to photograph the front of the eye for example, only the central portion is seen to be in focus. One of the biggest problems that faces retinal photographers is

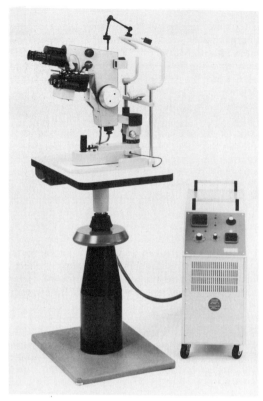

Figure 20.3 Typical fundus camera showing floor-standing power pack. The power pack, apart from providing illumination, also controls the exposure by increasing or decreasing the amount of light being discharged from the flash tube. (Photograph by courtesy of Carl Zeiss Oberkochen)

focusing and this results from the fact that the retinal camera has no significant depth of field. Consequently, unless focusing is critical, the resultant photograph will not be sharp. It is important, therefore, that the eyepiece is correctly focused. Below is a list of the main techniques that should be followed for the production of good photographs:

(1) Pupil dilatation—the pupil requires a dilatation of at least 5 mm if satisfactory results are to be produced.
(2) Eyepiece focusing—eyepiece focus should be checked every time the equipment is used. It is difficult to produce consistently sharp photographs and this is often due to accommodation; the photographer must therefore ensure that they are relaxed and comfortable.
(3) Preparation—the procedure should be explained and it should be ensured that the patient is comfortably seated at the camera.
(4) The photographer's seating should be adjusted to ensure that there is no strain; strain can lead to accommodation.

(5) Camera preparation—it is advisable to check that the correct film is loaded in the camera and the correct power setting has been selected.
(6) Focusing—the viewing lamp should be focused on the patient's cornea which is achieved by looking around the side of the camera.
(7) By looking through the focusing eyepiece, any final adjustments to alignment and focus can be made and the photograph taken.

Fluorescein angiography

The diagnostic procedure known as fluorescein angiography involves injecting sodium fluorescein intravenously and then photographing the passage of this dye as it flows through the retinal circulation. This procedure relies on the principle of fluorescence, which is the ability of a substance to absorb light of one wavelength and to readmit it at a longer wavelength. To achieve this an exciter filter (blue) which passes light no longer than 490 nm is placed in the light path of the flash source and this blue light is absorbed by the fluorescein in the blood vessel. It is then re-emitted as yellow–green light. This light then passes through a barrier filter (yellow) which will only pass light longer than 520 nm. This filter is placed just in front of the camera thereby allowing the camera to record the fluorescent image.

Conclusion

This chapter has endeavoured to give some guidelines on how acceptable clinical results are produced in this specialist field of ophthalmic photography. A list of some useful photographic definitions is included below.

Acutance	A numerical measurement of the photographic image at the division between a light and dark area.
Colour temperature	The temperature to which a full radiator must be brought in order to match visually the light from the source, measured in kelvins (K).
Contrast	The density range of a negative, also involving the tone scale of the subject.
Density (optical)	The light absorbing power of the photographic image and the quantity of deposited silver in a given area.

Depth of field	The distance between objects furthest and nearest to the lens which are in focus at the same time.
Depth of focus	The amount of distance which the film or lens can be moved without causing the image to appear out of focus.
Diaphragm	This is the adjustable aperture which controls the amount of light reaching the film.
Emulsion	A gelatin solution containing the light sensitive silver halides (in a colloidal suspension).
Exposure	The length of time the shutter is open thereby allowing light to reach the sensitized material (film).
f numbers	These are a measure of the light-passing power of a lens. The smaller the number the larger the amount of light passing through the lens and vice versa.
Focal length	The distance between the image of a distant subject and a standard point on the lens.
Graininess	The grainy appearance of a photographic image when it is magnified.
Latent image	The invisible image which is produced when the film is exposed to light.
Latitude	The range of exposures over which a film will give an acceptable result.
Orthochromatic	Film sensitive to ultraviolet, blue, green and yellow radiation.
Panchromatic	Film sensitive to ultraviolet, blue, green, yellow and red radiation.
Reversal	The production of a direct positive image.
Speed	The response of photographic film to light, normally expressed in an arithmetical form, i.e. ASA.

Reference

NOVOTNY. H.R. and ALVIS. D.L. (1961) A method of photographing fluorescein in circulating blood of the human retina. *Circulation*, **24**, 82

21

Ultrasonography of the eye

John Storey

Ultrasound may be defined as sound above the audible frequency, i.e. above a frequency of 20 kHz. In air, sound travels at 340 m/s, but its speed in water is much faster, being around 1500 m/s. Johnson (1979) in his book *The Secret War* draws attention to the work of the Allied Submarine Detection Investigation Committee (ASDIC) which was set up in 1915 by the Admiralty Board of Invention and Research. The French contribution was the application by Professor Langevin of Jacques and Pierre Curie's discovery earlier (1880) of the piezoelectric effect, which occurs when electric voltage is applied to a quartz crystal cut along its axis causing it to oscillate at a particular frequency to produce ultrasound waves.

The quartz crystal is acting as a loudspeaker but, on receipt of echoes it will convert them into a modified voltage for display on an oscilloscope or for processing by a computer. The term 'transducer' is applied to such a quartz crystal and currently transducers are made of ceramic materials, such as barium titanate, or from special polymers. Ultrasound is inaudible and can, therefore, be used at destructive levels for drilling teeth or cleaning industrial components. However, medical equipment is designed to work only at a very low level of output which is why, for example, it can be used safely to scan the fetus in pregnancy. Ultrasound exposure is not cumulative, unlike X-ray exposure, hence its great value in serial examinations. Mundt and Hughes (1956) were the first to use ultrasound for ophthalmic investigations. Baum found a maximum safe ultrasound level to be 0.25 W/cm^2 per 5 min to 1.0 W/cm^2 per 3 min, although most ophthalmic instruments work at about 10^{-4} W or less and depend on amplification to boost the echoes displayed. Output is pulsed at about 1000 pulses/s which reduces exposure further and, between pulses, the returning echoes are received, converted and displayed to give an apparently continuous picture. The outstanding value of ultrasonography lies in the visualization of optically inaccessible areas of the eye and orbit and the precise measurement (biometry) of the eye.

Transducers

Transducers are chosen to operate at a frequency that will give the greatest accuracy and yet function well. For the eye, a high frequency of 10–12 MHz is necessary to achieve anywhere near an accuracy of ±0.07 mm and then only if there is a uniform waveform produced. Coleman, Lizzi and Jack (1977) showed that echoes obtained with perfect matching have a total duration of $1.5/f$, where f is the resonant frequency. For work on the anterior segment, 20–30 MHz can be used, such very short wavelengths giving higher resolution but poorer penetration. Due to near field distortions, transducers must be at least 5 mm from the area under investigation. Fluid contact is essential as ultrasound travels better in fluids than in air, a very important factor with such low levels of output. Normally, saline is the correct coupling agent for studies on the eye direct, or a water-soluble jelly may be used on the eyelids if the eye is to be closed during examination. When scanning through the eyelids, anterior detail is distorted by the nearness of the transducer and the lid echoes. Consequently, this is valuable only for visualization of the posterior segment and beyond the globe. For good visualization of the whole eye in the supine position, a stand-off saline bath is used with Steri-drape fitted carefully to the area around the eye without pleating and secured further with Steri-strip. The periphery of the Steri-drape is drawn through a 16-mm metal ring which is supported on a stand just above the eye. It is folded over the ring and clipped. Saline at near body temperature is poured into this up to a suitable depth. An eye cup is easier to use for central A-scans of the eye.

Forms of display

B-scan

Should a section of the eye in more than one meridian be required, the transducer can be moved mechanically to generate a series of sections which may be shown together as a B-scan (intensity-modulated) display with spots for each echo. Baum and Greenwood (1958) pioneered this method which gives an approximate anatomical cross-section of the eye. Mechanical movement has draw-backs and, for real time scanning, it is better to have an array of transducers with electronic switching along adjacent cells. Such systems are entering the market and, with them, more detail is possible showing, for example, pulsation of the ophthalmic artery. Furthermore, the speed of such a scan can be enough to avoid discrepancies caused by unexpected movement of the eye. B-scanning provides qualitative information and the practitioner is able to identify the meridian of interest before a quantitative A-scan of that single section is carried out.

Oscilloscopes may produce a B-scan display which is grey scale similar to a black and white television picture, green scale or chromatic scale similar to a colour television picture. Grey scale has been used very successfully in the Bronson Turner B-scan ultrasonoscope which was the first commercially available equipment. The controls on this instrument permit the shift of the B-scan picture to the left, so that orbital echoes can be examined at the same magnification. This has some advantages, but it means that the eye and orbit cannot be seen together. Also the highest amplification gives very little scope for an analysis of orbital contents, because it is insufficient for deeper parts of the orbit. Stronger echoes are shown as brighter spots and this applies also on the green scale display of the Sonometric Ocuscan where an important facility is the vector A-scan display (*Figure 21.1*). Here there are simultaneous A- and B-scan displays with the A-scan corresponding to the position of the vector line on the B-scan. The vector line is set to cut any suspicious part of the B-scan for a more detailed A-scan assessment. Unlike the Bronson Turner equipment, magnifications of $\times 1$, $\times 2$ and $\times 4$ are provided, but the screen size is much smaller.

Chromatic scale is too expensive for most investigators, but Coleman and Katz (1974) have worked on this and gave their choice of colours to represent differing degrees of reflectivity. Red represented highest reflectance, green medium and blue lowest reflectance. Clearly there must be agreement between users of such equipment on the colour coding or the wrong conclusions can be drawn from the scan, but the advantage of a good colour system is easier detection of variation in echo amplitudes.

M-mode

Coleman and Weininger (1969) introduced an M-mode system or time motion (TM) system where the transducer remained stationary, while B-scan echo spots from the ocular interfaces were displayed in a sweep down the screen to produce parallel lines if principal structures in the eye remained static or wavy lines if their positions changed. With a sweep of 6 seconds, for example, movement of lens surfaces during accommodation was studied and even choroidal and retrobulbar vascular pulsation could be monitored.

Coleman, Katz and Lizzie (1975) superimposed the amplitudes of A-scan echoes on the B-scan picture to produce an isometric display, sometimes called D-mode (deflection modulation). The idea was to produce a simulated three-dimensional image, but despite its attractive appearance it is used little in most clinical evaluations.

Aldridge, Clare and Shepherd (1974) designed equipment which was capable of ophthalmic A-, B-, C- and M-scanning and was intended to provide holographic imaging as well. A 10-MHz focused transducer moved mechanically in a rectilinear fashion (C-mode) with the transducer shifted 1 mm after each 4-cm sweep. McLeod, Restori and Wright (1977) used this equipment at Moorfield's Eye Hospital and they showed that the rapid 7 B-scan/s gave the clinican enough time resolution to carry out dynamic studies on abnormalities. In these studies the direction of gaze is changed suddenly (0.15) and after-movements of echoes are observed for several seconds.

In advanced instruments of this kind, extra facilities can include digital image memory with a frame-freeze button which stops or freezes the image and a computer link which offers the opportunity for better three-dimensional imaging.

B-scan displays indicate well the position of a detachment, for instance a superior temporal detachment (*see Figure 21.1*), but the A-scan display is more useful for a critical study of the acoustic properties of the eye and measurement of the precise distances between the reflecting structures. This scan contrasts the presentations well, although some detail is lost when the A-scan occupies so little of the oscilloscope screen. Generally, a B-scan is performed first for a survey of the whole eye, so that the area of greatest interest can be pinpointed and inspected more closely with the A-scan. However, McLeod, Restori and Wright (1977) rely heavily on rapid B-scanning for dynamic vitreous studies and hardly use A-scanning at all.

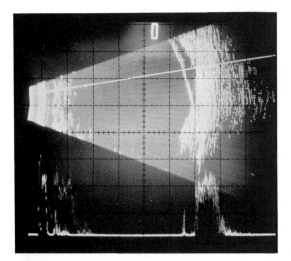

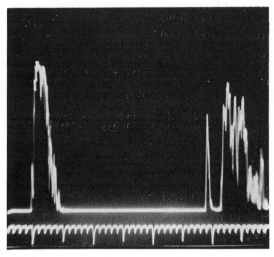

Figure 21.1 This shows the Sonometrics Ocuscan 400 trace with B-scan above and A-scan beneath it. The A-scan corresponds to the position of vector line on the B-scan. The probe is pointing through closed lids to the nasal sclera with A-scan going from sclera to sclera (diasclerally) behind the lens. This reveals a superior temporal retinal detachment

Figure 21.2   Kretz A-scan of same eye as in *Figure 21.1*, but here the probe is placed directly on nasal sclera and is not aimed through the lids. The superior temporal detachment is shown by an echo before the posterior complex. This scan was at a lowered amplification of 58 dB, to confirm the presence of a retinal detachment

A-scan

The A-scan (time-amplitude) display is formed when a static transducer is directed along a specific line in the eye. The resultant echoes from the interfaces between the various media appear as deflections on the time base of an oscilloscope screen, according to the positions of the reflecting surfaces. Echoes from the surfaces which are deeper within the eye take longer to return to the transducer for conversion back into electrical energy and so they appear further along the time base. The relative heights of the deflections along the time base give valuable information about the strength of the echoes and hence about the reflecting structures. In *Figure 21.2*, an A-scan trace is shown which was taken from the same eye as scanned in *Figure 21.1*, but the amplification is reduced to 58 dB from 80 dB. An A-scan probe has been used which is smaller than its B-scan counterpart, so it can be placed directly over any part of the visible sclera and, because the eye is open, the exact positions of eye and probe are evident. The best scan of the detachment has been photographed and, as the echo remains strong at less than 60 dB, it confirms a retinal detachment and does not indicate, for example, a vitreous haemorrhage.

If accurate biometry is to be performed, then the A-scan method is essential as the shape and size of these deflections is a guide to accurate centring with the appropriate axis of the eye.

Cataract, retinal detachment and vitreous haemorrhage

A- and B-scans facilitate the detection of retinal detachment in an eye with no view or a poor view of the fundus. In advanced cataract, or vitreous haemorrhage, apart from slitlamp biomicroscopy of the anterior segment and measurement of the ocular tension, there is little beyond an assessment of projection that can be performed optically to ensure that all is well behind the lens. Before referral for ophthalmic surgery, it is valuable to know as much as possible about the patient's eye. If a recent injury has caused a cataract or vitreous haemorrhage, then detection of a retinal detachment would necessitate urgent referral. However, retinal detachment behind a cataract may be of long standing, in which case the prospects for good vision after cataract extraction are very poor. A solid lesion under the detachment (*Figure 21.3*) would be another case for urgent referral, and normally the ultrasonic echoes would be very different from those of a simple detachment (*Figure 21.4b*).

Vitreous haemorrhage occurs also in some diabetic patients and more recently vitrectomy has been undertaken by some surgeons on the most seriously affected cases. Clearly, there is here a strong case for a search with ultrasound to rule out retinal detachment prior to such an operation. This may be difficult, as dense vitreous membranes can

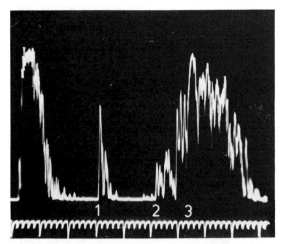

Figure 21.3 This man had reported pain in the right eye with serious visual loss. An A-scan at 70 dB behind the lens from the temporal sclera revealed an echo in the vitreous from the detached retina above point 1. The echo above point 2 is from a solid lesion beneath, which extends to the nasal sclera at point 3

be nearly as reflective as detached retinas. The Kretz A-scan procedure for the confirmation of retinal detachment is best illustrated as follows.

In *Figure 21.4a*, the A-scan is from inferior to superior sclera, i.e. diasclerally, for the affected left eye (injury caused by steel entering the eye). It was arranged so that the maximum amplitude of the superior scleral peak just reached a line placed arbitrarily about half-way up the screen. This occurred when the attenuator read 38 dB. With an increase in amplification to 50 dB on the attenuator, the echo (2) in the vitreous rose to meet this arbitrary line (*Figure 21.4b*). Because the increase in decibels was a good deal less than 18, there was a high degree of certainty that the echo was from a detached retina. This is supported completely by the vertical B-scan of that eye (*Figure 21.5a*) where the echoes (3 and 4) of the detachment converge on the optic nerve head. *Figure 21.5b* illustrates a B-scan in a similar position over the normal right eye. A modern alternative to the Kretz A-scan method is the rapid B-scanning method of McLeod, Restori and Wright (1977).

Preretinal or prepapillary proliferations are also quite reflective. Jerneld, Algvere and Singh (1980) have reported on 93 diabetics (168 eyes) with opaque ocular media and low visual acuities. They used the Coleman Ophthalmoscan 100 for ocular scans prior to vitrectomy. As a consequence, they were able to compare the results by ultrasound with the findings during vitrectomy. They deduced that the ultrasonic accuracy for retinal detachments was 78% and it was 67% for prepapillary and preretinal proliferations. They concluded that ultrasound helps

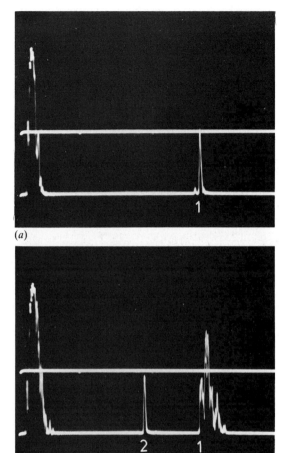

(a)

(b)

Figure 21.4 An illustration of a method to distinguish between echoes from a retinal detachment and organized vitreous haemorrhage or membranes. (a) A-scan directed from inferior to superior sclera, i.e. diasclerally, behind traumatic cataract. The maximum height of the scleral peak (1) just reaches the line at 38 dB. (b) The same position held as above with the A-scan increased in amplification to 50 dB. At this point the scleral peak (1) has increased in height above the line and an echo (2) in the vitreous (detached retina) reaches the line. The difference between the settings is 12 dB, i.e. well below 18 dB, which confirms the detached retina

to predict the prognosis after vitrectomy. It must be remembered that, as improvements in resolution of echoes from different membranes are occurring, so the accuracy of ultrasonic investigations is getting better. Generally, a total detachment is obvious apart from its reflectivity, because on the B-scan a pattern of echoes can be shown to converge on to the optic nerve. The accuracy of detection for a large retinal detachment in a normal vitreous is likely to be close to 100% provided diascleral A-

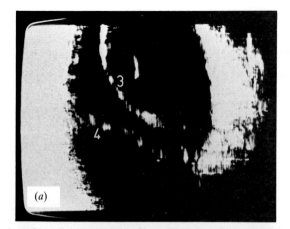

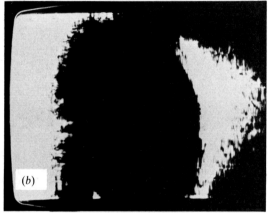

Figure 21.5 (*a*) Vertical B-scan at 80 dB of same left eye as shown in *Figure 21.4*. Echoes 3 and 4 are from the detached retina and they converge on the optic nerve head. (*b*) Vertical B-scan of normal right eye for comparison with scan of injured left eye of same patient

scans are carried out carefully in addition to scans through the cornea.

In diascleral A-scans (for example, see *Figure 21.4b*) the probe supports a drop of saline in contact with the sclera so that a sharp vertical echo can be obtained from the opposite wall of the eye. As the ultrasound is passing behind the lens, in a normal vitreous there should be an unobstructed passage of ultrasound transversely across the eye. More anterior detachments can be detected in this way. All meridians should be checked as a general routine. In passing, it is easy to detect vitreous floaters of any reasonable size if the amplification is turned up to maximum.

Frequently checks are carried out on axial lengths before cataract extraction to see whether myopia is due to the cataract or not. If an axial length is very long, posterior chamber implants only are used and then only with caution. A developing cataract causes

more obvious secondary echoes from the nucleus, which appear between the usual echoes from the anterior and posterior surfaces of the lens (*Figure 21.6a*). If the lens is intumescent, then on the B-scan the lens echoes form a well-defined, sharply curved surface and on the A-scan the lens thickness is excessive (*Figure 21.7*). An oedematous retina likewise shows an excessive retinal thickness on the A-scan and stronger echoes on the B-scan. When ocular implantation is likely after removal of cataract, it is recommended that biometry be carried out so that the correct implant power can be chosen.

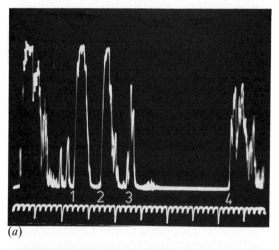

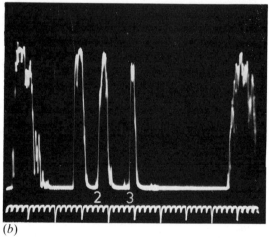

Figure 21.6 (*a*) An axial A-scan of the right eye of a man with advanced cataract in this eye. The transducer was dipped into a saline column held above the eye by an eye cup contact lens. Echoes beyond those off the transducer (far left) and bubbles in the saline are: (1) cornea, (2) anterior lens, (3) posterior lens, and (4) retina. Some extra echoes due to the cataract are seen between the principal lens echoes at 2 and 3. (*b*) Similar A-scan of the left eye which had very little cataract. Between lens echoes 2 and 3 there are virtually no extra echoes

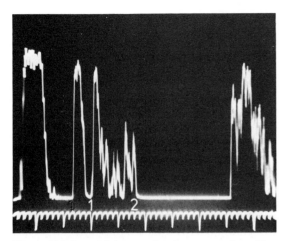

Figure 21.7 An axial A-scan of an intumescent lens. The anterior lens echo (1) is separated from the posterior lens echo (2) by multiple echoes from the oedematous tissue and the distance between these echoes is excessive

Biometry

A-scan ultrasonography is used for accurate measurement of the eye. With a double-beam oscilloscope (e.g. Kretz Ophthalmic A-scan), the lower trace carries a scale which is calibrated either in millimetres or microseconds. The latter is preferable as the speed of ultrasound (in m/s) is greater in the lens (1640 m/s) than it is in the aqueous or vitreous (1532 m/s), so the millimetre calibration would only apply correctly for the chosen medium. If the distance between echoes is read in microseconds (μs) this can be converted quickly with a conversion table or calculator for that medium. For example, in *Figure 21.6a*, the anterior chamber (AC) depth (1–2) is roughly 5 μs × 0.766 = 3.83 mm; the lens thickness (2–3) is roughly 6 μs × 0.82 = 4.92 mm; and the vitreous length (3–4) is 19 μs × 0.766 = 14.55 mm. On this basis the axial length would be 3.83 + 4.92 + 14.55 = 23.3 mm which appears quite reasonable. However, the velocity of ultrasound in the cataractous lens may be higher (shrunken lens) or lower (swollen lens) than the normal value.

For such eyes it is better to assume a velocity over the whole eye of 1550 m/s and simply measure from corneal apex to fovea. In this case, the result would be 30 × 0.775 = 23.25 mm and clearly this relates well to the first calculation. By comparison, the fellow eye (*Figure 21.6b*) has a similar axial length, but a different AC depth and vitreous length.

Eye cups

In these scans, the initial echo from the cornea is separated from the initial complex off the transducer because an eye cup has been used to support warm saline above the anaesthetized supine cornea. As the speed of ultrasound is temperature dependent, it is better to use saline at near body temperature, which warms up the anterior chamber to match the rest of the eye. The transducer is dipped into this saline at a minimum distance of 5 mm from the cornea which avoids near field effects, and it is angled to maximize the height of echoes so that they are vertical and 'clean' with the corneal peak being the highest followed by the lens peaks in descending order and the echo off the vitreous retina borderline as high as possible (*see Figure 21.6*). It is possible to measure the eye erect if a jacket is fitted over the transducer which holds a water delay path. A very thin membrane is placed over the far contact end of the jacket which may be permanent or disposable. It is important that most of the ultrasound passes through the membrane and little is lost by reflection at this point. Yamamoto *et al.* (1961), Leary *et al.* (1963) and Storey (1972) were among the early users of this technique. Although near field distortions are avoided, the corneal echo is not separated from the membrane echo and compression of the cornea is likely unless the device is moved to the eye on a spring-loaded mount. A way round this has been found by the Storz company with the probe which fits the Alpha 20/20 biometric ruler. Here the membrane is fitted and filled to produce a very soft balloon tip which does not compress the cornea when applied by hand gently. Furthermore, it does employ a central fixation light which is seen through a hole in the transducer and computer assistance makes electronic counting very quick indeed. So the tedium of measuring between echoes is removed and measurements are taken electronically only when the retinal echo reaches a preset height. This height needs to be at least one-quarter of the maximum height, but with absorption of ultrasound anteriorly due to cataract, for example, the amplification of posterior echo should still be enough to trigger a measurement.

Measurement

Clinically, the Kretz measurement from the initial rise of one echo to another is made from a polaroid photograph, but greater accuracy is achieved if a negative film of the trace is measured on a travelling microscope. Also it is very important to reduce the amplification to an absolute minimum (15–20 dB from maximum) so that measurements can then be made between peaks of echoes. This ensures that only the central beam of echoes is accepted and weaker peripheral ones are not included. Weaker ones return earlier and would give too short a measurement. A focused transducer is better than a plane one, in this respect, because the width of the beam at the retina is smaller. By analogy, it is more accurate to measure the depth of a cup with a narrow ruler than a wide one, as the wide one will underestimate the depth.

The Kretz A-scan has maintained its high reputation in biometry because it has good circuitry and any fluctuations in the display affect the A-scan and calibration trace equally. Before each eye is examined, a square wave is switched on to the calibration beam and 20-μs divisions are fitted into it exactly.

Rabie and Storey (1984) compared the Storz and Kretz intruments on 23 aphakic eyes. It was demonstrated that the Storz instrument was as reliable as the Kretz, even when measurements with the latter were taken from negative film with the travelling microscope. Further, calculation of axial length optically in the aphakic eye from refraction and corneal curvature related well to ultrasound measurements.

Accuracy of A-scan measurement can be improved in several ways, but one important point is to ensure that measurement is on or very near to the visual axis. Coleman, Lizzie and Jack (1977) considered this with transducers drilled with central sighting apertures and Storey (1982) has reflected ultrasound off a thin glass plate set at 45° to the line of vision. However, the examiner must be satisfied that echo peaks are up to standard objectively despite apparently good fixation and, if accommodation is to be controlled, the other eye must fixate accordingly.

Rabie (1986) has found pupil size to be of importance and, for anterior chamber depth, the pupil should be dilated, but for axial length it is better to be small. Coleman, Lizzie and Jack (1977) have considered at length other factors influencing accuracy including frequency and rectification.

Calculation of implant power

Shammas (1984) explained that, before 1975, the power of an intraocular lens to be inserted after cataract extraction was calculated from the equation:

$$P = 18 + (1.25 \times R)$$

where P = power of iris-supported intraocular lens for emmetropia and R = pre-operative refraction prior to cataract formation.

Shammas noted that with this method, errors exceeding 1 D occurred in over 50% of cases and some errors were so large that they have been referred to as the '9-dioptre surprise'. He considered many formulae in current use, but suggested that the SRK formula (Sanders, Retzlaff and Kraff, 1983), is the most popular regression formula. The formula for emmetropia is based on the following equation:

$$P = A - 2.5L - 0.9K$$

where P is the intraocular lens power (D) for emmetropia, L is the axial length (mm) and K is the mean corneal power (D). 'A' is the constant for the type of implant used and details are available from the manufacturers of the implant.

Modern instruments such as the Storz alpha 20/20 biometric ruler carry programmes for various formulae including the SRK formula and require only the 'A' constant, corneal radii, assumed refractive index for corneal power and axial length to give estimated implant power for emmetropia or any other post-operative refraction.

Most surgeons aim for emmetropia in eyes of normal length, −3 D for longer eyes with a history of myopia prior to cataract and +3 D for very short eyes with a history of at least this in the spectacles. Much depends on the refraction and the level of cataract in the contralateral eye. Future bifocal wear has to be considered with the avoidance of very different refractions for the two eyes. Some patients prefer to read without spectacles and wear them for the distance following the habit of a lifetime.

Aphakic refraction and contact lens power are predicted in case an implant is not inserted. Where an eye is measured with an implant *in situ*, marked reflection from the implant is to be expected.

Serial biometry of developing myopia is an interesting area of research and Storey and Rabie (1983) have measured the changes that occur when near emmetropic and highly myopic eyes accommodate. Storey and Rabie (1985) have determined for the first time the transverse diameter of the crystalline lens at rest and during accommodation in eyes with normal irides. Fincham (1935) achieved this optically *in vivo* on an aniridic subject as did Story (1924) and Grossman (1903). Ultrasound offers such exciting possibilities and is becoming an important tool for both the optometrist and the ophthalmologist.

Tumours contained within the eye

Vitreous haemorrhage is expected in some diabetics and following serious ocular trauma, but suspicions of an ocular tumour should be aroused otherwise, especially if there are signs of uveitis. Poor projection in any quadrant may point to a detachment which could have an underlying tumour (*Figure 21.8*). If the detachment is seen easily because the media are clear, ultrasonography can still be of value in the detection of a solid lesion beneath the retina. The practitioner is wiser to keep to facts, i.e. to describe the suspected lesion in terms of the echoes returned, so that opinions can be drawn from this on medical referral. Naturally, interpretation will be necessary during the examination, as this will

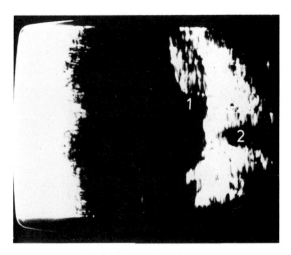

Figure 21.8 Large mass found temporal to the disc and near to the macular area. B-scan of retina detached by this tumour just above point 1 with the position of optic nerve shown clearly at point 2

aim the investigations in the correct way. Differentiation between lesions calls for a lot of experience.

Ultrasound is more reliable within the eye than modern forms of computerized X-ray tomography (CT scan), largely because the eye is fluid-filled without bones and the whole of the display screen can be covered with the eye alone, but the CT scan will be more informative in the orbit, most certainly towards the back of the orbit, where ultrasound penetrates but reverberates badly.

The B-scan should be carried out first so that the outline of the mass and its position can be determined. In *Figure 21.9a*, a large mass is outlined on the B-scan and, with the A-scan, it can be measured and examined more accurately. If the A-scan probe is directed more transversely along line X, then the A-scan appears as in *Figure 21.9b* with an area of clear vitreous between the tumour and retina, whereas along the line Y the more sagittal approach gives echoes from the tumour up to the underlying choroid and sclera (*Figure 21.9c*).

Alterations should be made to the amplitude of the echoes by adjustment of the attenuator in decibels (every 8 dB of increase doubles the amplification of the trace on the Kretz machine) and this conveys valuable information about the strength of echoes from the outside and inside of the tumour. A tumour that is quiet within may be absorbing ultrasound heavily if it is very solid, so there is a dampening effect on echoes from the orbit in comparison with the same area in the unaffected eye. Such shadowing is shown in *Figure 21.9a*. If a tumour does not absorb ultrasound heavily, it transmits well with good returns from beyond the tumour.

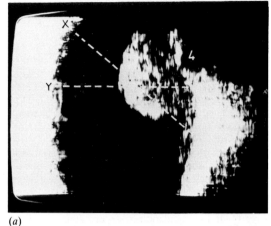

(*a*)

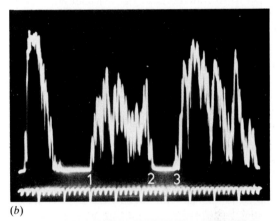

(*b*)

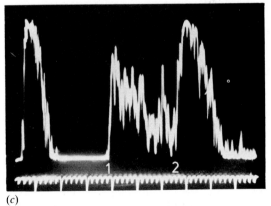

(*c*)

Figure 21.9 (*a*) B-scan through closed lids in the right vitreous of a man who said that his vision in that eye had been defective for 10–12 years. Shadowing in the orbit can be seen at point 4 beyond the echoes from this mass. (*b*) An A-scan that corresponds to line X on the B-scan in (*a*) with echoes from the tumour between points 1 and 2 and clear vitreous up to point 3. (*c*) An A-scan corresponding to line Y on the B-scan in (*a*) with the echoes from the tumour between points 1 and 2 after which they join the retina

Orbital work and the adnexa of the eye

Generally, a tumour in the orbit but near to the eye would absorb ultrasound in a way quite different to the orbital fat or the muscle near to it. B-scans are easier to interpret than A-scans and, for a deeper search, a lower frequency of transducer will help. However, deep surveys of the orbit can be inaccurate and a CT scan is likely to be more reliable. Proptosis is a major reason for an ultrasound investigation, although a fair proportion of these cases will not be due to a space-occupying lesion, but to swollen muscle. Shammas, Minckler and Ogden (1980) found that, in 14 patients with unilateral exophthalmos, the extraocular muscles were enlarged. Of these, 12 patients were found later to have thyroid dysfunction. The B-scan is not reliable for measurement, only for location of the muscle. So, with the A-scan, it is possible to demonstrate a relative difference in muscle thickness for corresponding areas in the affected and contralateral orbit. Ossoinig (1977) outlined his approach to this subject on which he has done much work.

Where a lesion of the lacrimal gland or some other mass under the eyelid is suspected, ultrasonography can be useful. For an investigation of the lacrimal gland, it is helpful to direct the probe up and out from the nasal sclera. In a patient with a palpable mass under the upper eyelid which was causing ptosis, the mass can be investigated simply with the probe on the eyelid. This case is illustrated in *Figure 21.10a* with the normal comparison in *Figure 21.10b*.

Anterior segment studies

Although ultrasonic investigation of the anterior segment would appear to be rarely needed, there are times when it is necessary. If the surgeon has a poor view of the anterior chamber prior to keratoplasty, it is useful to scan the area immediately behind the opaque cornea. However, an optical use for ultrasound in very severe cases where the corneal transparency has not remained after repeated keratoplasty is the calculation of the power for a corneal implant. Generally, the crystalline lens will be removed, so with a knowledge of the axial length only it is possible to calculate the power of the corneal implant. Another use of ultrasound anteriorly is a survey behind the iris. Because there are 'near field' problems with ultrasound, the patient should be examined under a saline bath so that the transducer is at least 5 mm from the cornea. In this way, the cornea is outlined as are the structures beneath it. Contact of the transducer with the eye or eyelids obscures anterior detail in the initial complex of echoes from the transducer.

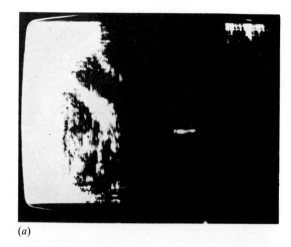

(*a*)

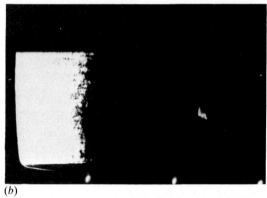

(*b*)

Figure 21.10 Patient with palpable mass under the upper eyelid. (*a*) B-scan directly against upper eyelid pointing above globe. Echoes from the mass are clearly seen by comparison with similar scan on normal eye. (*b*) B-scan above contralateral eye through upper eyelid

Anterior segment surveys are not always easy, but Le May (1978) appeared to do well with the Sonometric Ophthalmoscan 100 and a wire speculum to keep the eyes open. This may be partly because transducers of higher frequency (12–20 MHz) were employed which were most valuable for anterior work. Le May made the important point that the eye must be still for the few seconds of the B-scan.

Foreign bodies

Generally, removal of a foreign body is undertaken soon after an accident in a casualty department of an eye hospital with no need for an ultrasound examination, as the mode of entry for the foreign body betrays its location. However, when some old cases from elsewhere come to a hospital, apart from the need for a survey of the posterior eye if a view beyond the lens is impossible, there can be litigation pending for injury where an ultrasound scan is seen by a solicitor as an advantage for the plaintiff. In two such cases seen by the author, glass entered the eyes (and elsewhere) after an explosion in a laboratory. One man was left with such a large piece of glass in his vitreous that much of his central vision was through it. Although this could be seen clearly with the ophthalmoscope, to the layman an ultrasound scan was more tangible evidence. With the A-scan, the glass reflected ultrasound more than the retinal detachment and with the B-scan the echoes on the screen appeared to shimmer. Denser foreign bodies reflect ultrasound even more heavily as the next case shows. A young man had joined a pistol club. Unfortunately one of the members put a cocked and loaded pistol on the shelf and a tremor in the building caused the pistol to be fired at him. He was discharged after a week from a general hospital when he had been assured that the pellet was in one of his extraocular muscles. His vision reduced over the next 4 years, when a B-scan revealed the pellet on his retina (*Figure 21.11a*) and the A-scan showed such reflectivity that, in *Figure 21.11b*, only the echo from the pellet appears and it is only with further amplification that the retinal echo is seen (*Figure 21.11c*).

Other ultrasonic techniques

Ultrasonic Doppler systems have been employed to measure the velocity of red blood cells. A frequency shift occurs when ultrasound reflects off moving interfaces such as blood in the ophthalmic artery or carotid artery. Blood flow can be calculated once the vessel width is known.

Port (1976) measured the sags of soft contact lenses with ultrasound from which the radius of curvature could be deduced. Commercial equipment has been developed for this purpose.

References

ALDRIDGE, E.E., CLARE, A.B. and SHEPHERD, D.A. (1974) Scanned ultrasonic holography for ophthalmic diagnosis. *Ultrasonics*, **12**, 155–160

BAUM, G. (1956) The Effect of ultrasonic radiation upon the eye and the ocular adnexa. *Am. J. Ophthalmol.*, **42**, 696–706

BAUM, G. and GREENWOOD, I. (1958) The application of ultrasonic locating techniques to ophthalmology, part 1, reflective properties. *Am. J. Ophthalmol.*, **46**, 319–329

COLEMAN, D.J. and KATZ, L. (1974) Colour coding of B-scan ultrasonograms. *Arch. Ophthalmol.*, **91**, 429–431

COLEMAN, D.J., KATZ, L. and LIZZI, F.L. (1975) Isometric three dimensional viewing of ultrasonograms. *Arch. Ophthalmol.*, **93**, 1362–1365

COLEMAN, D.J., LIZZI, F.L. and JACK, R.L. (1977) *Ultrasonography of the Eye and Orbit.* Philadelphia: Lea and Febiger

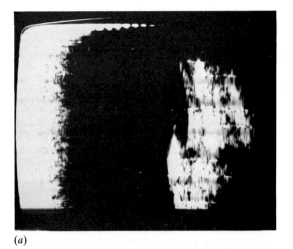

(a)

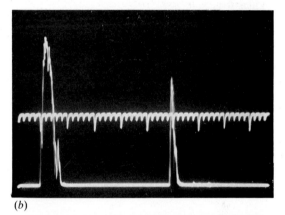

(b)

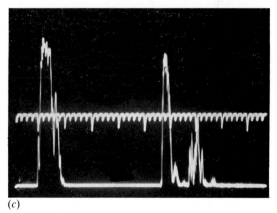

(c)

Figure 21.11 A lead pellet was detected within the left eye of this young man. An optical view of his eye beyond the crystalline lens was impossible. (*a*) B-scan shows the foreign body sitting on the retina; (*b*) A-scan from superior sclera at 40 dB where only the echo from the lead pellet is seen. This demonstrates the high reflectivity of the foreign body. (*c*) An increase in amplification to 50 dB reveals a smaller echo from the retina beyond

COLEMAN, D.J. and WEININGER, R. (1969) Ultrasonic M-mode technique in ophthalmology. *Arch. Ophthalmol.*, **82**, 475

CURIE, J. and CURIE, P. (1880) *Comptes Rendus*, p. 204 and other papers cited by A.B. Wood (1955)

FINCHAM, E.F. (1935) A Study of accommodation by photography of the living lens and ciliary body in a case of aniridia. *Trans. Ophthalmol. Soc. UK*, **55**, 145–158

GROSSMAN, K. (1903) The mechanism of accommodation in man. *Br. Med. J.*, **2**, 726–731

JERNELD, B., ALGVERE, P. and SINGH, G. (1980) An ultrasonographic study of diabetic vitreo-retinal disease with low visual acuity. *Acta Ophthalmol.*, **58**, 193–201

JOHNSON, B. (1979) *The Secret War*, p. 222–228. London: Arrow Books

LEARY, G., SORSBY, A., RICHARDS, M.J. and CHASTON, J. (1963) Ultrasonographic measurement of the components of ocular refraction in life. 1. Technical considerations *Vision Res.*, **3**, 487–498

LE MAY, M. (1978) B-scan ultrasonography of the anterior segment of the eye. *Br. J. Ophthalmol.*, **62**, 651–656

MCLEOD, D., RESTORI, M. and WRIGHT, J.E. (1977) Rapid B-scanning of the vitreous. *Br. J. Ophthalmol.*, **61**, 437–445

MUNDT, G.H. and HUGHES, W.F. (1956) Ultrasonics in ocular diagnosis. *Am. J. Ophthalmol.*, **41**, 488–498

OSSOINIG, K. (1977) Echography of the eye, orbit and periorbital region. In *Radiology of the Orbit*, edited by P.H. Arger, p. 229–233. New York: John Wiley

PORT, M. (1976) New methods of measuring hydrophillic lenses. *Ophthalmol. Opt.*, **16**, 1079–1082

RABIE, E.P. (1986) Biometry of the crystalline lens during accommodation, *PhD Thesis*, Manchester

RABIE, E.P. and STOREY, J.K. (1984) The reliability of ultrasonic axial length measurements. *Transactions of the First International Congress*, Vol.2, pp. 51–57. London: British College of Ophthalmic Opticians (Optometrists)

SHAMMAS, H.J. (1984) *Atlas of Ophthalmic Ultrasonography and Biometry*. St Louis: C. V. Mosby Co.

SHAMMAS, H.J.F., MINCKLER, P.S. and OGDEN, C. (1980) Ultrasound in early thyroid orbitopathy. *Arch. Ophthalmol.*, **98**, 277–279

SANDERS, D.R., RETZLAFF, J. and KRAFF, M.C. (1983) Comparison of empirically derived and theoretical aphakic refraction formulas. *Arch. Ophthalmol.*, **101**, 965–967

STOREY, J.K. (1972) The use of ultrasonic equipment for the measurement of intraocular distances. *Transactions of the International Ophthalmic Optical Congress.* pp. 255–272. London: British Optical Association

STOREY, J.K. (1982) Measurement of the eye with ultrasound. *Ophthalmol. Opt.*, **22**, 150–160

STOREY, J.K. and RABIE, E.P. (1983) Ultrasound—research a tool in the study of accommodation. *Ophthal. Physiol. Opt.*, **3**, 315–320

STOREY, J.K. and RABIE, E.P. (1985) Ultrasonic measurement of the transverse lens diameter during accommodation. *Ophthal. Physiol. Opt.*, **5**, 145–148

STORY, J.B. (1924) Aniridia; notes on accommodation changes under eserine. *Trans. Ophthalmol. Soc. UK*, **44**, 413–417

WOOD, A.B. (1955) *A Textbook of Sound*. London: G. Bell & Sons

YAMAMOTO, Y., NAMIKI, R., BABA, M. and KATO, M. (1961) A study of the measurement of ocular axial length by ultrasonic echography. *Jap. J. Ophthalmol.*, **5**, 58

Part 6

Further investigative techniques

22

Visual fields

Elizabeth McClure

There are few aspects of ophthalmic investigation more neglected than visual field examination. Many optometrists and ophthalmologists regard the field test as a boring and time consuming part of their routine commitment and as a result it is often omitted.

Perimetry undertaken without knowledge of the overall ocular status is unrewarding since intelligent, informed interpretation of findings as they evolve during the test is an essential part of achieving useful results. Approaching a case of unexplained visual loss or visual symptoms armed with confidence in technique, equipment and a depth of knowledge in the subject make the task more interesting and certainly a more effective exercise.

Practitioners should aim to produce repeatable responses even with uncooperative subjects so that they can achieve reliable results, relate findings to the overall ophthalmic examination, and proceed to follow up any abnormality detected. Cases can then be authoritatively referred with clinical findings expressed in the correct terminology.

The purpose, therefore, of the field examination is to supply confirmation of normality, or evidence of specific abnormality.

The field of vision

The appreciation of the surrounding world in extent, form, detail and colour is a projection of the visual pathway in space. The macular region which is the point of fixation has maximum visual acuity, all other areas being less able to perceive detail. Euclid's analogy (developed by Traquair, *see* Scott, 1957) of an island of seeing in a sea of blindness is an ideal way to imagine the varying sensitivity of visual function (*Figure 22.1*). The shoreline of the island, which is ovoid in shape, represents the extreme limit of visual sensation. From here a gradual sloping hill

rises just as retinal function improves, reaching a maximum at the peak of the island hill—the point of fixation (*Figure 22.2*). On its less steep slope every island has a deep pit dropping to sea-level where the projection of the optic nerve head (devoid of visual receptors) results in a physiological blind spot. On the shore of the island, only large objects can be seen and colour cannot be distinguished, but nearer the summit greater detail is gradually appreciated, reflecting the increased density of the retinal receptors in the more central retina and improved efficiency due to greater neural representation.

The practitioner's task is to assess the island's dimensions, to explore its surface and coastline for irregularities or erosion, and to display the findings like a contour map (*see Figure 22.2*).

Measuring the field

The map is drawn by establishing how far distant from the point of maximum acuity the eye responds to a particular size or brightness of sensation. The response depends on the area under test, but normally the further from fixation the lower the sensitivity.

Lines joining points of equal sensitivity are known as isopters; each *isopter* represents the distance from fixation at which an observer becomes aware of a specific testing target, while maintaining steady fixation. These isopters simulate the contour lines of the island map. Normally, an extremely large or bright stimulus will be recognized by the most peripheral receptors and the isopter obtained with such a target will map the shoreline or extreme limit of the field of vision. Reducing the stimulus size by making it smaller or dimmer means the target must come nearer to the fixation point before the eye responds to it thus producing a smaller field. The part of the

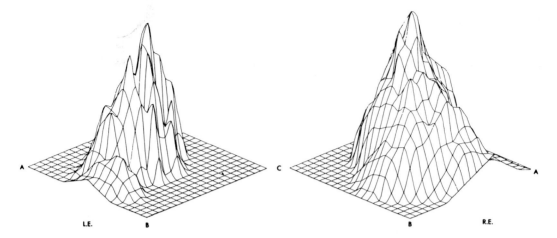

Figure 22.1 Three-dimensional representation of the island of vision obtained from multiple retinal threshold readings of a normal right eye and a left eye with defective lower field. The same fields are charted in conventional fashion in *Figure 22.2*. The islands are viewed from point B. (Plots were produced by Glasgow University Computing Service (GCL 2988 Computer) using routines from the GHOST package)

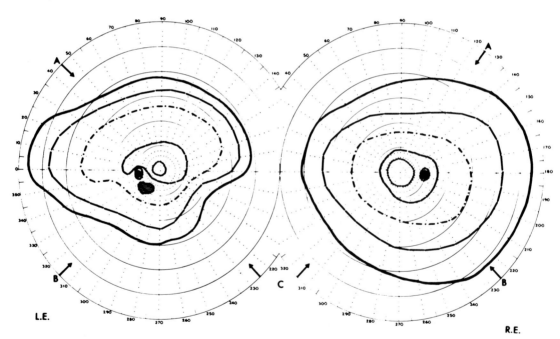

Figure 22.2 Charts of kinetic fields recorded in the usual way. These show the normal right eye and depressed lower left field displayed in *Figure 22.1*.

Tubingen targets: 1.0 (white) at 00, 05, 10, 15 dB

field of vision enclosed by a particular isopter is said to be above threshold and any point within the isopter is supraliminal, i.e. that target will be seen, unless, of course, it happens to coincide with the physiological blind spot.

Dimensions of the visual field are dependent, not only on the size of the testing target, but on a host of other variable factors, and especially on the level of the ambient illumination used during the examination.

The contrast between the target and its background governs its visibility and the target's effect on the retina depends on the state of adaptation of the retinal receptors. Maximum cone response (represented by the summit of the island hill) is greatest in photopic conditions. A reduction to mesopic levels reduces cone activity and flattens the peak of the hill. With scotopic conditions the external isopter may widen due to increased rod response in the peripheral retina, and a physiological central depression will be found, caused by the absence of rods in the foveal area (*Figure 22.3*). Despite these variations, normal average statistics have been established by such authorities as Traquair (1938) and Harrington (1981).

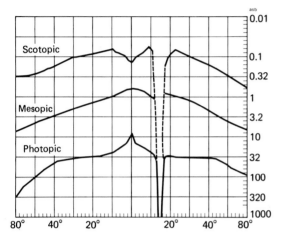

Figure 22.3 Static perimetry of horizontal meridian of the same eye showing alteration of retinal receptor thresholds under different background illuminations.

However large or bright the stimulus, a limit to the extent of the island is imposed by the physical boundaries of the eye and the facial structure.

The visual field is defined as that area in space within which the eye can perceive a visual stimulus without altering its position of gaze. It has maximum normal limits of 100° temporally, 60° upward, 60° nasally and 75° downwards. Strictly speaking this is the *relative* field. The *absolute* field is found by altering the angle of the head without changing fixation in order to eliminate the field restrictions caused by the bony prominences of the orbit and nose.

The optic disc through which the nerve fibre bundles pass to the optic nerve has no receptors and projects in the field a physiological blind spot which is a vertical oval approximately 8.5° × 5.5°, found 15.5° out in the temporal field one-fifth above and four-fifths below the horizontal midline. Around this central absolute area is a much less constant relative scotoma, the extent of which will depend on the refractive condition of the eye and the target employed.

Establishing normality

Factors influencing the field of vision

Familiarity with all the possible causes of variation of field measurements is essential in the recognition of a significant abnormal finding.

Physical factors

Overall measurement of the field is limited by facial contours. The patient with deeply set eyes or who habitually narrows the palpebral aperture will show a smaller field than a patient with exophthalmos. Note should be taken of an overhanging brow, lid or hairstyle. The elderly patient may have a drooping lid, often more noticeable at the end of an examination when the patient is tired or bored. It may be necessary to have an assistant hold the lid up or to raise it with adhesive tape. Frequently, artefacts are produced by a spectacle frame or a trial lens which sits too low. If the nose is large and interferes with the field, the patient can be asked to angle the head while maintaining central fixation.

Care must be taken to ensure sequential tests are carried out under the same conditions. Ambient lighting (which affects the state of adaptation of the eye), the rate of presentation of stimulus, its actual size and brightness must all be kept constant throughout the test sequence.

Physiological factors

Variations of normal are also to be expected because of the refractive state of the eye.

Myopia

The highly myopic eye has a large blind spot.

Aphakia

The aphakic eye has a reduction in overall size of the field and the blind spot is displaced slightly towards fixation.

Ametropia

Uncorrected refractive errors can induce 'refractive scotomata' and so the greatest care should be taken to eliminate refractive errors by full correction, including appropriate positive addition for the testing distance. To do this without restricting the field, it may be necessary to use full aperture trial case lenses. When the patient requires a high-powered spectacle correction, and particularly aphakic patients, the best solution is a contact lens. Anderson (1981) advocates a high near addition to ensure no stress on accommodation reserve which in turn helps maintain steadier pupil size.

Pupil size

Miosis reduces overall field by reducing the apparent brightness of the stimulus, but has the advantage of compensating for small refractive errors. Recording the pupil size is of particular importance when monitoring a glaucoma patient in whom changes of treatment may significantly alter pupil size and refraction with resulting changes in apparent visual field.

Media

Patients who have reduced clarity in the optical media often have a smaller field and an apparent increase in depressed areas. This is because the stimulus reaching the retina is less bright and so the test is rendered more sensitive. Glaucoma patients who have cataract extractions with or without lens implants show dramatic improvement in field status (*Figure 22.4*).

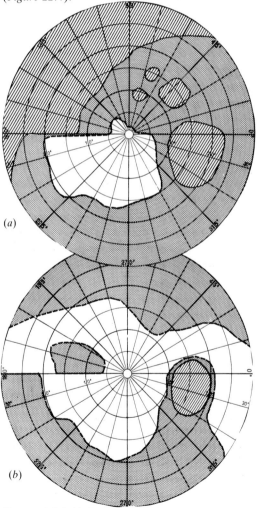

Targets: 1.0 (white) at 00 and 05 dB

Figure 22.4 (*a*) Visual field of patient prior to cataract surgery when visual acuity is 6/24. (*b*) The same eye following cataract extraction and lens implant procedure showing apparent improvement of field. The visual acuity was than 6/9+

Ageing

Reduction in isopter size in the ageing eye is said to be normal. This is possibly due to the less clear media combined with slower reaction time and a general reduction in overall efficiency, both physical and mental.

Psychological factors

The quality of results obtained depends greatly on the practitioner's ability to assess the patient's physical and mental limitations correctly. An unwell, elderly, fatigued or anxious person will be unable to concentrate, slow to respond, and will often become less helpful as anxiety increases with the examiner's persistence. Changing to a different investigative method, for instance from kinetic to multiple stimulus presentation, may reduce stress and improve cooperation. Encouragement and reassurance may not be sufficient to relax the patient and so, on occasion, a return visit may be required to achieve useful results.

Even when complete compliance and cooperation are obtained, two sequential fields may appear different (although the status of the eye remains unchanged) due to patient and examiner variations. Different examiners, despite taking care to standardize their techniques, will produce results which are not identical because of the subjective element inherent in the practice of perimetry. Allowances must be made for such variations when charts are interpreted.

Perimetry is a subjective investigation and cannot be expected to achieve findings of absolute consistency.

Establishing abnormality

Terminology

An area of loss of sensitivity surrounded by normal field, i.e. a *scotoma*, is easily recognized as abnormal. Problems arise when the changes are more subtle—when, for instance, an irregularity in the shape of an isopter may be the only indication of reduced function. This is a *depression*. On closer examination, a depression may be found to include or surround a scotoma or may, by the next examination, have developed into a scotoma. The term 'depression' can also be applied to the entire field when the area within the isopters are all smaller than usual or when internal isopters are missing. An overall depression indicates general loss of function such as may occur gradually as an eye develops opacities in the media. The effect on the island of vision is as though it were sinking into the sea, losing not only part of its shoreline but also some of its height above sea-level. The common analogy, of the shores of the island being eroded away, is inaccurate.

When the peripheral boundary alone is lost the field is said to be *contracted*. True contraction consists of total blindness to any stimulus such as may be found in a hemianopia. The different isopters in contraction are superimposed and the area of deficit is the same to all stimuli (*Figure 22.5*). The term 'relative' applied to a depression is superfluous, because all depressions are areas of relative loss.

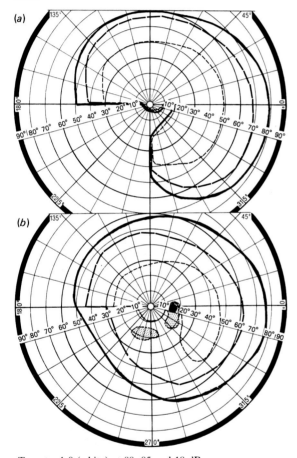

Targets: 1.0 (white) at 00, 05 and 10 dB

Figure 22.5 (*a*) Steep-edged contracted lower nasal field due to retinal vascular occlusion. (*b*) Sloping edged lower nasal field defect due to glaucoma enclosing a depressed area

Locating the abnormality

Defects of the visual field are manifestations of a disease process or injury either in the eye itself or in the higher visual pathways.

Retinal distribution of nerve fibres is symmetrical, arching from the fovea and the nasal retina each side

of the horizontal midline to join the temporal fibres (which follow a more direct route) at the optic nerve head (*Figure 22.6*). The major retinal blood vessels have a similar distribution pattern.

Each optic nerve carries fibres from the entire retina to the chiasma where the nasal fibres cross to the opposite side to join the temporal fibres from the other eye. The image received by the temporal retina (of the nasal half of the field) is relayed by uncrossed fibres to the cortex on the same side, whereas the image of the temporal half of each field is transmitted to the opposite cortex. Thus fibres from the right half of each retina pass from the chiasma by way of the right optic tract, lateral geniculate nucleus and optic radiations to the right visual cortex, and those from the left side of each retina are processed on the left side of the brain (*Figure 22.6*).

Furthermore the fibres alter their relative position along the entire pathway. For example, the macular fibres start together on temporal section of the nerve head as they leave the globe and gradually move to the centre of the nerve as they approach the chiasma (*Figure 22.6*) (*see* also Chapter 1).

Relating observed details of field defects to known anatomy and physiology of the visual system helps locate the abnormality and thus facilitates diagnosis.

Identification of abnormality

Certain important characteristics of field defects should be obtained to establish as much information as possible and to allow detailed description of the field deficit. These characteristics are: position, size, density and margins, development, and shape. Shape can be more easily dealt with when subdivided into central and peripheral.

Position

The field is divided into upper and lower nasal, and upper and lower temporal quadrants. 'Peripheral' applies to the extreme boundaries, 'central' to the area within 30° of fixation.

The term 'Bjerrum region' is used frequently and describes the areas 10–15° from fixation particularly above and below the blindspot. The field is drawn as the patient sees it, so a scotoma in the right (temporal) upper field of the right eye reflects damage in the right lower (inferonasal) retina and should be shown on the right side of the matching diagram of the fellow eye and vice versa (*Figure 22.7*).

Size

The overall extent of the field and the size of a scotoma depend on the intensity of the stimulus and are much less important for diagnosis than shape,

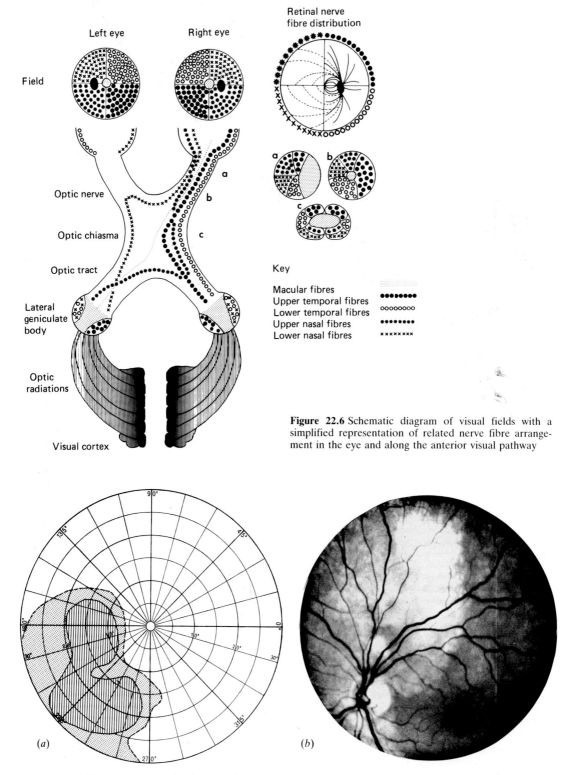

Figure 22.6 Schematic diagram of visual fields with a simplified representation of related nerve fibre arrangement in the eye and along the anterior visual pathway

Figure 22.7 (*a*) Scotoma below left blind spot due to choroidal melanoma seen as depigmented area above disc in accompanying retinal photograph (*b*)

except when looking for evidence of progression. A large area of depression discovered using a difficult target may be of less diagnostic value than smaller scotomata with more definite shapes or distributions (*Figure 22.8*). Conversely, a group of small patches of loss found with a large target may assume a more characteristic shape when the area is retested with a more difficult stimulus.

Density and margins

Sensitivity levels within a field defect may not be uniform. This can be demonstrated by using different testing targets as an area of field loss discovered with a particular stimulus may have patches within it which are scotomata to a bigger or brighter target (*see Figure 22.8*). These are described as being denser than the surrounding deficit. The margins of a defect, or the gradient of loss of sensitivity, are described as 'sloping' when the isopters are widely

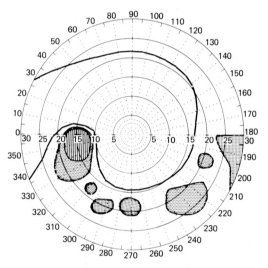

Figure 22.8 A target of 5/2000 shows a normal blind spot only. An isopter of 2/2000 indicates a depressed lower field. Further examination with 3/2000 reveals multiple scotomata in the Bjerrum area and a nasal step

spaced, and 'steep' when the isopters crowd together closely. When steep edged, the area of loss is almost the same no matter which testing stimulus is employed. A sloping edge indicates gradually changing sensitivity and is said to be found when a disease process is active. A steep-edged defect is more common in long-standing, passive or healed conditions, indicating a sudden alteration of function. For example, the visual field loss due to a retinal vascular lesion, has steep margins while the similar defect found in glaucoma has sloping margins (*see Figure 22.5*).

Development

Comparison of the field loss of one eye with that of its fellow may also indicate the likely pattern of development which would otherwise be unknown without sequential plots. In the same way, monitoring improvement during treatment confirms diagnosis and informs about the healing process.

Shape

Central

Scotomata are most common in the central field where the nerve fibres and receptors are more numerous and vulnerable. It is important to select the best stimulus to allow the patient to give reliable responses and the practitioner to recognize the shape of an evolving defect (*see Figure 22.8*). The terminology applied to the shape of scotomata is largely self-explanatory:

(1) Circular or irregular—usually due to a local lesion within the eye or optic nerve.
(2) Oval—usually centrocaecal, i.e. affecting the papillomacular bundle between the macula and disc.
(3) Ring—complete or partial, equidistant from fixation.
(4) Arcuate—a nerve fibre bundle defect following the path of the nerve fibres arching around fixation to the blind spot.

A complete upper and lower arcuate may look like a ring scotoma. An incomplete arcuate may appear as a series of round, oval, sausage or scimitar-shaped patches scattered anywhere in the 'Bjerrum' region. They may also be called Bjerrum scotomata. When these extend to the horizontal in the nasal field, they will end with a sharp horizontal margin forming Seidel's sign or Roenne's step at the junction of the upper and lower fibre bundles along the horizontal raphe. These defects occur both in glaucoma, where there is a nerve fibre bundle defect due to disturbance at the optic disc, and following occlusion of the retinal vessels which, like the nerve fibres, do not cross the horizontal midline.

When a central scotoma has a straight margin along the vertical meridian, it is a central hemianopic defect. It will almost certainly be bilateral and due to interference with the pathway at the chiasma or beyond. Its characteristics should be explored and described in exactly the same way as a peripheral sector defect.

As central scotomata increase in size, they may eventually reach the peripheral limit of the field and 'break through' to involve the shoreline of the island of vision of Traquair's analogy.

Peripheral

Because of the anatomical arrangement of the nerve fibres already mentioned, defects of the peripheral field are frequently manifest in both eyes and have well-defined and characteristic shapes described as sector defects. Those which affect the nasal or the temporal side of each field are termed binasal or bitemporal defects. A defect which affects both right or both left sections of a field is known as a right or left *homonymous* sector defect. If the complete half of a field is involved it is known as a *hemianopia*, when less as a partial hemianopia or as a *quadrantanopia*. Such defects are described as *congruous* when identical in shape in each eye and *incongruous* if of different shapes. Not all peripheral defects are bilateral. A reduced field in one eye only, perhaps due to a retinal disorder such as a detachment, can be described easily by location and extent.

A less common condition is when a hemianopia is horizontal, affecting only the upper or lower, right or left eye.

General techniques

Best results are obtained from patients who are comfortable and relaxed and who understand why they are doing and why. Concentration is aided by eliminating distractions such as noise or interruption. The better seeing eye is examined first allowing for adaptation to ambient lighting while an explanation is given of what is required. Use of a translucent rather than a black occluder facilitates adaptation of the second eye. The patient's eye should be level with the fixation target and, if necessary, the fixation size, brightness or colour should be adjusted. If a central scotoma is present, it may be useful to fix a large ring or a cross in the middle of the screen and to ask the patient to look where the centre should be.

The patient should be shown the test target and others of various sizes and brightnesses, presenting them in different parts of the field for familiarization with what may be required later. Any refractive error should be corrected accurately for the testing distance, particularly when exploring the central area. The patient must be reminded of the paramount importance of maintaining steady fixation.

Kinetic method

As an introduction to check both the accuracy of patient's position and his cooperation the blindspot is demonstrated with a very easily detected target. Then, with the stimulus selected for the test, the blindspot is plotted and an isopter established by moving from the non-seeing periphery towards the fixation point with a smooth movement at 10–15° intervals around the circumference of the field.

Further isopters may be plotted using targets of increasing difficulty to provide a full survey of the island. Irregularity of isopter spacing indicates possible areas of depression which should be searched for scotomata with a target of suitably adjusted sensitivity.

When examining the central field in detail, a useful 'rule of thumb' is to select a target which brings the isopter to 25°. Areas of deficit are detected by moving across the field radially outlining any scotoma discovered by repeatedly moving from blind to seeing each time aiming to cross the suspected border at a right angle to show as definite a contrast as possible, thereby enhancing the patient's reactions. If the target travels along the edge of a scotoma through areas of varying sensitivity, the responses will be less reliable and the task unnecessarily difficult. Radial movement of the target is preferable because meridional searching follows the path of the retinal vessels and increases the chance of plotting angioscotomata which can be mistaken for early arcuate defects. (In theory, however, the true arcuate scotoma should be narrower nearer the disc due to the close arrangement of the fibres and should broaden further from the disc as the fibres fan out across the retina. Angioscotomata should be wider nearer the disc where the vessels are of greater calibre.)

The speed of presentation is important (5°/s is about the correct maximum rate). Too slow a movement will tempt the patient to search and lose fixation, too fast a movement will reduce the apparent field size. It is helpful to tell the patient from which direction the target will first appear and, occasionally, to break the rhythm of presentation to ensure that he is attentive and alert.

If the initial survey of the field proves unsatisfactory, the selected test conditions should be altered and the test repeated with the aim of obtaining a more decisive picture. The temptation to prompt or anticipate responses should be avoided.

Static, profile, contrast threshold or light sense perimetry

In kinetic field testing, evaluation of sensitivity is achieved by varying the size or colour of the testing target but, since the advent of electrically operated perimeters with luminous targets and controlled background brightness, it has been possible to measure sensitivity by establishing the differential light threshold for a given size of spot at any one fixed location. This 'static' test may be employed in two ways:

(1) By 'spot' checking—a target of selected sensitivity is used to establish whether it can be seen in a series of fixed positions. This provides a useful screening method, the Armaly tech-

nique (Rock, Drance and Morgan, 1973). Though somewhat more laborious, spot-checking using reversible black/white targets can also be attempted on a tangent screen.

(2) To quantify a specific area of field—an individual threshold value is obtained for a series of locations chosen to examine sensitivity in areas where a field defect is expected. Thus, by plotting in graphic form the thresholds of neighbouring areas of the field, it is possible to build up a picture of the sensitivity giving, in effect, a cross-sectional diagram of the island of vision (*see Figure 22.3*).

Most static profiles are taken over the central area, 30° each side of fixation and across the 180° meridian as this provides information on the comparative sensitivity of macula, optic nerve head and centrocaecal area. However, any meridian may be selected, for example, when the kinetic method fails to confirm an area of suspected deficit above the blind spot, then an oblique meridian cutting through the Bjerrum area would be chosen (*see Figure 22.19*). Static profiles need not be meridional. Threshold values taken at points equidistant from fixation (known as a circular static) should, of course, remain constant if visual function is intact.

Static perimetry provides a method of assessing the depth of scotoma (*Figure 22.9*) and has the added advantage of monitoring recovery or regression even in an eye with very severely reduced visual function, since it can be carried out with a large target. This also helps compensate for small refractive errors. Furthermore, since static modes eliminate successive lateral summation (a major unavoidable cause of loss of fixation in kinetic methods), it often proves more successful with an uncooperative patient.

A particularly useful application of this technique is the macular profile (*Figure 22.10*), in which detailed evaluation of the central 10° can be obtained with a very small target at 1° intervals. The full near refractive correction is essential.

Flicker

Another method of assessing sensitivity utilizes measurement of the flicker fusion frequency. This depends on the ability of the visual system to recover from the inhibitory phase following one stimulus and to become receptive to another. The ability of the eye to recognize a light of decreasing frequency of flicker is poorer when the retinal receptors are damaged or the visual pathway embarrassed.

Since this technique is independent of variation of acuity, media changes, age, amblyopia, and refractive blur, it proves useful in many difficult cases and has the added advantage of being easily understood.

It is a particularly useful and quick method of demonstrating a difference in sensitivity each side of the midline when an optic tract or a cortical disorder is suspected, but not confirmed, by kinetic methods.

Colour

The use of coloured targets is another method of altering stimulus sensitivity.

Disease processes which affect specific colour function, such as retrobulbar neuritis or tobacco amblyopia (*see Figure 22.9*), result in a marked reduction in the red isopter or a very noticeable enlargement of the scotoma to colour in comparison to that of a white target. This is known as *disproportion*. The practical aspects of colour perimetry present some problems, since the peripheral retina is comparatively insensitive to colour, the patient is

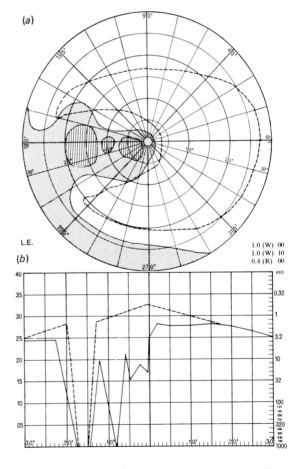

Figure 22.9 (*a*) Kinetic field in a case of tobacco amblyopia. The larger shaded area of field loss was found using a red target. (*b*) Static perimetry across the 180° meridian of the same eye showing the relative density of the centrocaecal scotomata. (Dotted line shows normal profile)

aware of the target at its *visibility* threshold before being aware of its hue, i.e. at the *recognition* threshold and this concept, beyond the grasp of many patients, adds an unnecessary complication which, however, can be avoided if a sufficiently difficult white stimulus is chosen.

The advent of projection perimeters with luminous targets increased the popularity of colour perimetry, but the problems of standardization of wavelength and intensity and the subsequent difficulty in establishing normal colour isopters prevent its widespread application. The size of the field obtained by a particular hue and brightness is difficult to interpret and it is more useful to employ colour targets for specific comparison of function in the four quadrants of the field in an attempt to detect subtle changes.

Illumination

Ambient illumination affects the field results by altering the state of adaptation of the eye. Dim background illumination reducing cone function and increasing rod activity flattens the profile of the island (*see Figure 22.3*).

In practical terms, these features affect patient response during kinetic perimetry as the reaction to stimuli is more accurate and consistent when the isopters are close together and responses indecisive when the slope of the hill is gradual.

However, the standard background illumination of the Tubingen instrument is near mesopic level and so activates both rods and cones and this can be advantageous because reduced background brightness does not alter the integrity of the field of a healthy eye, but does help show up any early defects. It is also useful in demonstrating abnormal retinal function in cases of shallow retinal detachment, when the unusually slow recovery of rod and cone activity after the stress of photopic exposure will help reveal the full extent of the retinal area affected.

Extra care must be taken, therefore, to ensure accuracy of calibration and to avoid inadvertent changes in background illumination, particularly if working with a larger target and reduced background brightness.

Dark adaptation

Although not usually thought of as part of perimetry, dark-adaptation testing follows in natural sequence in this discussion. Most bowl perimeters can be used for dark-adaptation measurement by pre-adapting the eye to very bright light ensuring maximum cone activity and thereafter monitoring the eye's adjustment to total darkness and maximum rod activity. The dark-adaptation curve is obtained by taking threshold values at one retinal location at 1 or 2-minute intervals for at least 30 minutes. The normal eye produces a biphasic curve reflecting first cone, then rod, response. Most retinal disorders which cause poor dark adaptation also damage the visual field so, although practitioners are unlikely to have equipment to undertake dark-adaptation studies in their consulting rooms, they can alter the room lighting and, bearing in mind points mentioned above, can add another useful variation to their normal perimetric routine.

Instruments and techniques

Reliable results depend on the examiner's skill with a variety of instruments and techniques and on the correct selection of the type of test for a particular patient or a particular condition. No one instrument suits all cases, each having advantages and limitations. Some of the newest utilize the latest in microchip technology and are rapidly superseded by 'improved versions'. Some are time honoured, simple and much less expensive. The basic universal test is the confrontation test.

Confrontation

Confrontation techniques are seldom given the time or care which, in the hands of a well-practised exponent, make the test much more than a screening routine.

The patient and examiner sit facing one another half a metre apart, their eyes at the same level. The patient is required to stare into the examiner's eye so even the smallest change in fixation when the target is noticed will be seen immediately by the examiner. Where reactions are poor, as with children or less alert adults, this observed reaction can be taken as signifying threshold. The patient should be placed with his back to the light, one eye occluded and facing a uniform dark background against which the targets can be detected. When the defect is gross, a pen torch or ophthalmoscope bulb may be used. Welsh (1961) suggested a finger counting method described well by Anderson (1981), who also advocates the additional use of colour identification to demonstrate variation of function either side of the vertical midline.

Spherical targets ranging from 10 mm to 2 mm on a short wand should be adequate in most cases. The peripheral limits of the visual field should be examined by moving the target in an arc from behind the patient's head until it is just seen. The central quadrants can then be explored for scotomata.

As with all field tests, it is usual to judge reliability of response by locating the blind spot and assuring the patient that it is a normal finding. Failure to demonstrate the blind spot reflects inadequate technique on the examiner's part or lack of comprehension or compliance by the patient. Whatever the reason it almost certainly invalidates the results.

Once proficiency with the basic test has been acquired, further detail can be added by altering the room illumination, the target colour or size or particularly by Bender's (Bender and Tenber, 1946) application of the extinction phenomenon. This is described as the instant disappearance of a stimulus in one half of the field when another is presented on the opposite side, or may also be observed as a fading of a stimulus when another is presented simultaneously. It is a frequent though not universal characteristic of hemianopia, and is very valuable clinically in identifying parietal lobe damage. This technique is not confined to confrontation and can be applied by two examiners on the tangent screen or arc perimeter. Multiple pattern display instruments are ideal vehicles for demonstrating this phenomenon.

In summary, the confrontation test should be regarded not only as the basic screening method, but as a useful adjunct to more detailed investigations. It is also the most suitable bedside method of checking the field.

Amsler grid

The patient should be wearing the near spectacle correction as this test is specifically designed to detect macular and paramacular pathology. It consists of a series of plates of various patterns of grid which, when viewed at 30 cm, cover the central 10° of field each side of fixation. The patient stares at the centre spot and is asked specific questions about each plate in order to determine any break or irregularity of the grid. The patient can be asked to draw on reproductions of the grid any patches of loss or distortion of pattern (*see Figure 22.10*; Amsler. 1953).

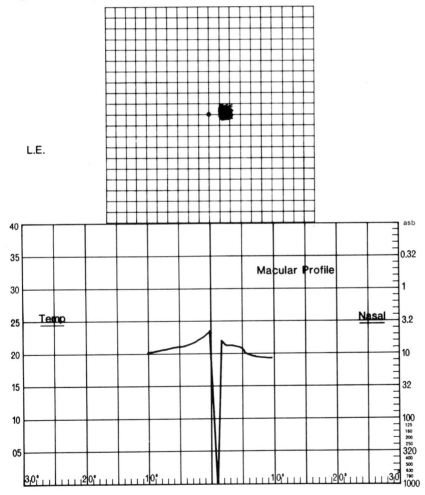

Figure 22.10 Patient's drawing of a very small paramacular scotoma on an Amsler recording chart. Macular profile static perimetry across the horizontal meridian of the same area confirms the position and shows the density of the deficit

Oculokinetic field test

The success of all perimetric tests depends on a stationary eye. This requires constant supervision by the observer and, above all, considerable concentration and self-control on the part of the patient. Such restraints have been reduced by the introduction of a novel test which, as its name indicates, uses a moving eye and a fixed target.

The charts present a pattern of points or a page of script at the centre of which is a spot—the test stimulus. The subject concentrates his gaze systematically on each area marking off any number, letter or word which causes the central spot to disappear. By inverting the plan obtained, the results can be read in the same way as a conventional field diagram (*Figure 22.11*). The sensitivity of the test may be altered by changing the size or colour of the central

point (Damato, 1985).

This test, by providing a more repeatable and flexible alternative to the Amsler chart, may prove useful for self-monitoring by hospital patients living in outlying districts and for screening by family doctors or healthcare personnel. The practitioner can have the test completed by the patient prior to his appointment thereafter verifying any defect detected if necessary.

The tangent screen

The most versatile of all field testing methods involves the use of a black or grey flat felt screen which is usually 1 m square. At its centre, an easily seen white spot serves as fixation point, from which radiate faint black stitched lines indicating meridians and circular lines showing degrees from fixation for a set viewing distance. Most screens also have the position of the physiological blind spot marked on each side. Where space permits, a 2-m screen has the advantage of projecting a defect on a larger area thereby allowing a more accurate outline to be drawn, while in addition, introducing flexibility by varying the patient's viewing distance. The nearer is the screen to the patient, the larger the overall area plotted. Conversely, the further apart are the eye and fixation point, the smaller the field area covered. When required to investigate a peripheral defect with only a tangent screen available, the simplest method is to bring the patient closer to the screen. Moving the fixation point to the edge of the screen and plotting half the field at a time is another way of tackling the problem.

The screen should be evenly illuminated, 100 lm/m^2 being the usual recommended level. Overhead tubular fluorescent lights parallel with the screen and deflector shades directing the light evenly over the whole screen area are satisfactory. A rheostat or diffusing shade is an optional extra which, since it allows investigation of mesopic field, is a useful way of adding increased sensitivity. Even illumination is more easily maintained if the surface of the screen is stretched taut. This can be achieved either by mounting the whole screen on a rigid frame or by arranging fixing points to the floor if a retractable type of screen is required. If not fixed firmly, the screen is likely to waver when it is touched by the practitioner's hand and such distraction will disturb the patient's concentration.

The choice of the correct target to produce the correct sensitivity is essential if accurate results are to be obtained. Targets are available in flat or spherical form in sizes from 30 mm down to 0.5 mm, and in various colours. The size chosen depends on the patient's visual status but, for most purposes, white (W) targets of 3 mm and 1 mm on a 1-m screen, and 5 mm and 2 mm on a 2-m screen prove best. The isopters obtained are expressed as the (3/1000) W,

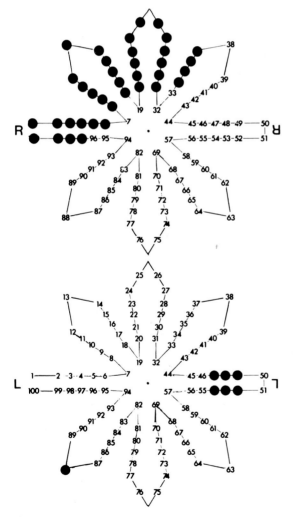

Figure 22.11 Oculokinetic visual field test. Lower temporal defect right eye, and enlarged blind spot left eye detected by unsupervised patient

(1/1000) W, (5/2000) W and (2/2000) W isopters, respectively.

Flat targets are preferable as they can be more accurately measured and, as they are usually coloured on the reverse side, they can be quickly flipped over to present a much more sensitive or invisible spot, thereby providing a simple check on the patient's concentration and reliability.

The target is attached to a long thin handle finished in matt black and should be 0.66–1 m in length. No shiny surface must be allowed to show, nor must the targets be allowed to become chipped or dirty, as this will lead to spurious results.

Instruments are available that project an illuminated target onto a screen. The Autoplot and the Lumiwand are examples and for these a grey screen is advisable.

Method

If the screen is rigidly fixed as suggested, the height of the patient's chair must be adjustable to ensure the eye is level with the fixation dot. The patient is instructed carefully and settled comfortably. The poorer seeing eye is covered and a simple response such as 'gone' and 'back' used to reduce confusion and conversation once the test has begun. A decision must be made about correction of the refractive error depending on the distance at which the test is being carried out. The aim must be to reduce refractive artefacts at all times by correcting as accurately as possible for the appropriate distance. If the patient wears spectacles with large lenses, these may be used during the test. Some of the practical problems posed by the aphakic or highly myopic patient wearing lenticular lenses or bifocals or both, may be overcome by the use of a full aperture trial set, a selection of ready glazed spectacles with spherical corrections, or a selection of contact lenses specially retained for this purpose.

Dedicated practitioners wear a black sleeve and glove, avoid light-coloured clothes (especially white coats) and distracting jewellery. A constant watch on the reliability of fixation is facilitated by standing facing the patient, the wrist being used to move the target wand, the forearm supported on the side of the wall or screen.

A large target 10–20 mm is first used in the area of the blind spot, moving the target from seeing to non-seeing and back so that the required responses may be demonstrated and the accuracy of the patient's position checked. Once it is evident that the patient understands the process, an isopter is plotted with a smaller target (5 mm on a 2-m screen, 2 mm on a 1-m screen), bringing the stimulus in from the non-seeing periphery and inserting a black-headed pin with the other hand as soon as the spot is perceived. It is best to begin somewhere midway between the vertical and horizontal midlines and to avoid the 90° and 180° meridians altogether, approaching either side of the midlines as this increases the chance of demonstrating a difference in sensivity at these junctions. Having outlined the isopter, the plot of the blind spot area is repeated recording the point where the patient sees the target reappearing. A systematic search should be made within the isopter with the same target for any area of depressed sensitivity, moving at an even, regular pace with occasional variation in rhythm to avoid automatic time-related responses from the patient. It should not be oscillated as this increases its effective size.

When this initial survey has been completed, the pin plot on the screen is transferred to a diagram. In most cases, further detail will be required to complete the plot thoroughly, another target being selected, the blind spot replotted, and the search repeated. Experience and practice provide the best basis for reliable results.

The illuminated projection target already mentioned has proved popular as it can be used on a tangent screen or on a Fincham–Sutcliffe-type screener board to obtain more detailed information. The Juler scotometer is a hand-held torch-like projector capable of presenting a target of ranging colour, size, and brightness. It can also be used to present single flash stimuli to check the integrity of particular points on the retina, employing a spot sampling method to detect areas of deficit. This static (as opposed to kinetic) method is more effectively used with the automatic or electronic equipment discussed below.

Arc perimeters

These instruments are used for plotting the peripheral field. They consist of a rotating arm some 100–150 mm (4–6 inches) wide with a chin rest at the centre of the arc. The arm is placed at various angles around the eye and a testing target moved from the edge towards the central point, where the fixation spot is placed. Targets may be on short wands or may be projected illuminated spots. Most arc perimeters have an automatic pantograph arrangement to facilitate the charting of results. The simplest of the arc perimeters are portable and may be used at the bedside. None, however, is capable of great accuracy due to the difficulty in maintaining constant ambient illumination. They are best used in a dimly lit room to reduce distraction (*Figure 22.12*).

Bowl perimeters

Introduced as long ago as the 1940s, the hemispherical projection perimeter is still considered the most accurate method of perimetry. The most widely used are the Goldmann perimeter made by Haag-Streit and the Harms Tubingen instrument marketed by Oculus.

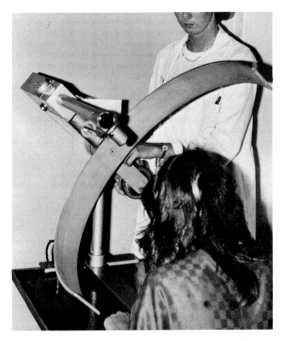

Figure 22.12 The Aimark arc perimeter

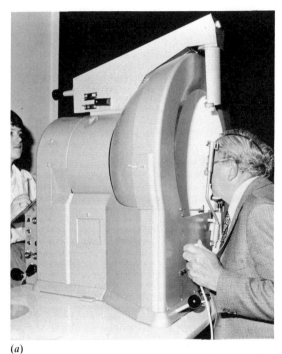

(*a*)

Each of these machines consists of a matt white, evenly illuminated bowl with a central fixation point. Targets of various size, wavelength and brightness can be projected on the surface of the bowl. An electronically operated hand switch controls a series of neutral density filters in 0.1 log unit steps so that static perimetry may be conveniently performed (*Figure 22.13*).

Simple adjustment of the projection system enables the instruments to explore both central and peripheral fields with equal ease and accuracy either by kinetic or static methods. Although the standard background illumination on the Tubingen is at mesopic level, and on the Goldmann at photopic level, these may be altered if required.

The short distance of 0.33 m between the patient's eye and the bowl necessitates critical control of fixation and position, but this is readily monitored by means of a telescopic viewing device. It is also necessary to ensure accurate correction of refractive errors for this distance either with spectacles or an appropriate supplementary lens.

The bowl perimeter is, therefore, a most versatile piece of field equipment and it can be used for flicker fusion tests, colour perimetry and dark-adaptation tests in addition to the conventional techniques. The cost of such instruments and the need for skill in their operation to ensure good results mean that they are not widely available in general optometric practice, being more suitable for hospital or research work.

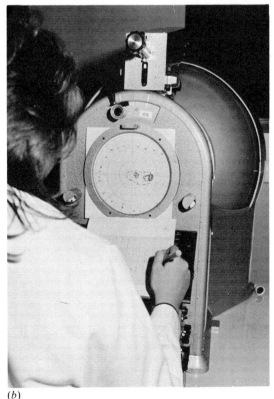

(*b*)

Figure 22.13 (*a*) Tubingen projection perimeter, (*b*) operator's view

Screening devices

Visual field examination carried out by the tangent screen, arc or bowl perimeter requires the attention of trained informed personnel, and is so expensive in terms of time and capital cost that it is not practicable for large numbers of patients. In an attempt to overcome these difficulties, screening instruments have been developed which employ static spot checking. These present in rapid succession a single stimulus or patterns of stimuli in those parts of the field most likely to develop defects.

If it were possible to establish static thresholds for every main area of the field, a three-dimensional model of the hypothetical island of vision would result, but this is clearly an unrealistic objective. A test which uses a limited series of static presentations is of necessity a sampling or screening technique only, and usually the quicker the test is to complete the less accurate are the results.

Harrington–Flocks screener

The earliest type of screening device such as the Harrington–Flocks screener (Harrington and Flocks, 1959), consists of a series of cards placed at 33 cm from a chin rest and illuminated from below by an ultraviolet light source. Fluorescent spots in patterns of different sizes and positions are illuminated for 0.25 s. This test requires minimum time and examiner skill, and its simplicity makes it useful for the inattentive subject.

Space permits mention of only some of the screeners available. Best known are the Fincham–Sutcliffe and the Friedmann visual field analyser, the latter being available in an improved form 16 years after its original introduction.

Fincham–Sutcliffe screener

The Fincham–Sutcliffe screen consists of a grey matt finished, wall-mounted board with apertures through which are presented a series of groups of flashed stimuli—the brightness and duration of which may be adjusted as required. The patient reports the number and location of stimuli seen and so the pattern of field loss is established. If required, the screen may then be used as a tangent screen by using a hand-held target projector torch to plot kinetically the extent of the area of reduced sensitivity discovered. The results can be combined and presented on a single chart.

Friedmann visual field analyser

The Friedmann visual field analyser has proved to be an efficient, convenient and popular screening device. The patient is accurately positioned on a chin and head rest 0.25 m from a black, circular, evenly illuminated screen in a darkened room. Simultaneous presentation of timed flashes allow quick coverage of the central 25° over which uniform threshold value is achieved as the apertures through which the stimuli are presented increase in size by a carefully calculated amount as they become more peripheral. The single light source ensures a uniform level of brightness at all points and a series of easily controlled neutral density filters allows the intensity of the target light to be adjusted.

When the instrument was first introduced, 'normal' standard levels of threshold were recommended based on the patient's age group (Friedmann, 1966, 1979), but various researchers claim improved specificity by establishing threshold at a paracentral location in each eye and then running the test at a filter setting 0.4 log units brighter (Gutteridge, 1983). Points missed at this working threshold are re-presented at still brighter levels until all are recognized thus providing limited analysis of the depth of the deficit.

Unfortunately, the interpretation of charts can be difficult because of the numerous threshold values possible at each of 98 points making comparison of sequential charts most awkward. One solution is to quantify the result by calculating an error score, the sum of each point missed at each brightness setting. Specific alteration in error score from one field check to the next is chosen to indicate a significant loss of field (*Figure 22.14*).

Despite these disadvantages the Friedmann visual field analyser is the first choice of many optometrists and ophthalmologists because of its dependability and ease of use.

Automated perimetry

In the last decade, advances in electronics and microchip technology have been successfully applied to visual field instrumentation, but already many of the earlier designs have been withdrawn or superseded and so it would be unwise to dwell on any one in this text. Most are based on the bowl perimeter design employing either projection, fibreoptics or light-emitting diode systems to randomly present stimuli of preselected brightness and distribution. Most computerized perimeters have automatic calibration, automatically monitored fixation, arrhythmic presentation and a variety of examination routines designed to place emphasis on the areas vulnerable in particular disease processes. The operator chooses the basic parameters, the test pattern and the complexity of approach he considers appropriate. Interruption, false replies to 'trick' tests or loss of fixation initiate repeats to check patient compliance.

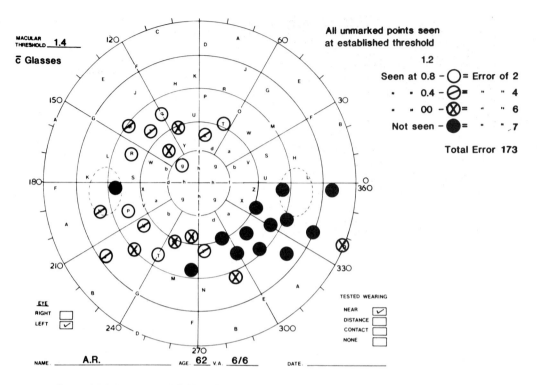

Figure 22.14 Chart of Friedmann visual field analyser
Mark II showing points missed and a method of coding
and numerically evaluating the deficit

The more sophisticated instruments establish
thresholds for each retinal location by what is known
as the 'staircase' method, presenting in gradually
smaller steps, supra- and subliminal levels of target
brightness until the precise threshold is found. The
program is entirely random and the responses are
processed by the computer which can produce
a printout showing the field evaluation either numerically annotated or on a pattern coded chart (*Figure
22.15*).

Of particular interest to optometric practitioners
in general practice is the recently introduced Henson Hamblin CFS 2000. This compact design reminiscent of the Friedmann visual field analyser in
appearance and approach presents groups of points
at a time, the more peripheral being brighter to
compensate for the normal slope of retinal sensitivity. Results and an assessment of significance are
displayed on an integral visual display unit (VDU)
or may be stored or printed by connection to
standard computer post.

Advanced systems such as the Octopus by Inter-
zeag of Switzerland (Frankhauser, Spahr and Bebie,
1977), the Dicon 3000 made by Coopervision Ltd and
Allergan's Humphrey Vision Analyser, store all
patient data on floppy disk facilitating comparison
and analysis by the computer of sequential results.
The Dicon system allows the operator to observe the
plot as it evolves and to interrupt, amend or augment the program if appropriate (*Figure 22.16*).

Many comparative studies of the results of automated instruments and those of trained perimetric
practitioners using Goldmann and Tubingen
machines have shown a very high degree of success
in the detection of defects (Heigl and Drance, 1981).
There is no doubt that for screening of specific
groups of patients, automatic systems are most
efficient in terms of time saved and standards of
results obtained. All can be operated by relatively
unskilled persons under supervision.

Despite the important points in favour of automated perimetry, there are those with reservations
about the wisdom of its universal application.
Certainly, for basic screening routines on essentially
healthy alert people, the systems are superb and can
even be self-operated. However, when the more
complicated programs are used the routine is necessarily longer, which reduces patient compliance and
often gives rise to spurious results. When the
patients' responses are variable, repeats are automa-

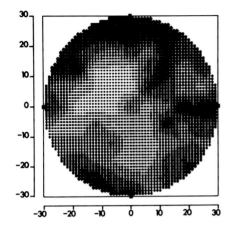

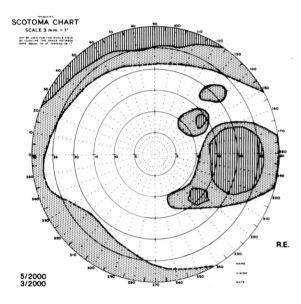

SCOTOMA CHART
SCALE 3 mm. = 1°

5/2000
3/2000

R.E.

Figure 22.15 Printout of interpolated results obtained by the Octopus system and the same field plotted and displayed in conventional fashion

some of the problems encountered with the longer automated programs.

Most difficulties arise because the computer-assisted perimeters, however sophisticated, can only follow through the program which has been initiated. A skilled perimetric practitioner, in contrast, learns to cut short the routine or vary the emphasis of the investigation as the results evolve. Using knowledge of the case, effort will be concentrated on obtaining specific information to demonstrate a diagnostically positive result. So far, no automated perimeter can operate in this way, and so is less effective when it comes to detailed diagnostic field evaluation.

Common causes of visual field defects

Central defects

Any eye with reduced visual acuity will have a depressed central field. Sometimes this is very difficult to demonstrate or demarcate and can be found only with most sensitive targets or by a macular profile test. Reduced central vision also occurs due to hazy media or macular pathology, which may be confirmed by ophthalmoscopy.

Among the most common *macular* disorders causing central scotomata are macular degeneration, macular haemorrhage, macular oedema, central serous retinopathy, eclipse burns and retinal vein occlusion (*Figure 22.17*). *Vascular* incidents affecting any vessel serving the visual pathway may cause isolated central scotoma, but more usually precipitate widespread loss of retinal function.

In addition, central scotomata may be due to *optic nerve* disturbances, by far the commonest being optic neuritis which, in its acute form, causes pain on movement of the eye and, when the axial portion of the optic nerve is involved, a dense central scotoma The attack may resolve within days only to recur in the same eye or the fellow eye days, weeks or even years later.

Optic atrophy subsequent to optic neuritis or in any of its congential or hereditary forms may also lead to central loss of field though this is usually extensive and dense.

Compression of one *optic nerve* within the orbit can produce unilateral central scotomata of varying sensitivity depending on the site of pressure.

Central field loss may be caused by a wide range of *toxins* (the pathogenesis of which is seldom understood, although some probably affect the optic nerve). In these cases the scotomata are usually dense and always bilateral.

tically initiated. Therefore the test is prolonged, sometimes more than doubled in duration, and the advantage of rapid patient processing is lost. The test may even have to be repeated by conventional methods to obtain satisfactory results. A recent publication by Heijl and Drance (1983) shows that repeated presentation of stimuli, particularly in areas adjacent to scotoma, increases the contrast threshold, so enlarging the apparent defect. The longer the testing continues the more widely spread this response becomes. These facts may account for

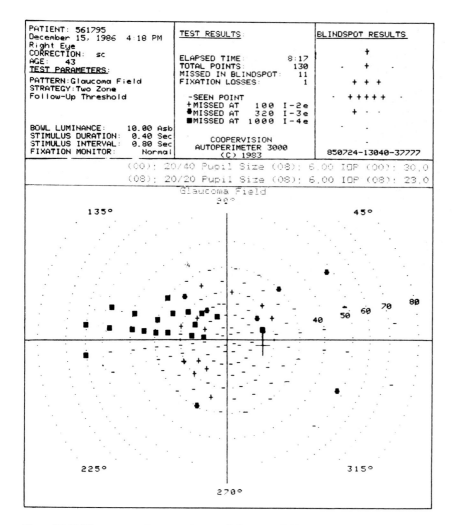

Figure 22.16 Dicon autoperimeter: printout of glaucoma field

The most common toxins causing field loss are:

(1) Drugs: ethambutol; chloramphenicol; digitalis; perhexiline maleate (Pexid).
(2) Chemicals such as methyl alcohol.
(3) Excess of alcohol associated with dietary deficiencies.

Malnutrition, systemic disorders causing malabsorption and liver disease also damage retinal function and cause central scotomata.

Disturbance of the *optic chiasma* may result in central scotomata (often hemianopic) if the pressure on the chiasma interferes with the decussating macular fibres. This type of defect is usually associated with similar symmetrical peripheral field loss.

Paracentral defects

These are patches of isolated defect which can be described by their position relative to fixation. They may be very small and shallow or they may be larger patches of loss due to such major incidents as occlusion of a branch retinal vein.

Most causes of multiple small patches of field loss are evident with an ophthalmoscope and include choroiditis, macular degeneration, myopic degeneration, hypertensive retinopathy and diabetic retinopathy. Glaucoma and optic neuritis may also cause patchy loss.

Pericentral defects

A pericentral scotoma is a form of paracentral scotoma which is annular or horseshoe shaped.

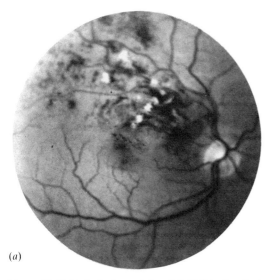

(a)

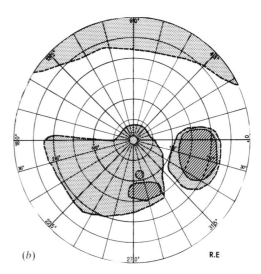

(b)   R.E

Figure 22.17 Retinal picture (*a*) and field (*b*) of patient
with branch retinal vein occlusion and associated macular
oedema

1.0 (W) 00
1.0 (W) 05

The ring scotoma of chloroquine (an antimalarial
drug also used in the treatment of discoid lupus
erythematosus and arthritis) is unique, detectable in
its earliest stage with a red target. It takes the form
of a pericentral ring usually found first around 4–8°
from fixation. In its advanced stage it expands
outwards, breaking through to the periphery (*Figure
22.18*).

Centrocaecal defects

(1) Centrocaecal defects of sudden onset are most
probably due to occlusion of a cilioretinal artery
which produces a dense centrocaecal loss within
an otherwise normal full field.
(2) Inflammation of the nerve head in optic neuritis
may cause centrocaecal defects spreading from
the disc towards fixation.

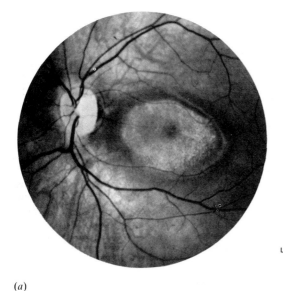

(a)

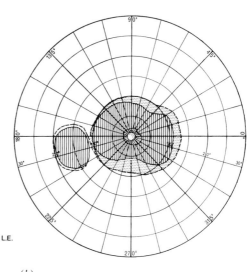

L.E.

(b)

1.0 (W) 00
1.0 (W) 10

Figure 22.18 Doughnut-shaped defect due to chloroquine
retinopathy. (Fundus as seen by direct ophthalmoscopy)

(3) Inherited juvenile optic atrophy causes enlarged blind spots and centrocaecal damage.
(4) Patients with toxic amblyopia due to tobacco have a characteristic centrocaecal defect of irregular density between disc and macula (*see Figure 22.9*). In addition they have severely impaired colour discrimination which accounts for the defect misleadingly being described as a 'scotoma to red.' The disease is complex and its aetiology still not fully understood, but it is often associated with metabolic disorders or dietary deficiencies.

Enlargement of blind spot

Papilloedema associated with inflammation of the nerve head or increased intracranial pressure gives overall symmetrical enlargement of the blind spot. Myelinating nerve fibres, myopia and colobomata will produce more specific enlargement. Enlargement or, more accurately, extension of the blind spot frequently described in glaucoma is discussed below.

Sector-like defects emanating from the blind spot along the nerve fibre bundle and frequently breaking through to the periphery are found in juxtapapillaris choroiditis.

An atrophic disc will usually produce an enlarged blind spot.

Glaucoma

Most of the causes of field defects discussed so far have other detectable clinical abnormalities. This is frequently the case in glaucoma as well, the combination of raised intraocular pressure, a pathologically cupped disc and characteristic field defect being diagnostic. It is of the greatest importance, however, to detect the earliest signs of field loss before any serious damage develops and so a high percentage of any practitioner's patients will be glaucoma 'suspects'.

Acute closed-angle glaucoma

Dramatic and sudden increased intraocular pressure of acute closed-angle glaucoma causes extreme discomfort and needs urgent medical attention. An eye under such stress may have acuity reduced to light perception only, but in many cases nearly normal vision is recovered after timely medical attention, although there may be residual field defects.

Chronic simple glaucoma

There is a wealth of published material on this subject and authorities agree that the earliest signs of field damage in glaucoma are attributable to loss

of function in specific nerve fibre bundles producing combinations of the following:

(1) Isolated paracentral patches in the Bjerrum area.
(2) Depression of peripheral isopters most common in the upper nasal quadrant.
(3) Difference in sensitivity above and below the horizontal midline in the nasal field (nasal step) which reflects the anatomical arrangement of the nerve fibre bundles.
(4) Gradual increase in size and number of the scotomata as more fibres are involved progressing to a continuous arc of damage. This subsequently joins the blind spot and may also break through to the periphery. Lower and upper arcs may then combine to reduce the field to a tiny central area of vision and a peripheral temporal island (*see Figures 22.4, 22.5b, 22.8, 22.14, 22.15, 22.16, 22.19, 22.22*).

It is frequently said that enlargement of the blind spot is the earliest sign of glaucomatous field damage, but it has been shown conclusively that,

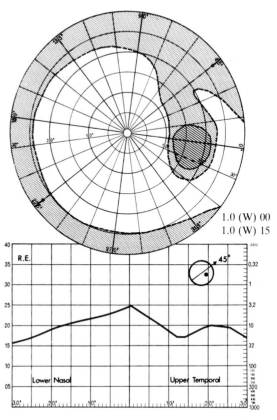

Figure 22.19 Oblique static profile confirms very early nerve fibre bundle defect in glaucoma 'suspect'

where elongation of the blind spot is found, the extended area has differences in density of damage—the patch of maximum density being adjacent to but not continuous with the blind spot. The importance of this is underlined by Armaly (1969) who examined the blind spot area in a large number of normal eyes, and found that many exhibited an extensive area of reduced sensitivity around the nerve head much in excess of the 1° relative blind spot usually quoted. He showed that a very small alteration of target brightness, such as would be caused by early lens opacities or by inadequate correction of refractive error, produces enlargement and elongation of the blind spot simulating arcuate loss. The detection of a discreet area of denser depression within an extension scotoma distinguishes pathological loss due to raised intraocular pressure.

Early depressions of sensitivity may be more easily demonstrated or verified with bi-oblique static profiles (*Figure 22.19*).

Although field damage is generally regarded as irreversible, the very earliest depressions may disappear when treatment is instigated and the intraocular pressure controlled.

Eyes predisposed to glaucoma, even those which are well monitored, are vulnerable to sudden field loss due to retinal vein occlusion.

Peripheral field defects

Defects of the peripheral field may not be noticed by the patient for they cause little inconvenience when patchy (as in choroiditis) or when they affect only one part of one field as in a case of retinal detachment. Most unilateral causes of loss of peripheral field should be detectable with the ophthalmoscope because they are due to retinal or choroidal problems; they may be described by the area of field lost. The ring scotoma found in cases of retinal pigmentary degeneration is unusual and unique as the earliest signs of reduced sensitivity are found in the midperiphery around the 30–40° meridian. Small patches of field damage join into a ring-shaped scotoma which then spreads inwards and outwards in due course causing extreme handicap to the afflicted individual (*Figure 22.20*). Since the rods are primarily affected, the field loss is accompanied by abnormal dark adaptation and the patient's first complaint may be of night blindness.

However, most peripheral field defects are bilateral due to the anatomical arrangement of the nerve fibre pathways and so they tend to affect large portions of the coastline of the island. Patients may report such difficulties as bumping into furniture, having difficulty moving along a crowded pavement, or locating the beginning of a line of print.

Peripheral defects are described as homonymous or heteronymous defects.

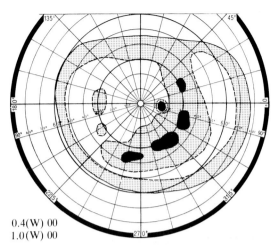

0.4(W) 00
1.0(W) 00

Figure 22.20 Incomplete ring scotoma due to retinitis pigmentosa. Note the most dense areas are in the midperiphery where the earliest loss of retinal function is found

Homonymous defects

Total homonymous hemianopia

This describes complete loss of function in the temporal field of one eye and the nasal field of the fellow eye. The cut-off is sharp at the vertical midline and may either 'spare' or 'split' the macular area. Total homonymous hemianopia is caused by severe interference with the visual pathway on one side posterior to the chiasma and is commonly the result of a vascular incident (*Figure 22.21*).

Partial homonymous hemianopia

This is incomplete loss of half the field, frequently asymmetrical (known as incongruous). One section of the border follows the vertical midline, the remaining part is irregular. Detailed analysis of such defects with different sizes of stimuli will show a wide variety of shapes; the characteristic details of a particular chart may enable the examiner to locate the cause of the defect. For example, the greater the incongruity of the two charts, i.e. the more dissimilar in shape, size, density and position, the more anterior the cause of the problem.

Homonymous quadrantopia

This may be a partial homonymous hemianopia and should also be described as congruous or incongruous (*Figure 22.22*).

Homonymous hemianopia in a young patient is usually congruous and is often due to a cerebral

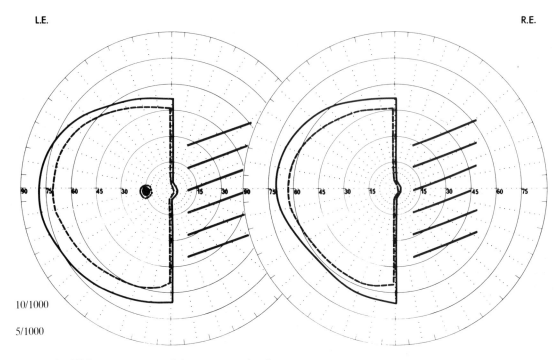

Figure 22.1 Right congruous total homonymous hemi-anopia

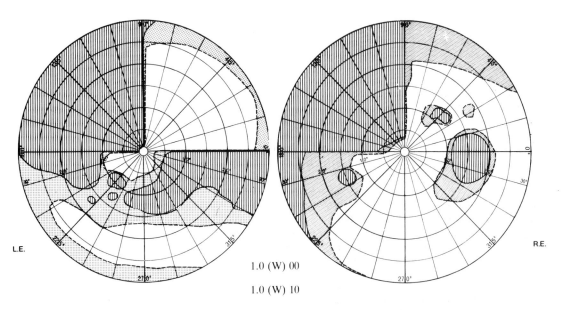

Figure 22.22 Left upper incongruous homonymous quadrantopia due to retrochiasmal vascular incident probably in the right optic tract. The congruity of the defect can be judged only on the difference in macular sparing as the picture is complicated by extensive glaucomatous field loss including a large nasal step left eye

tumour. A congruous hemianopia in an older patient is more likely to be vascular in origin and, if located in the occipital lobe, it may also produce paracentral areas of damage.

Heteronymous defects

These are more commonly described as bilateral defects and may be bitemporal or binasal.

Bitemporal hemianopia

This is comparatively common and may affect only a very small slice of the field. Often first detected at the vertical midline, it progresses clockwise in the right field and anticlockwise in the left to become a hemianopic type loss. Sometimes the defect is very incongruous, requiring the greatest perseverance to reveal the earliest changes in the second eye. Bitemporal hemianopia is due to damage to the complicated nerve fibre interchange at the chiasma. The complexity of anatomy and physiology of this region (particularly the area below where the pituitary gland rests in the sella turcica and the internal carotid arteries pass on the lateral borders) produces considerable variation in development of visual loss. Furthermore, the growth of a tumour is not necessarily regular and the relative positions of the chiasma and the gland not identical in all patients, features which also contribute to the variety of field defects discovered. However, interference by pituitary gland enlargement and the resultant upward pressure is the most common cause of bitemporal field loss although damage can also be indirect due either to embarrassment of the vascular supply or to an aneurysm. In the former case the onset is sudden; in the latter it is more gradual (*Figure 22.23*).

Binasal hemianopia

This is very rare. It is unlikely that one incident could affect the uncrossed fibres of both retinas or both optic nerves. Nevertheless, it is possible for a sphenoidal ridge meningioma to put pressure on one side of the chiasma, causing a small displacement of the whole structure, which in turn compresses the fibres or their vascular supply at the other side. It is more probable, however, that an apparent binasal quadrantopia is actually symmetrically advanced nasal steps of glaucoma.

Crossed quadrantopia

This is also very rare. It can be due to unusual retinal lesions or glaucomatous defects, but in the absence of retinal disease must be attributed to asymmetrical interference at the chiasma.

Altitudinal hemianopia

This is loss of the upper or lower half of the visual field. It is often vascular in origin. When unilateral, the problem must be prechiasmal, probably either retinal detachment or vascular occlusion or perhaps interference with the vascular supply at the optic nerve.

It is usual and useful to expand on the description of a hemianopic defect by adding macula 'spared' or

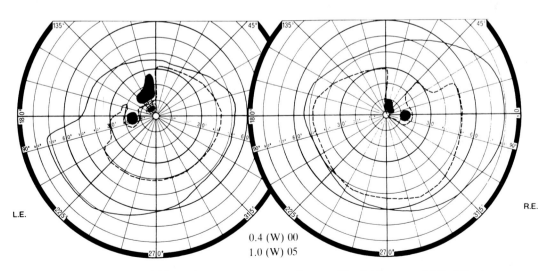

L.E.

0.4 (W) 00
1.0 (W) 05

R.E.

Figure 22.23 Bitemporal upper field loss due to pressure at the optic chiasma caused by a pituitary chromophobe adenoma. The field recovered fully following surgery

'split'. In some cases, the patient's observations will be enough to determine macular function although it is uncommon to find severely reduced visual acuity even when the macular area is split, and it is very difficult to establish by testing as the patient quickly learns to compensate by minute alteration in fixation position. Macular sparing is found, however, in most postchiasmal lesions. The area spared may vary from 0.5° to wide sparing; the more posterior the lesion the smaller and more regular the edge of the spared area.

Interpretation of results

Charting the visual field defect is only part of the practitioner's task. Equally important is the correct interpretation of results. In some cases, the cause of the problem is obvious from the overall ocular investigation and the field plot is required to confirm the diagnosis or to watch for progression. On occasion, however, the practitioner's findings are the sole indication of a disorder and are, therefore, of paramount importance.

The interpretation of results can be approached by asking the questions as set out in *Figure 22.24*.

The final possibility is that spurious results may be functional in origin, i.e. may be caused by an hysterical or malingering individual. The so-called hysterical field may have a very irregular star shape with overlapping isopters, a grossly constricted tubular field or it may have an inward or outward spiral. Such results can be due to apprehension or lack of comprehension and may disappear at subsequent examinations. Detailed enquiry into the patient's symptoms or observation of mobility may help establish the validity of an unexpected severe field loss. It may also prove useful to repeat the test by another method or to introduce different test conditions (particularly to alter the distance when using a tangent screen) to reveal inconsistency of response or contradictory results. When all subjective investigations fail to give satisfactory conclusions, it may be necessary to perform electrophysiological tests to eliminate the possibility of cryptic pathology.

Acknowledgements

The author wishes to acknowledge the support and encouragement given to her in the preparation of this text by Professor W.S. Foulds and the rest of her colleagues at the Tennent Institute and in particular for the advice and guidance of Dr J.L. Jay.

The author is most grateful to Dr D. Allan, Departmental Physicist, for his work computing the three-dimensional diagrams, to Mrs M. Reilly (Medical Illustration), Mrs A. Currie and the photographic staff and lastly Mrs J. Murray for her patience and secretarial skill.

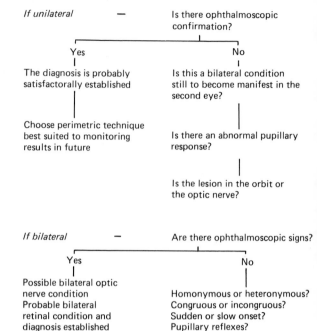

Is the field loss affecting both eyes or confined to one eye?

If unilateral — Is there ophthalmoscopic confirmation?

Yes — The diagnosis is probably satisfactorally established — Choose perimetric technique best suited to monitoring results in future

No — Is this a bilateral condition still to become manifest in the second eye? — Is there an abnormal pupillary response? — Is the lesion in the orbit or the optic nerve?

If bilateral — Are there ophthalmoscopic signs?

Yes — Possible bilateral optic nerve condition Probable bilateral retinal condition and diagnosis established

No — Homonymous or heteronymous? Congruous or incongruous? Sudden or slow onset? Pupillary reflexes?

No conclusion?   Then:

Are the results reliable?

Could they be artefactual?

Can the investigation be supplemented to add more information?

What other tests might be helpful?

Figure 22.24 Questions for interpretation of results of visual field defect investigations

References

AMSLER. M. (1953) Earliest symptoms of disease of the macula. *Br. J. Ophthalmol.*, **37**, 521–537

ANDERSON. D.R. (1981) *Testing of the Field of Vision*. St Louis: C.V. Mosby Co.

ARMALY. M.F. (1969). The eye and location of the normal blind spot. *Arch. Ophthalmol.*, **81**, 192–201

BENDER. M.B. and TENBAR. H.L. (1946) Phenomenon in visual perception. *Arch. Neurol. Psychiatr.*, **55**, 627–631

DAMATO. B.E. (1985) A simple field test for use in the community. *Br. J. Ophthalmol.*, **69**, 927–931

DRANCE. S.M. and ANDERSON. D.R. (1986) *Automated Perimetry. A Practical Guide*. Orlando: Grune & Stratton

FRANKHAUSER. F.. SPAHR. J. and BEBIE. H. (1977) Three years of experience with the Octopus automatic perimeter. *Doc. Ophthalmol. Proc. Ser.*, **14**, 7–15

FRIEDMANN, A.I. (1966) Serial analysis of visual field analyser Mark. *Ophthalmologica*, **152**, 1–12

FRIEDMANN, A.I. (1979) Outline of visual field analyser Mark II. *Doc. Ophthalmol. Proc. Ser.*, **22**, 65–67

GUTTERIDGE, I.F. (1983) The working threshold approach to Friedmann Visual Field Analyser Screening. *Ophthal. Physiol. Opt.*, **3**, 41–46

HARRINGTON, D.O. (1981) *The Visual Fields*, 5th edn. St. Louis: C.V. Mosby Co.

HARRINGTON, D.O. and FLOCKS. M. (1959) the multiple pattern method of visual field examination—a five year evaluation. *Arch. Ophthalmol.*, **61**, 755–765

HEIJL, A. and DRANCE. S.M. (1981) A clinical comparison of three computerised automatic perimeters in the detection of glaucoma defects. *Arch. Ophthalmol.*, **99**, 832–836

HEIJL, A. and DRANCE, S.M. (1983) Changes in the differential threshold in patients with glaucoma during prolonged perimetry. *Br. J. Ophthalmol.*, **67**, 512-516

ROCK, W.J., DRANCE, S.M. and MORGAN, R.W. (1973) Visual field screening in glaucoma. An evaluation of the Armaly technique for screening glaucomatous visual fields. *Arch. Ophthalmol.*, **89**, 287–290

SCOTT, G.J. (1957) *Traquair's Clinical Perimetry*, 7th edn. St Louis: C.V. Mosby Co.

TRAQUAIR, H.M. (1938) *An Introduction to Clinical Perimetry*, 6th edn. London: Henry Kimpton

WELSH, R.C. (1961) Finger counting in the four quadrants as a method of visual field gross screening. *Arch. Ophthalmol.*, **66**, 678-679

23

Tonometry

Michael Wolffe

Tonometry is one of a number of methods of investigating whether glaucoma is present in a particular eye. Although it provides a means of measuring intraocular pressure at a single point in time, it is not an infallible technique for detecting glaucoma. While an eye with a very elevated intraocular pressure is undoubtedly glaucomatous, there are eyes having intraocular pressures which are well within 'normal' limits and yet which display all of the other changes associated with glaucoma.

Duke-Elder, in 1940, described glaucoma as embracing a collection of pathological conditions where the clinical manifestations are to a greater or lesser extent dominated by an increase in the intraocular pressure and its consequences. It was suggested that the increase in intraocular pressure was a symptom not a disease process in itself. Smith (1965) argued that it is understating the case to dismiss intraocular pressure as a symptom unless it is transient and non-recurrent. In recognizing the difficulty of defining glaucoma, he suggested: 'An ophthalmic disease characterised by persistent or repeated elevation of the intraocular pressure which eventually causes certain pathological changes in the affected eye; or by a state in which it is known that under certain physiological conditions a pathological rise in intraocular pressure can be induced; or by a state in which the eye, in the absence of demonstrably raised intraocular pressure, shows signs indistinguishable from those usually resulting from raised intraocular pressure and for which no reason can be found.' This definition clearly illustrates the problems that glaucoma presents; while at one end of the scale it may be characterized by elevated intraocular pressure, at the other end it may be characterized by all the changes that are associated with such increases in pressure, although the pressure remains within apparently normal limits. It can be seen, therefore, that intraocular pressure cannot be used as an infallible means of detecting whether glaucoma is present. While not unreasonable to assume, until proven otherwise, that an elevated intraocular pressure is indicative of glaucoma, a normal or even low intraocular pressure does not necessarily mean that glaucoma is absent. With this reservation, tonometry is an invaluable method of investigating both suspected and diagnosed cases of glaucoma.

The clinical problem remains to determine when an individual patient is glaucomatous. Before deciding whether a pressure is raised, the 'normal' level must be determined. This may vary between individuals and may include an overlap between the higher levels of normal and the lower levels of abnormal. Diurnal variation changes the pressure measured throughout the day and some pressures remain consistently high without any of the characteristic field loss associated with glaucoma.

Measurements of intraocular pressure

All clinical methods of measuring intraocular pressure are indirect rather than direct. Generally, the intraocular pressure is assessed by means of taking measurements either through the cornea or through the sclera. In doing so, attempts are being made to assess the extent to which these structures can be indented or applanated. The higher the intraocular pressure the greater the resistance to such attempts and, therefore, the harder the eye will appear. Of the two structures, i.e. cornea and sclera, it is preferable and more accurate to take measurements through the cornea because corneal characteristics vary little between one eye and another whereas considerable variations exist between the scleral characteristics of different eyes. The only direct means of measuring intraocular pressure is by manometry, which entails penetrating the eye, clearly not a viable technique for functioning eyes and therefore with no clinical application.

Tonometry can be broadly classified into instrumental and non-instrumental techniques. The main non-instrumental technique is digital tonometry—a qualitative means of assessing intraocular pressure which has been used clinically since the last century. It involves placing the two hands on the patient's forehead, the two index fingers being used to palpate the patient's eye through the upper lid. The patient is directed to look downwards and not to close the eye so that the palpation takes place through the upper sclera. It is important that any pressure is applied above the tarsal plate. The simplest approach is to keep one forefinger still while lightly pressing in with the other. Assessment is then made of the lightest force that is required to produce a sense of fluctuation in the stationary finger. The very fact that this assessment of intraocular pressure is taking place through two fairly thick structures, i.e. the lid and the sclera, means that at best it can only be described as inexact, but it does allow a means of grading the pressure on the basis of high, low or normal. The standard method of classifying pressure recorded by digital tonometry is using the following symbols: Tn (normal), T+, T++ (raised pressure), T−, T−− (low pressure). Digital tonometry should be regarded as no more than a coarse screening technique. Priestley Smith (1891) observed that, as far as digital tonometry is concerned, it is a technique which leaves the clinician in the position where 'we cannot state with precision the resistance we feel, and we cannot rely upon the constancy of our sense of touch'. Nevertheless, digital tonometry is a useful screening method, but, if it is to have any value at all it needs to be carried out regularly so that the degree of sensitivity is improved and refined by experience. Even with experience it has been suggested that the level of accuracy by palpation is about ± 10 mmHg (Draeger, 1966).

Instrumental methods—general

Instrumental methods of measuring intraocular pressure can be divided into two groups: indentation and applanation. Both techniques, being based on an indirect method of assessing pressure, have their own sources of error which must be recognized.

Apart from the very specific problems associated with each particular type of instrument and technique, there are a number of problems and sources of error which are common to all techniques of tonometry. Contraction of the intraocular muscles, associated with accommodation, lowers the intraocular pressure by approximately 1 mmHg, although this is variable. The patient should, there-

fore, ideally fixate a distant object, but this is not always possible, either because the patient's fixating eye has poor visual acuity or because a distant object is not visible. This is particularly the case when carrying out applanation tonometry using a slitlamp. Steady fixation is particularly important and, if this can only be achieved by fixating an object which stimulates accommodation, then this is preferable to attempting measurements on an unsteady eye. The small reduction in intraocular pressure thus produced should, however, be borne in mind when interpreting the results. Contraction of the extraocular muscles, in contrast, raises intraocular pressure. This can be very marked indeed and can lead to rises of pressure of 10 mmHg and even more. If such contraction is associated with lid squeezing, then intraocular pressure may be raised by 20 or 30 mmHg.

Apprehension and nervousness on the part of the patient will also raise intraocular pressure above the normal level, again the increase being quite pronounced and commonly of the order of 4 mmHg.

It is therefore important to try to reassure the patient in order to aid relaxation. Failure to do this can result in incorrect readings. In order to assess the level of apprehension, it is necessary to repeat the measurements, reassuring the patient after the first reading is taken. Unfortunately, repetition of the measurements can in itself produce false results by artificially lowering the pressure due to an increase in the rate of aqueous outflow. This is certainly the case with indentation tonometry, while with applanation tonometry it is generally possible to repeat the readings without affecting the rate of aqueous outflow and this should be done until a plateau is reached.

Other factors which can increase intraocular pressure artificially are associated with the patient's head position. If the patient is not comfortable in the supine position, due to the head rest being badly adjusted, or alternatively if the chin rest is too high when readings are taken on the slitlamp, then pressures may well be elevated substantially. Equally, the patient with a tight collar could have the intraocular pressure artificially raised for the same reason.

Indentation tonometry

There are a number of different indentation tonometers available on the market but the most commonly used are the Schiötz tonometers. There are two versions of this tonometer—the 'X' or unweighted tonometer and the weighted model. There are many manufacturers but all models are based on the original design of Schiötz. Both types of instrument are used to measure the extent to which a movable plunger of known weight indents the (anaesthetized) cornea. Both instruments are almost identical in appearance, the only difference being found in the shape of the end of the movable plunger; the end of the X plunger is convex as opposed to concave in the weighted instrument. In terms of function and capability, the two instruments differ considerably, despite the fact that both are based on the same principle.

The weighted tonometer has a standard plunger weight of 5.5 g which can be increased with additional weights to 7.5, 10 and 15 g. The 5.5 g weight covers pressures ranging from less than 4 mmHg to 40 mmHg, the 7.5 g weight increasing the range up to almost 60 mmHg, the 10 g weight extending this to 80 mmHg, while the 15 g weight will measure up to 127 mmHg (*Table 23.1*). The X tonometer has a single plunger weight of 5.2 g and this is calibrated to cover a range of pressures from approximately 8 mmHg up to 90 mmHg. Although the X tonometer was introduced many years after the weighted tonometer, it is the weighted instrument that is by far the most accurate and reliable and hence the one

that was most commonly used. The reasons for this are directly related to the inherent problems associated with indentation tonometry (Kronfeld, 1957).

Source of errors

Indentation tonometry is subject to a considerable number of errors specific to the particular technique which can be grouped as follows: instrument errors; scale errors; those related to the method itself.

Instrumental errors are associated with the problems of control and tolerances in manufacture. All tonometers are currently manufactured according to standards laid down by the American Academy of Ophthalmology and Otolaryngology and should be issued with a certificate specifying the tolerances under which they are manufactured. Even instruments manufactured to such tolerances can still show variations of ± 3 mmHg between one instrument and another for the same eye.

The second group of errors arises from simply reading the 20 division scale—they can be divided into two aspects: the first is due to the fact that the pointer does not in fact make contact with the scale and therefore slight parallactic movements can produce an error in the reading. The second problem arises from the fact that the needle may be moving during the reading due to the variation in intraocular pressure associated with the cardiac cycle. The scale should be read at the midpoint of the pulsation and errors can clearly arise from incorrectly reading the midpoint.

The technique of indentation introduces its own inherent errors associated with the structure of the eye itself. The Schiötz tonometer is used for patients in the supine condition, the cornea having been anaesthetized. It basically measures the depth of corneal indentation produced by the known weight of the movable plunger.

The tonometer is a relatively heavy instrument; that part which sits on the eye and is not supported by the fingers is just over 16 g in weight. Since the effective weight of the plunger without any additional weights is 5.5 g, the eye itself is supporting a constant weight of 11 g or more. Placing the tonometer on the eye will, in itself, raise the intraocular pressure considerably, above the level that existed prior to the measurement being taken. This fact is taken into account in converting the arbitrary scale readings into millimetres mercury; the reading itself, therefore, is essentially an estimation of the pre-tonometric value. The measurement that is actually recorded, however, is the depth to which the plunger sinks into the eye, having taken into account the fact that intraocular pressure is raised prior to the plunger sinking in. In sinking into the eye, an appreciable volume of aqueous fluid is displaced.

Table 23.1 Conversion tables for the Schiötz standard tonometer Friedenwald, 1955 scale (Friedenwald, 1957)

Scale	5.5 g	7.5 g	10 g	15 g
0.0	41.4	59.2	81.6	127.5
0.5	39.3	55.2	75.2	117.9
1.0	34.6	49.7	69.3	109.2
1.5	31.7	45.6	64.0	101.3
2.0	29.0	42.1	59.1	94.4
2.5	26.6	38.8	54.7	88.1
3.0	24.4	35.8	50.6	82.2
3.5	22.4	33.0	46.9	76.5
4.0	20.6	30.4	43.4	71.1
4.5	18.9	28.1	40.2	66.3
5.0	17.3	25.8	37.2	61.8
5.5	15.9	23.7	34.6	57.5
6.0	14.6	21.8	31.8	53.6
6.5	13.4	20.2	29.5	50.0
7.0	12.2	18.5	27.2	46.5
7.5	11.2	17.0	25.1	43.2
8.0	10.2	15.6	23.1	40.1
8.5	9.3	14.3	21.3	37.3
9.0	8.5	13.1	19.5	34.6
9.5	7.7	11.9	17.9	32.1
10.0	7.1	10.9	16.5	29.6
10.5	6.5	10.0	15.3	27.4
11.0	5.9	9.1	13.8	25.2
11.5	5.3	8.2	12.4	23.2
12.0	4.8	7.5	11.5	21.4
12.5	4.4	6.8	10.4	19.7
13.0	4.0	6.2	9.5	18.0
13.5	3.6	5.6	8.6	16.5
14.0	3.2	5.1	7.8	15.1
14.5	2.9	4.6	7.1	13.8
15.0	2.6	4.1	6.4	12.6

This displacement gives rise to a considerable number of problems and errors, all of which are directly related to the method being used. The volume of fluid displaced must go somewhere. It could theoretically all be pushed out of the eye (via the canal of Schlemm), assuming that the valve mechanism offered no resistance to outflow. In such a case, the eye would be unaffected by this displacement. Alternatively, taking the other extreme, if no fluid could escape, the displaced fluid would remain within the eye and the pressure would rise considerably. The extent of this rise would depend on how flexible the walls of the globe happen to be and, therefore, how much they could expand to accommodate the displaced fluid. In reality the exit routes are neither fully open nor fully closed, there being a resistance to outflow which varies from one eye to another.

Aqueous displacement

Due to the volume of fluid displaced by the tonometer (*Figure 23.1*) there is initially a rise in intraocular pressure. This in turn triggers off a safety mechanism which leads to an increase in the rate of aqueous outflow from the eye (compensatory outflow) and a consequent reduction in pressure—the massaging effect. The extent of the fall will depend on the resistance to outflow that exists. The more readings that are taken or the longer the

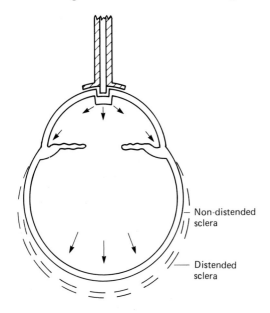

Figure 23.1 Indentation (Schiötz) tonometry displaces a large volume of fluid within the eye. Some of this fluid leaves the eye through the anterior angle due to compensatory outflow, while the remainder produces a distension of the scleral coats, thus bringing the factor of ocular rigidity into play

Non-distended sclera

Distended sclera

tonometer is left on the eye, the greater the reduction in pressure. This, therefore, militates against accuracy and is clearly a source of error because the technique itself reduces the intraocular pressure artificially below its normal pre-tonometric value. It is essential, therefore, to take the minimum number of readings and to carry out the procedure as quickly as possible.

It is not possible, in these circumstances, to assess the effect of patient apprehension by repeating the readings because any fall in pressure will in fact be due to the increase in the rate of aqueous leaving the eye as well as patient relaxation.

Only a small proportion of the displaced aqueous actually leaves the eye as a result of the increased rate of outflow. The major part is displaced backwards together with the other contents of the eye, distending the sclera and thus raising the intraocular pressure in the process. The extent to which the pressure will rise depends on how flexible the ocular walls happen to be. Unfortunately, flexibility of the sclera may vary considerably from subject to subject. If the ocular walls are very rigid, the displaced fluid will produce a greater increase in pressure than in an eye with very flexible walls. The difficulty lies in assessing this factor—known as ocular rigidity—yet without such an assessment the results obtained may be meaningless.

Investigations into ocular rigidity have been carried out by Schiötz and by Friedenwald, as a result of which an average value of ocular rigidity has been calculated (expressed as $K = 0.0215$). The tables for converting the 20 division tonometry scale units into millimetres mercury are based upon this average value. If the ocular rigidity of the eye being measured is outside normal limits, the standard conversion tables are no longer valid. In such circumstances, it will be necessary to use a special nomogram to determine the intraocular pressure (*Figure 23.2*).

In order to assess whether ocular rigidity is within normal limits, the Schiötz-weighted tonometer must be used. The pressure is first recorded without using any additional weights *in situ*, the effective weight therefore being 5.5 g. A second reading is then taken with an additional weight—increasing the effective weight to 7.5 or 10 g. If the scleral walls have a normal degree of flexibility, then the two readings will convert to approximately the same intraocular pressure. If the two values do not agree, then ocular rigidity is either below or above the average value. For example, if the pressure found with the heavier weight is higher than that obtained initially, the eye is more rigid than normal; both values obtained from the standard tables are incorrect, the true pressure being lower than the lowest pressure obtained. If the second reading shows a lower pressure than the first, the eye is more elastic than normal and the true

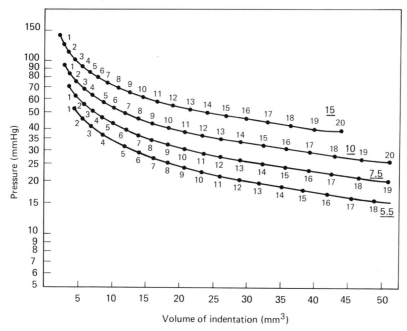

Figure 23.2 Nomogram for indentation tonometry
—based on Friedenwald (1955) calibration
(Friedenwald, 1957)

pressure will be higher than the highest value obtained. In such a case, therefore, a specially prepared nomogram must be used. This will provide a single value for the intraocular pressure which will differ from either of the values obtained using the standard conversion tables. This nomogram contains four curves, each one relating to one of the four weights used with the Schiötz tonometer and each divided into 20 divisions representing the tonometer scale units. The scale values obtained using the two different weights are plotted on the appropriate curves; the intraocular pressure is found by noting where the straight line joining these two points crosses the vertical axis. In addition it is possible to obtain an ocular rigidity value for the eye in question from the nomogram. It should be noted that this nomogram, which was designed by Friedenwald, is based on the assumption that ocular rigidity for a particular eye will remain constant irrespective of the pressure within that eye. This has been shown to be incorrect; it is now known that rigidity increases as pressure increases. Nevertheless, this source of error is clinically insufficient to invalidate the intraocular pressure (IOP) values obtained.

Method of use

Indentation tonometry should always be carried out with the patient supine. The tonometer must be cleaned prior to use, ideally using an agent which evaporates rapidly, thus avoiding the risk of damaging the cornea with the chemical used. Ether is particularly suitable. It is important not only to clean the tonometer footplate, but also the plunger and the tube in which it fits. Prior to use, the tonometer should be placed upon its test block to check that it is reading correctly; it should produce a scale reading of either zero or −1, depending upon the radius of curvature of the test block. (Each test block is usually engraved with the reading it should produce.) Failure to clean the plunger and its tube regularly is the most common reason for the tonometer reading incorrectly on its test block.

The cornea must be anaesthetized using a topical anaesthetic, such as oxybuprocaine (Benoxinate) 0.4%. The patient should be directed to look at a point on the ceiling such that the cornea is in the centre of the palpebral aperture. In order to allow easy access of the tonometer, the palpebral aperture should be widened, by lightly pulling the upper lid against the upper orbital margin usually with the index finger of the free hand, while, if necessary, pulling the lower lid lightly in the opposite direction with the thumb. It is essential to avoid resting the fingers on the globe when pulling the lids apart because even the lightest touch will raise the intraocular pressure considerably. Should the patient's skin be wet or damp through lacrimation, it may be difficult to maintain a grip on the lids. The use of a small piece of paper tissue on the skin will usually solve this problem.

The tonometer should be lowered vertically onto the centre of the cornea, making sure that the cornea is supporting the full weight of the tonometer by sliding the finger support towards the footplate, but carefully avoiding making contact with the footplate itself. If the tonometer is not held vertically, the footplate may lose full contact with the cornea resulting in an incorrect reading. When the tonometer is correctly positioned, the lever will be seen to pulsate against the scale. This is due to the change in intraocular pressure associated with the cardiac cycle. The scale should be read at the midpoint of the pulsation.

The tonometer should be removed, an additional weight added and the procedure repeated. Care must be taken to take the minimum number of readings and to leave the tonometer on the eye for as short a time as possible in order to keep the effect of compensatory outflow to a minimum.

The scale readings in each case should be converted into millimetres of mercury either from the appropriate tables or, if necessary, from the nomogram. Care must be taken to ensure that the conversion tables and the nomogram are the correct ones for the instrument being used since calibration standards have altered over the years. For example the upper limit of normality for the Friedenwald (*see* Friedenwald, 1957) scale is 22 mmHg whereas on the old Schiötz (1928) scale, it is 28 mmHg. Tonometry readings should therefore always indicate the tonometer and calibration tables used. In addition the time of day at which the readings were taken should always be recorded, so that diurnal variations can be taken into account, e.g. Schiötz (1957) weighted 18 mmHg 15.30 h.

The unweighted Schiötz tonometer cannot be used to assess the extent to which ocular rigidity is affecting the recorded values of intraocular pressure. Its conversion tables are valid only for those eyes having an average ocular rigidity. Since there is no way of cross-checking the results with this tonometer, the results therefore will be in error for those eyes whose ocular rigidity is above or below the average. This tonometer is also less accurate than the weighted version because the 20-division scale covers such a wide range of pressure; thus errors in reading the scale will result in quite significant variations in intraocular pressure values particularly for those eyes with raised pressure, the relationship between the scale values and intraocular pressure being curvilinear. The only advantage of the unweighted tonometer is that it produces less massaging than the weighted version since only one reading per eye is required.

Conclusions

It is quite clear that indentation tonometry is subject to many sources of error all of which militate against accuracy. It is no longer the method of first choice having been replaced by applanation tonometry. It does, however, still have a place as a preferred method in certain cases, in particular in cases of nystagmus and corneal scarring.

Applanation tonometry

Applanation tonometry differs from indentation tonometry in as much as the corneal surfaces—anterior and posterior—are flattened as opposed to being indented. Its advantage stems from the fact that normally the volume of aqueous displaced is very small being approximately 0.5 mm^3 with an applanated diameter of approximately 3 mm. At this level, there is no significant distension of the ocular coats nor any increase in the rate of aqueous outflow from the eye. Providing that the applanated area is kept small, therefore, the reading can be repeated without any risk of artificially reducing the intraocular pressure. Thus the two major sources of error in indentation tonometry—ocular rigidity and compensatory outflow—do not normally arise in applanation tonometry.

There are two basic methods of approach in applanation tonometry:

(1) The weight or force applied to the cornea is kept constant, the variable area or diameter flattened being measured.
(2) The weight or force applied to the cornea is varied in order to applanate a constant fixed area.

Fixed force applanation tonometry

The Maklakow tonometer, introduced originally in 1885, and the later Tonomat tonometer, employ a fixed weight to applanate the eye, the diameter flattened being measured in order to determine the pressure. The Maklakow tonometer consists basically of a hollow dumb-bell-shaped cylinder, the ends of which are sealed by polished milk glass plates 10 mm in diameter. Within the cylinder is a freely movable lead weight which serves to lower the centre of gravity of the instrument, thus making it more stable when positioned on the eye. A simple wire loop handle is attached to the cylinder to hold the tonometer vertically on the eye. In order to measure the diameter of applanation, the end plates, which have been previously sterilized, are coated evenly with a water-soluble dye (Argyrol). When the tonometer is placed on the cornea, the dye is removed over the area that is applanated and the diameter is measured using a specially designed ladder gauge which is directly calibrated in terms of pressure. There are four different weighted Maklakow tonometers: 5 g, 7.5 g, 10 g and 15 g. Normally, the two lower weights are used, the lightest tonometer being employed for pressures up to approximately 35 mmHg and the 7.5 g tonometer for higher pressures. The two heaviest tonometers generally are only used when a measurement of ocular rigidity is required. Ocular rigidity, however, does not significantly affect the results when using the lightest tonometers, because the volume of displaced fluid is very small.

Nevertheless, the Maklakow results may be incorrect. The source of the errors is related to the way in which the conversion scales were prepared by Kalfa. Like Friedenwald, he assumed that scleral rigidity remained constant irrespective of intraocular pressure, whereas in fact rigidity increases with pressure. These errors are only likely to arise when the heavier weights are used and in any event their magnitude is likely to be small.

Care must be taken to avoid the tonometer drifting around on the cornea because this will result in an excessive amount of dye being removed and a false low reading being obtained. It is essential that the tonometer is placed vertically and steadily on the apex of the anaesthetized cornea, the patient being supine. It is important that the coating of dye on the end plates should not be too thick, otherwise a clear imprint will not be obtained. If the cornea being measured is very astigmatic, an oval imprint may be obtained; in such a case the shortest diameter should be measured.

Readings may be repeated when using the lightest tonometers with little risk of lowering the pressure through massaging. Errors tend to arise mostly in measuring the diameter of imprints, the edges of the dye-free area in some cases being rather ill defined.

The Maklokow tonometer is not suitable for use on subjects with nystagmus and irregular corneas.

Constant area applanation

It has already been shown that errors associated with ocular rigidity and compensatory outflow do not arise if the volume of fluid displaced within the eye is very small. This state of affairs exists when the area applanated is small. As the applanated area increases, a point is reached where the fluid displacement becomes sufficient to introduce the same ocular rigidity and massaging errors that arise in indentation tonometry. This then is the inherent problem associated with fixed weight variable area Maklakow-type tonometry, because in a very soft eye, even the 5 g tonometer may flatten a relatively large area. By using a variable force to flatten a constant predetermined area, the introduction of

these errors can be avoided. This represents the major advantage of this group of tonometers.

It has been shown (Smith, 1965) that if the applanating force or weight (W) used to flatten a fixed corneal area (A) is being used solely to counterbalance the intraocular pressure (P), then under these conditions, $P = W/A$. For this simple state of affairs to apply, it is necessary to eliminate some residual errors related to the cornea itself and the layer of tears.

When a rigid flat surface is applied to the cornea in an attempt to measure the IOP, it is essential that sufficient force is applied to flatten the posterior corneal surface. The cornea itself has its own elasticity or rigidity; this differs from scleral rigidity in two important aspects:

(1) It does not vary significantly from eye to eye.
(2) It represents a much smaller source of error than scleral rigidity.

Nevertheless, the cornea does have a resistance to being flattened and would on its own inflate the measured IOP value. An additional source of error arises due to the collection of a pool of tear fluid around the applanating surface. This pool stays *in situ* due to surface tension which acts as an attracting force pulling the tonometer onto the eye and, as such, depresses the true IOP value. In flattening the cornea, however, the tear layer is squeezed, there being an inherent resistance to such squeezing; this has the effect of inflating the IOP value. Goldmann (1955) discovered, however, that when a corneal diameter of approximately 3 mm is flattened, the attracting force of surface tension (ST) is cancelled out by the corneal rigidity (CR) and the squeezed tear layer (TL): ST = CR + TL. He also showed that when the applanated diameter is exactly 3.06 mm, a linear relationship exists between the force applied and pressure in millimetres of mercury, 1 g force equalling 10 mmHg.

The Goldmann tonometer based on these principles was introduced in 1954 and has become the standard against which all other tonometers are judged. It consists essentially of a sealed hollow conical-shaped cylinder, containing a pair of prisms, apices together (*Figure 23.3*). The prisms have the effect of shifting the upper half of the field of view to the left, and the lower half to the right, so that the centres of the two halves are separated by a distance of exactly 3.06 mm. The applanated cornea is viewed directly through the cylinder or probe itself. The area of corneal contact, which, without the prisms, would have appeared as a circle, is seen as two semicircles, the centres of which are separated by 3.06 mm. When the applanated diameter is exactly 3.06 mm, the inner edges of the semicircles will just be in contact. The variable force required to

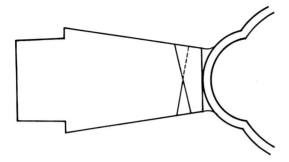

Figure 23.3 Goldmann tonometer head showing arrangement of prisms and tear accumulation around applanated zone

flatten the cornea is applied by means of a simple lever system employing an eccentrically placed weight as opposed to a spring system, thus avoiding the problem created by variations in spring tension due to wear and tear (Draeger, 1966).

Procedure

The tonometer unit is usually used in conjunction with a slitlamp and is mounted so that it is positioned in front of either the right or left eyepiece, a full binocular view not being possible. The magnification should ideally be set at × 10–12. The slitlamp beam fully open should be positioned at about 60° on the temporal side of the tonometer, such that the leading edge of the circular patch of light just reaches the tip of the tonometer cone. The blue filter should be used. The tonometer drum should be set at approximately 1 g prior to commencing measurement, in order to avoid the tonometer making and breaking contact with the cornea which will occur if the drum is set at zero.

Having sterilized the tonometer cone, the cornea being anaesthetized, a small amount of fluorescein is instilled in each eye to colour the tears. Ideally, a paper strip should be used; this should be moistened prior to application. It is essential that only a trace of fluorescein is applied because, if a full drop is instilled, the concentration may be too high to allow adequate fluorescence to be produced.

With the patient fixating straight ahead, the tonometer is positioned approximately along the visual axis so that corneal contact is made initially at the approximate centre of the applanating surface. The patient should be instructed to blink a few times prior to applanation in order to moisten the cornea properly, to keep the head pressed against the headrest and to keep the eyes wide open, trying not to blink while the measurements are being taken. In bringing the tonometer into contact with the eye, care must be taken to avoid trapping any eyelashes

between the tonometer and the cornea because this will have the effect of inflating the IOP results. It may be necessary, therefore, particularly if the lashes are long, to lower the tonometer to avoid trapping the upper lashes, and then raising the tonometer when *in situ* on the cornea.

When the point of contact has been made, forward movements of the slitlamp should cease, although it is important to ensure that the cornea is fully supporting the tonometer cone. If contact is minimal then every small movement of the patient will lead to a loss of contact.

Vertical centration is critical; if the two half circles are not of equal size, the IOP values obtained will be incorrect. The tonometer must therefore be vertically adjusted on the cornea to ensure that the semicircles are matched (*Figure 23.4*). Once this has been done, the weight being applied should be adjusted until the inner edges of the semicircles are just in contact. In order to avoid drying of the

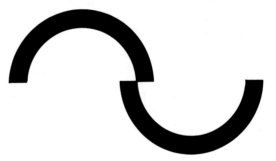

Figure 23.4 View through the Goldmann tonometer head when a diameter of 3.06 mm is applanated.

corneal epithelium and subsequent staining, the tonometer should then be removed from the eye so that it is just clear of the lashes and the patient asked to blink again to moisten the cornea. The procedure is then repeated until two readings within 0.5 mmHg of each other are obtained.

Apprehension on the part of the patient will raise IOP. Once the patient realizes that the procedure is painless, pressure usually falls; a reduction of 4 mmHg from the initial reading is quite common. The lowest reading obtained is the value recorded. As with other tonometers the time of day should always be noted. It will be found that the semicircles pulsate. This is due to the effect of the cardiac cycle. Goldmann (1955) recommends that the value recorded is the lowest point, i.e. the diastolic value. This differs from the approach used for the Schiötz tonometer where the average value is taken. There is, therefore, a case for recording the midpoint value which is where the inner edges of the circles underlap and overlap each other by the same amount.

If a high degree of corneal astigmatism is present (usually more than 3 D), the applanated area will be oval rather than round. In order to ensure that measurements are correct in such cases, the two semi-ovals must be equal in shape and size. To achieve this, the dividing line of the prisms must be rotated to bisect the short axis of the oval.

Problems can arise if the fluorescein pool is too wide or too narrow. Ideally, the width of the circle should be about one-tenth the final applanating diameter (0.3 mm), i.e. with × 10 magnification it should appear to be approximately 3 mm wide. The major problem arises if the tear pool circle is much wider than this, which occurs if the patient is lacrimating heavily. As a result, the large pool begins to drain across the applanated cornea and can affect the readings. In such cases, the tonometer must be removed, its surface wiped dry and the measurements repeated. If the same problem recurs, it may be necessary to lift the upper lid so that it no longer makes contact with the bulbar conjunctiva, thus avoiding the tears pooling under the upper lid and flooding down when the tonometer touches its edge.

A number of problems can arise with this form of tonometry which prevent a satisfactory result being obtained. This is usually due to errors in procedure as shown in *Table 23.2.*

The normal range of pressures recorded with the Goldmann tonometer falls between 10 and 18 mmHg, while values below 10 mmHg are not uncommon. The upper limit of normality is re-garded as 20 mmHg. Pressures above 22 mmHg should be regarded with suspicion and investigated further. Borderline pressures should be rechecked earlier on the following day if possible.

This type of tonometry is regarded by many clinicians as the method of choice because of its reliability and repeatability. It is applicable in all cases with the exception of nystagmus and gross corneal scarring.

Hand-held constant area tonometers

A number of hand-held optical applanation tonometers have been produced. Their advantage lies in their portability. They are not, initially, as easy to use as their slitlamp counterparts, but once the handling technique has been mastered, they provide a similar level of accuracy.

The Perkins tonometer is a good example of a hand-held instrument. It is nicely balanced and uses the Goldmann probe. It is completely self-contained with its own power supply for the illuminating source. Although it incorporates a forehead rest which enables the tonometer to be pivoted onto the cornea, difficulty may be experienced in judging the proximity of the probe to the cornea, prior to contact. Greater control can be achieved by extending the forefinger of the hand holding the tonometer so that digital contact is made with the patient's cheek before corneal contact is achieved. The pro-

Table 23.2 Errors in procedure for applanation tonometry

Problem		Cause—solution
(1) Semicircles keep appearing and disappearing		Patient not pressing head against headrest
	or	Tonometer only just barely in contact with cornea—push tonometer slightly closer to cornea using joystick
(2) Semicircles very indistinct		Eyepiece incorrectly focused. Adjust eyepiece so that circular edges of prism are clear
(3) No semicircles visible		Tonometer not in contact with the eye
	or	Fluorescein washed out of eye due to excessive lacrimation
	or	Too much fluorescein in eye (most likely cause). Add a drop of saline in lower sac

cedure in all other respects is identical with that used for the slitlamp version.

Electronic tonometers

The first electronic tonometer, introduced in 1950, was basically a standard weighted Schiötz tonometer which incorporated an electronic recording device in order to eliminate the scale reading errors which arise with the mechanical versions of such tonometers. These instruments, which are particularly suitable for tonography, nevertheless, present the same errors associated with ocular rigidity and compensatory outflow that arise with their mechanical counterparts. The introduction of digital displays in laters years added little to their accuracy.

Mackay Marg tonometer

The electronic tonometers that were subsequently introduced have all been based on the applanation principle. The Mackay Marg tonometer was the first such tonometer to be marketed (Mackay and Marg, 1959). It utilizes a rigid stainless steel applanation probe 5 mm in diameter, in the centre of which is a fused quartz rod which acts as a flat plunger, this being held in position within the probe by a silicone rubber or steel web spring. Movements of the plunger, which is 1.5 mm in diameter and surrounded by a non-sensitive flat steel plate, activate a linear transducer which is sensitive to movements of less than 1 μm. As the probe is pressed horizontally against the cornea, micromovements of the plunger occur, the resultant signal being amplified and the pressure recorded on heat sensitive paper.

The typical pressure curve shows an initial peak followed by a temporary trough or dip. This trough, which represents the intraocular pressure exclusive of corneal rigidity and surface tension, occurs when the corneal flattening exceeds the 1.5 mm diameter of the plunger and spreads onto the non-sensitive probe shoulder. As the probe is removed from the cornea, a mirror image of the trace will be produced.

Readings from the Mackay Marg have been shown to be higher than Goldmann values (Moses, 1962; Tierney and Rubin, 1966). Although the upper limit of normality was found to be 29 mmHg compared to 20 mmHg with the Goldmann tonometer, on average the Mackay Marg values were 2 mmHg higher than those of Goldmann. The Mackay Marg probe is very sensitive to small hand movements and tremor, as a result of which a reasonable degree of skill is required in application. In the hands of an unskilled practitioner the results can be unreliable (Petersen and Schlegel, 1973). Nevertheless, this tonometer has been found to be of particular value in cases of scarred and irregular cornea (Kaufmann, Wind and Waltmann, 1970). The Mackary Marg is regarded as a useful screening tonometer rather than being an alternative to the Goldmann tonometer (Moses, Marg and Oechsli, 1962).

It was originally thought that the diameter of cornea applanated when the Mackay Marg is used correctly, would be between 2 and 3 mm, bearing in mind that the plunger is only 1.5 mm in diameter. Two independent studies have shown however, that the trough, representing the actual IOP, occurs when the diameter of the corneal flattening is between 5 and 6 mm (Stepanik, 1970; Moses and Grodzki, 1971). In view of the fact that, before the probe is removed from the cornea, manual pressure often continues beyond the point at which the trough is reached, it is certain that, in many cases, measurements of IOP with this tonometer involve flattening the cornea considerably more than 6 mm in diameter. There is a strong possibility, therefore, that this technique will displace sufficient aqueous to introduce errors associated with ocular rigidity and compensatory outflow.

Owing to difficulties in satisfactorily sterilizing the plunger, it is recommended that sterile disposable sheaths are used to cover the probe. Although measurements can be taken without the use of anaesthetics, it is preferable to anaesthetize the cornea. The probe should be held between the thumb and forefinger, care being taken to apply it horizontally and to avoid handshake.

Mackay Marg readings represent the intraocular pressure at a single point in time and, therefore, the values obtained may be anywhere within the ocular pulse cycle. Consequently it is recommended that approximately 10 simultaneous readings are taken on each eye, each reading taking about 0.25 second. The lowest consistent repeatable value recorded is taken as the IOP.

Digilab tonometer

The Digilab tonometer (Durham and Langham tonometer), in contrast to the Mackay Marg, provides a continuous measurement of intraocular pressure as it varies with the cardiac cycle. In using gas pressure to achieve this, it is similar in some respects to the Tonair applanation tonometer—a non-electronic instrument in which air is pumped into a small pressure chamber contained in the tonometer probe, the pressure increasing until it equals the IOP when a small movable plunger is unseated thus allowing the pressure to escape (*Figure 23.5*). Whereas the Tonair instrument uses a rigid plunger against which air is pumped, the Digilab pumps inert bottled gas against a flexible Silastic membrane. This membrane, 5 mm in diameter, forms the tip of the tonometer probe. When in contact with the cornea, it forms an airtight seal allowing the gas

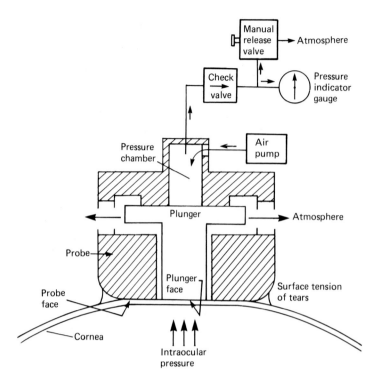

Figure 23.5 Diagram of the Tonair probe tip in situ on the cornea showing the plunger position when the IOP exceeds the pressure in the air chamber. At the point of equilibrium, the plunger will be minimally displaced allowing the air to escape to the atmosphere, the pressure in the chamber dropping below that of the IOP. The cycle will be repeated as long as the probe remains on the cornea

pressure to increase until it balances the intraocular pressure. At this point the membrane is minimally displaced, allowing the excess pressure to escape; the seal is immediately reformed and the cycle repeated as long as the probe remains in contact with the cornea (Langham and McCarthy, 1968).

The probe employs a frictionless bearing which allows the sensor to float freely on a cushion of gas. A pneumatic force of approximately 2 g gently holds the tonometer against the cornea, thus overcoming the effect of hand movements; applanation is, in this way, automatically maintained. The gas bearing allows measurements to be taken with the patient in any position between the vertical and supine (*Figure 23.6*).

Readings can only be obtained if the tonometer is correctly applied to the eye, i.e. the axis of the probe must be perpendicular to the eye at the intended point of contact. At this point, when the cornea is supporting the probe, an audible signal, varying in pitch with the pulse beat, is emitted.

The results, traced on pre-calibrated heat sensitive paper, represent a record of the continuous changes in intraocular pressure that occur due to the cardiac cycle. Apprehension may produce an initially elevated trace and, therefore, the lowest traces obtained are regarded as representing the IOP. The midpoint of the lowest trace is taken as the true IOP value. (Walker, Compton and Langham, 1975; Walker and Langham, 1975.)

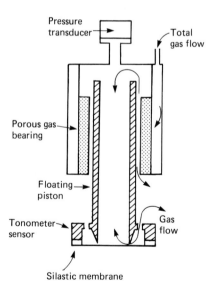

Figure 23.6 Diagram of the Digilab floating tonometer probe. (From Langham and McCarthy, 1968, by permission)

The volume of aqueous displaced with this tonometer is insufficient to bring into play errors associated with ocular rigidity and compensatory outflow. The results obtained have been shown to closely correlate with the Goldmann tonometer (Quigley and Langham, 1975), although they tend to be higher. Its accuracy has, however, been questioned (Moses and Grodski, 1979).

Non-contact tonometers

The American Optical non-contact tonometer involves no mechanical contact with the eye. It applanates the cornea by means of a controlled pulse of air which linearly increases in force until the cornea is just flattened. The pulse is carefully collimated to ensure that the applanated area does not significantly exceed 3 mm in diameter.

The instrument, which incorporates its own small computer, consists of three main components. The first comprises a pneumatic system which, when the instrument is at the correct distance from the cornea, produces an air pulse which reaches its peak in about 12 ms. As it increases in force, it reduces the corneal curvature until it is flattened and then

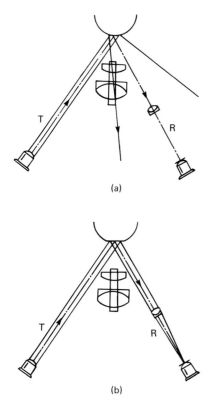

(a)

(b)

Figure 23.7 (*a*) Diagram of light rays emitted from non-contact tonometer transmitter (T), reflected from undisturbed cornea and received by receiver (R). (*b*) Diagram of light rays emitted from cornea applanated by the non-contact tonometer air pulse and totally received by receiver (R). (From Forbes, Pico and Grolman, 1974, p. 136; copyright 1974, American Medical Association by permission)

becomes minimally concave (*Figure 23.7*). The second component monitors the state of the corneal curvature. It consists of a transmitter, which directs a collimated beam at the corneal apex, and a telecentric receiver symmetrically positioned to the transmitter. As the corneal curvature decreases, the received signal increases in strength reaching its maximum when the cornea is flat. When the cornea becomes minimally concave there is a marked reduction in the reflected signal and at this point the air flow is shut off. The third component is a modified spherometer, similar to the Radiuscope, which enables the instrument to be correctly aligned and positioned. A fail-safe system ensures that a measurement cannot be made unless the instrument is correctly positioned. The results are displayed on a digital screen, the time taken to applanate being automatically converted into intraocular pressure.

This tonometer has a number of advantages and disadvantages. The volume of aqueous displaced is insufficient to introduce any significant errors associated with the compensatory outflow and ocular rigidity. As a result, measurements can be safely repeated. Because no physical contact is made with the cornea, anaesthetics are not required. The air pulse, however, may dry the corneal epithelium and this may lead to corneal staining. It is essential, therefore, to keep the cornea moist by blinking between measurements. The triggering of the air pulse is relatively noisy; this has the effect of increasing apprehension in some patients which, on repeating the measurements, increases the IOP. The pulse produces a displacement of the eyelashes and a subsequent sensation. While not painful, some patients find this disagreeable, thus adding to the sense of apprehension while waiting for repeat measurements to be undertaken (Pina and Martins, 1978).

The non-contact tonometer measurements represent a single value for the IOP which can be anywhere within the ocular pulse cycle. Repeated readings are likely to vary for this reason, if for no other.

The non-contact tonometer was primarily designed for use on eyes with a clear cornea and good fixation. It has been shown that it is not the best instrument to use on dry eyes, and those with corneal oedema and scarring, as well as those with poor acuity (Forbes, Pico and Grolman, 1974).

The results obtained with this tonometer show reasonably good correlation with the Goldmann tonometer for the lower range of pressures but, as the pressure increases, the correlation decreases, the non-contact tonometer values being higher than the true values. Since the non-contact tonometer was originally calibrated against the Goldmann tonometer, it must be regarded as inaccurate whenever it deviates from these values. For this reason, there is a very strong case for cross-checking both borderline and raised non-contact tonometer values

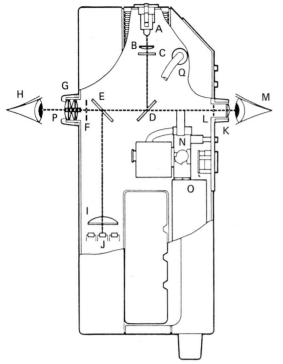

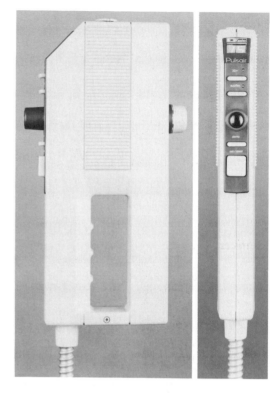

Figure 23.8 Keeler Pulsair tonometer. (Reproduced with permission from Keeler Ltd)

with a Goldmann tonometer (Brooser, Anda, Ahi and Papp, 1978; Shields, 1980).

The Keeler Pulsair tonometer is a hand-held instrument which, like the American Optical non-contact tonometer, uses air pressure to applanate the cornea. Its measuring range is 0–55 mmHg, but for intraocular pressures up to 30 mmHg, it uses a lower pulse air pressure than the American tonometer. Rather than measuring pressure indirectly by recording the time taken to applanate the cornea, the Pulsair uses a transducer to directly measure the air pressure at the point at which the cornea becomes flattened. The mechanism by which this is achieved can be seen from *Figure 23.8*.

Light from bulb A passes through condenser lens B, filter C and on to the beam splitter D. Part of this light is then projected forward through beam splitter E and mask F. Mask F produces the target image which is projected by an objective lens system onto the patient's cornea.

Part of the reflected corneal image is diverted by beam splitter E via a 'contrast lens' I onto a set of three photodetectors J. Some of the light also passes through beam splitters E and D through viewing lens K, forming an image which the operator uses for alignment.

Only when the tonometer is at the right distance and correctly aligned with respect to the patient's cornea, will the image of the corneal reflex fall onto the three photodetectors J in such a way that more light falls onto the two outer detectors than the centre one. At the moment, the instrument senses that the contrast between the sum of the outer and the centre detectors is correct, a valve N on the air reservoir O automatically opens releasing a pulse of air via tube P onto the patient's eye.

The increasing pulse of air decreases the cornea curvature until it is eventually flattened. This changes the characteristics of the corneal reflex such that more light now falls on the centre detector than the sum of the outer two: a contrast reversal thus occurs. When this happens the pressure transducer Q, which is connected directly to the pneumatic system, samples the pulse pressure and the result is digitally displayed in millimetres of mercury. The measurement process from the moment of correct alignment takes only a few milliseconds.

A facility exists for taking measurements on scarred, irregular and dry corneas.

Preliminary results with this tonometer indicate that it does not produce any significant errors associated with ocular rigidity and compensatory outflow. As it is relatively noiseless, it does not cause significant problems associated with patient apprehension. Like the American Optical non-contact tonometer, the measurements may be anywhere within the ocular pulse, and repeated readings may vary due to this factor.

Conclusions

Applanation tonometry is unquestionably the method of choice in terms of reliability and repeatability. The Goldmann tonometer is the most universally accepted form of applanation tonometry and still remains the norm against which all other methods are judged. Nevertheless, the interpretation of all tonometer results must be made in the context of the wide variation in normal (and abnormal) values seen in the population, and can therefore rarely be diagnostic in their own right.

References

BROOSER, G., ANDA, L., AHI, O. and PAPP, L. (1978) Experience with the non contact tonometer. *Szemeszet*, **115**, 129

DRAEGER, J. (1966) *Tonometry, Physical Fundamentals, Development of Methods and Clinical Application.* Basel: S. Karger

DUKE-ELDER, W.S. (1940) *Textbook of Ophthalmology*, Vol. 3. London: Henry Kimpton

FORBES, M., PICO, G. and GROLMAN, B.(1974) Non contact applanation tonometry. *Arch. Ophthalmol.*, **91**, 134

FRIEDENWALD, J.S. (1957) Tonometer calibration. *Trans. Am. Acad. Ophthalmol. Otolaryngol.*, **61**, 108

GOLDMANN, H. (1955) Un nouveau tonomètre à aplanation. *Bull. Soc. Fr. Ophtalmol.*, **67**, 474–478

KAUFMANN, H.E., WIND, C.A. and WALTMANN, S.R. (1970) Validity of the Mackay Marg electronic applanation tonometer in patients with scarred irregular corneas. *Am. J. Ophthalmol.*, **69**, 1003

KRONFELD, P.C. (1957) Tonometer calibration. *Trans. Am. Acad. Ophthalmol. Otolaryngol.*, **61**, 123

LANGHAM, M.E. and McCARTHY, E. (1968) A rapid pneumatic applanation tonometer. *Arch. Ophthalmol.*, **79**, 389

MACKAY, R.S. and MARG, E. (1959) Fast automatic electronic tonometers based on an exact theory. *Acta Ophthalmol.*, **37**, 495

MOSES, R. (1962) The Mackay Marg tonometer. A report to the Committee on Standardisation of tonometers. *Trans. Am. Acad. Ophthalmol. Otolaryngol.*, **66**, 88

MOSES, R.A. and GRODSKI, W.J. (1979) The Pneumotonograph—A laboratory study. *Arch. Ophthalmol.*, **97**, 547

MOSES, R.A. and GRODSKI, W.J. (1971) The Mackay Marg tonometer—a note on calibration methods. *Acta Ophthalmol.*, **49**, 800

MOSES, R., MARG, E. and OECHSLI, R. (1962) Evaluation of the basic validity and clinical usefulness of the Mackay Marg tonometer. *Invest. Ophthalmol.*, **1**, 78

PETERSON, W.C. and SCHLEGAL, W.A. (1973) Mackay Marg tonometry by technicians. *Am. J. Ophthalmol.*, **76**, 933

PINA, M.L. and MARTINS, J.F. (1978) Our experience with the non contact tonometer. Act 3 Luso – Hisp – Braz. Congress of Ophthalmologists, 421, 1976

QUIGLEY, H.A. and LANGHAM, M.E. (1975) Comparative Intraocular Pressure Measurements with the Pneumotonograph and Goldmann Tonometer. *Am. J. Ophthalmol.*, **80**, 266

SMITH, P. (1891) *On the Pathology and Treatment of Glaucoma.* London: J & A Churchill

SMITH, R.J.H. (1965) *Clinical Glaucoma.* London: Cassell

SHIELDS, M.B. (1980) The non contact tonometer—its value and limitations. *Surv. Ophthalmol.*, **24**, 211

STEPANIK, J. (1970) The Mackay Marg tonometer—correlation of the tonogram to the corneal applanations induced by the tonometer. *Acta Ophthalmol.*, **48**, 1140

TIERNEY, J.P. and RUBIN, M.L. (1966) A clinical evaluation of the Electronic Applanation tonometer *Am. J. Ophthalmol.*, **62**, 263

WALKER, R.E., COMPTON, G.A. and LANGHAM, M.E. (1975) Pneumatic applanation tonometry studies 4. Analysis of pulsatile response. *Exp. Eye Res.*, **20**, 245

WALKER, R.E. and LANGHAM, M.E. (1975) Pneumatic applanation tonometry studies 3. Analysis of floating tip sensor. *Exp. Eye Res.*, **20**, 167

24

Gonioscopy

Sarah Janikoun

Gonioscopy is a difficult, specialist examination where interpretation is often a subject for discussion and consultation. It should be emphasized that many normal eyes should be examined before any reliable results or observations can be obtained.

Applications

The gonioscope is used to examine the recess of the angle of the anterior chamber.

Primary glaucoma

In the diagnosis of primary glaucoma, the state of the angle is important to determine whether it is 'open' or 'closed'. In addition, other contributory factors in the diagnosis of secondary glaucoma may be seen. These include abnormally large quantities of pigment (pigmentary glaucoma), peripheral anterior synechiae (either secondary to iritis or injury) and blood vessel proliferation as occurs in diabetic or post-thrombotic conditions.

Other pathology

Abnormal angle structures may only be visible through the gonioscope and among these are peripheral iris or ciliary body tumours or intraocular foreign bodies.

Structural changes

Changes in the normal anatomy of the angle or the peripheral iris can also more easily be viewed. Some peripheral iridectomies can be effective while invisible on direct viewing. Iris dialyses as a result of trauma may only be inferred by a D-shaped pupil, but is seen clearly with a gonioscope.

Principles of gonioscopy

Method of examination

The patient should be positioned comfortably at the slitlamp and the cornea anaesthetized. A lubricant contact fluid such as saline or hypromellose is dropped into the concave surface of the gonioscope lens. The eyelids should be held apart gently with one hand, while the patient looks down and the lens is gently applied to the exposed upper bulbar conjunctiva. When the patient then looks straight ahead, the lens will be in the correct position over the cornea. Any bubbles between the lens and the cornea will necessitate removal and reapplication of the lens.

It is much easier to insert a lens into a relaxed, reassured patient who should be informed that the examination is not painful, although not entirely comfortable and that the fluid which may run down the face is merely the liquid put into the lens.

It may be necessary to hold the lens in position throughout the procedure, although sometimes it may be retained on its own. Any eyelid squeezing will dislodge the lens.

If the mirror is positioned first at the top, the inferior angle can be viewed. Gentle twisting of the lens clockwise through 360° will allow each part to be observed in a routine and methodical manner, the angle viewed always being opposite to the mirror. Orientation can be difficult and is best achieved by scanning the iris from the pupil, into the mirror. When the peripheral iris is identified, close examination of the area anterior to it is important.

The gonioscope lens may be removed by eyelid squeezing, otherwise the globe should be supported below with the thumb of one hand, and the lens carefully prised off with the thumb and forefinger of the other hand.

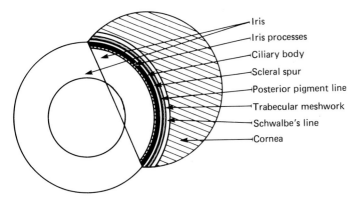

Figure 24.1 Diagram illustrating the structures of the angle

Anatomy *(Figure 24.1)*

Iris

This should appear flat. If there is any bowing, its site and extent should be noted. At the extreme periphery, iris processes may be seen in wide open angles.

Ciliary body

This may be seen as a narrow dark band beyond the iris.

Scleral spur

This is seen as a bright white band. It is an extension of the sclera which forms part of the wall housing the canal of Schlemm. It also provides insertion for fibres of the longitudinal muscle of the ciliary body which may be significant in the opening of the pores of the trabecular meshwork.

Trabeculum

This is seen as a greyish band anterior to the scleral spur from which it may be divided by a line of pigment on its posterior edge. In some conditions, this pigment may affect the whole band.

Canal of Schlemm

This is not normally visible. In some cases, however, it may be seen as a dark band within the trabeculum if it fills with blood, which can be induced by pressure on the episcleral vessels.

Schwalbe's line

This is a white line anterior to the trabeculum. It can be glistening white or rather dull and is a continuation of Descemet's membrane.

Blood vessels

It is quite normal to see a few blood vessels in the angle. (Rubeosis implies fronds of new vessels which course haphazardly over the angle and iris.)

Estimation of the angle

If the trabeculum can be seen, the angle is open, but it is then necessary to determine how open it is or whether there is any danger of it closing. There are two main methods of estimation of the angle which should be carried out in each quadrant:

(1) Gauging the angle by the number of structures visible—if all the elements, including the ciliary body can be seen, the angle is ·wide open. If those up to the scleral spur are seen, which is very common, it is moderately open. If the trabecular meshwork is not seen, the angle is closed.
(2) Gauging the angle between the flat iris and the curved cornea *(Figure 24.2)*.

For comparative purposes, grading or lettering of the estimated angles has been advocated, but all methods are subjective.

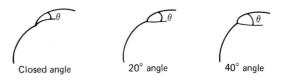

Closed angle   20° angle   40° angle

Figure 24.2 Gauging the angle between the flat iris and the curved cornea

Hazards and implications

(1) The angle can be artificially opened by pressure on the gonioscope lens.
(2) Any bubbles in the contact medium will distort the focus and make accurate examination impossible.
(3) It is always important to direct a good strong beam of light into the angle and it is necessary to reorientate the beam column using a horizontal as well as vertical beam.
(4) High microscope magnification is required.
(5) It is difficult to assess the significance of small areas of angle closure because normal intraocular pressures can be maintained with such angles.

Referral

In general, the angle is only examined where glaucoma is suspected. If open, in a case of raised intraocular pressure with disc cupping and a field defect, then chronic or simple open-angle glaucoma may be diagnosed.

In acute glaucoma, the presentation is usually of an acute episode which requires urgent attention.

Problems arise when routine inspection with a slit-lamp reveals an abnormally shallow anterior chamber. In these cases, gonioscopy will help in determining whether there is truly a narrow angle. If the angle is closed all round to a large degree, it may be necessary to refer the patient even if there are no symptoms. This is, however, a very rare occurrence. A finding of borderline narrow angle is a more difficult consideration and, where there are no symptoms, its management will depend upon several factors which may or may not warrant referral.

Conclusions

Gonioscopy is a very useful diagnostic aid and tool for management but it is a difficult procedure to execute and interpret, and caution is needed in the early stages of its use.

Further reading

DUKE-ELDER. W.S. (1969) *System of Ophthalmology*, Vol. XI, p. 597. London: Henry Kimpton
DUANE. T.D. (1985) *Clinical Ophthalmology*, Vol. 3, pp. 1–19. Philadelphia: Harper & Row
MILLER. S.J.H. (1984) *Parson's Diseases of the Eye*, 16th edn, p. 110. Edinburgh: Churchill-Livingstone
WOLFE. E. (1976) The eyeball. In *Anatomy of the Eye and Orbit*, 7th edn, edited by R. Warwick, pp. 57–59. London: H.K. Lewis & Co. Ltd

25

Sphygmomanometry and ophthalmodynamometry

Simon Barnard

Sphygmomanometry

The optometric practitioner is generally responsible for detecting, not only ocular disease, but also systemic disease with ocular manifestations. Vascular hypertension falls into both of these categories. Not only can it seriously affect vision, but it may be a threat to life itself, with a potential for damage to the cardiovascular system, kidneys, and brain.

It is relatively easy to detect hypertension of retinal grades 3 and 4 because retinopathy is present (Keith, Wagener and Barker, 1939). Careful ophthalmoscopy may detect some cases of retinal grades 1 and 2, but will miss others, and also give rise to incorrect referrals. The final arbiter in the detection of vascular hypertension is the measurement of the systemic blood pressure, i.e. sphygmomanometry. Elmstrom (1974) has urged all optometric practitioners to adopt the practice of routine sphygmomanometry.

History

While the unpleasant consequences of vascular hypertension have been recognized from the earliest times, the recognition of high blood pressure demanded the means to measure it. This was first achieved in horses by Stephen Hales in 1733 who was one of the pioneers of experimental physiology. He inserted a vertical tube into the artery of a horse and measured the height to which the blood in the tube rose. Nearly a century later Poiseuille used a 'U' tube filled with mercury to measure the blood pressure of an animal.

It was not until the latter part of the nineteenth century that reasonably accurate instruments were developed to clinically estimate blood pressure in man. One instrument of the period was Gaertner's

digital manometer which measured blood pressure by inflating a pneumatic cuff to cut off flow to the finger and the pressure at which flush occurred was observed during cuff deflation. This method is similar to a flush method currently used to determine the blood pressure in infants (Goldring and Wohltmann, 1952).

Estimation of blood pressure by palpation of the first radial pulse following arm cuff inflation and deflation was introduced by Riva-Rocci in 1896. The use of mercury column oscillation was introduced by Erlanger in 1904, and the use of sound or auscultatory manometry was advocated by Korotkoff in 1905.

Measurement of blood pressure

The most accurate procedure for measuring blood pressure is to place a cannula in a large artery such as the brachial and to connect the tube to an electronic pressure transducer. This technique is called direct blood pressure determination and is limited to rare hospital situations.

By far the most common method of determining blood pressure is by the indirect method utilizing an inflatable cuff connected to a measuring device, and used in association with a listening device. The cuff is placed around the arm and inflated until the pressure causes collapse of the artery below the cuff. The air is then slowly released and, when the pressure in the cuff is just below the systolic pressure, blood will spurt through the vessel with each systolic rise. This movement of blood produces *Korotkoff* sounds which may be picked up with a listening device such as a stethoscope. When the air pressure in the cuff has reduced to below diastolic pressure, there is no embarrassment to flow and there is a cessation of these sounds.

Measurement devices

There are two commonly used pressure measurement devices: mercurial and aneroid.

Mercurial

The mercurial type of pressure measurement equipment is the oldest and simplest type. It consists of a simple glass tube graduated in millimetres connected to a reservoir of mercury. As the cuff is inflated the pressure created is conducted simultaneously to the reservoir. The mercury is forced out of the reservoir and up the vertical tube as the pressure increases. The pressure in the cuff is determined by the level of mercury in the vertical glass tube. The number of millimetres that the mercury is raised above its resting level indicates the pressure in the cuff in millimetres of mercury (mmHg). The advantage of this type of device is that it is simple to operate.

As long as the air-conducting tubes are free of leaks and clear of obstruction, the air vent at the top of the mercury column is open, the column is vertical and the mercury level is at zero before the cuff is inflated, then the accuracy and reliability of this instrument is as good as or better than any other of the devices available.

The disadvantage of the mercury unit is that it is somewhat bulky and therefore marginally less portable for domiciliary visits.

Aneroid

The aneroid type of measurement device makes use of air pressure and a diaphragm. The diaphragm is connected to a series of springs and gears which move an indicator needle over a dial face. The mechanical nature of the device makes it more prone to errors, and it is, therefore, wise to check an aneroid sphygmomanometer against a mercurial one once or twice a year.

The advantages of the aneroid over the mercurial sphygmomanometer are that it is compact, it is easy to use and its portability makes it useful for domiciliary visits.

In recent years a variety of electronic pressure transducers have been incorporated into sphygmomanometers. An advantage of these is that an automatic zeroing device can be incorporated.

Pressure cuff and bladder

The pressure cuff and bladder of the sphygmomanometer are most important for accurate blood pressure determination. The cuff and bladder should be of the appropriate size and it is recommended that the width of the bladder and cuff should be 25% wider than the diameter of the limb on which it is to be used. If the cuff and bladder are excessively wide, then the measured pressure will be erroneously low; conversely, if the cuff and bladder are excessively narrow, the measured pressure will be erroneously high (Kaplan, 1973); Kirkendall *et al.*, 1977).

The length of the air bladder in the cuff should be more than one-half the circumference of the limb. To allow for variation in limb sizes a variety of cuff sizes should be available to the practitioner.

Methods of determining end-points

Stethoscopes

Stethoscopes vary considerably in their construction and design. Most are designed to allow practitioners to hear various sounds emitted at the surfaces of the body and are not specifically designed for indirect determination of blood pressure (*auscultatory technique*).

The Korotkoff sounds that are of interest during blood pressure determination are low frequency sounds from 20 to 300 Hz, with the highest sound energy being produced in the lower end of the range. As a result, the practitioner should select an instrument which can receive and conduct these low frequency sounds efficiently.

The selection of the appropriate stethoscope is a personal decision depending upon demands of comfort, desirable working distance from patients, and variations in auditory acuity. For practitioners with a degree of hearing impairment, there are a number of different types of amplified stethoscopes which enhance the Korotkoff sounds.

Electronic listening devices

In these instruments, a sensitive microphone replaces the stethoscope and is set into the cuff. The practitioner carefully places the microphone over the brachial artery and the Korotkoff sounds may be detected.

The piezoelectric ceramic microphones used in many of these instruments are fragile and care should be taken not to apply any digital force to its surface when adjusting the cuff.

Doppler systems

Doppler systems utilize ultrasound echoes to evaluate sources in motion (e.g. flowing blood cells in vessels). The frequency of such echoes will differ from that of the emitted ultrasound.

The echo frequency varies depending on the direction and speed of blood flow. The strength of echo depends upon the volume of blood flow. Systolic and diastolic pressures may then be assessed by observing the flow characteristics during the sphygmomanometric procedure.

Such techniques are especially useful in cases where it is difficult to assess the Korotkoff sounds, particularly in children.

Palpatory method

Some physicians use the first pulsation felt at the radial artery as the indicator of systolic pressure. Although the method often gives comparable results to the auscultatory method, there can be variations between the two as, in some cases, the pulse can be felt before any sound is heard.

Oscillatory method

In this method, the oscillations of the column of mercury or the aneroid gauge needle are used to indicate systolic and diastolic pressure. As the air pressure is reduced, the first oscillations signify systolic pressure, and the disappearance of the oscillations shows the diastolic pressure.

Korotkoff sounds

In 1905, Korotkoff described a series of arterial sounds which could be heard below an inflated cuff during partial compression of the vessel within a limb. Korotkoff sounds are divided into five phases (phases I–V) and these five phases can be directly related to the *distal* intra-arterial pressure.

When a cuff is placed around an arm and inflated to a pressure greater than the systolic blood pressure of the artery beneath it, then the arterial walls will collapse and there will be no flow of blood through the vessel. As the air pressure in the cuff is reduced there will come a moment when the systolic blood pressure is slightly greater than the cuff pressure and a 'tap' will be heard (phase I). The pressure in the cuff at this point is recorded as the systolic blood pressure. As the air in the cuff continues to be released, the regular tapping sound becomes associated with, and is often dominated by, a regular murmur with each systolic rise (phase II). Continued deflation of the cuff gives rise to the regular murmur being replaced with a series of tapping sounds (phase III). With further depressurization of the cuff, the regular tapping sound suddenly loses its volume and becomes muffled (phase IV). The first muffled sound is indicative of the diastolic blood pressure. These regular muffled sounds suddenly stop and all sound ceases (phase V). This cessation of sound is also indicative of diastolic pressure, and the cuff pressure at which the sound ceases should be recorded.

There is no absolute agreement as to which of the two phases is the best indicator of the 'true' diastolic pressure.

The pressure taken on the right arm of a sitting person would be recorded as follows: right arm 120/80/75 sitting. The first number indicates the systolic pressure and the latter two numbers indicate diastolic I and diastolic II, respectively.

General technique for indirect sphygmomanometry

Whatever method the practitioner adopts for measurement of blood pressure, the following should be noted:

(1) The patient should be seated comfortably and relaxed.
(2) Any loose clothing around the arm should be rolled up to allow correct positioning of the cuff. Any tight items of clothing should be removed.
(3) The cuff is then positioned on the arm and, in the case of an electronic instrument incorporating a microphone, the latter is carefully positioned over the brachial artery. The cuff should be neither too tight nor too loose and of the correct size.
(4) The arm of the patient should be placed on the armrest of the chair. The elbow should be slightly bent, the palm of the hand open and facing upwards, and the arm otherwise relaxed. The patient should be reclined slightly to bring the cuff position level with the patient's heart.
(5) The examiner should have a relaxed and unhurried attitude.
(6) Cuff inflation to above the systolic pressure should be carried out quickly and deflation commenced immediately, as pain and discomfort increase blood pressure. Most electronic instruments incorporate an automatic valve release which releases the air at some 2–3 mmHg/s. During routine screening it is reasonable to initially inflate the cuff to 180 mmHg. If the systolic pressure turns out to be higher than this the air pressure may be increased further.

Erroneous measurements

Patient discomfort or anxiety may give rise to higher readings than expected. In addition, the position of incorporation in the optometric routine should be considered carefully. For example, it is possible that there would be a variation in blood pressure following certain stressful techniques such as non-contact tonometry or after a complex and difficult refraction.

Other erroneous measurements that can occur are:

(1) If the cuff is not inflated sufficiently then the systolic pressure may be underestimated.
(2) Cardiac arrhythmias can cause difficulties in determining end-points.

(3) Careful positioning of the stethoscope or microphone is important, and location of the artery may sometimes be difficult with obese patients.

Whenever possible, more than one reading should be taken, but if the measurement is going to be repeated on the same visit, at least a few minutes should be allowed between readings.

Hypertension and normotension

Much research has been carried out to determine a dividing line between 'hypertension' and 'normotension'. Pickering (1968) pointed out that there was, in fact, no dividing line. If the population were made up of two groups with regard to blood pressure, frequency distribution curves would be expected to be bimodal, and this is definitely not the case. However, the higher the blood pressure the worse the prognosis.

Although there is no clear pathophysiological dividing line, practitioners have had to decide on theoretical dividing lines above which they start treatment, refer for further investigation or, in the case of surveys, to enable them to categorize the patient.

In the past, suggested dividing lines between normotension and hypertension have been: 120/80 mmHg (Robinson and Brucer, 1939), 130/70 mmHg (Browne, 1947), 140/80 mmHg (Ayman, 1934), 150/90 mmHg (Thomas, 1952), 160/100 mmHg (Bechgaard, 1946), 180/100 mmHg (Burgess, 1948), and 180/110 mmHg (Evans, 1956).

More recently a number of studies have set such a dividing line at 160/95 mmHg (Elek, 1970; Fowler, 1970; Kannel et al., 1970; Veterans Administration Co-operative Study Group, 1970; Abernathy, 1974; Christie, McPherson and Vivian, 1976).

Prevalence and screening

Vascular hypertension has long been known as a major community and individual health problem. Although the disease is the most chronic condition seen by physicians, the majority of hypertensives remain undetected except when community surveys are made (Wilbur and Barrow, 1974).

Hart (1970) screened 912 patients aged 20–64 years in his general medical practice and found 38 patients required consideration for treatment. The Australian National Blood Pressure Survey (Abernathy, 1974) estimated that 3% of Australians had diastolic blood pressure greater than 110 mmHg and 9–10% between 90 and 114 mmHg. The Queenscliff study (Christie, McPherson and Vivian, 1976) showed that in their population, 13.9% had casual blood pressures greater than 160/95 mmHg or were already on hypertensive treatment. The American Heart Association estimated that 23 million Americans (or 1 in 7 adults) are hypertensive (Page and Sidd, 1972). Using a criterion of 160/95 or higher, Laragh (1974) estimated that approximately 20% of the American population has vascular hypertension and that more than half of these have hypertensive heart disease. In a small survey of consecutive patients in an optometric practice, 13.3% were referred on the basis of casual blood pressure measurements (Gutteridge, 1978). Daubs (1974) estimated that, with proper screening, the optometric practitioner could expect to discover, for the first time, one new hypertensive for each 14 adult patients seen in the practice.

Mass screenings employing blood pressure readings frequently result in 25–30% referral rate. Usually about half of these referrals are later confirmed as hypertensives. Although this high 50% over-referral rate may seem excessive to the practitioner, it is probably about the best that could be expected of a single parameter mass screening performed by laymen or technicians (Daubs, 1973 a,b). Ayers et al. (1974) recommended that all physicians should routinely screen all their patients for hypertension. The physician, regardless of speciality, should record each patient's blood pressure at least once a year if he is the only physician following the patient. For children between the ages of 6 and 14 years, a reading should be taken every 2 years; for younger children, at least one reading should be taken before the age of 6 years.

In the USA, dentists have developed screening programmes for their practices (Berman, 1972; Berman, Guarino and Giovannoli, 1973; Abbey, 1974; Abbey, Keenes and Roper, 1976) and the pharmaceutical profession have also developed plans for involvement (Mattei et al., 1973; McKenny, Jennings and White, 1976).

Hollenhorst (1974) has urged all ophthalmologists to take an active role in the detection of vascular hypertension.

General effects of hypertension

Hypertension is not only the most common chronic disease, but also the biggest single causative factor of death (Laragh, 1974) and there is considerable evidence that elevated systolic or diastolic pressure is associated with increased morbidity and mortality (Law, 1959a, b; Kagan et al., 1962; Breslin, Gifford and Fairnbairn, 1966; Beard et al., 1967; Smirk, 1967; Johnson, Yano and Kato, 1968; Flora, Cmae and Nishimor, 1969; Kannel, Schwartz and McNamara, 1969; Hayden, et al., 1969; Kannel et al., 1970; Cassell, 1971; Heyman et al., 1971; Julius and Schork, 1971; Nagle, 1971; Paul, 1971; Schoenberger, 1971).

One study failed to show this relationship for borderline elevation (Mathieson et al., 1965). Increased morbidity and mortality from stroke (Paul,

1971; Kannel *et al.*, 1970), congestive heart failure and ischaemic heart disease (Kagan, *et al.*, 1962; Paul, 1971), and from renal failure (Fejfar, 1967) have clearly been demonstrated. The Framingham study (Kannel *et al.*, 1970) shows that other morbid events such as arrhythmias are more common in the hypertensive than in the normotensive population. Quoting actuarial data for men (without regard for age). Pickering (1968) demonstrated that mortality ratios increased with both increasing systolic and diastolic pressure readings.

Vascular accidents can seriously affect vision leaving the patient partially sighted or even blind, or they may affect ocular motility with subsequent visual problems.

Effects of treatment on hypertensive morbidity and mortality

Discovering the unknown hypertensive patient is of limited value unless the patient is referred and receives effective treatment (Stokes, Payne and Cooper, 1973) and clearly there would be very little advantage to the patient in the early detection unless the condition could be easily treated.

In the 1950s, it was conclusively demonstrated that therapy with antihypertensive drugs reverses the manifestation of malignant hypertension and that long-term survival could be obtained if renal damage was not advanced at the time treatment was begun (Dunstan *et al.*, 1958; Harrington, Kincaid-Smith and McMichael, 1959).

In the case of essential hypertension, the first controlled study did not take place until 1964 (Hamilton, Thompson and Wissniewski, 1964) when it was shown that treatment clearly benefited men with uncomplicated diastolic hypertension of 110 mmHg and over. Wolff and Lindemann (1966) showed over a 2-year study that the incidence of morbid events was one-third that observed in the group treated with placebos. In the Veterans Administration Co-operative Study (1967, 1970) one group of patients with initial diastolic levels of 90–114 mmHg and another group with 115–129 mmHg were studied. In both groups there was a clear benefit to those patients who were treated compared to those in the control groups. The Framingham Study (Kannel *et al.*, 1970) showed that the control of hypertension, labile or fixed, systolic or diastolic, at any age, and in either sex, appears to be central to prevention of atherothrombotic brain infraction (stroke).

Prognosis in untreated retinal grade 3 and 4 patients

The classic paper of Keith, Wagener and Barker (1939) mentions a mean survival time of 10.5 months in grade 4 patients and 27.6 months in retinal grade 3 patients. At 5 years, 99% of grade 4 and 80% of grade 3 patients had died. The mean age of the patients studied was 40 years for the grade 4 and 42 years for the grade 3 patients.

Frant and Groen (1950) found that 60% of untreated grade 3 patients had died after 5 years.

Results of treatment for hypertension of retinal grades 3 and 4

Breckenbridge, Dollery and Parry (1970) reviewed the progress made with treated malignant hypertensive and retinal grade 3 patients. The overall mortality rate after 5 years was 66%. Simpson and Smirk (1962) showed a 58% mortality rate over 5 years in treated retinal grade 4 patients.

Prognosis in untreated retinal grade 1 and 2 patients

Keith, Wagener and Barker (1939) found a mean 5-year mortality rate of 46% for retinal grade 2 patients, and 30% of grade 1. The mean ages of the grade 1 and 2 patients were 55 years and 41 years, respectively. The authors did not compare the ages of those who had died to those who had survived, and they also included deaths which may not have been secondary to hypertension. Smirk (1964) found a combined mortality rate in retinal grades 1 and 2 of 44% in males and 25% in females. It should be noted that in this study there was a higher proportion of older patients in the untreated group than in the treated group (this was, however, compensated for in the comparison of mortality rates between the two groups).

Results of treatment for hypertension of retinal grades 1 and 2

There is evidence (Hamilton, Thompson and Wissneiwski, 1964; Smirk, 1964; Hood, *et al.*, 1966; Veterans Administration Study Group, 1967, 1970) that, in addition to reducing overall mortality rates, effective antihypertensive measures at an early stage of hypertension and before advanced retinal changes have developed, reduce the risk to the patient of developing severe hypertension with exudative retinopathy (grades 3 and 4).

Sphygmomanometric criteria for referral by practitioners

The theoretical dividing line between 'high' and 'normal' blood pressure has already been discussed. The diagnostic criteria used in the Framingham Study (Kannel *et al.*, 1970) were that hypertension was arbitrarily designated as present when at least two blood pressures during a clinic visit were recorded at 160/95 mmHg or greater. Normotension was considered present at pressures under 140/90 mmHg. The remainder were considered to be borderline.

Maxwell (1974) recommended similar criteria to those used in the Framingham Study but with a number of alterations which make the scheme unnecessarily complex for optometric use.

Grosvenor (1978) suggested a simpler screening system:

(1) All patients having findings of 150/90 mmHg or greater should be referred for medical evaluation.
(2) Patients with readings between 140/90 mmHg and 150/90 mmHg should be scheduled for rescreening and referred for medical evaluation if findings remain in this range.

Daubs (1975) suggested a referral system based on age. Gutteridge (1978) utilized Daub's criteria but suggested three casual blood pressure readings. He also included referral for any patient with one diastolic reading of 115 mmHg or above, and he suggested further modifications in the presence of fundus signs or associated risk factors.

Barnard (1983) suggested slight modifications to this scheme. Both Maxwell (1974) and Grosvenor (1978) suggested two readings for borderline patients rather than the three of Gutteridge (1978). Repeated sphymomanometric measurements of patients having borderline blood pressure may not always assist a referral decision, and the author feels it is reasonable to refer to the general medical practitioner for evaluation any patient who exhibits two or more readings over and above the levels suggested by Daubs (1975) as follows:

(1) Age 18–44 years   140/90 mmHg.
(2) Age 45–64 years   150/90 mmHg.
(3) Age 65 years and older 160/90 mmHg.

The practitioner may also consider referring a patient exhibiting one diastolic reading of 110 mmHg.

It is important to use additional clinical judgement and to modify the referral scheme in the presence of other factors including:

(1) Relevant symptoms, e.g. headaches that are present on awakening.
(2) Fundus signs, e.g. arteriolar narrowing.
(3) Family history of cardiovascular disease.
(4) Non-compliance with hypertensive therapy.
(5) Diabetes mellitus.
(6) Obesity.
(7) Smoking.

As in screening for the glaucomas, each practitioner must decide on whether all patients over a certain age (e.g. 35 years) are routinely screened or whether the technique is reserved for selected patients.

The relationship between systemic blood pressure and the optic disc capillary perfusion pressure must be considered and the latter's relationship with some types of glaucoma and related ischaemic conditions of the optic nerve head (*see below*).

Ophthalmodynamometry

The presence of a cardiac cycle in the eye is often apparent during Goldmann applanation tonometry. Visible pulsation of the central retinal artery is not usually considered normal when observed by ophthalmoscopy, although Duke-Elder (1966) suggested that it may be observed in the great majority of patients if instruments providing higher magnification are used.

However, if while carrying out ophthalmoscopy the practitioner simultaneously applies digital pressure on the globe, a more pronounced arteriolar pulsation will be observed on the disc. This is a rather crude way of assessing the blood pressure of vessels within the eye—ophthalmodynamometry.

History

Soon after the introduction of the ophthalmoscope, spontaneous venous pulse was noted by Coccius in 1853 and van Trigt in 1854. Arteriolar pulse was noticed in the retinas of normal eyes by Donders in 1855 and Becker in 1872.

One of the first workers to describe a device for making measurements of the blood pressure of the ophthalmic artery was Henderson in 1914, but the first instrument with adequate sensitivity was described by Baillart in 1917. He originally claimed that the technique of ophthalmodynamometry, which he described, measured the pressure of the central retinal artery of the retina. Numerous authors have since pointed out that this is not the case, and that the pressure being measured is that of the ophthalmic artery.

Measurement of blood pressure

The manometric method

A manometer is connected to the interior of the eye and, while the intraocular pressure is raised by an injection of saline, the pulsatory behaviour of the retinal arterioles or the amplitude of the associated rhythmic changes of intraocular volume is studied, the points of maximum oscillation and cessation of oscillation being taken as the diastolic and systolic pressures, respectively. This is the only reliable technique (Duke-Elder, 1966), but being invasive it has no clinical applications.

Ophthalmodynamometry

The technique of ophthalmodynamometry utilizes the eye as a natural sphygmomanometer. Increasing force is slowly applied to the eye while the observer views the optic disc with an ophthalmoscope. As the force applied approaches and then exceeds the diastolic pressure of the ophthalmic artery, the central retinal artery will intermittently collapse. The dynamometric force applied is noted. Further force is applied until total and persistent collapse of the artery is observed, which will occur when the intraocular pressure has just exceeded the systolic pressure in the ophthalmic artery, and at that point the second dynamometric reading is taken.

Instruments and techniques

The Baillart ophthalmodynamometer consists of a piston, one end of which carries a foot-plate which can be pressed against the bulbar conjunctiva, so raising the intraocular pressure, while the other end works against a standardized compression spring, the excursion being indicated by a pointer. The force required to elicit maximal pulsation and to cause complete collapse of the retinal artery is noted. Tonometry is performed and the forces producing maximal pulsation and collapse may be deduced.

Kukan (1936) described a system whereby the intraocular pressure was raised by applying suction to the eye and other workers, including Galin, Baras and Cavero (1969), have improved this technique. Friedman (1966) reported the observation of pulsating arterioles of the optic disc as seen through the Goldmann fundus lens at the slitlamp, when mechanical pressure was applied against the globe of the eye by digital pressure on the Goldmann lens.

Sisler (1972a) devised an optical–corneal pressure ophthalmodynamometer that applies Friedman's principle quantitatively and this instrument is now produced as the 'Dynoptor' (American Optical Company) as a slitlamp attachment. The Dynopter is basically an adaption of the applanation tonometer. The spring resistance of the applanator box is increased to deliver graded pressures via the control dial from zero to 150 g. The entire applanator head is replaced by a small (8 mm in diameter) −60 D fundus lens that is rigidly affixed to the support post by means of which graded pressures are delivered anteroposteriorly against the cornea when the dial of the weight-spring box is advanced.

Sisler claimed that, since the axes of global pressure application are essentially coincident with the visual axis of both the examiner and the patient, and since the fundus lens applicator tip is concave, conforming to the cornea, there is a minimum of global distortion as pressure is applied. He argued that both the Baillart and suction type instruments cause deformation of the globe and therefore introduce inaccuracies.

Sisler (1972b) compared diastolic readings using scleral pressure, suction, and corneal pressure units, in 56 normal subjects. His analysis of standard deviations and correlation coefficients between the two eyes of each subject showed greater accuracy with the corneal pressure technique than with the other instrument.

Kaufman (1965) modified two Baillart instruments and yoked them by means of a geared separator bar which permitted adjustments in lateral separation. He was able to simultaneously apply equal force to each eye. As force is applied to the globe and the intraocular pressure nears the ophthalmic artery pressure, the visual field shrinks in from the periphery, leaving a small central island of vision. This island then fades out as pressure is maintained. Kaufman considered the eye losing vision first was reflecting the presence of a lower internal carotid or ophthalmic artery pressure homolaterally.

Another subjective technique has been developed by Henkind and Chambers (1978), who noted that by using the Hadinger Brush Phenomenon, the level of systole in the ophthalmic artery could be determined. As pressure was increased on the eye with a standard Baillart ophthalmodynamometer, the visualized 'brushes' seemed to slow and stop just as systole was reached. This technique may be of value in patients with cataracts or hazy media, as they will still be able to perceive the Hadinger brushes when adequate ophthalmoscopy is not possible.

Ophthalmodynamometric results

A number of workers have measured the pressures on healthy human eyes and common values are 35–45 mmHg for the diastolic and 65–75 mmHg for the systolic pressure in the ophthalmic artery. However, what is most important is the comparison of the two eyes (Duke-Elder, 1966). Duke-Elder also deduced that the pressure in the intraocular portion of the central retinal vein is 17–18 mmHg, and that the capillary pressure within the eye may be as high as 45–50 mmHg.

Clinical applications

Ophthalmodynamometry is of ophthalmological value as a non-invasive technique to corroborate carotid occlusive disease.

Glaser (1978) pointed out certain reservations: flow characteristics in the carotid are not necessarily altered until there is 70–90% stenosis; collateral circulation may support flow and pressure in the opthalmic artery in high grade carotid stenosis or even complete occlusion; and symptomatic carotid embolic disease may occur with minimal stenosis. Therefore, in the symptomatic patient, the absence of ophthalmodynamometric abnormality does not mitigate against carotid atheromatous disease.

Galin, Baras and Cavero (1969) suggested that a difference in ophthalmic artery diastolic pressure between the two eyes of more than 20% should give rise to suspicion of carotid insufficiency.

A number of workers have studied the relationship between ophthalmic artery pressure and intraocular pressure in glaucomatous patients. Lobstein and his co-workers estimated the 'efficient gradient', i.e. the mean pressure in the ophthalmic artery less the intraocular pressure. The greater this difference the more copious is the blood flow in the cribriform plate (Lobstein, Bronner and Nordmann, 1960; Lobstein and Herr, 1966).

A fall in the systemic blood pressure, particularly its diastolic reading, in patients with simple glaucoma, and thus a reduction in the 'efficient gradient', has been shown to result in a deterioration in the visual field (Harrington, 1959; Lobstein, Bronner and Nordmann, 1960; Lobstein and Herr, 1966).

Although it is unlikely that an ophthalmodynamometric instrument will be used in practice, simple digital ophthalmodynamometry is a most useful technique and can give additional information. The practitioner must, however, be aware of the inherent dangers in the measurement of the systolic pressure.

References

ABBEY, L.M. (1974) Screening for hypertension in the dental office. *J. Am. Dental Assoc.*, **88**, 563

ABBEY, L.M., KEENES, L.M. and ROPER, A.J. (1976) A dental school hypertension screening program. *J. Dental Educ.*, **40**, 287

ABERNATHY, J. (1974) The Australian National Blood Pressure Survey. *Med. J. Aust.*, **1**, 821

AYERS, C.R., SLAUGHTER, A.R., SMALLWOOD, H.D., TAYLOR, F.E. and WEITZMAN, R.E. (1974) Standards for quality care of hypertension patients in office and hospital practice. In *Hypertension Manual*, edited by J. H. Laragh, pp. 683–710. New York: Yorke Medical Books.

AYMAN, D. (1934) Heredity in arteriolar (essential) hypertension: a clinical study of blood pressures of 1524 members of 277 families. *Arch. Intern. Med.*, **53**, 792

BARNARD, N.A.S. (1983) and Screening by optometrists *Ophthal. Physiol. Opt.*, **3**, 365

BECHGAARD, P. (1946) Arterial hypertension: a follow up study of one thousand hypertonics. *Acta Mad. Scand. Suppl.*, 172

BEARD, O.W., HIPP, H.R. ROBINS, M. *et al.* (1967) Initial myocardial infraction among veterans. *Am. Heart J.*, **73**, 317

BERMAN, C.L. (1972) Screening by dentists for hypertension.

N. Engl. J. Med., **286**, 1416

BERMAN, C.L., GUARINO, M.A. and GIOVANNOLI, S.M. (1973) High blood pressure detection by dentists. *J. Am. Dental Assoc.*, **37**, 359

BRECKENBRIDGE, A., DOLLERY, C.T. and PARRY, E.H.O. (1970) Prognosis of treated hypertension *Q. J. Med.*, **39**, 411

BRESLIN, D.J., GIFFORD, R.W. and FAIRNBAIRN, J.F. (1966) Essential hypertension. A twenty year follow up study. *Circulation*, **33**, 87

BROWNE, F.J. (1947) Chronic hypertension and pregnancy. *Br. J. Med.*, **2**, 283

BURGESS, A.M. (1948) Excessive hypertension of long duration. *N. Engl. J. Med.*, **239**, 75

CASSELL, J.C. (1971) Summary of major findings of the Evans County cardiovascular studies. *Arch. Intern. Med.*, **128**, 887

CHRISTIE, D., McPHERSON, L. and VIVIAN, V. (1976). The Queenscliff Study: a community screening programme for hypertension. *Med. J. Aust.*, **2**, 678

DAUBS, J.G. (1973a) The influence of prevalence on screening test validity. *Opt. J. Rev. Optom.*, **110**(24), 15

DAUBS, J.G. (1973b) Basic concepts in optometric screening. *Opt. J. Rev. Optom.*, **110**(20), 29

DAUBS, J.G. (1974) Cost efficiency of optometric screening. *Opt. J. Rev. Optom.* **111**(6), 9

DAUBS, J.G. (1975) A protocol for hypertension screening and referral. *Am. J. Optom. Physiol. Opt.*, **52**, 351

DUKE-ELDER, S. (1966) *System of Ophthalmology*, pp. 4, 14–31. London: Henry Kimpton

DUNSTAN, H.P., SCHNECKLOTH, R.E., CORCORAN, A.C. and PAGE, I.H. (1958) The effectiveness of long term treatment of malignant hypertension. *Circulation*, **18**, 644

ELEK, S. (1970) *Classification of Hypertension; Monographs on Hypertension*. Rahway, NJ: Merck and Co.

ELMSTROM, G. (1974) Examining the 're-examination'. *Opt. J. Rev. Optom.*, **111**(15), 9–12

EVANS, W. (1956) *Cardiology*, 2nd edn. p. 386. London: Butterworths

FEJFAR, S. (1967) Some aspects of epidemiology of arterial hypertension. The epidemiology of hypertension. Proceedings of an International Symposium, edited by J. Stamler, R. Stamler and T.N. Pullman, p. 188. New York: Grune & Stratton

FLORA, G.C., CMAE, T. and NISHIMOR, U. (1969) Stroke: U.S. and Japan. Clinical profile of the stroke patient. *Geriatrics*, **24**, 95

FOWLER, N. (1970) *Prognosis in Systemic Hypertension Monographs in Hypertension*, Rahway, NJ: Merck and Co.

FRANT, R. and GROEN, J. (1950), Prognosis of vascular hypertension. *Arch. Intern. Med.*, **85**, 727

FRIEDMAN, B. (1966) A new apparatus and technique for ophthalmodynamometry. *ENT Monthly*, **45**, 72

GALIN, M.A., BARAS, I. and CAVERO, R. (1969) Ophthalmodynamometry using suction. *Arch. Ophthalmol.*, **81**, 494

GLASER, J.S. (1978) Topical diagnosis: prechiasmal visual pathways. In *Clinical Ophthalmology*, edited by T. Duane, pp. 2, 5, 7. New York: Harper & Row

GOLDRING, D. and WOHLTMANN, H. (1952) Flush method for

blood pressure determination in new born infants. *J. Pediatr.*, **40**, 285

GROSVENOR. T.. (1978) The prelininary examination. Part 12. Blood pressure measurement. *Optom. Monthly*, March, 105

GUTTERIDGE. I.F. (1978), Hypertension—Referral criteria for optometrists. *Aust. J. Optom.*, **6**, 133

HAMILTON, M., THOMPSON. E.M. and WISSNIEWSKI. T.K.M. (1964) The role of blood pressure control in preventing complications in hypertension. *Lancet*, **i**, 235

HARRINGTON. D.O. (1959) The pathogenesis of the glaucoma field. *Am. J. Ophthalmol.*, **47**, 177

HARRINGTON, M.. KINCAID-SMITH. P. and McMICHAEL. J. (1959) Results of treatment in malignant hypertension. *Br. J. Med.*, **2**, 969

HART. J.T. (1970) Semicontinuous screening of a whole community for hypertension. *Lancet*, **ii**, 223

HAYDEN, S., BARTEL. A.G.. HAMES, C.G. *et al.* (1969) Elevated blood pressure levels in adolescents. Evans County, Georgia: seven year follow up of 30. *J. Am. Med. Assoc.*, **209**, 1683

HENKIND. P. and CHAMBERS. J.K. (1978) In *Clinical Ophthalmology*, edited by T. Duane, pp. 3, 14, 6. New York: Harper & Row

HEYMAN, A.. KARP. H.R.. HENDY. S. *et al.* (1971) Cerebrovascular disease in the biracial population of Evans County, Georgia. *Arch. Intern. Med.*, **128**, 949

HOLLENHORST. R.W. (1974) Vascular hypertension and the ophthalmologist. *Am. J. Ophthalmol.*, **77**, 275

HOOD, B.. AURELL. M. FAIKHEDEN, T. and BJORK. S. (1966) Analysis of mortality in hypertensive disease. In *Antihypertensive Therapy*, edited by F. Gross, p. 370, Berlin: Springer Verlag

JOHNSON, K.G.. YANO K. and KATO. H. (1968), Coronary heart disease in Hiroshima, Japan. A report of a six year period of surveillance, 1958–1964. *Am. J. Publ. Hlth*, **58**, 1355

JULIUS. S. and SCHORK. M.A. (1971) Borderline hypertension. A critical review. *J. Chron. Dis.*, **23**, 723

KAGAN. A.. DAWBER. T.R.. KANNEL. W.B. *et al.* (1962) The Framingham Study. A prospective study of coronary heart disease. *Fed. Proc.* **21** (Suppl. 2), 52

KANNEL. W.B.. SCHWARTZ, M.J. and McNAMARA. P.M. (1969) Blood pressure and risk of coronary heart disease. *Dis. Chest*, **56**, 43

KANNEL. W.B.. WOLF. P.A.. VERTER. J. and McNAMARA. P.M. (1970) Epidemiologic assessment of the role of blood pressure in stroke—The Framingham Study. *J. Am. Med. Assoc.*, **214**, 301

KAPLAN. N. (1973) *Clinical Hypertension*. New York: Medicom Press

KAUFMAN. J.H. (1965) Instrument for conjugate opthalmodynamometry. *Am. J. Opthalmol.*, **60**, 527–528

KEITH. N.M.. WAGENER. H.P. and BARKER. N.W. (1939) Some different types of essential hypertension: Their course and prognosis. *Am. J. Med. Sci.* **197**, 332

KIRKENDALL. W.M.. BURTON. A.C.. EPSTEIN. F.H. and FREIS. E.D. (1977) Report of a sub-committee of the Postgraduate

Education Committee, American Heart Association. *Circulation*, **36**, 980

KUKAN. F. (1936) Erg ebnisse der blutdruckmessung en mit einem neuen ophthalmodynamometer. *Z. Augenheilk.*, **90**, 166

LARAGH. J.H. (1974) Evaluation and care of the hypertensive patient, *Hypertension Manual*, pp. 673–781. New York: York: Medical Books

LEW. E.A. (1959a) *Build and Blood Pressure Study*, Vol. 1, p. 1. Chicago: Society of Actuaries

LEW. E.A. (1959b) *Build and Blood Pressure Study*, Vol. 2, p. 1. Chicago: Society of Actuaries

LOBSTEIN. A.. BRONNER. A. and NORDMANN. J. (1960) De L'interet de la dynamometrie dans glaucome simple. *Ophthalmologica*, **139**, 271

LOBSTEIN. A. and HERR. F.J. (1966) L'ophtalmodynamometrie dans le glaucome. *Ann. Oculist (Paris)*, **199**, 38

McKENNY. J.H.. JENNINGS. W.B. and WHITE. E.V. (1976). Blood pressure screening in community pharmacy. *J. Am. Pharm. Assoc.*, **16**, 4

MATHISEN. H.S.. LOKEN. H.. BROX. D. *et al.* (1965) The prognosis of essential hypertension. *Scand. J. Clin. Lab. Invest.*, **17** (Suppl. 84), 257

MATTEI. T.J.. BALMMER. J.A.. CORBIN. L.A. and DUFFY. M.D. (1973) Hypertension: a model for pharmacy involvement. *Am. J. Hosp. Pharm.*, **30**, 683

MAXWELL. M.H. (1974) Hypertension, a fundamental approach to screening. In *The Hypertension Handbook*. West Point, Pa.: Merek, Sharp, and Dohme

NAGLE. R. (1971) Prognosis of hypertension. *Practitioner*, **207**, 52

PAGE L. and SIDD. J. (1972) Medical management of primary hypertension. *N. Engl. J. Med.*, **287**, 960

PAUL. O. (1971) Risks of mild hypertension: a ten year report. *Br. Heart J.*, **33** (Suppl.), 116

PICKERING. G. (1968) *High Blood Pressure*. London: J. & A. Churchill Ltd.

PICKERING. G. (1974) Hypertension: Definitions, natural histories, and consequences. In *Hypertension Manual: Mechanisms and Management*. edited by J.H. Laragh. New York: Dunn-Donnelly Publishers

ROBINSON. S.C. and BRUCER. M. (1939), Range of normal blood pressure. A statistical and clinical study of 11, 383 persons. *Arch. Intern. Med.* **64**, 409

SCHOENBERGER. J.A. (1971) Management of essential hypertension. *Med. Clin. North. Am.*, **55**, 11

SIMPSON. F.O. and SMIRK. F.H. (1962) The treatment of malignant hypertension. *Am. J. Cardiol.*, **9**, 868

SISLER. H.A. (1972a) Optical–corneal pressure ophthalmodynamometer. *Am. J. Ophthalmol.*, **74**, 987

SISLER. H.A. (1972b), Comparative ophthalmodynamometry using scleral pressure, suction, and corneal pressure units. *Am. J. Ophthalmol.*, **74**, 964

SMIRK. F.H. (1964) Observations on the mortality of 270 treated and 199 untreated retinal grade 1 and 2 hypertensive patients followed in all instances for five years. *N.Z. Med. J.*, **63**, 413

SMIRK. F.H. (1967) The pathogenesis of hypertension. In

Antihypertensive Agents, edited by E. Schlittler, p. 1. New York: Academic Press

STOKES. J.. PAYNE. G. and COOPER. T. (1973) (Editorial) Hypertension control—the challenge of patient education. *N. Engl. J. Med.*, **289**, 1369

THOMAS. C.B., (1952), The heritage of hypertension. *Am. J. Med. Sci.*, **224**, 367

VETERANS ADMINISTRATION CO-OPERATIVE STUDY GROUP ON ANTI-HYPERTENSIVE AGENTS (1967) Effects of treatment on morbidity in hypertension: (1) Results in patients with diastolic blood pressures averaging 115 through 129 mmHg. *J. Am. Med. Assoc.*, **202**, 1028

VETERANS ADMINISTRATION CO-OPERATIVE STUDY GROUP ON ANTI-HYPERTENSIVE AGENTS (1970) Effects of treatment on morbidity in hypertension: (2) Results in patients with diastolic blood pressure averaging 90 through 114 mmHg. *J. Am. Med. Assoc.*, **213**, 1143

WILBUR. J.A. and BARROW. G. (1974) Hypertension, a community problem. In *Hypertension Manual,* edited by J.H. Laragh. New York: Yorke Medical Books

WOLFF. F.W. and LINDEMANN. R.D. (1966) Effect of treatment on hypertension. *J. Chron. Dis.*, **19**, 227

Further reading

SWALES. J.D. (1979) *Clinical Hypertension*. London: Chapman and Hall.

26

Colour vision assessment

Jennifer Birch

All visible hues can be matched by an additive mixture of three primary colours taken from the long wave 'red', the medium wave 'green' and short wave 'blue' parts of the spectrum. The three types of cones contain photopigments which have maximum absorption in these spectral regions. The trichromatic theory of colour vision was proposed by Thomas Young in 1801 and elaborated by Hermann von Helmholtz 50 years later. The three photopigments are not present in equal amounts and the blue receptors are almost absent from the central fovea. This gives rise to the phenomenon of 'small field tritanopia' if colour matches are made within an area subtending less than 0.5°. The size of the field of view is important in colour vision examination. A field size of approximately 2° is preferred as this also ensures that very few rod receptors are stimulated. Red–green vision remains stable throughout life, but threshold blue sensitivity decreases with age due to greater absorption of shorter wavelengths within the crystalline lens. Differences in density of the macular, or lutean, pigment also causes individual variations in threshold blue perception in people with normal colour vision.

Electrical signals from the three types of cone receptor are coded within the neural layers of the retina into three opponent channels. Colour opponent theory, based on colour appearance phenomena such as complementary colours and after images, was first proposed by Ewald Hering in 1870. The coding of signals at the retinal ganglion cell level is extremely complex but Hering's idea of a luminance channel (light opponent to dark) and two colour opponent channels (red opponent to green and blue opponent to yellow) is an acceptable simplification. Opponent channels are maintained in the visual pathway and in the visual cortex. Therefore both the Young–Helmholtz and the Hering theories are necessary to explain the process leading to colour perception.

Defective colour vision

Defective colour vision is characterized by abnormal colour matching and colour confusions. There is a reduction in the number of separate hues that can be distinguished and changes in the relative luminous efficiency of the eye. Colour deficiency is usually congenital but can be acquired.

Congenital colour vision defects

Congenital colour deficiency arises from abnormal cone photopigments. The retina may be lacking in functional cone receptors or there may be only one or two photopigments instead of three. Although three photopigments may be present, one of them may have abnormal absorption characteristics.

Colour vision defects are classified according to the number of primary colours required to match all the spectral hues and thus to the number of photopigments present. The terms used are monochromats, dichromats and anomalous trichromats (*Table 26.1*). Monochromats are of two types: typical or rod monochromats have no functioning cone receptors and in consequence have poor visual acuity (6/60 or 6/36), photophobia and nystagmus; cone monochromats are extremely rare—they have a single cone response and otherwise normal visual function. Dichromats and anomalous trichromats can be further classified according to which of the three photopigments is affected, and whether a pigment is absent or has abnormal absorption characteristics. The collective terms used are 'protan', 'deutan' and 'tritan'. For example, protanopia refers to absence of the 'red' photopigment and protanomalous trichromatism to the presence of a 'red' photopigment with abnormal absorption. These defects are in the protan category: they are similar in type but different in degree. Deuteranopia and deuteranomalous trichromatism are defects of the

Table 26.1 Classification of congential colour vision defects

Type of vision	Subdivision	Colour matching variables	Approximate incidence (%)	
			Male	Female
Normal trichromatism		3	92	99.5
Anomalous trichromatism	Protanomalous	3	1	0.02
	Deuteranomalous	3	5	0.40
	Tritanomalous	3	Unknown	
Dichromatism	Protanopic	2	1	0.02
	Deuteranopic	2	1	0.02
	Tritanopic	2	0.001	0.001
Monochromatism	Cone	1	Unknown	
	Rod (typical)	1	0.003	0.003

'green' photopigment. Tritanopia and tritanomalous trichromatism are defects of the 'blue' photopigment. Protan and deutan defects are sometimes described collectively as red–green defects because they share a tendency to confuse these colours. The hue discrimination ability of anomalous trichromats varies from near dichromatism to nearly normal vision (Wright, 1946). For convenience, some clinical tests differentiate slight, moderate and severe categories. The severe category usually includes dichromats and the most extreme anomalous trichromats.

Protan and deutan defects are inherited in a sex-linked manner (*Figure 26.1*). In males the incidence is approximately 8%. The different types of defect do not occur with the same frequency. Deuteranomalous trichromatism is more common and is found in about 5% of men. Protanopia, protanomalous trichromatism and deuteranopia are each found in about 1% of men, respectively. In communities which are isolated by geographical location or religious practice, the incidence of colour deficiency may differ from the accepted figure. Approximately 0.4% of females are colour defective. The lesser defect is dominant over severe defects.

Congenital tritan defects are inherited as an autosomal dominant trait. An equal number of men and women are affected. The incidence of congenital tritanopia is not thought to be greater than 1 in 13 000, but no reliable estimate of the incidence of tritanomalous trichromatism is available. Normal variations in blue perception make it difficult to distinguish these defects but improvements in tritan screening tests may yield new data shortly.

Congenital colour deficiency is binocular, present at birth and stable throughout life, with no other visual function being affected. Normal colour vision cannot be restored by any known treatment, but the prescription of a coloured filter may assist an individual to complete a particular task or to pass a colour vision test while not implying normal colour vision or correction of the defect (Taylor, 1983). If an aid is prescribed in the form of a monocular contact lens, the practitioner should satisfy himself that the tint is appropriate for the type of defect. Instruction in colour naming should be given and long-term effects monitored. Practitioners should also bear in mind possible legal obligations before prescribing an aid for professional use.

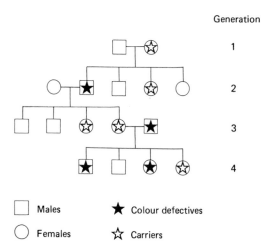

Generation

1

2

3

4

☐ Males   ★ Colour defectives

◯ Females   ☆ Carriers

Figure 26.1 Sex-linked inheritance of red–green colour vision defects. In each generation there are four possible combinations of X and Y chromosomes. Women are able to 'carry' the defect and to pass it to 50% of their sons. Women are only colour defective if they inherit genes for colour deficiency from both parents

Acquired colour vision defects

Acquired colour vision defects occur as secondary features to pathological states. The pathology can be ocular or systemic. Some drugs may produce colour vision defects if given in excessive amounts or if an allergic response occurs. The prolonged use of chloroquine and ethambutol may produce toxic effects on the retina and optic nerve which are responsible for acquired colour deficiency.

Acquired defects fluctuate in severity and are associated with loss of visual acuity and visual field defects. Monocular differences frequently occur. Three types of defect can be distinguished (*Table 26.2*). Acquired defects often show a combination of characteristics associated with more than one type, but dichromatic and anomalous trichromatic stages occur. The perception of blue is particularly vulnerable to pathology and type III defects are found most frequently. Because a neutral zone occurs in the yellow part of the spectrum, these are sometimes erroneously described as 'blue–yellow' defects.

Acquired colour vision defects are of particular interest if they are found to be an early symptom of the causative pathology or can be used to monitor the pathology. Acquired red–green defects do not generally occur without obvious ill health or loss of visual acuity. The exception is in the early stages of Stargardt's disease where the appearance of a red–green defect, in a previously colour normal family member, can be the first easily recognized feature of the disease. The onset of type III defects can be insidious and the defect may be severe before other symptoms are noticed. Type III defects occur in a variety of diseases which either affect the peripheral retina or cause macular oedema. Defects increase in severity with increased loss of visual field or reduction in visual acuity.

In some patients, an initial deterioration in colour vision is followed by a recovery. Patients having

Table 26.2 Classification of acquired colour vision defects

Type

I Red–green
Similar to a protan defect
Found in macular dystrophy

II Red–green
Similar to a deutan defect
Found in retrobulbar neuritis

III Blue
Similar to a tritan defect
Found in many central and peripheral retinal lesions and in lesions of the visual pathway, e.g. senile macular degeneration, central serous retinopathy, retinitis pigmentosa, diabetic retinopathy

disseminated sclerosis can suffer unilateral attacks of retrobulbar neuritis; acuity is greatly reduced and recovers slowly. As vision recovers a type II red–green defect occurs and this may improve from apparent dichromatism to anomalous trichromatism. Even when visual acuity is apparently within normal limits, a slight unilateral colour vision defect may remain (Cox, 1961). Attacks of central serous retinopathy can be monitored in the same way. The type III defect may recover spontaneously as interstitial fluid is reabsorbed, but in severe cases photocoagulation is required. The benefit of this treatment can be assessed according to the improvement in colour vision (Leaver and Williams, 1979).

Non-specific defects can occur. Chronic alcoholics are often malnourished and deficient in vitamin A. Visual acuity is normal but rod function is affected and there is gross constriction of the visual field and an overall reduction in hue discrimination (Bronte-Stewart and Foulds, 1972). Dramatic improvement in colour vision follows oral doses of vitamin A; the field loss recovers more slowly.

Unfortunately the tendency in ocular pathology is towards deterioration of colour vision. Diabetic retinopathy has been studied extensively in this respect. In the early stages of background retinopathy, there is a slight type III defect accompanied by a slight overall reduction in hue discrimination. The colour defect increases in severity as the retinopathy develops (Birch, Hamilton and Gould, 1980). Acquired tritanopia can occur in proliferative retinopathy and in maculopathy. Overall hue discrimination may be so poor that colour-coded methods for assessing glycosuria cannot be interpreted correctly. Panretinal photocoagulation causes a deterioration in colour vision. This can either be permanent or transitory according to the treatment style and extent. However, the loss of colour vision following photocoagulation is not greater than would occur in the non-treated eye.

Colour vision can be disturbed as a result of lesions in the central nervous system. Episodes of coloured vision (coloropsia) may be reported. Alternatively, the patient may have almost complete loss of hue discrimination or may suffer from colour agnosia, the inability to remember colour names (Pearlman, Birch and Meadows, 1979).

Colour vision tests

Clinical colour vision tests are simplified versions of psychophysical measurements which employ spectral stimuli. Only spectral tests, such as the Nagel anomaloscope, are able to distinguish between dichromats and anomalous trichromats. Clinical tests have different aims and functions. Different tests are designed primarily for screening, diagnosis of the type of defect and for grading the degree of the defect. No single test performs all these functions. A battery of tests is recommended for a complete colour vision examination or if occupational advice is to be given.

The efficiency of individual tests depends on good design and on appropriate administration. The design parameters can be analysed in terms of the colour differences employed and whether intended confusion colours are situated within isochromatic zones for each type of defect (Lakowski, 1969). These data, alone, are not sufficient to establish the efficiency of an individual test. This should be confirmed in a clinical trial.

Recommendations for test administration include the viewing time, viewing distance and the lighting conditions. A short viewing time is desirable as this limits colour adaptation effects and a set viewing distance is required in order to control the angular subtense of individual elements of the test. Most tests are designed for use in natural daylight corresponding to overcast north-sky illumination. This is equivalent to standard illuminant C as recommended by the Commission Internationale d'Eclairage. If this is not available in the consulting room, it is best to aim for good blue-white illumination provided by high quality fluorescent lamps. Test performance is stable if the illumination is selected with reasonable care. For many years, the illuminant of choice has been the MacBeth Easel lamp.

The colour vision examination is made at the end of the routine examination when the refractive error and optimum visual acuity have been established. The appropriate refractive correction is worn for the test. The standard of visual acuity is relevant to performance on many clinical tests and is an important consideration when studying acquired defects. If the defect is a congenital one, binocular testing, followed by a brief monocular check, is satisfactory. If an acquired defect is suspected, a monocular examination must be made. It is useful to record the colour vision status of all new patients; thereafter additional examinations will depend on the patient's symptoms and history.

Pseudoisochromatic plates

Pseudoisochromatic plates are the most popular screening tests for defective colour vision. They are quick and easy to use and are inexpensive. There are many different tests available and some appear in several editions. Not all pseudoisochromatic tests are equally efficient.

Most tests are designed to be viewed at 0.66 m. The MacBeth Easel lamp is ideal for this as it incorporates a tray in which the book is placed (*Figure 26.2*). Alternatively, the examiner can give the patient the book to hold. The patient is instructed to indicate the numbers that are seen as

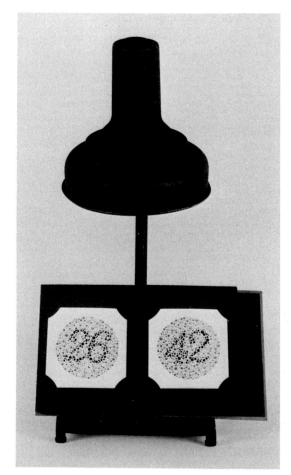

Figure 26.2 The Ishihara pseudoisochromatic plates illuminated with the MacBeth Easel lamp

the page is turned. The examiner turns the pages in order to control the viewing time. About 4 seconds is allowed for each plate. If the figure is not seen in this time, the examiner turns to the next design. Undue hesitation can be a symptom of slight colour deficiency. Cut-out figures can be used to help young children to identify what they see. If illiterate plates are used, the patient should be provided with a clean brush with which to trace the figure.

The Ishihara pseudoisochromatic plates

The Ishihara test is the most popular screening method for red–green defects and clinical trials have shown that it is the most efficient. The full version of the test consists of 25 plates containing numerals. Twenty plates are for screening (plates 2–21) and four for protan/deutan diagnosis:

(1) Plate 1—this is an introductory plate which is correctly seen by all patients. It is useful for

demonstrating the visual task and for detecting malingerers.

(2) Plates 2–9—transformation or confusion designs. One number is seen by colour normals and a different number by colour defective patients. Sometimes colour defective patients see no number.

(3) Plates 10–17—vanishing number designs. A number is read by colour normals but cannot be seen by colour defective patients.

(4) Plates 18–21—hidden digit designs. A number cannot be seen by colour normals but can be read by most colour defective patients.

(5) Plates 22–25—diagnostic designs. Two numbers are presented; only the right hand number can be seen by protan observers and only the left hand number by deutan observers. Sometimes neither number can be seen. This suggests that the patient has a severe red–green defect coupled with a high density of macular pigment. If both numbers are seen, but significant errors have been made on the screening plates, the examiner should ask if one number looks clearer than the other. This often enables the differential diagnosis to be made.

A tentative estimate of the degree of the defect can be made from the number of errors. However, it is important to note what actually constitutes an error. Slight topographical misinterpretation should not be included with these. The test can be abbreviated to a small selection of the most efficient plates, if desired, but it is unwise to rely on a single plate.

The Ishihara plates can be used to examine acquired red–green defects. They are also useful for showing poor overall hue discrimination in some patients with acquired type III defects. These patients cannot read the plates correctly, but cannot see either the confusion or hidden digits.

The American Optical Company (Hardy, Rand and Rittler) plates

The Hardy, Rand and Rittler test is a grading test and is used with the Ishihara test whenever possible. Mild, medium and severe categories are distinguished. Tritan and 'tetartan' plates are included. The 'tetartan' plates were designed when a fourth type of defect involving a possible 'yellow' sensitive pigment was considered possible. It is best to consider these designs as additional tritan plates. Unfortunately, the Hardy, Rand and Rittler plates are no longer available.

The City University test

The City University test is another grading test and is a possible alternative to the Hardy, Rand and Rittler plates. The test is derived from the Farnsworth DI5 panel (Fletcher, 1972). There are two editions of the test and these have similar accuracy (Birch, 1984). Each test consists of 10 charts. These display a central colour and four peripheral colours. The patient is asked to select which of the outer colours looks most like the central colour. A normal selection and diagnostic protan, deutan and tritan colours are displayed. Unfortunately, the differential protan/deutan diagnosis is poor and patients tend to select colours in both diagnostic categories. This is an artefact of the test design and should not be interpreted as a 'mixed' defect. The majority diagnostic response is usually correct but it is probably better to consider that the test indicates red–green defects only. Three categories of red–green defect can be distinguished if the Ishihara plates and the City University test are used together. Significant tritan defects can be detected:

Red–green defect	Ishihara plates	The City University test
Slight	Fail	Pass
Moderate	Fail	Fail with less than 4 red–green errors
Severe	Fail	Fail with more than 4 red–green errors

Farnsworth-Munsell tests

The Farnsworth–Munsell tests were developed to assist in vocational guidance. The standard tests are the Farnsworth DI5 panel and the Farnsworth–Munsell 100-hue test (Farnsworth, 1943). Other tests have been developed from these but are not widely used.

The D15 test is not a screening test. It is designed to indicate 'significant' defects which might lead to occupational difficulties. However, its relevance to occupational needs has not been established. About 5% of men fail the test. The patient arranges the 15 colours in what he considers to be a natural order starting from the reference colour, and the sequence of colours is then plotted on a circular diagram. Typical results are obtained in protan, deutan and tritan defects. The number of errors indicates whether the defect is either moderate or severe (*Figure 26.3*).

The 100-hue test is designed to test hue discrimination ability in normal patients and to examine hue discrimination losses in colour defective patients. The test consists of 85 colour samples representing a complete hue circle in approximately equal steps. The colours are placed in four boxes and the patient is required to arrange the colours, in each box, between two reference colours. The patient is allowed to review the initial colour sequence and to correct any errors. The final arrangement is then

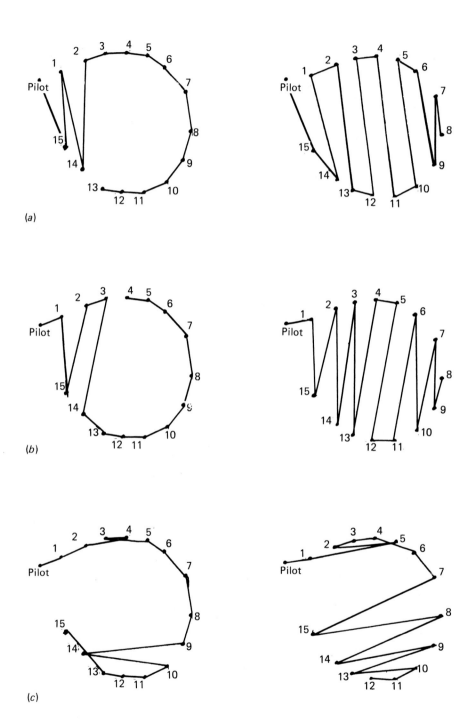

Figure 26.3 Diagnostic results for the Farnsworth D15 panel. (*a*) Moderate and severe protan defects; (*b*) moderate and severe deutan defects; (*c*) moderate and severe tritan defects

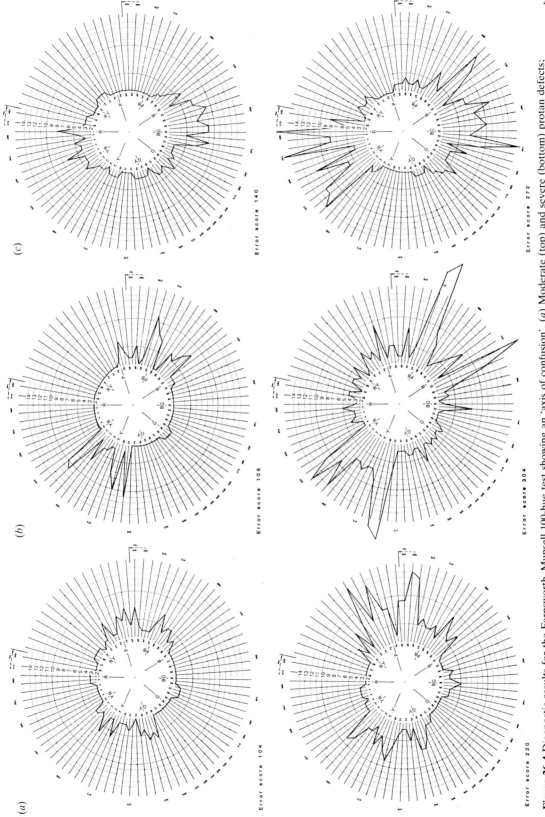

Figure 26.4 Diagnostic results for the Farnsworth–Munsell 100-hue test showing an 'axis of confusion'. (*a*) Moderate (top) and severe (bottom) protan defects; (*b*) moderate (top) and severe (bottom) deutan defects; (*c*) moderate (top) and severe (bottom) tritan defects

Error score 104

Error score 108

Error score 140

Error score 220

Error score 304

Error score 272

recorded. An error score is calculated for each colour by obtaining the sum of the numerical differences of the adjacent colours. This is represented on a radial line, designated for that colour, in a polar diagram. A total error score is then calculated. On-line computers are available which can compute and plot the 100-hue chart automatically.

The 100-hue test is not a screening test. Moderate and severe congenital colour vision defects are demonstrated by a concentration of errors in two well-defined poles which are diametrically opposite in the hue circle. The combined effect is to produce an 'axis of confusion' (*Figure 26.4*). The degree of the defect can be estimated from the total error score.

The 100-hue test is very useful for examining acquired defects. Non-specific defects can be distinguished and fluctuations with time can be monitored (*Figure 26.5*).

The boxes of the 100-hue test should be attempted in order so that either fatigue or learning effects can be recognized. Good results depend on the use of standard lighting conditions and on the skill and motivation of the patient. Intelligent patients can improve their error score on re-test due to familiarity with the test format. The 100-hue test is used in some industries to select recruits with normal colour vision and very good hue discrimination. Deterioration of hue discrimination in the blue part of the hue circle occurs with age. This must be taken into account when examining older patients.

The Nagel anomaloscope

The Nagel anomaloscope is not generally used in optometric practice, but it is an ideal colour vision test for protan and deutan defects. It can be used to show whether a patient has normal or defective colour vision, whether the defect is protan or deutan and whether the patient is a dichromat or an anomalous trichromat. Its use is essential in clinical trials to categorize the colour defective patients taking part. The examination relies on the fact that an additive mixture of monochromatic red and green light appears the same as a yellow light (the Rayleigh match). Individuals with normal colour vision make precise colour matches within a small range of red/green ratios. Anomalous trichromats match outside this range. Deuteranomalous trichromats require more green in their mixture and protanomalous trichromats more red. The range of acceptable matches indicates the severity of the defect. Protanopes and deuteranopes are able to match any red/green ratio, from pure red to pure green, with yellow because they have only one photopigment in this range. They are distinguished by the relative luminance needed in the yellow comparison field (Schmidt, 1955; Birch, 1982).

The test procedure is as follows: the patient adjusts all the matching controls to obtain three precise colour matches; in between matches the patient looks away from the instrument and the examiner resets the scales with the matching field firstly too red and then too green. No more than 10 seconds should be allowed for each match. The second part of the examination is to explore the matching range. To do this the examiner sets the red/green mixture in steps. At each setting the patient establishes whether a precise colour match is possible by altering the luminance of the yellow field only. The aim is to determine the limits of the matching range using the patient's previous matches as a guide.

There is no comparable colour match capable of distinguishing tritan defects. The use of selective colour adaptation holds more promise as a diagnostic test.

The Pickford–Nicolson anomaloscope is a filter instrument and does not have the same efficiency either for screening or for diagnosis of the type of defect. Three colour matches can be obtained, a red/green match with yellow, a blue/green match with blue-green and a blue/yellow match with white. The results are treated statistically and are recorded in terms of standard deviations.

Colour vision lanterns

The use of colour names is avoided in a colour vision examination. Tests rely on the recognition of a figure, the ability to arrange colours in order or the ability to match colours together. Correct colour names for familiar objects are learned in childhood and it is only if shape and location clues are removed that false colour naming can be revealed.

Colour vision lanterns are vocational tests. They are designed to assess signal recognition in military, maritime, aviation and transport services. Lanterns can be used either for protan/deutan screening or as a grading test to distinguish severe red–green defects only. There are two types displaying either pairs of colours or single colours. Instruments which display pairs of colours, such as the Holmes–Wright lantern, are restricted in availability—only white, red and green colours are used. The presentation is automatic and the results are treated statistically. Prolonged dark adaptation is sometimes used prior to the test. Lanterns which show single colours include yellow as well as white, red and green. This is particularly helpful for demonstrating false colour naming in anomalous trichromats (Giles, 1960). The colour sequence and speed of presentation is critical to the efficiency of the test (Birch, 1974).

There are two Giles–Archer lanterns. The Aviation model contains two extra colours 'light green' (LG) and 'signal yellow' (SY). These are named

415

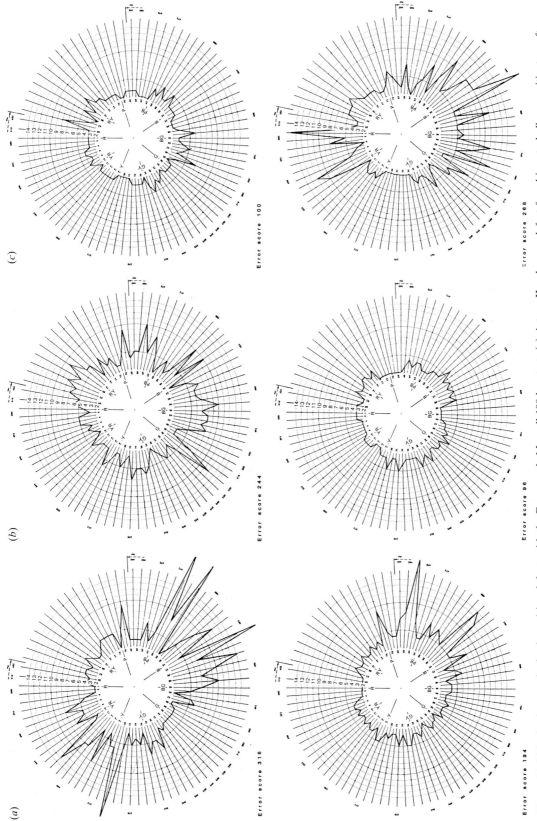

(a)

Error score 316

Error score 194

(b)

Error score 244

Error score 96

(c)

Error score 100

Error score 268

Figure 26.5 Monitoring acquired colour vision defects with the Farnsworth–Munsell 100-hue test. (*a*) A type II red–green defect found in retrobulbar neuritis; top: after attack V/A 6/12; bottom: 1 year later V/A 6/9. (*b*) A non-specific loss of hue discrimination found in vitamin A deficiency (from Bronte-Stewart and Foulds, 1971 with permission); top: before treatment V/A 6/9; bottom: 1 week later following oral doses of vitamin A V/A 6/6. (*c*) A type III blue defect found in proliferative diabetic retinopathy. Top: before treatment V/A 6/9; bottom: after Argon laser panretinal photocoagulation V/A 6/9

incorrectly by normal observers and should not be used. For a routine examination the lantern should be positioned adjacent to the test chart and viewed by the patient at 6 metres. No extra dark adaptation is required. There should be just sufficient ambient illumination to enable the examiner to adjust the lantern and write down the results. It is best to work out the colour sequence beforehand, so that a score sheet can be prepared and errors recorded quickly. The colours should be exposed for a matter of a few seconds, just giving the patient enough time to name the colour. The aperture is then covered by the examiner's hand while the next colour is selected and then presented. The patient should be instructed that only the colour names red, yellow, green and white are allowed. Care should be taken to interpose either yellow or white between the red and green colours in the order of presentation. The sequence must be repetitive and should consist of at least 20 presentations. The large aperture is used initially and the test repeated with smaller apertures only if the results are indecisive.

Errors are as follows:

(1) Any misnaming of red.
(2) Any misnaming of green.
(3) Yellow called either red or green.
(4) Inability to distinguish red at large aperture, i.e. called 'no light.'

The following are not errors:

(1) White called yellow.
(2) Yellow called white.
(3) Inability to distinguish red at small aperture.

The type of error is informative (*Table 26.3*). If the requirements of a particular occupation are that only red and green must be correctly named, about 20% of patients with defective colour vision are able to pass the test—these are usually slight anomalous trichromats. Good screening efficiency is obtained if the incorrect naming of yellow is included as an error. The inability of protanopes to see dark red because of 'shortening of the red end of the spectrum' is a diagnostic feature.

Occupational requirements

Normal colour vision is generally required for the following occupations: the armed services; the merchant navy; customs and excise officers; electrical and electronic engineering; transport services (aviation, railways and bus driving); the police and fire services; chemistry (including chemical engineering, pharmacy and laboratory technology); textile and printing trades.

There are many other occupations, such as horticulture and cartography, in which defective colour vision is a handicap. Colour coding is used widely in business and industry and complex codes are sometimes used in learning systems for reading and mathematics. It is important that children should be examined for defective colour vision at an appropriate age so that areas of potential difficulty can be identified and last minute career disappointments avoided. The degree of difficulty experienced will depend on the type of defect and its severity. Protans are likely to experience more practical difficulties than deutans because of the reduced visibility of reds. This may cause problems in the identification of traffic lights, especially at night. Clinical tests designed for grading the severity of colour deficiency successfully indicate patients who are most at risk in the use of colour codes.

Table 26.3 Typical errors in colour naming with the Giles–Archer lantern

| Colour order | | | | | | | | | | | | | | | | | | | |
G	W	DR	R	Y	SG	Y	R	W	G	Y	DR	W	SG	Y	R	G	Y	G	W
Protanope	(W)	W	—	R	Y	(W)	(G)	R	W	(R)	Y	—	W	(W)	Y	R	(Y)	(R)	G	W
Deuteranope	(Y)	W	R	R	Y	G		(R)	R	W	(R)	(R)	R		W	(W)	(R)	R	(R)	(G)	(R)	W
Protanomalous trichromat	(Y)	(G)	R	R	Y	G	Y	R	W	(Y)	Y	R	W	G	Y	R	(Y)	(G)	(Y)	W
Deuteranomalous trichromat	(W)	W	R	R	Y	G	(R)	R	W	G	(G)	R	W	G	Y	R	(W)	Y	G	W

G = green.   SG = signal green.
R = red.   DR = dark red.
Y = yellow.   W = white.
— = nothing seen.

Errors in colour naming are bracketed.

References

BIRCH. J. (1974) Colour vision tests and colour vision advice. *Br. J. Physiol. Opt.*, **29**, 1–29

BIRCH. J. (1982) Diagnosis of defective colour vision using the Nagel Anamaloscope. *Doc. Ophthalmol. Proc. Ser.*, **33**, 231–235

BIRCH. J. (1984) The contribution of the City University test (first and second editions) in a clinical test laboratory. *Doc. Ophthal. Proc. Series*, **39**, 193–198

BIRCH. J. HAMILTON, A.M. and GOULD. E.S. (1980) Colour vision in relation to the clinical features and extent of field loss in diabetic retinopathy. *Colour Deficiencies* V, pp. 83–88. Bristol: Adam Hilger

BRONTE-STEWART. J. and FOULDS. W.S. (1972) Dyschromatopsia in vitamin A deficiency. In *Modern Problems in Ophthalmology*, edited by G. Verriest, Vol. II, pp. 168–178. Basel: Karger

COX. J. (1961) Unilateral colour deficiency. *J. Opt. Soc. Am.*, **51**, 992–999

FARNSWORTH. D. (1943) The Farnsworth–Munsell 100-Hue and Dichotomous tests for colour vision *J. Opt. Soc. Am.*, **33**, 568–578

FLETCHER. R.J. (1972) A modified D15 test. In *Modern Problems in Ophthalmology*, edited by G. Verriest, Vol. II, pp. 22–24. Basel: Karger

GILES. G.H. (1960) *Principles and Practice of Refraction*, p. 366, London: Hammond

LAKOWSKI. R. (1969) Theory and practice of colour vision testing. *Br. J. Industr. Med.*, **26**, 173–189, 265–288

LEAVER. P.K. and WILLIAMS. C.M. (1979) Argon laser photocoagulation in the treatment of central serous retinopathy. *Br. J. Ophthalmol.*, **63**, 674–677

PEARLMAN. A.L.. BIRCH J. and MEADOWS. J.C. (1979) Cerebral colour blindness, an acquired defect in hue discrimination. *Ann. Neurol.*, **15**, 253–261

SCHMIDT. I. (1955) Some problems relating to testing vision with the Nagel Anomaloscope. *J. Opt. Soc. Am.*, **45**, 514–522

TAYLOR. S.P. (1983) The X Chrom lens—a case study. *Ophthal. Physiol. Opt.*, **2**, 165–170

WRIGHT. W.D. (1946) Researches on normal and defective colour vision, p. 304, London: Henry Kimpton

Further reading

BOYNTON. R.M. (1979) *Human Colour Vision*. New York: Hart, Rinehart & Winston

POKORNY. J.. SMITH V.C.. VERRIEST. G. and PINCKERS. A.J.L.G. (1979) *Congenital and Acquired Colour Vision Defects*. New York: Grune & Stratton.

27

Aniseikonia—a classical and clinical review

Kenneth Harwood

Early history

Donders (1864) first postulated that inequality of image size must often result from the correction of refraction which was unequal between the eyes. He recognized that in small inequalities binocular vision is hardly affected, but that in larger inequalities confusion and diplopia may result. He even suggested that to employ lenses of different specification (for example, to reverse one of a periscopic pair so that the more strongly curved surface is nearer the eye for the more hyperopic eye of the anisometropic pair) would diminish, if not fully correct, the difference of image size.

Lancaster (1938) first appreciated that unequal image size is not always or wholly due to unequal refraction; he suggested that it might arise from an unequal distribution of the retinal receptors—as in the slightly stretched retina of a lengthened myopic eye—or from an inequality of the cortical representation of two equal optical images. He first used the term 'aniseikonia', which is derived from the Greek: *an* (not), *iso* (equal), *eikon* (image), *ia* (state of), and it is clear from later work that aniseikonia may indeed arise in emmetropia or isometropia, although this is uncommon, while occasionally in the anisometropic case, where a size difference would be expected, nothing measurable may be detected. A typical example is quoted by Gillott (1956–57).

The symptoms of aniseikonia

Most aniseikonic symptoms are indistinguishable from those associated with uncorrected refractive errors and uncompensated phorias; complaints of the actual distortion of visual space, persisting after a period of adaptation to a new correction, are rare, except in the higher disparities. Asthenopia, head-aches and reading difficulties are the most common. For an early list, graduated by relative frequency, *see* Bannon and Triller (1944).

Because the symptoms are not pathognomonic, the assessment of a case must always commence with the elimination of more general pathological and ocular causes. An accurate refraction is required, and an inspection of the current correction to make certain that it is accurately dispensed for centration and vertex distance. Uncompensated phoria should be dealt with by orthoptics or prismatic relief before embarking upon size measurements. However, it is not uncommon for a patient to present with aniseikonic symptoms wearing an accurate, well dispensed correction; indeed the aniseikonic clinic tends to become the last resort of the 'grief case'.

Instrumentation

Direct comparison eikonometer

This first, practicable instrument (*Figure 27.1*) for measuring size difference was developed at the Dartmouth Eye Institute, Hanover, New Hampshire, by Ames, Gliddon and Ogle during many years of classic research into problems of vision. In its final form, it depended upon the then recently invented polarizing film to differentiate the images seen by the two eyes. Odd numbered images were perceived by one eye, even numbered by the other. The images were equalized by variable size lens cells which produced magnifications over a ±5% range, with horizontal effect before one eye and vertical effect before the other.

However, this instrument proved limited in its usefulness to measurements in the horizontal and vertical only; its accuracy was established by taking measurements with plano size lenses of known effect

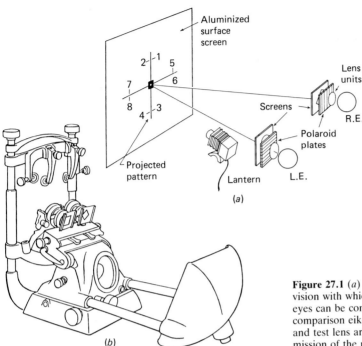

Figure 27.1 (*a*) Scheme of the eikonometer for distant vision with which the relative sizes of images in the two eyes can be compared directly. (*b*) The direct comparison eikonometer showing details of the headrest and test lens arrangement. (From Ogle, 1950, with permission of the publishers, W.B. Saunders, Philadelphia)

and using several observers. In size disparities at oblique axes, such as often occur with oblique cylinders, the fixation disparity, among other factors, proved too disturbing for useful measurement.

The space eikonometer

This instrument was also developed at Dartmouth, in succession to the direct comparison eikonometer. It made use of a target comprising four vertical strings in two frontoparallel planes, with a rectangular oblique cross between and equidistant from these pairs. *Figure 27.2* shows the layout of the target and the appearance of the measuring head, which uses the same variable magnification cells as the direct comparison eikonometer.

Method of measurement

To measure horizontal magnification, the horizontal magnifying cell before the right eye is adjusted to give either positive or negative magnification, until the vertical strings appear aligned in the frontoparallel plane. *Figure 27.3* shows the relationship between the direct comparison and the stereoscopic, space eikonometer methods of determining the sensitivity to size difference in the horizontal.

Now, if the cross appears vertical in the fronto-

parallel plane, horizontal size difference only is present. If not, the correcting horizontal size difference is left set up and the patient's attention is directed to the cross. If this appears to be rotated about a vertical axis, because horizontal differences have been corrected, it must be due to a vertical magnification which appears to stretch the cross vertically in the image of one eye, so that relative vertical magnification, using the left magnifier, must be applied to the eye away from which the cross appears to be twisted. Both cells have a range of $\pm 5\%$, and the sign convention is that right eye magnifications are positive and left eye negative.

If both the vertical lines and the cross appear to lie in the frontoparallel plane, the total size difference is a combination of exactly horizontal and vertical elements. But if the axes of the magnification ellipse are not horizontal and vertical, the vertical line through the cross undergoes a rotary deviation making the cross appear to be tilted towards or away from the observer. This obliquity is measured by the rotation of an equal pair of meridional magnifiers set at 45° and 135° in front of the other cells, geared together so that they rotate in equal and opposite directions; hence the horizontal and vertical components of the pair are always equal, and do not disturb the horizontal and vertical components already measured. This deviation angle, δ, is considered positive if the axes must be rotated tops towards each other to restore the cross to the vertical plane, and negative if rotated away. The

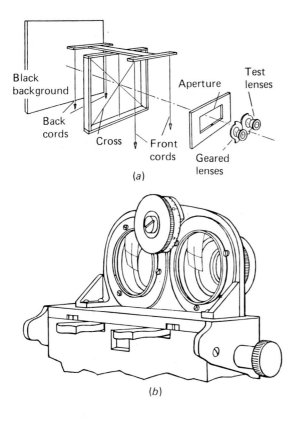

(a)

(b)

Figure 27.2 (*a*) Perspective drawing showing essential features of the space eikonometer. (*b*) The declination device used on the space eikonometer. Also shown is the location of the adjustable magnification units and cells for holding lenses. (From Ogle, 1950, with permission of the publishers, W.B. Saunders, Philadelphia)

relation is given by:

$$\delta = 0.57m\sin2\rho$$

where *m* is the percentage magnification of the paired lenses, and ρ is the actual angle through which the lenses have been rotated. A fuller explanation and analysis of the above is given by Ogle (1950).

This last setting should complete the measurement. Each setting will, however, have a small effect on the others, and therefore it is best to return to the horizontal setting and adjust each in a succession of approximations.

Patients vary widely in their accuracy of observation. Quite often the stereoscopic effects are not at first distinguished, and some practice, using extreme variations of settings, is necessary to demonstrate what is required. A 'bracketing' system is the most effective, showing the effect first of +4%, then −4%, and then slowly reducing the spread. For example, the next settings might be +3% and −3%, at which the effect of the first might be less distinguishable than the second. This suggests +2.5% followed by 0%, arriving finally at perhaps 1.5%. It is usual to add the range over which change cannot be detected; ±0.2% would indicate a satisfactory accuracy for the horizontal element (HOR), ±0.4% for the vertical (VER), 0±10 for δ. A similar routine is followed for the vertical and declination components.

The process is visually tiring, and several sets of readings should be made with substantial rest periods between each set. Furthermore, it is often wise to repeat the measurements on another occasion if an expensive pair of lenses is to be ordered. If

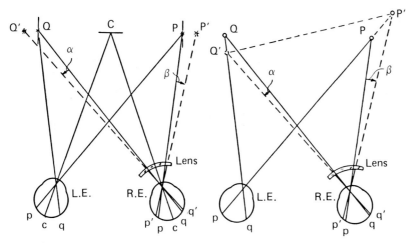

Figure 27.3 Relationship between the direct comparison and the stereoscopic space eikonometer methods of determining sensitivity to size difference in the horizontal. (From Ogle, 1950, with permission of the publishers, W.B. Saunders, Philadelphia)

readings of 0.5% HOR ±1.0%, or +1.5% VER ±2.0% are recorded repeatedly, the readings are probably worthless, and such an inadequate observer is unlikely to be troubled by a size difference of this amount, even if it does exist.

A very good observer may be expected to set the horizontal element within ±0.2%, the vertical component within ±0.4%, and declination within 5° or 10°. This greatly depends on acuity, and is unlikely to be true of patients with less than 6/6 acuity in each eye. Measurements can be made with acuities as low as 6/18, in the opinion of Bannon (1965), but in the present author's experience reliability falls off very rapidly as acuity decreases from 6/6. Distortion of the cross sometimes occurs, so that one limb only may appear 'towards'. A careful correction of phorias, especially the vertical, will often minimize this effect, but sometimes it must be accepted and the patient asked to assess the cross 'as a whole'.

The notation may be written in different ways. For example: R +1.5% ±0.4% HOR, L −2.2% ±0.6% VER, may be written R +1.5% HOR, +2.2% VER with sufficient accuracy. This would involve magnification of the right eye only, although the form of the left lens must be taken into account when designing the right lens.

It is usually most convenient to correct the refraction with thin flat trial case lenses in the cells of the instrument to minimize shape effect, but with lenses of higher powers, curvatures and thicknesses must be taken into account and the relative magnifications calculated. This is even more important with the patient's curved lens correction.

Prescribing

Having arrived at an assessment of size difference which seems likely to have clinical significance, Berte and Harwood (1961) have found it very useful, when the magnification is essentially uniocular, to tape a plano magnifying lens over the appropriate lens of the spectacles. This should be worn for a week and, if increased comfort is reported, the lens should be taped to the other eye as a provocative test. If increased discomfort is reported, or the lens removed before reporting, the need of a size correction is endorsed in a most satisfactory way. However, if equal comfort is reported it may be assumed that the response is psychological only. Size corrections should always be conservative and undercorrected, rather than fully corrected.

The equations for the aniseikonic ellipse are given by Ogle (1950):

$$\tan 2\phi = 3.5\delta \,/(v-h)$$
$$f = 3.5 \,(v-h) \cos 2\phi$$
$$o = 0.5 \,(v+h-f)$$
$$m_0 = o + f$$
$$m_{0+90} = o$$

where h and v are the measured horizontal and vertical components, ϕ the major axis of the ellipse (when δ is positive, 2ϕ is less than 180°, and when negative, between 180° and 360°), o the magnification along the short axis of the ellipse, and $o+f$ that along the long axis.

The most useful guide to the clinician is Bannon's *Clinical Guide to Aniseikonia*. This describes the space eikonometer, giving much sound advice on measurement and its interpretation and including suggestions on cases where size correction is inappropriate, and a long series of case reports. Ogle's equations above may, of course, be used to obtain the magnification ellipse. However, an alternative and quicker method is to use the tables published by The American Optical Company (1957).

Iseikonic lenses were discussed by Bennett (1937) and by Linksz and Bannon (1965). The design of correcting lenses to include the required magnification makes use of the formula:

$$M = \frac{1}{1 - F_1 \,(t/n)}$$

where M is the magnification, F_1 the front surface power, t the thickness in cm, and n the refractive index. Percentage magnification m is given by

$$m = 100(M - 1)$$

or, with sufficient accuracy:

$$m = F_1 \,(t/n)$$

As a general rule for glass with an approximate refractive index of 1.5, m increases by 0.1% for each 1.5 mm increase in thickness, and is proportional directly to F_1. Thickness and curvature may therefore be juggled to give the best cosmetic result, but, on the whole, increases in curvature are preferable to increases in thickness.

However, A.G. Bennett (1961, personal communication) has designed a very useful chart which enables the effects of curvature and thickness to be appreciated at a glance (*Figure 27.4*).

The aniseikonic pair usually comprises two bitoric lenses. The axes of back and front toric surfaces must be placed with great accuracy, since very small departures from parallelism causes large changes in the powers and axes of the correction. It frequently occurs that the axes of the aniseikonic ellipse are not identical with the axes of astigmatism, and then it is necessary to compromise. Where the astigmatism is of low degree, it may be necessary to rotate its axis to that of the ellipse, but where of higher degree it is better to adjust the ellipse axis to the astigmatic.

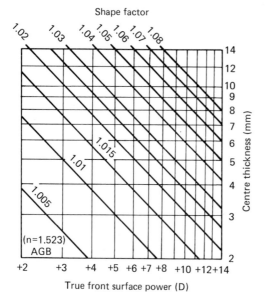

Shape factor

True front surface power (D)

Figure 27.4 Chart to facilitate design of aniseikonic lenses. Each point on a diagonal line represents a possible combination of front surface power and centre thickness that would produce the given magnification. For example, a 4% (shape) magnification would be obtainable with a front surface power of +10 D and a centre thickness of 5.9 mm or, alternatively, with +8 D at 7.4 mm. (Reproduced by courtesy of A.G. Bennett)

Other methods of assessing size difference

The space eikonometer occupies a great deal of room, and the American Optical Company produced a compact instrument, the Office Model Eikonometer, which is about the size of a synoptophore. This makes use of photographic transparencies which are fused binocularly for stereoscopic vision. Projection lenses of about 6 D are used to project the image to a distance of about 3 m. Horizontal magnification is controlled by a variable magnifier before the right eye, and vertical magnification by a similar device before the left eye. As in the original instrument, declination is measured by a matched pair of meridional size lenses mounted so that these can be rotated by equal and opposite amounts.

The result is a small compact instrument which gives good results, although its users find that it should be moved some way from any wall to avoid proximity effects. This instrument is no longer manufactured.

The Charnwood stereograms represent the space eikonometer target as seen with several differing magnifications, and is intended as a screening device to be used in a stereoscope. Charnwood

(1952) noted that a very high quality stereoscope is required without which the results tend to be inconclusive.

The Simplified Space Eikonometer of Malin (1955) represented an attempt to adapt normal consulting room equipment to the task. A Stevens phorometer head was modified to contain the geared declination lenses, with the gearing altered to rotate the lenses in equal and opposite directions. Loose meridional size lenses measured *H* and *V*. Despite the rather crude system, the author was able to prescribe 28 corrections (63 were examined) and claimed definite benefit for 28 patients.

Pedersen (1958) adopted an entirely different approach. Rather than use measuring lenses, the targets were arranged to be movable so as to bring the image into the frontoparallel plane. The overall length of the instrument is 93 cm. A frame holding the front vertical cords pivots about a vertical axis, the central cross pivots about both horizontal and vertical axes, and the back vertical cords are fixed. A range of ±6% is attainable. Pedersen has published tables to convert rotations to percentage magnifications, and reliability was tested with loose size lenses and was found to be good.

Hawkswell (1974, 1975) constructed an instrument on similar lines with an overall length of 60 cm. He investigated 1000 'measurable cases' seen in hospital practice. It was observed that of 409 patients with some degree of aniseikonia, 373 were symptom free. Analysis of the symptoms reported by the remaining 36 patients was:

Symptoms	No. of cases	Percentage size difference
Vertigo	5	2–7
Vertigo with disordered spatial judgment	9	2–7
As above, and headache	2	3–5
Vertigo and diplopia	20	8–18

This lists the more extreme symptoms of the condition. It does not include the milder discomforts of asthenopia and reading difficulty which are generally regarded (Bannon, 1965) as associated with aniseikonia. This is possibly due to the hospital conditions of the survey, and the difficulty of ensuring that patients with such lesser symptoms were, at the time of measurement, adequately corrected. Hawkswell's final conclusion was that some 3.6% of his patients had symptoms of aniseikonia, as defined above.

Gillott (1956) constructed a space eikonometer of the original design, and made careful measurements of 100 subjects comprising a normal cross-section of the population, chosen 'on a basis of their availability'. One person was checked over a one-month period for repeatability, and was found to be satisfactory. Of 17 emmetropic patients, 10 were found to have negligible size difference, defined as less than 0.8% (in common with Bannon). But the other seven had size errors of between 0.8 and 3.0%.

Of 43 isometropic subjects, 11 showed size differences, none more than 2.0%, but none reported symptoms of the commonly associated type.

A particular study of 40 anisometropic subjects was made—60% were aniseikonic (24). Of these, 17 displayed size difference which corresponded with the anisometropia, i.e. that the larger retinal image corresponded with the more hyperopic eye. The anisometropes ranged from a refractive difference of 0.5 D upwards, but among those with more than 1 D differences, there was better correspondence between refraction and size. Of the subjects showing greater levels of aniseikonia, six were anisometropic and one emmetropic. His results on anisometropia seem to suggest that, in the absence of actual measurement, some approximation and correction of assumed size difference based on the degree of hyperopia is justified and this may be important in the treatment of squint. However there are exceptions.

Gillott considered that four of his 100 subjects would have benefited from size correction but was not in a position to prescribe.

Other publications and surveys

Ogle (1952) investigated the size effect of prisms. Fisher and Ludlow (1963) proposed and used afterimages for measuring size difference in squint; this was a laborious method with uncertain results. Burian and Ogle (1952) reported two cases of increasing myopia: one due to nuclear sclerosis of the crystalline lens, which showed increasing size difference, and one due to axial lengthening, which showed none. Troutman (1963) discussed size difference in relation to postcataract implants. Davis (1959) proposed an approximate rule for estimating and correcting size differences in the pre-school anisometrope. He followed Bannon in adding 1% magnification for each 1 D of anisometropia. This simple rule is easily applied clinically. Margach (1964) attacked the same problem analytically and produced rather complex rules. Brown and Enoch (1970) proposed rules for an approximate correction by changes in thickness, power, and vertex distance. Keating (1982) formulated a matrix method for considering aniseikonia, for which many advantages were claimed. Bannon *et al.* (1970) reviewed the history of aniseikonia and space perception over the last 50 years.

Conclusion

The history of aniseikonia is long, and much effort and ingenuity has been expended on its problems. It has never attained much importance in the consulting room, and the manufacture of the Office Model Eikonometer has ceased. Comparative lack of clinical interest may be due, in part, to more accurate methods of refraction and correction, and more advanced orthoptic treatment, which have rendered fewer the grief cases which are the eikonometrist's parish.

However, those who have practised the art will confirm that there are still some cases for which size lenses are the only solution to the problems of discomfort, and these are often some of the more observant and rewarding patients.

The field of the child anisometrope, with amblyopia and with or without a squint, could be better explored, and approximate estimated size corrections undoubtedly have a place.

Malin (1955) and Hawkswell (1974, 1975) have shown what can be done with simple instruments, and with these perhaps lies the future.

References

AMERICAN OPTICAL COMPANY (1957) *Magnification Tables for use with the Space Eikonometer*. New York: American Optical Company

BANNON, R. E. and TRILLER, W. Aniseikonia — a clinical report covering a ten year period. *Am.J.Optom.*, **21**, 171–182

BANNON, R.E. (1964, 1965) *A Clinical Manual on Aniseikonia*. American Optical Co.

BENNETT, A.G. (1937) The fundamental principles of aniseikonic lenses. *Optician*, Jan., Feb.

BERTE, A.P. and HARWOOD, K.A. (1961) The clinical correction of aniseikonia. *Br. J. Physiol. Opt.*, **18**, 108–116

BROWN, R.M. and ENOCH, J.M. (1970) Combined rules of thumb in aniseikonia. *Am. J. Ophthalmol.*, **69**, 118–126

BURIAN, H.M. and OGLE, K.N. (1952) Aniseikonia with increased unilateral index myopia. *Am. J. Ophthalmol.*, **26**, 480–489

BANNON, R. E., NEUMUELTER, J., BOEDER, P. and BURIAN, H. M. (1970) Aniseikonia and space perception – after 50 years. *Am. J. Ophthalmol.*, **42**, 423–441

CHARNWOOD, LORD (1952) A new test for measuring aniseikonia. *Optician*, Dec 26th

DAVIS, R.J. (1959) Empirical correction of aniseikonia in preschool anisometropia. *Am. J. Optom Physiol. Opt.*, **36**, 351–364

DONDERS, F.C. (1864) *The Accommodation and Refraction of the Eye*, translated by W.D. Moore, pp. 565–566. The New Sydenham Society

FISHER, H.M. and LUDLOW, W.M. (1963) An approach to

measuring aniseikonia in non-fusing strabmismus. *Am. J. Ophthalmol.*, **40**, 653–655

GILLOTT, H. F.. (1956) The effect on binocular vision of variation in the relative sizes and levels of illumination of the ocular images. *Br. J. Physiol. Opt.* **13**, 122–146.

GILLOTT, H.F. (1957) The effect on binocular vision of variation in the relative sizes and levels of illumination of the ocular images. *Br. J. Physiol. Opt.*, **14**, 43–58

HAWKSWELL, A. (1974). Routine aniseikonic screening. *Br. J. Physiol. Opt.*, 126–129.

HAWKSWELL, A. (1975). The development of a portable space eikonometer. *Br. J. Physiol. Opt.*, **30**, 25–33

KEATING, H. (1982) A matrix formation of spectacle magnification. *Ophthal. Physiol. Opt.*, **2**, 145–158

LANCASTER, W.B. (1938) Aniseikonia. *Arch. Ophthalmol.*, **20**, 907–912

LINKSZ, A. and BANNON, R.E. (1965) Aniseikonia and refractive problems. *Int. Ophthalmol. Clin.*, **5**, 515–534

MALIN, A.H. (1955) Testing anisekonia with a simplified space eikonometer. *Am. J. Optom. Physiol. Opt.*, **32**, 30–40

MARGACH, C.B. (1964) Aniseikonia in anisometropia. *Aust. J. Optom.*, **XLVII**, 299–304

OGLE, K.N. (1950) *Researches in Binocular Vision.* New York: W.B. Saunders & Co.

OGLE, K.N. (1952) Distortion of the image by ophthalmic prisms. *Arch. Ophthalmol.*, **47**, 121–131

PEDERSEN, M.R. (1958) The construction of a space eikonometer and the correction of aniseikonometer. *Aust. J. Optom.*, **XII**, Nov.

TROUTMAN, R.C. (1963) Artiphakia and aniseikonia. *Am. J. Ophthalmol.*, **56**, 602–639

Part 7

Ocular pharmacology

28

Pharmacological principles

Janet Vale

Whenever drugs are used for therapeutic, prophylactic or diagnostic purposes the important principle is to get sufficient drug to the site of action (wherever that is) and to keep it there sufficiently long to exert the required action. The drug level achieved and the time for which this level is maintained are determined by factors such as administration (route and frequency), absorption from the site of administration, distribution within the body and elimination. Elimination in this context is taken to include both excretion (mainly through the kidneys) and the conversion of the active drug to inactive products (mainly by metabolism in the liver).

The route of administration may be chosen for convenience, dictated by stability of the drug and the ease (or lack) of absorption from certain sites and influenced by the desire for a systemic or local, e.g. ocular, effect. Absorption, distribution and metabolism are determined by two main properties of the drug molecule in question, namely the lipid/water solubility ratio and the degree of ionization. This is because absorption, distribution and the relative need for metabolism are all concerned with the ability of drug molecules to cross biological membranes passively, i.e. not involving any specialized active transport mechanisms. This movement may be from the site of administration, e.g. the gastrointestinal tract, from one 'compartment' to another in the body, or across the membranes of the kidney tubule during excretion.

Lipid/water solubility ratio

All biological membranes have a similar basic structure, namely a biomolecular layer of lipids containing protein and small water-filled 'pores' or channels. This membrane is impermeable to water-soluble molecules unless they are sufficiently small to pass through the pores in the lipid material (molecular weight of 100 or less), whereas it is readily permeable to lipid-soluble molecules. Few water-soluble drugs have a molecular weight below 100, and so most drugs with a high water solubility cross biological membranes only poorly. Those with high lipid solubility cross readily and those with intermediate properties show intermediate behaviour. As a consequence of this behaviour at biological membranes, lipid-soluble drugs are well absorbed from the site of administration, e.g. the gastrointestinal tract, are distributed outside the vascular system, cross the blood–brain barrier into the CNS and are metabolized, mainly in the liver, before being excreted by the kidneys. Metabolism converts the drug into metabolites with increased water solubility which are more readily excreted. Without this metabolism, lipid-soluble drugs would be reabsorbed from the kidney tubule after filtration at the glomerulus (because of the ease with which they cross membranes). Water-soluble drugs are only poorly absorbed from the site of administration, are largely restricted to the vascular system, do not cross the blood–brain barrier and do not undergo metabolism before excretion. Many drugs fall into an intermediate category and are handled in a manner between the two extremes.

Degree of ionization

The second factor which largely determines the handling of a drug by the body is the degree of ionization. Many drugs are weak acids or weak bases and, therefore, can exist in both a non-ionized and an ionized form. The ratio of the two forms, the degree of ionization, is determined by the pH of the media in which the drug is present, e.g. solution, stomach contents, kidney tubule, and the pK_a. The pK_a is an inherent, immutable property of the drug and indicates its tendency to ionize. The degree of ionization of a drug molecule is important because the ionized form is generally water soluble and, therefore, only crosses biological membranes poorly, whereas the non-ionized form is usually lipid soluble and readily crosses membranes. Thus the ease with which weak acids and bases are absorbed, distributed and eliminated will be influenced by the degree of ionization. Within limits, the pH may be changed to influence the degree of ionization and, therefore, the absorption or elimination of a drug.

Ophthalmic drugs

Drugs used by the optometric practitioner are applied topically to concentrate the drug in the eye and prevent unwanted systemic effects. In this situation, absorption must take place across the cornea. When considering the absorption of drugs applied to the cornea, the situation is slightly different to that above because the structure of the cornea is somewhat different from other biological membranes. From the point of view of drug absorption the cornea may be considered to have three layers: the epithelium, the stroma and the endothelium. The epithelium and endothelium both have a high lipid content while the stroma has a high water content. Thus, the epithelium and endothelium are readily penetrated by lipid-soluble molecules and the stroma by water-soluble molecules. In order for a drug to penetrate through all layers of the cornea to reach a site of action in the anterior chamber, it must possess a degree of both lipid and water solubility. Solubility in only lipid or water will limit the absorption of the drug. This may occasionally be useful, as with the water-soluble stain fluorescein which is unable to penetrate the lipid epithelium while it is intact. One explanation for the poor performance of procaine as a corneal anaesthetic, compared with amethocaine for example, is that it is both less lipid soluble and less water soluble.

The majority of the drugs employed by the practitioner are weak acids and bases, so that the degree of ionization is also important in determining absorption across the cornea. However, while a low degree of ionization favours drug absorption across most biological membranes, the situation is more complex at the cornea. The lipid–aqueous–lipid nature of the cornea requires a molecule to have both lipid and water solubility, which in the case of weak acids or bases may require the drug to be present in both the non-ionized (at the epithelium and endothelium) and the ionized form (at the stroma). It is envisaged that weak acids and bases applied topically will establish an equilibrium between the ionized and non-ionized forms at each surface or interface between different layers of the

cornea. The degree of ionization at each point will be dictated by the pH and the pK_a of the drug (*Figure 28.1*). Thus, after application to the corneal surface, the non-ionized form will cross the epithelium and re-establish equilibrium within the stroma. The ionized form will most readily cross this layer, but the non-ionized form will be required for penetration of the endothelium into the anterior chamber. The situation must be seen as a dynamic one—at each point when molecules diffuse away, the equilibrium will be disturbed in favour of producing more of that form (ionized or non-ionized). It can then be imagined, theoretically, that virtually all the drug could eventually cross the cornea, but in practical terms this is less likely to occur because, once applied to the cornea, some of the drug will be lost (in the nasal canthus, by overspill and through the conjunctiva). At the same time, any drug which has crossed the cornea will drain away with the aqueous, so that the levels required at the site of action may not be achieved. What is important is a rapid initial penetration of the drug across the epithelium. This is favoured by poor ionization of the drug. However, if the tendency to ionize is very low then, although there is rapid movement across the epithelium, movement across the stroma and therefore into the aqueous may be slow. This will not be a problem with drugs, such as local anaesthetics, which exert their action within the epithelium and are not required to enter the aqueous. If drugs are more highly ionized at the epithelial surface then even initial penetration will be slow. One of the reasons for the poor anaesthesia produced at the cornea by procaine is that it is more highly ionized than lignocaine or amethocaine at any pH. It is possible to alter the pH of eye drops to influence the degree of ionization, but the extent to which this may be done is limited by the induced irritation and damage to the cornea (most eye drops are within the pH range 5–9), by the stability of the drug at different pH values (cyclopentolate is less stable above pH 6) and by the buffering ability of the tears.

(1) Surface action—surface active agents, such as benzalkonium chloride, will increase the permeability of the cornea by reducing the surface tension. Such agents have been used with some drugs, e.g. carbachol and neostigmine (both quaternary ammonium compounds which are highly ionized), to increase absorption.

(2) Viscosity—the use of oily preparations rather than aqueous drops may improve absorption of drugs because of prolonged contact time and reduced loss through the canthus. Such preparations tend to interfere with vision and there is the chance that lipid-soluble drugs may be held

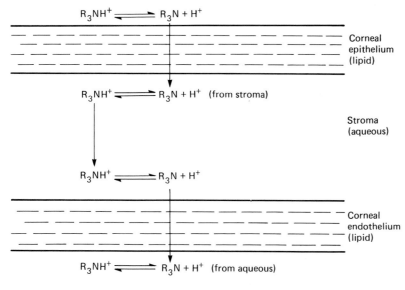

Corneal surface

Figure 28.1 Diagrammatic representation of the possible method of absorption of a weak base (e.g. atropine, R_3N) across the cornea following topical application

preferentially in the preparation rather than being absorbed into the cornea. The use of eye drops containing viscosity increasing agents, such as hypromellose, will also keep the drug in contact with the cornea longer and improve absorption.

(3) Corneal integrity—damage to the corneal epithelium will allow water-soluble, ionized drugs to penetrate more rapidly to the stroma. This is not made use of except in the case of fluorescein which is used specifically to detect such damage.

The main factor tending to reduce drug levels within the anterior chamber is drainage away with the aqueous humour.

Site of drug action

As stated earlier, the aim of all drug administration is for sufficient drug to arrive at the site of action and the location of this site should be considered for drugs used by optometric practitioners.

The main sites of action are components of the autonomic nervous system in the case of cycloplegics, mydriatics, miotics and vasoconstrictors, and the membrane of excitable cells in the case of the local anaesthetics.

The antibacterial compounds do not act at either of these sites, but on the metabolism or the integrity of bacterial cells. Staining agents may be regarded as having no action in the sense that this is discussed here.

The autonomic nervous system

This is defined as that peripheral, efferent system innervating those tissues and organs not generally under conscious control, e.g. the heart, secretory glands and the smooth muscle of the blood vessels, bronchioles and gastrointestinal tract. Its relationship to other sections of the nervous system is shown in *Figure 28.2*. A typical pathway of the autonomic nervous system is shown in *Figure 28.3*. The cell body of the preganglionic nerve (or neurone) lies within the brain or spinal cord. The axon of this neurone forms a synapse with the cell body of the postganglionic fibre in the ganglion. The postganglionic fibre makes a synapse with the cell innervated at the neuroeffector junction. Transmission along the nerve is by electrical changes (*see* Excitable cells) and across the synapses by chemical means.

The autonomic nervous system has two subdivisions—parasympathetic and sympathetic—distinguished partly on anatomical grounds (point of outflow from the central nervous system and posi-

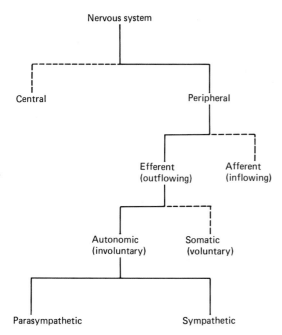

Figure 28.2 Subdivision of the nervous system on anatomical basis. (Adapted from J. Vale and B. Cox (1985) *Drugs and the Eye*)

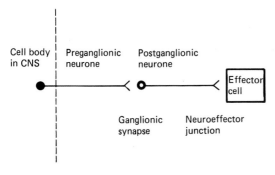

Figure 28.3 A typical autonomic neuroeffector pathway

tion of the ganglion in the pathway) and partly on the nature of the transmitter at the neuroeffector junction (the transmitter at the ganglion is the same in both the parasympathetic and the sympathetic systems). Many structures are innervated by both divisions of the autonomic nervous system, stimulation of the two pathways usually producing opposite effects. The parasympathetic division is regarded as being most concerned with the control of 'normal' day-to-day functions, whereas the sympathetic division enables the body to respond to abnormal, stressful situations.

Neurohumoral transmission and receptors

Impulses are transmitted along nerve fibres by changes in electrical properties. This cannot occur across the small, but finite, gap between nerve cells (as in the ganglion) or between a nerve cell and the structure it innervates (the neuroeffector junction). At these two points transmission is achieved by chemical means. A chemical, the transmitter, is synthesized within the nerve and stored, usually in vesicles or special cellular compartments, within the nerve endings. The arrival of an electrically transmitted impulse (action potential) produces changes in the permeability of the membrane at the nerve endings which result in the movement of ions into the nerve. This influx of ions, particularly Ca^{2+}, causes migration of the vesicles towards the cell membrane and the release of the transmitter into the synapse. From here, the transmitter diffuses down its concentration gradient towards the membrane of the postsynaptic cell (a postganglionic neurone in the case of the ganglion or various types of cells at the neuroeffector junction). The transmitter interacts with receptors located on the postsynaptic membrane and this interaction results in a response in the postsynaptic cell. This response may be the generation of an action potential in the postganglionic nerve and increased (or decreased) activity in muscle or secretory cells. After interaction, the transmitter diffuses away from the receptor and is inactivated, usually either by enzymic destruction or active re-uptake into its storage sites in the presynaptic nerve endings.

Receptors are envisaged as specialized areas on the membranes of cells having chemical groupings, spatial configurations and charge distributions which are complementary to the transmitter. The transmitter is thus able to 'occupy' the receptor. During this occupation, and subsequent interaction, the receptor and transmitter are held in proximity only by weak bonds, such as van der Waal's forces, hydrogen bonds etc. It is, therefore, necessary for the transmitter to be able to approach very closely to the receptor and the 'fit' of the two must be very good. Slight changes in the structure of the transmitter can result in this 'fit' being lost. Although each receptor is specific for one transmitter only, the same transmitter may interact with more than one receptor. For example, acetylcholine interacts with receptors known as nicotinic and muscarinic which are not identical. This does not negate the statement that structure is important, but probably reflects the ability of acetylcholine, which is a flexible molecule, to assume different spatial configurations.

Interaction of the transmitter with the receptor leads to changes in the postsynaptic cell, but the detailed mechanisms are not fully understood. In some cases, the interaction of the transmitter with the receptor causes a change in the conformation of the cell membrane resulting in changes in permeability, ion movements and electrical behaviour of the cell. In others, the interaction appears to influence membrane and/or intracellular enzymes resulting in biochemical changes which produce the final result.

Occupation of, and interaction with, a receptor is not limited to the natural transmitter. Drugs which are able to act in the same way, i.e. occupy and interact to produce a response, are known as agonists. They may be more specific than the transmitter. For example, pilocarpine acts at the muscarinic receptor for acetycholine with little or no activity at the nicotinic receptor. Compounds which are able to

occupy a receptor, but do not interact to produce the response are antagonists. Most of those in clinical use are competitive—they simply occupy the receptor and prevent access of the transmitter. A few antagonists produce changes in the receptor and are classed as non-competitive.

The parasympathetic division of the autonomic nervous system

The fibres of the parasympathetic nerves leave the central nervous system at the cranial and sacral levels and the ganglia are located close to, or within, the structures innervated (*Figure 28.4*). The transmitter is acetylcholine at both the ganglion and the neuroeffector junction.

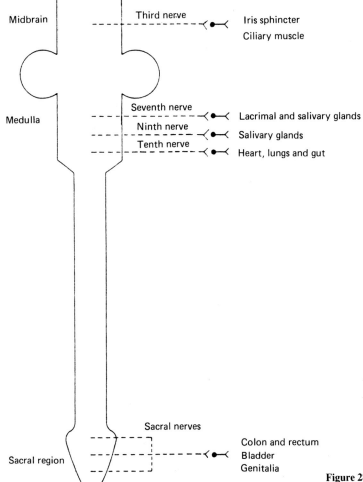

Figure 28.4 The parasympathetic nervous system. (From J. Vale and B. Cox (1985) *Drugs and the Eye*)

Acetylcholine is synthesized within the nerve endings in a series of steps as outlined below:

$$Pyruvate + AcetylCoA \longrightarrow Citrate + CoA$$

This takes place in the mitochondria from where the citrate and coenzyme A (CoA) diffuse into the cytoplasm.

$$Citrate + CoA \longrightarrow AcetylCoA + Pyruvate$$

$$AcetylCoA + Choline \longrightarrow Acetylcholine + CoA$$

The choline, present in the diet, is actively taken into the neurone by a relatively selective 'choline pump' located in the membrane. The final stage of the synthesis is catalysed by the enzyme choline acetyltransferase. The acetylcholine is stored, together with adenosine triphosphate (ATP), in membrane-bound vesicles within the nerve endings. On arrival of an action potential at the nerve endings, the permeability of the neuronal membrane is changed, various ions, including Ca^{2+}, enter the cell and cause the acetylcholine-containing vesicles to migrate to the neuronal membrane where the transmitter is released into the synaptic cleft by a process known as exocytosis. The vesicles are retained within the nerve and refilled with acetylcholine. The released acetylcholine diffuses to the postsynaptic membrane where it occupies and interacts with the receptors. At the ganglion, the receptors are known as nicotinic (the natural alkaloid nicotine initially produces the same response at these receptors as acetylcholine). The interaction of acetylcholine with these receptors results in the depolarization of the post-ganglionic neuronal membrane and the generation of a nerve action potential which is conducted the length of the nerve. At the neuroeffector junction, acetylcholine interacts with receptors known as muscarinic (the natural alkaloid muscarine produces the same effect here as acetylcholine). The response depends on the structure innervated (*Table 28.1*), but includes contraction of the sphincter muscle of the iris and the ciliary muscle giving miosis and accommodation for near vision. Action at muscarinic receptors in the lacrimal gland causes increased secretion. Secretion by other glands, for example the salivary and bronchial glands and those of the gastrointestinal tract, is also increased. In addition the heart is slowed, the bronchioles are constricted and the propulsive muscle of the gut is contracted. Most blood vessels are unaffected as they receive no innervation although they have muscarinic receptors.

After interaction, the acetylcholine diffuses away from the receptor and is rapidly hydrolysed by the enzyme acetylcholinesterase which is found in association with the nerves. This enzymes splits the molecule at its ester link yielding acetate and choline. The acetate can be used in the general metabolic pool and the choline is actively taken back into the nerve and reused in synthesis.

Obviously, there are a number of points at which the system can be interrupted or implemented, but

Table 28.1 Effector cells innervated by postganglionic parasympathetic nerves and the effects of nervous activity

Tissue/structure	*Effect of parasympathetic activity*
Ciliary muscle	Contraction
Iris sphincter muscle	Contraction
Lacrimal glands	Secretion
Salivary glands	Secretion
Heart rate	Decrease
Bronchiolar muscle	Contraction
Bronchiolar glands	Secretion
Propulsive muscle of gut	Contraction
Glands of the gastrointestinal	Secretion
Glands of the gastrointestinal tract	Contraction
Most blood vessels	No effect
Blood vessels of erectile tissue	Dilatation

not all of these are utilized in clinical practice. Thus, it is possible to interfere with the synthesis of acetylcholine by the use of hemicholinium, which blocks the choline pump, or with triethylcholine. This latter differs only slightly in structure from choline (ethyl instead of methyl groups) and is, therefore, able to use the choline pump to gain entry to the nerve, enter the synthetic pathway and be converted to acetyltriethylcholine. This is stored and released like acetylcholine but has less activity at the receptor, and is known as a false transmitter. These compounds are used only as experimental tools. Botulinus toxin, produced by *Clostridium botulinum*, prevents the release of acetylcholine from all sites and is only used experimentally, but can occur in contaminated tinned food producing serious or fatal effects.

Of more relevance are the agonists and antagonists at the receptors, particularly the muscarinic receptor. Antagonists at the nicotinic receptor in the ganglion have been used in the past, mainly for their ability to reduce blood pressure, but they are now rarely used because of frequent side-effects.

Agonists at the muscarinic receptor, such as pilocarpine, will act at the sphincter muscle of the iris and the ciliary muscle. At both sites the result of agonist–receptor interaction is contraction of the smooth muscle. In the iris, this results in the constriction of the pupil because of the circular arrangement of the muscle fibres and, in the ciliary muscle, again because of the mainly circular arrangement of the muscle fibres, the tension on the capsule of the lens via the suspensory ligaments is reduced allowing the lens faces to assume a greater curvature and altering the focal length for near vision. Secretion from the lacrimal gland is increased and relaxation of the smooth muscle in the conjunctival blood vessels results in vasodilatation (these vessels have muscarinic receptors even though they do not have a parasympathetic nerve supply). The use of antagonists, such as atropine, cyclopentolate and tropicamide, prevents the access of acetylcholine to the receptors in the sphincter and ciliary muscles and removes the parasympathetic-induced tone normally present in these muscles. The sphincter muscle thus relaxes resulting in mydriasis and an inability to respond to increased light intensity. The ciliary muscle also relaxes, pulling on the suspensory ligaments, reducing the curvature of the faces of the lens and accommodating the eye for distance vision only (cycloplegia). The secretion of the lacrimal gland is reduced. As there is no parasympathetic nerve supply to the blood vessels there is no direct effect on them from the blocking of the receptors.

A further means of influencing the activity of acetylcholine is to prevent its breakdown by the use of anticholinesterase drugs. These inhibit the activity of the acetylcholinesterase enzyme normally responsible for the inactivation of the transmitter.

Thus, any acetylcholine released from nerve endings remains in the vicinity of the receptor longer and can undergo more transmitter–receptor interactions, producing a response similar to stimulation of the parasympathetic nerves. In the eye this will cause miosis and spasm of accommodation. As acetylcholine is released at sites other than the muscarinic receptor, the results of acetylcholinesterase inhibition are complex but topical use more or less restricts the effects to the eye.

The sympathetic division of the autonomic nervous system

The fibres of the sympathetic nerves leave the central nervous system at the thoracic and lumbar levels and the ganglia are generally located close to the spinal cord. The structures innervated are shown in *Figure 28.5*. The transmitter at the ganglion is acetylcholine (as in the parasympathetic system) but at the neuroeffector junction the transmitter is noradrenaline.

The noradrenaline is synthesized within the nerve endings in a series of steps as shown below:

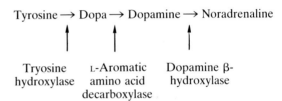

Tyrosine, present in the diet or produced from phenylalanine, is taken into the nerve endings by an active pump mechanism. The first two stages occur within the cytoplasm. The dopamine is then actively taken up into the storage granules where the conversion to noradrenaline takes place. Only in the adrenal medulla and at a few sites within the central nervous system does the synthesis proceed to adrenaline. The noradrenaline is stored in the granules in a complex with ATP, Mg^{2+}, Ca^{2+}, Cu^{2+} and proteins known as chromogranins. Release of noradrenaline appears to be effected by the same mechanism as that of acetylcholine. Thus, the arrival of the action potential at the nerve endings increases the entry of a number of ions, including Ca^{2+}, which cause migration of the granules to the neuronal membrane. Here, noradrenaline is released into the synaptic cleft and the granules are retained within the nerve. The noradrenaline diffuses to the postsynaptic membrane where it occupies and interacts with the receptors. Adrenoceptors located at the neuroeffector junction are not all identical and are classed as α or β. The β-receptors are further subdivided into β_1, found in cardiac tissue, and β_2, found elsewhere in peripheral tissues. Most tissues have either α- or β-receptors

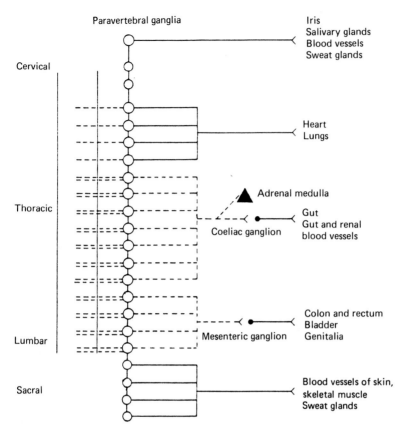

Figure 28.5 The sympathetic nervous system. (From J. Vale and B. Cox (1985) *Drugs and the Eye*)

(although there are exceptions). The interaction of noradrenaline with the receptors produces a number of responses (*Table 28.2*) including contraction of the radial muscle in the iris, giving mydriasis, contraction of the smooth muscle in the upper lid and blood vessels of the conjunctiva resulting in widening of the palpebral aperture and blanching of the conjunctiva, an increase in the rate and force of cardiac contraction, dilatation of the bronchioles and relaxation of the propulsive muscle of the gastrointestinal tract.

There may also be presynaptic receptors, both α and β, which are located on the nerves releasing noradrenaline. Interaction of the transmitter with these receptors may control further release of the transmitter.

After interaction with the receptors the noradrenaline diffuses away. Most of it is inactivated by uptake from the synaptic cleft into the cytoplasm of the presynaptic nerve ending. This uptake is brought about by an active mechanism, located in the membrane, which is dependent on Na$^+$ ATPase, requires energy, is saturable and shows a relative selectivity for noradrenaline. The major portion of

the noradrenaline is then actively transported into the storage granules, and small amounts are metabolized to inactive compounds by monoamine oxidase (MAO) located in the cytoplasm. Any noradrenaline which is not taken back into the nerve endings is converted to inactive metabolites by monoamine oxidase and/or catechol-*O*-methyl transferase.

Again there are many points within the process where drugs may either implement or interfere with transmission. Not all of the possible mechanisms are utilized in clinical practice and only a few are of direct use to the optometric practitioner.

The drugs most likely to be used by the optometrist are either agonists or antagonists at the α-receptor. These receptors are present in the radial muscle, the conjunctival blood vessels and the smooth muscle of the upper lid. Use of an α-agonist, such as phenylephrine, will cause contraction of the smooth muscle at all these sites giving a dilated pupil, vasoconstriction (seen as a blanched conjunctiva) and a widening of the palpebral aperture as the upper lids is raised. An α-antagonist such as thymoxamine, when used alone, will prevent access of neuronally

Table 28.2 Effector cells innervated by postganglionic sympathetic nerves and the effects of nervous activity

Tissue/structure	Receptor	Effects of sympathetic activity
Radial muscle of iris	α	Contraction
Smooth muscle of lids	α	Contraction
Heart, rate and force	β	Increase
Bronchiolar muscle	β	Relaxation
Propulsive muscle of gut	α, β	Relaxation
Seminal vesicles and vas deferens	α	Contraction
Uterine smooth muscle	β	Relaxation
All blood vessels	α	Contraction
Blood vessels in skeletal muscle	Muscarinic*	Relaxation
Pilomotor muscles	α	Contraction
Eccrine sweat glands	Muscarinic*	Secretion

*Acetylcholine is released to act on muscarinic receptors at these sites although the innervation is sympathetic.

released noradrenaline to the receptor and thus remove the effects of sympathetic activation. This will be seen as miosis (usually slight as there is not normally a great deal of sympathetic activity), vasodilatation and ptosis, a drooping of the upper lid. In optometry, the thymoxamine is likely to be used only after an α-agonist mydriatic when the effects will simply be to return the eye to its premydriatic state.

Effects similar to those obtained by the use of α-agonists or stimulation of the sympathetic nervous supply to the eye may be achieved by two indirect mechanisms. Some drugs, for example ephedrine, are sufficiently similar to noradrenaline in structure to successfully compete with it for the neuronal uptake mechanism. Thus ephedrine is able to enter sympathetic nerve endings and the storage granules and displace noradrenaline from storage into the synaptic cleft. The noradrenaline so displaced will then interact with the postjunctional receptors. Used systemically, the effects of ephedrine would not be the same as those produced by an α-agonist since the displaced noradrenaline would be able to interact with both α- and β-receptors. Used in the eye, which appears to have only α-receptors, the effects of ephedrine are the same as those of phenylephrine, namely mydriasis, raised upper lid and vasoconstriction. A second way in which drugs may indirectly produce effects the same as or similar to those resulting from stimulation of sympathetic

nerves is the block of noradrenaline re-uptake following release. The drug working by this mechanism, which has been used in the eye, is cocaine. The ability to block noradrenaline uptake (without itself utilizing the pump) is shown by non-anaesthetic concentration of cocaine and is a property not shared with the other local anaesthetics.

Instillation of cocaine causes mydriasis, vasoconstriction and, possibly, elevation of the upper lid (together with local anaesthesia). However, because of its stimulant effect on the cortex (and therefore abuse potential), its use is restricted by the Misuse of Drugs Act and it is not available to the optometric practitioner (Chapter 31). Compounds such as imipramine and amitriptyline, used as antidepressants, block noradrenaline uptake in a similar manner to cocaine and the practitioner may encounter patients using these drugs (*see* Chapter 30).

Drugs interacting with the sympathetic nervous system by two other mechanisms may be used by patients with glaucoma. Guanethidine is an adrenergic neurone blocking drug. It interferes with the release of noradrenaline from the nerve ending in response to nerve stimulation and also blocks the uptake mechanism. In glaucoma, it is most often used to potentiate the effects of adrenaline (by blocking its neuronal uptake), but it may also be used alone. In this situation, the patient may experience ptosis and miosis (due to a reduction in sympathetic activity) in addition to the fall in intra-ocular pressure. Also used in glaucoma is timolol, a β-adrenoceptor antagonist (both β_1 and β_2) which most probably causes a reduction in the formation of aqueous humour. There are no effects on the upper lid or the dilator muscle as these structures have only α-adrenoceptors.

Other interactions with the sympathetic system are not of direct importance to the optometric practitioner, although some, for example inhibition of monoamine oxidase, should be borne in mind because of possible interactions with drugs the optometric practitioner may wish to use (Chapter 30).

The excitable cell

When considering the excitable cell as a site of action in connection with drugs used by the optometric practitioner, we are concerned with the effects of local anaesthetics on sensory nerve fibres. The function of these fibres is to transmit information concerning sensory stimuli (pain, touch, pressure, heat, cold) from the point of the stimulus to the central nervous system. For the optometric practitioner, the sensory nerves in question are branches of the trigeminal nerve located in the corneal epithelium.

The essential function of any nerve is the generation and conduction of nerve impulses in response to the appropriate stimulus. Most of the information known about this function has been gained from studies on large, myelinated nerve fibres. The fibres innervating the cornea are small and non-myelinated, but it is assumed that they behave in an essentially similar manner.

A nerve fibre (of which there will be a number in a nerve, not necessarily of the same size), consists of a core of cytoplasm, the axon, surrounded by the plasma membrane. Like other membranes, this is a bimolecular layer of phospholipids with scattered proteins. The membrane is broken at intervals by pores, or channels, through which ions can pass, although not freely in all cases. Some fibres are further surrounded by a myelin sheath interrupted by the nodes of Ranvier (*Figure 28.6*). As with all excitable cells, the inside of a nerve cell is negative with respect to the outside. In the case of nerve cells this potential, the membrane potential, is in the range of 50–85 mV. The potential arises because the membrane shows differing permeabilities to various ions, in particular the permeability to Na^+ is low in the resting state and Na^+ does not easily enter the cell despite the concentration gradient in its favour. In addition there is a Na^+/K^+ pump (Na^+/K^+ ATP-ase) which utilizes the energy from ATP to actively transport Na^+ out of the cell and bring K^+ in, both against the prevailing concentration gradients. Finally, the membrane is totally impermeable to the large, organic anions within the cell. If a stimulus is

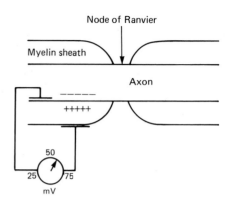

Figure 28.6 Diagrammatic representation of a myelinated nerve fibre. (From J. Vale and B. Cox (1985) *Drugs and the Eye*)

applied to a nerve cell, there is a small localized depolarization, i.e. the membrane potential becomes less negative. As the magnitude of this stimulus is increased, the resulting depolarization is also increased, but the response remains localized and non-propagated unless the membrane is depolarized to its threshold potential. If this potential, some 15 mV less negative than the resting potential, is reached an action potential is generated: as the potential reaches the threshold there is a large increase in the permeability of the membrane to Na^+ which enters the cell through the Na^+ channels.

The Na^+ channel in the membrane is believed to have two 'gates', one towards the outer surface (closed during the resting phase) and one at the inner surface (open during the resting phase). When the cell is depolarized to its threshold potential, the outer gate opens producing the large increase in the entry of Na^+. This is the activated phase. The influx of Na^+ produces a marked depolarization, such that the membrane potential becomes progressively less negative until it reaches approximately +30–40 mV which is the Na^+ equilibrium potential. At this point, the inner gate closes and the permeability to Na^+ falls thus decreasing its entry. This is the inactivated phase for the Na^+ channels. Separate K^+ channels open and K^+ leaves the cell resulting in a return of the membrane potential to its resting state. During this phase of repolarization, the Na^+ channels return to their resting state. The balance of Na^+ and K^+ ions within the nerve is restored by the Na^+/K^+ pump. The depolarization and repolarization constitute the nerve action potential. Once a stimulus is sufficient to cause depolarization to the threshold and produce an action potential, further increase in the magnitude of the stimulus produces no change in the magnitude of the individual action potential.

An action potential generated in response to a stimulus must be conducted along the length of the fibre. This is achieved by local circuit currents: the action potential generated at one point of the membrane gives a suprathreshold stimulus to the adjacent section of the membrane, which is depolarized to its threshold and generates an action potential that, in turn, gives a suprathreshold stimulus to the next section of the nerve fibre. The speed of this conduction varies in different fibres and, in those which are myelinated, the depolarizations occur only at the nodes of Ranvier where the myelin sheath is absent. This results in more rapid conduction known as saltatory conduction.

Theoretically, the generation of nerve impulses could be prevented or made more difficult in three ways. First, the membrane could be hyperpolarized, i.e. rendered more negative. In this situation there would be a greater difference between the resting potential and the threshold and a greater stimulus would be required to produce the necessary depolarization to the threshold. Second, persistent depolarization of the membranes on the 'wrong' side of the threshold would render the cell unresponsive to stimuli. Thus, although a stimulus might produce some further decrease in membrane potential, there would be no crossing of the threshold value and no action potential would be generated. Such cells would remain unresponsive to stimuli until the membrane potential had returned to the 'right' side of the threshold. Third, the generation and conduction of action potential may be affected by membrane stabilization. In this situation, the resting membrane potential remains normal, there is no hyper- or depolarization but the ability of the cell to be depolarized is lost. Membrane stabilization is the mechanism by which local anaesthetics act. They are able to block the generation and conduction of impulses in sensory fibres, not only in response to pain, but also to heat, cold, touch and pressure. They can also produce block in motor fibres and all other excitable cells.

All nerve fibres (and excitable cells) are not equally sensitive to blockade by local anaesthetics, cell diameter appearing to be the most important determining factor. Thus, nerve fibres are blocked before other types of cells and smaller nerve fibres are more readily blocked than larger ones. Also important is the firing rate of the cells. Nerve fibres with a higher firing rate are more easily blocked than those with a lower firing rate. This means that fibres subserving pain, which are of small diameter and high firing rate, are more easily blocked in a mixed nerve bundle than are other sensory fibres (for cold, warmth, touch or pressure) or motor fibres (large diameter and lower firing rate). The range of fibres or cells affected is usually restricted by the method of application.

The basic way in which local anaesthetics prevent the generation and conduction of action potentials in excitable cells is to prevent the essential large increase in membrane permeability to Na^+ which occurs when the cells are depolarized to the threshold. From studies on artificial membranes and various nerve preparations, a number of suggestions have been made in attempts to explain this action of the local anaesthetics. One suggestion is that the drug (in its non-ionized and lipid-soluble form) dissolves in the lipid layers of the plasma membrane and increases its surface pressure. The would distort the membrane and close the channels through which Na^+ enters the cell. It has also been suggested that local anaesthetics compete for binding sites in the membrane normally occupied by Ca^{2+} and that the freeing of these sites is essential for the increase in permeability to Na^+. Any Ca^{2+} bound to these sites is suggested to be readily released, but this is not the case with the local anaesthetics. A more recent suggestion is that the local anaesthetics (in their cationic form) bind to a receptor in the Na^+ channels and increase the probability of the inner gate closing and preventing the movement of Na^+ through the channels. The affinity of local anaesthetics for this receptor is higher when the gate is open (the activated state) than when it is closed in the resting state. Thus cells with a high firing rate are more easily blocked.

This last action of local anaesthetics is limited to the cationic ionized form of the drug molecule, whereas the suggested effect on surface pressure is attributed to the non-ionized form. Thus the degree of ionization of a local anaesthetic may influence, not only its absorption from the site of administration, but also its ability to exert its actions.

Selective toxicity

One group of drugs used by the optometric practitioner which does not exert its action at the membranes of excitable cells, through interaction with the autonomic nervous system, nor via receptors is the antibacterial/antibiotic group. Drugs of this group exert their action against microorganisms, generally bacteria. The principle crucial to their successful use is that of selective toxicity. By this is meant the ability of a drug to destroy or damage bacterial (or other parasitic) cells with little or no damage to the cells of the host tissue. The selective action may be qualitative, meaning that the host cells are unaffected at any concentration of the drug, or quantitative, meaning that drug concentrations exerting a toxic effect on the microorganisms are without marked effect on the host cells, but that host toxicity could occur if the drug concentration was increased.

To achieve selective toxicity it is necessary to exploit some difference, absolute or relative, between the bacterial and the human or host cells. One obvious difference between such cells is a structural one. Bacterial cells possess a rigid cell wall in addition to the cell membrane, human or mammalian cells do not. This cell wall maintains the shape of the bacterial cell and is important because of the high osmotic pressure within the cells. Any drug which can damage the cell wall or interfere with the synthesis of its components may cause lysis of the cell. The penicillins are one of the major groups of antibiotics which exert their action by interfering with the synthesis of components of the cell wall. They prevent the formation of murein, an insoluble mucopeptide which is one of the major components of the cell wall in a number of both Gram-positive and Gram-negative bacteria. Lack of susceptibility to the penicillins may be due to a lack of the specific proteins to which the penicillins initially bind, or to difficulties in penetrating to the site of these proteins, particularly in Gram-negative bacteria which have an outer phospholipid membrane. Resistance to the penicillins may develop through the production by bacteria of an enzyme, β-lactamase, which can metabolize and inactivate some members of the group.

Because the antibacterial action is dependent on a qualitative difference there is usually little direct host toxicity. The antibacterial drug most likely to be used in optometry is probably sulphacetamide. This, like all members of the sulphonamide group to which it belongs, exploits a qualitative biochemical difference between bacterial and human (or mammalian) cells. Many bacterial cells require *p*-aminobenzoic acid. This is utilized in the first stage of a biochemical pathway which leads finally to the formation of nucleic acids. In the presence of the enzyme dihydrofolate synthetase, *p*-aminobenzoic acid is converted to dihydrofolate and subsequently to tetrahydrofolate. The sulphonamides are closely related in structure to *p*-aminobenzoic acid (*Figure 28.7*) and compete with it for the enzyme producing non-functional analogues of dihydrofolic acid. Thus the synthesis of nucleic acids is reduced and the growth of the bacteria is prevented (bacteriostasis). Human and animal cells are unaffected as they use dihydrofolate directly and are not dependent on its production from *p*-aminobenzoic acid. Some bacteria also use dihydrofolate directly and are not sensitive to the sulphonamides. Bacteria which produce a large excess of *p*-aminobenzoic acid are less sensitive to the action of the sulphonamides as this depends on a competition for the enzyme. This competition, and the effect of raising *p*-aminobenzoic acid concentrations, is the basis for the concern sometimes expressed about the use of sulphacetamide in the eye following the use of certain local anaesthetics, particularly amethocaine.

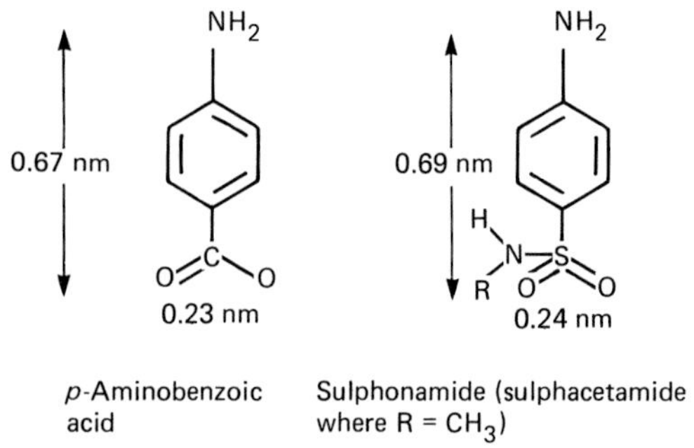

Figure 28.7 The molecular structure of *p*-aminobenzoic acid compared with that of the sulphonamides

Metabolism of the anaesthetic may produce *p*-aminobenzoic acid which could compete with the sulphonamide and impede its activity. As a result of mutation in some resistant bacteria, the enzyme, dihydrofolate synthetase, has developed a higher affinity for *p*-aminobenzoic acid than for the sulphonamides (normally the reverse is the case).

As the synthetic step inhibited by the sulphonamides is absent in human and other mammalian cells, there is no toxicity related to the mode of action of the drugs but there are other, unrelated toxic effects.

Another antibacterial compound available to the optometric practitioner is framycetin which, together with gentamicin and neomycin (used by the medical) profession in the treatment of ocular infection), belongs to the group known as the aminoglycoside antibiotics. Members of this group, together with chloramphenicol and the tetracyclines, all produce their effects by inhibiting protein synthesis (although the detailed mechanism varies). The biochemical selectivity is usually quantitative, synthesis in bacterial cells being inhibited at concentrations which have less effect on human cells. With the tetracyclines, the selectivity is reinforced by concentration of the drug within susceptible cells by an active transport mechanism. Resistant bacteria, and mammalian cells, do not concentrate the drugs. Resistance to chloramphenicol and the aminoglycosides may result from a variety of mechanisms, for example, bacteria resistant to chloramphenicol produce an enzyme which metabolizes it. This is true of bacteria resistant to the aminoglycosides, although resistance may also be due to a lack of specific sites to which the drugs bind.

Whatever the mechanism of the selective toxicity of antibiotics this is reinforced for the drugs used in optometry by their topical administration.

Further reading

See end of Chapter 31.

29

Drug use in optometry

Janet Vale

In the normal course of practice, drugs are used for diagnosis or prophylaxis. In the first case, the drugs are used to enable the best possible examination to be carried out and to gain information which might not otherwise be readily obtained. The drugs used to this end may include cycloplegics, mydriatics, local anaesthetics and staining agents. In the case of prophylaxis, the optometric practitioner is seeking to prevent the possible occurrence of events detrimental to the patient, such as corneal infection or a rise in intraocular pressure following the use of mydriatics. The drugs used here are the antimicrobials and the miotics.

In addition, emergency situations may arise where action must be taken to reduce patient discomfort and minimize subsequent damage as far as possible. Some of these situations may require the use of drugs and virtually any of the drugs mentioned in Chapters 28 and 31 may be required depending on the nature of the problem.

In any of these situations, it is important that there is an awareness of the reasons for using a drug and the factors influencing the selection of any particular drug from the group available. For this a clear understanding of the mechanism by which drugs produce their effects is needed (*see* Chapter 28) together with a knowledge of how the individual members of a group differ from each other. These two will aid the rational choice of drug and also alert the practitioner to any possible problems, side-effects or interactions which could occur.

Cycloplegics

The cycloplegics are the group of drugs which result in paralysis of accommodation and thus prevent the eye from bringing close objects into clear focus.

They all act by the same mechanism, but vary in the magnitude and duration of the effect they produce.

As detailed in Chapter 28, cycloplegics exert their action at the muscarinic receptors of the ciliary muscle where they act as competitive antagonists of the neurotransmitter acetylcholine. Thus, although the transmitter continues to be released from the parasympathetic nerve endings during attempts to accommodate, it cannot gain access to its receptors to bring about contraction. The smooth muscle fibres are thus relaxed which, because of their arrangement, increases the tension on the suspensory ligaments and flattens the lens, thereby fixing it for distance vision.

Because of this mechanism of action, cycloplegia is always accompanied by mydriasis and loss of the light reflex (the converse however is not true—*see* Mydriatics). Thus muscarinic antagonists will also prevent the access of acetylcholine to its receptors in the sphincter muscle of the iris. The removal of parasympathetic tone will cause the sphincter to relax giving mydriasis and preventing any response to increasing light intensity.

In addition, tear production will be reduced due to the antagonism of acetylcholine at muscarinic receptors. Conjunctival blood vessels are not affected by muscarinic blockade *per se* (they are not controlled by parasympathetic nerves), although individual cycloplegics may result in dilatation through other mechanisms.

Associated with the dilatation of the iris and the relaxation of the ciliary muscle is the possibility of an increase in intraocular pressure in susceptible patients. This is due mainly to the possible block of the angle by the dilated and immobile iris and the removal of the pumping action of the ciliary muscle which, during the normal contraction and relaxation associated with accommodation, encourages the drainage of aqueous humour via the canal of Schlemm and trabecular meshwork. Both these factors can reduce the outflow of the aqueous humour but whether or not a rise in pressure will occur will depend on the particular drug used (being most likely in those with an effect of high magnitude and prolonged duration) and the potential predisposition or otherwise of the patient. It is, however, improbable that the patients most likely to be at risk, i.e. those over 40 years old, would be exposed to the most active, long-lasting cycloplegics.

Cycloplegics are used in any situation where it is felt that the best answer regarding the refractive error cannot be obtained while the accommodation remains fully active. This may include difficult patients (who will not, or cannot, cooperate in subjective tests), in cases of convergent squint, high esophoria, latent hypermetropia, pseudomyopia and any other situation where the findings are not in agreement with the symptoms described by the patient. The depth of cycloplegia desirable may range from complete, in accommodative squint when it is desired to determine the role of accommodation in the problem or other situations where knowledge of the full correction is required, to simply a quietening effect on restless and spasmodic accommodation or to break down the spasm in pseudomyopia. It is unlikely that any one cycloplegic will be suitable in all situations.

Available cycloplegics

Those most easily available are:

(1) Atropine as 1% ointment and drops (including single dose units).
(2) Cyclopentolate as 0.5 and 1% drops (including single dose units).
(3) Homatropine as 1 and 2% drops (single dose units at 2% only).

Other cycloplegics, such as hyoscine 0.25% and lachesine 1%, are only available in multidose containers with the attendant problems of possible bacterial contamination and wastage through infrequent use and the need to discard opened bottles in a relatively short time.

Atropine

Atropine is the only readily available cycloplegic which will reliably produce full cycloplegia. When instilled as 1% drops, the maximum cycloplegic effect is usually only achieved after several hours. At this point, the pupil is widely dilated (an effect which reaches a maximum in about 30–40 minutes) and is unresponsive to light. If complete cycloplegia is required, for example in young children with accommodative squint, it is more often obtained by

the use of atropine ointment at home. A small quantity is applied to each eye 2 or 3 times daily for 3 days. None is applied on the day of the examination because of the greasy film left on the cornea which may interfere with refraction. While some recovery from the cycloplegia may occur within 2 or 3 days, full recovery is likely to take up to 10 days and the child may experience some problems during this period. Likewise the pupil may take several days to return to normal size and responsiveness to increased light intensity. This again may be distressing. Opinions vary on the question of using atropine in a child with intermittent squint, because the prolonged paralysis of accommodation may convert the squint from an intermittent to a permanent condition. Because of the complete cycloplegia produced it may be necessary to make an allowance for ciliary muscle tonus when deciding the correction to be used. The value of the allowance applied, if any, will vary from patient to patient, but may be up to 2 D.

Problems associated with atropine usage

For the situations in which atropine is used the main problems, other than those associated with the duration of action, are possibly poisoning and allergy. Poisoning is most likely to occur from incorrect usage of the ointment at home and it is essential that the practitioner ensures a clear understanding on the part of the parent of the drug's use and associated dangers. Instructions, preferably written, should be given to the parent outlining the way the ointment is to be used, the need to wipe away any excess ointment after application (to prevent accidental ingestion via the fingers), to keep the ointment in a safe place and to dispose carefully of any remaining after treatment, or to return it to the practitioner for disposal. The toxic effects of atropine result from both block of peripheral parasympathetic neuroeffector junctions and a central effect, initially stimulant and then depressant. The most striking peripheral effects would probably be a rapid pulse, a hot dry skin and a dry mouth associated with difficulty in speaking or swallowing. These effects are understood by considering the results of parasympathetic stimulation (*Table 28.1*, Chapter 28). The central stimulant effects may be manifested as excitement, incoherence or delirium replaced, if sufficient has been ingested, by central depression and respiratory paralysis causing death. Deaths from poisoning in children have been reported from as little as 10 mg and thus a 3 g tube of atropine ointment does contain a potentially fatal dose should the whole quantity be ingested.

The second problem which may arise is that of allergy, although this is not common and is normally only associated with prolonged or repeated usage.

Because of the magnitude and duration of atropine's effect on the ciliary and sphincter muscles, and the great difficulty in reversing these effects, atropine is theoretically the most likely of the cycloplegics to induce a rise in intraocular pressure in susceptible patients. However, such patients do not require a cycloplegic (or mydriatic) of the strength of atropine and this particular side-effect is not a practical worry, unless the drug has been inadvertently used in elderly patients.

Cyclopentolate

Cyclopentolate is the cycloplegic most frequently used in optometric practice and, in all but those situations where complete cycloplegia is required, it is probably the nearest approach to the ideal.

The onset of cycloplegia occurs a few minutes after instillation of the drops and the amplitude of accommodation falls rapidly, even in children, such that the maximum effect is usually achieved in 30 minutes. Mydriasis follows a similar time course and the pupil is widely dilated and unresponsive to light in approximately 30 minutes. Although the two effects do follow a similar time course, it cannot be assumed that attainment of maximum mydriasis is an indication that maximum cycloplegia has also been obtained and steps should be taken to determine when this point has been reached. The residual accommodation is of the order of 1–1.5 D. It has been claimed that repeated instillations, three drops of 1% cyclopentolate at 10-minute intervals, will produce complete cycloplegia. Recovery from the cycloplegic effect is more rapid than with atropine. The maximum cycloplegia lasts some 45 minutes, close work is usually possible within 4 hours and full recovery takes 12–24 hours. The pupil may take longer to return to its normal state, i.e. some 24–48 hours.

Problems with cyclopentolate

Cyclopentolate does not have the toxic potential of atropine, particularly as it is not normally used at home. There have, however, been reports of CNS disturbances (hallucinations, ataxia, incoherent speech etc.) following the instillation of cyclopentolate drops. This temporary disturbance, which recovers in a few hours with no apparent lasting effects, has usually been associated with the use of higher concentrations (2%) than normally employed.

The melanin pigment in dark irides is able to bind cyclopentolate, thus there is less available to interact with the receptors in the ciliary and sphincter muscles and it may be more difficult to achieve cycloplegia. If this is found to be the case, shown as little or no effect on accommodation (or pupil size) in 20 minutes or so, an additional drop may be instilled.

Allergic responses to cyclopentolate are even less common than to atropine and cyclopentolate may be used in patients who are allergic to atropine. The difference in structure between the two avoids the possibility of cross allergy.

The risk of a rise in intraocular pressure following the use of cyclopentolate is lower than with atropine because of the less drastic effects and the shorter duration of action. It is also easier to reverse the effects of cyclopentolate if this is thought to be desirable.

Cyclopentolate is used in older children (over 6 years) at 1% and in young adults (over 15–16 years) and older patients in whom a cycloplegic is felt desirable at 0.5% (or 1% if the irides are very dark).

Other cycloplegics

The remaining cycloplegics find little use in current practice.

Homatropine

This generally produces a cycloplegia which is less complete than with cyclopentolate giving a residual accommodation of approximately 2 D. The maximum effect is usually achieved in 45–90 minutes, at which point the pupil is already maximally dilated and unresponsive to light. Close work may usually be undertaken in approximately 6 hours. Full recovery of accommodative ability may require 24 hours, with 24–48 hours being required for full return to normal pupil size.

Because of its longer duration of action, and difficulty of reversal, the risk of a rise in intraocular pressure is greater with homatropine than cyclopentolate (although less than the risk with atropine). Homatropine should thus be avoided in any patients in whom a predisposition to glaucoma is demonstrated or suspected.

Homatropine is very similar in structure to atropine. Any patient allergic to atropine is thus likely to be allergic to homatropine because of cross allergy.

The main application of homatropine is to produce a quietening of a restless and spasmodic accommodation or to break down the spasm in pseudomyopia to reveal the true error. However, even here cyclopentolate may be preferred as providing a faster recovery for an equal or greater degree of cycloplegia.

Hyoscine

This is rarely used, particularly as single dose units are no longer available. It produces maximum cycloplegia, which is incomplete, in approximately 40 minutes with recovery taking 24 hours or more. Systemically it is more potent, and potentially more toxic, than atropine and CNS disturbances can occur from topical instillation. It would seem to offer no advantage over cyclopentolate.

Lachesine

This has been suggested as an alternative to atropine in patients who show allergic responses. The maximum cycloplegia is achieved approximately one hour after the instillation of 2% drops. As the cycloplegia is less complete than with atropine, lachesine would seem to offer no advantage over cyclopentolate in this situation, particularly as only multidose containers are available.

Mydriatics

Obviously any drug producing cycloplegia will also produce mydriasis as detailed in the previous section. There are, however, situations where dilatation of the pupil is required but accompanying cycloplegia is both unnecessary and an inconvenience to the patient. In these circumstances, it is possible to achieve a good mydriatic effect with little or no accompanying cycloplegia. The drugs employed are either weak muscarinic antagonists (i.e. cycloplegics), where the split between mydriasis and cycloplegia is only relative, or sympathetic agonists where the split is absolute.

Muscarinic antagonists

The mechanism of action is as described in the previous section. The separation of mydriatic and cycloplegic effects is achieved by the use of antagonists at low concentration or with weak activity. The most likely explanation for the relative effects at the muscles is that the pathway to the ciliary muscle is longer than that to the sphincter and, with weak solutions or antagonists, the majority of the drug interacts with receptors in the iris leaving insufficient for marked drug/receptor interactions at the ciliary muscle. Thus, only a moderate or short-lived change in accommodation occurs. Another possible explanation is a differing sensitivity of the two receptors to block. Such a difference is exhibited by muscarinic receptors elsewhere. It follows from the mechanism of action that the pupillary response to light is abolished and that drugs of this group have the potential to block the angle of the anterior chamber and precipitate a rise in intraocular pressure in susceptible patients.

Sympathetic agonists

These are compounds which produce the same end result as the natural transmitter noradrenaline when interacting with α-receptors. They are, however, better absorbed across the cornea than noradrenaline and are not as susceptible to the inactivation process. They are thus able to produce clinically useful effects. Within the eye, the structures receiving sympathetic innervation and having α-receptors are the dilator muscle and conjunctival blood vessels. The smooth muscle in the upper lid also possesses a sympathetic innervation and α-receptors. The effects of instilling an α-agonist will, therefore, be contraction of the dilator muscle, giving mydriasis, constriction of the conjunctival blood vessels and elevation of the upper lid. The reason for the lack of cycloplegia is the absence of the physiologically important α-receptors in the ciliary muscle. Although the sphincter muscle is not affected directly by the presence of an α-agonist, the light response is slow, or absent, as the muscle is required to pull against the fully contracted dilator.

Mydriatics of either type are used in optometric practice so that a more complete examination of the fundus, the vitreous and the periphery of the lens may be carried out. Although they may be required in younger patients because of congenital cataracts for example, they are more likely to be required in elderly patients who have smaller pupils and a greater incidence of opacities. This group of patients is more likely to have, or be predisposed to, glaucoma and no mydriatic should be used in elderly patients until some steps have been taken to ensure that they are not at risk. Such investigations could include a history, not forgetting any family history of problems, an assessment of the angle and depth of the anterior chamber, a plot of visual fields and a measurement of the intraocular pressure. If after this, it is felt that there is no obvious cause for concern the mydriatic may be instilled, but suitable miotics should be available (*see* later). The main worry is that the dilated pupil will block a narrow angle, but it must also be remembered that any drugs exerting an effect on the ciliary muscle may also contribute to the reduction in outflow. This is an additional reason why drugs with a marked cycloplegic effect should be avoided when mydriasis alone is required.

Available mydriatics

The two most easily available are: tropicamide, a muscarinic antagonist, as 0.5 and 1% drops including single dose units, and phenylephrine, an α-agonist, as 10% drops including single dose units.

Ephedrine and low strength, i.e. 0.1%, cyclopentolate are no longer readily available.

Tropicamide

Instillation of 0.5% drops produces a mydriasis which commences in a few minutes and usually reaches a maximum within about 30 minutes, at which point the pupil is widely dilated and unresponsive to light. Full return to normal occurs in around 9 hours. The effect on accommodation varies between patients, but is usually only slight and transient, and should cause no difficulties to the majority of patients.

Problems with tropicamide
The only likely problem with tropicamide is that common to all mydriatics, or cycloplegic/mydriatics, namely a rise in intraocular pressure. This, however, is minimized by the careful selection of patients and the availability of suitable miotics should reversal be felt desirable.

Phenylephrine

Maximal mydriasis may be achieved 30–60 minutes following the instillation of 10% drops, but difficulty may be experienced in patients with heavily pigmented irides or in elderly patients with sclerosed iris blood vessels. Here the relatively weak dilator muscle, although stimulated by the phenylephrine, may not succeed in pulling the iris back towards the periphery. Once achieved, the mydriasis lasts for several hours. There is no true effect on accommodation although some patients may complain of blurring. This is probably due to spherical aberration resulting from the wide dilatation of the pupil and passage of light through the peripheral parts of the cornea and lens. The light response is slowed if not absent.

Problems with phenylephrine
As with tropicamide, the possibility of a rise in intraocular pressure should not be a problem if the patients are carefully selected. The pressure may in fact fall because of the effect of phenylephrine on aqueous formation.

The high concentration of phenylephrine normally used results in drops which are markedly hypertonic. This causes stinging with possible reflex increase in tear production and resultant loss of the drug.

The high concentration may also result in systemic effects and drug interactions following absorption through the conjunctiva and nasolacrimal ducts. Steps should always be taken to reduce absorption via the canaliculi and the use of the lower strength (2.5%) considered in patients with known cardiovascular problems. The lower strength is recommended for mydriasis in children. Phenylephrine should be avoided in patients with hyperthyroidism as they show excessive reactions to sympathetic drugs.

Comparing the two mydriatics, tropicamide would seem to give the more reliable mydriasis in a shorter time with the complete abolition of the light response which may be desirable in some circumstances. However, it may be more likely to raise intraocular pressure and is perhaps not so easily reversed should this be subsequently felt to be desirable.

Phenylephrine has the advantage that it produces no change in accommodation, can be reliably reversed with thymoxamine and possibly carries less risk of a rise in intraocular pressure. However, production of mydriasis is less reliable in some patients and some light response may remain.

Miotics

Miotics are those drugs which produce reduction in the size of the pupil. This is most usually achieved by activation of the muscarinic receptors in the smooth muscle of the sphincter pupillae, causing it to contract. Because the ciliary muscle also possesses muscarinic receptors, it too will contract resulting in accommodation for near vision. The pupillary response to light is unaffected unless the sphincter muscle is fully contracted by the miotic. The conjunctival blood vessels may dilate as they also possess muscarinic receptors which cause relaxation of the smooth muscle.

Activation of the muscarinic receptors is brought about by two different classes of drugs: muscarinic agonists and anticholinesterases.

Muscarinic agonists

These are compounds which mimic the action of the natural transmitter acetylcholine at the muscarinic receptors of the parasympathetic neuroeffector junction. Because they are better absorbed than acetylcholine and relatively or completely resistant to breakdown by acetylcholinesterase, they produce effects which are clinically useful.

Anticholinesterases

Anticholinesterases prevent the breakdown of released acetylcholine by inhibiting the acetylcholinesterase enzyme; the acetylcholine is thus able to take part in more transmitter–receptor interactions. In this case, the interaction will be not only at the muscarinic receptors causing pupil constriction, but also at the nicotinic receptors in skeletal muscle causing lid and facial muscle twitching. Inhibition of acetylcholinesterase does not, in itself, cause dilatation of the conjunctival vessels. These do not receive parasympathetic nerves and acetylcholine is not normally present at this site.

Sympathetic antagonists

Miosis, particularly as required by the optometric practitioner, may also be produced by the use of an α-antagonist. This will block α-adrenoceptors and prevent the access of the normal transmitter, noradrenaline, to its receptors. In the eye, these are present in the dilator muscle, and in the smooth muscle of the blood vessels and the upper lid. These three muscles all relax causing miosis, dilatation of the blood vessels and ptosis. When applied to the normal eye, there is usually only a slight effect on pupil size as there is not normally much sympathetic tone, but use of an α-antagonist will result in a reduction in the size of a pupil previously dilated with sympathetic agonists.

Miotics are normally used in optometry in an attempt to return the pupil size (and possibly accommodation) to normal after the use of a mydriatic or mydriatic/cycloplegic. The most likely patients in whom reversal of mydriasis is attempted are the elderly. In some cases, despite preliminary investigations showing no obvious contraindication to the use of a mydriatic, it may be felt that it would be preferable, and possibly safer, to return the pupil size to normal. If miotics are used for this reason the patients should be kept in the practice until some signs of reversal are evident and instructed to return or seek medical advice should there be any subsequent redilatation, pain, difficulty with vision or any other untoward reaction. It is perhaps better if elderly patients are dilated early in the day, thus allowing more time for reversal and return to the practice should this become necessary.

Occasionally, reversal may be required or requested by younger patients who are troubled by the lack of light response, or in the case of cycloplegics/mydriatics, by the lack of full accommodative ability if they need to attempt close work during the remainder of the day. One possible drawback is that the effect of the miotic on the ciliary muscle may be excessive causing spasm and pseudomyopia which can be more troublesome than the original disturbance of accommodation.

Available miotics

There are three miotics readily available, one example from each of the groups described. They are:

(1) Physostigmine, an anticholinesterase, 0.25% and 0.5% drops (multidose only).
(2) Pilocarpine, a muscarinic agonist, 0.5%, 1%, 2%, 3% and 4% drops (including single dose units of 1%, 2% and 4%).
(3) Thymoxamine, an α-receptor antagonist, 0.5% drops in single dose units only.

Carbachol 3%, available only in multidose bottles, is rarely used as a miotic. Neostigmine and bethanecol, although appearing on the list of prescription only medicines that an optometric practitioner may possess, are not in fact easily obtainable, while the long-acting anticholinesterases, such as demecarium and ecothiopate, are not available for optometric use.

Physostigmine

Used in the non-dilated eye at 0.5%, physostigmine induces miosis which begins in about 10 minutes and reaches a maximum in approximately 30 minutes; at this time the pupil is very small and no further response to light may be seen as the sphincter is fully contracted. Normal pupil size is regained in some 12 hours. A marked spasm of accommodation, which lasts 2–3 hours, is also produced and may result in brow-ache and discomfort. Attempts at close work once the spasm has worn off may cause it to return, since there is still sufficient inhibition of acetylcholinesterase activity to allow the persistence of acetylcholine liberated during the attempts to focus.

When instilled into eyes previously dilated with tropicamide (the most likely antimuscarinic mydriatic), physostigmine, 0.25 or 0.5%, should usually begin to return the pupil towards normal size in about 30 minutes. The cycloplegia, if any, is more easily overcome and the patient may experience difficulties due to ciliary spasm. Lid twitching may also be experienced.

Pilocarpine

Instilled into an eye which has not previously been dilated with mydriatics, pilocarpine 1% produces a miosis which begins in a few minutes, is maximal in about 30 minutes and lasts approximately 6 hours. The effect on accommodation is not usually as marked as with physostigmine, lasts 1–2 hours and does not return with subsequent attempts at close work (because of the direct action of pilocarpine not involving protection of acetylcholine). For the same reason there is no lid twitching.

When used after tropicamide, pilocarpine may not be as reliable as physostigmine in returning the pupil size to normal. Even if some reversal is achieved, the pupil may subsequently redilate because of the longer persistence of tropicamide at the site of action. The effect on accommodation may be more noticeable than that on pupil size and may cause the patient some short lived difficulty.

Thymoxamine

Instilled into an eye previously dilated with phenylephrine, 0.5% thymoxamine rapidly produces a reduction in pupil size with normal size being achieved in approximately 30 minutes. There is no effect on accommodation but the conjunctival vessels may dilate and the patient may complain of initial stinging.

Choosing a miotic for reversal of mydriasis

The aim of using a miotic after mydriasis is to return the pupil size to as near normal as possible, as rapidly as possible, without undue effect on accommodation, particularly if this was previously unaffected by the mydriatic. The choice of miotic will depend largely on the mydriatic used.

In the case of mydriasis achieved by stimulating the sympathetic system, the problem has been simplified by the availability of the specific antagonist thymoxamine. Other than some stinging on instillation, there should be no problem of either failure to reverse or disturbance of accommodation. The use of thymoxamine is to be much preferred to the previous method used for the reversal of phenylephrine mydriasis, namely pilocarpine. While this did reliably reverse the mydriasis, the pupil size was often reduced to smaller than normal, accommodation was disturbed as the previously unaffected ciliary muscle went into spasm, the simultaneous contraction of both the sphincter and the dilator muscles could cause discomfort and there was the possibility of pupil block and a rise in intraocular pressure. With thymoxamine which competes with phenylephrine for the α-receptors present in only the dilator muscle, these problems are generally avoided. The contracted dilator muscle is simply made to relax.

Not unexpectedly thymoxamine will not overcome the mydriasis produced by the muscarinic antagonists. Physostigmine or pilocarpine must be used for this. When either of these is instilled following a muscarinic antagonist, there is competition for the muscarinic receptors between the antagonist and either pilocarpine or acetylcholine (in the case of physostigmine). The outcome in terms of pupil size will depend on whether the receptors are occupied mainly by the agonist (miosis) or the antagonist (mydriasis). This, in turn, will depend on the relative concentrations of the two (which will change with time as they are either metabolized or diffuse away from the site) and the relative affinities for the receptor. (Atropine has a very high affinity which explains why its effects are so difficult to overcome.) Because the relative concentrations can change with time, there is the possibility that the pupil may constrict and subsequently redilate.

While tropicamide should be reversible by pilocarpine, this cannot always be relied upon (although the ciliary muscle may have been put into spasm) and physostigmine is perhaps the more reliable of the two. Patients, however, may find it less pleasant, experiencing brow-ache, more disturbance of accommodation and lid twitching. It also suffers the disadvantage of being available only in multidose containers. Physostigmine is rather unstable, breaking down to an irritant compound, rubreserine, and preparations thus have a relatively short shelf life.

Local anaesthetics

These reversibly block pain and other sensations in the sensory nerves of the cornea by preventing the generation and conduction of nerve impulses. They are used for contact tonometry, gonioscopy, moulding techniques, foreign body removal and possibly in other emergency situations where blepharospasm makes examination of the eye and determination of the problem difficult.

Available local anaesthetics

Local anaesthetics are all prescription only medicines and the Medicines Act allows the optometric practitioner to possess four such drugs. It must be remembered that, unlike the drugs discussed so far, the local anaesthetics may not be supplied to a patient, nor a supply arranged from a pharmacy. This is partly because there is no justification for home use, any problem warranting repeated local anaesthetic instillation warrants medical attention, and partly because of the dangers of corneal damage from prolonged and repeated use.

The four preparations available are: amethocaine 0.5% and 1% drops; oxybuprocaine 0.4% drops; proxymetacaine 0.5% drops; lignocaine 4% drops (with fluorescein 0.25% in single dose units). With the exception of proxymetacaine the drops are all available in single dose disposable units as well as multidose containers.

The four drugs are all similar in their mechanism of action and time courses. Local anaesthesia is normally produced within 60 seconds of instillation and recovery takes 20–30 minutes with the exception of lignocaine which is longer acting and may take 45 minutes. During the local anaesthesia, the corneal blink reflex is absent. The longer action of lignocaine is due to its different structure, lignocaine having an amide rather than an ester link in the chain. This, together with the substituents on the benzene ring (not possessed by the other compounds) makes enzymic breakdown more difficult. The other local anaesthetics have an ester link and are metabolized by pseudocholinesterase enzymes. The duration of the anaesthesia produced by any of the compounds may be extended by instillation of further drops.

Although some comments can be made about the individual drugs, the actual choice of local anaesthetic agent will be very much a matter of personal preference and experience on the part of the practitioner.

Oxybuprocaine

This is probably now the most popular of the local anaesthetics. It causes little initial stinging and there is no evidence of corneal epithelial damage following its use. In common with the other preparations used in optometry, oxybuprocaine (Benoxinate) causes no changes in pupil size.

Amethocaine

This is very similar to oxybuprocaine in terms of onset and duration of action, but it does normally sting immediately following instillation. Some evidence of superficial corneal damage may be seen on examination, but is more likely to occur after repeated or prolonged anaesthesia.

Proxymetacaine

Local anaesthesia may be achieved slightly more rapidly with proxymetacaine, but as all the drugs are effective in less than 60 seconds this is probably not a significant advantage. There is no evidence of corneal damage or stinging on instillation. However, the fact that proxymetacaine is not available in single dose units and requires storage in a refrigerator (being unstable at room temperature once the bottle has been opened), makes its use somewhat less convenient.

Lignocaine

Because lignocaine in single dose units is available only with fluorescein, its use is restricted to those situations where both local anaesthesia and staining or fluorescence are required. Such situations include applanation tonometry and foreign body removal. The combined preparation is useful because it necessitates only one instillation and there is less chance of drug loss (as can occur when multiple drops are instilled if insufficient time is allowed between them). In tonometry, it also avoids the use of the more concentrated fluorescein solutions. The combined preparations should not be used in the presence of soft contact lenses because of possible lens staining. Some patients experience stinging when lignocaine is instilled. The longer duration of action may be a drawback requiring the patient to remain longer in the practice after examination.

Problems associated with local anaesthetics

The patient should not be allowed to leave the practice until the normal corneal blink reflex has returned. This is to avoid the possibility of damage due to the undetected entry of a foreign body or rubbing of the eye. It is best to test for the return of the reflex by gently touching the cornea with a wisp of cotton wool or tissue rather than simply to assume that it will have returned once the usual time for recovery has elapsed. If the patient is unable to remain in the practice until the reflex has returned,

some protection may be offered by the instillation of viscous drops such as hypromellose, other artificial tears or contact lens wetting preparations. This will also reduce the drying of the cornea.

Although repeated or prolonged anaesthesia can cause damage to, and desquamation of, the corneal epithelium (which requires normally functioning nerves for its survival), this is unlikely to be seen in the situations in which the optometric practitioner normally uses local anaesthetics. If possible, local anaesthetics are best avoided if there are corneal abrasions present or suspected as repair may be delayed.

Allergic responses can occur to local anaesthetics, but they are not common and will only be seen in patients who have previously been exposed to the drugs. They are more likely to occur with the ester-linked compounds (amethocaine, oxybuprocaine and proxymetacaine) than with lignocaine.

Another possible problem is that of interaction between certain local anaesthetics, especially amethocaine, and sulphacetamide (*see* Antimicrobial drugs). If it is necessary to use both a local anaesthetic and an antimicrobial, it is probably advisable to avoid this particular combination.

Antimicrobial drugs

The term 'antimicrobial' covers drugs that are effective not only against bacteria but also against fungi and other microorganisms and includes the antibiotics, the sulphonamides and other compounds.

Drugs of this category are used in optometry as a prophylactic measure following certain procedures. The normal eye harbours potential pathogens on its surface, but these are usually without harm as they are unable to gain access to intact structures such as the cornea. However, should the corneal epithelium be damaged, as for example by a foreign body or following tonometry or contact lens work, it may not remain such an effective barrier and opportunist pathogens may gain access to the tissues and result in infection. Thus, following the potentially damaging procedures listed above, or if there is evidence of some breakdown of corneal integrity, antimicrobials may be used to reduce the chances of an infection developing. If the corneal damage detected is very superficial, it may be expected to heal within 24 hours and, after the instillation of the prophylactic, the patient may be requested to return the next day. Anything more serious should suggest referral of the patient to a hospital outpatient department following such prophylactic measures.

Available antimicrobials

The relevant antimicrobials are: sulphacetamide,

drops and ointment; mafenide, drops; framycetin, drops and ointment; propamidine, drops; dibromopropamidine, ointment.

Sulphacetamide and framycetin are prescription only medicines, but the Medicines Act specifically allows optometric practitioners to possess and use them. Additionally, in the case of sulphacetamide, a supply to the patient may be arranged from the pharmacy (for home use) or made direct by the practitioner in an emergency. This may not be done for framycetin whatever the circumstances—because framycetin is a true antibiotic, it might be construed that repeated instillation constituted treatment rather than prophylaxis, and that medical attention should be obtained in such a situation. Propamidine and dibromopropamidine are pharmacy medicines and may thus be purchased by a patient if required, the optometric practitioner only making a direct supply in an emergency.

Sulphacetamide

This is available as both ointment (2.5, 6 and 10%) and drops (10, 20 and 30%). The drops are available in single dose units only at 10%, the concentration most likely to be used for prophylaxis. Sulphacetamide in solution is the least alkaline (pH 7.4) of all the sulphonamides and it is for this reason that it was selected for use in the eye. Its mechanism of action, as discussed in Chapter 28, is to compete with *p*-aminobenzoic acid and inhibit the formation of nucleic acids by the bacteria. The spectrum of activity is fairly broad including both Gram-positive and Gram-negative bacteria.

Even the 10% drops used for prophylaxis are hypertonic and may thus cause stinging on instillation, together with some loss of the drug following increased tear production. The ointment causes less discomfort, and has the advantage of a longer contact time, but the greasy film it produces may be troublesome. There is also a preparation containing sulphacetamide 5% together with zinc sulphate 0.1%, which exerts an astringent action. This is available only in multidose containers.

As mentioned in the previous section, there is the theoretical possibility of interaction between sulphacetamide and some local anaesthetics such as amethocaine. These are metabolized to *p*-aminobenzoic acid or related structures which can be utilized by the bacteria in the production of nucleic acids. As sulphacetamide competitively inhibits the use of *p*-aminobenzoic acid, the presence of additional *p*-aminobenzoic acid could reduce the effectiveness of the antimicrobial. While it is difficult to evaluate how much of a real problem this is, if both a prophylactic and a local anaesthetic are to be used, it would perhaps be preferable to use either a different prophylactic or lignocaine, which is not metabolized in the same way, should be substituted as the local anaesthetic.

Mafenide

This may be used at 5%. It is very similar to sulphacetamide (belonging to the sulphonamide group) in terms of mechanism of action and spectrum and will have the same possible interaction with local anaesthetics. It is available only in multidose preparations and would seem to offer no advantage over sulphacetamide.

Framycetin

This is an antibiotic of the aminoglycoside group. Members of this group all have high potential systemic toxicity, involving damage to hearing and balance and to the kidneys. When used topically on the cornea, there is insufficient absorption of these extremely water-soluble compounds to cause systemic problems. Framycetin has a broad spectrum of activity being bactericidal to both Gram-positive and Gram-negative bacteria by inhibition of protein synthesis. It is available as both drops and ointment at 0.5%, but unfortunately there are no single dose units.

Propamidine and dibromopropamidine isethionate

These exert (by an unknown mechanism) both antibacterial and antifungal effects. There is a wide spectrum of activity including some Gram-negative organisms. They are available as drops in multidose units (propamidine) and as ointment (dibromopropamidine) and may provide a suitable alternative to sulphacetamide.

Some query might be raised about the value of a single instillation of an antimicrobial drug. If such drugs are used, together with working practices which minimize the chances of bacterial contamination of contact lenses, tonometer heads etc., then all reasonable measures have been taken to protect the patient against infection.

Staining agents

Stains are used to determine the integrity of the corneal epithelium, to demonstrate the presence of abnormal keratoconjunctival tissue and for a number of other purposes, for example applanation tonometry. Two stains are used for these different purposes: fluorescein sodium and rose bengal.

Fluorescein sodium

Fluourescein sodium is a water-soluble salt fully ionized at any pH. For this reason, it is unable to cross intact biological membranes. When applied to the eye, it will colour the tears and will be detected wherever the tears are present. The stain appears yellow or orange-yellow but shows a green fluorescence in alkaline conditions. The fluorescence is best visualized with cobalt blue light.

Fluorescein is available alone at 1 and 2% and together with lignocaine at 0.25%, all in single dose units. It is also available as sterile strips prepared by soaking filter paper in 20% fluorescein before packing and sterilizing. The choice of preparation will depend partly on the reason for using fluorescein, some procedures requiring greater quantities of the stain than others. For tonometry, the combined preparation is useful as only a small amount of fluorescein is needed. Larger amounts make the clear visualization of the annular pattern difficult. Alternatively, sufficient fluorescein may be obtained by the use of the strips. When placed in contact with the conjunctiva, with or without additional fluid, such as sterile saline or local anaesthetic drops, sufficient fluorescein is washed from the strip into the tears. If higher concentrations are required, when testing the patency of the nasolacrimal ducts for example, the higher strength drops (1 or 2%) may be preferred. Multidose containers of fluorescein drops are available but should be avoided. The solution makes a good growing medium for some bacteria including *Pseudomonas aeruginosa*, despite the presence of preservatives aimed at preventing the contamination of the drops. Should such a contaminated solution be introduced into an eye, where the integrity of the cornea is disturbed, the possible outcome for the patient is very serious. Fluorescein is often used in precisely such situations, for example looking for corneal damage, applanation tonometry and contact lens work. For this reason single dose units or sterile strips should always be used.

Fluorescein is used for a number of reasons.

Detection of corneal epithelial damage

If the corneal epithelium is damaged, fluorescein (in the tear film) will gain access to Bowman's membrane and the stroma. Irrigation of the eye with saline will wash away excess fluorescein and the damage will be seen as areas of green fluorescence when viewed under blue light. Because of the tear film surrounding mucus threads, these will also fluouresce but they may be distinguished from damage by their shape and movement on irrigation or when the eye is opened and closed. Fluorescein may be used to check for epithelial damage following removal of a foreign body, contact lens work or tonometry.

Detection of a foreign body

On occasions, it may be difficult to locate a foreign body in the eye. This can be made easier by the use of fluorescein and blue light. The stain will be seen as a green fluorescent outline around the foreign body. Any damage due to the movement of the foreign body across the cornea will also be seen as a fluorescent area. This will be the case even if the foreign body itself has already been washed out of the eye by tears, blinking of the lids and movement of the eye.

Applanation tonometry

Fluorescein, in low concentration, is instilled together with a local anaesthetic and the cornea viewed with a slitlamp using blue light. The fluorescence seen is due to the presence of tears around the flattened area of the cornea.

Contact lens fitting

Instillation of fluorescein will enable the fit of contact lenses to be determined. When viewed under blue light, areas of contact between the lens and cornea will appear purple (due to the absence of tears and fluorescein). Spaces between the lens and cornea will fluorese due to the presence of tears, the amount of fluorescence giving an indication of the dimension of the spaces. Obviously, the fluorescein will also detect any epithelial damage occurring during fitting. Because hydrophilic lenses will absorb the stain, it should not be used to assess their fit. A high-molecular-weight fluorescein, fluorexon, was produced to combat the problem. As the fluorescence produced is not very good and some lenses do absorb it, fluorexon has not found widespread use.

Tear flow and tear break-up time

These two can be assessed with the aid of fluorescein. For tear flow the stain is instilled and the time taken for the subsequent colour of the tears to fade is determined. To assess tear break-up time, fluorescein is instilled and the patient asked to blink (and then to refrain from further blinking). After blinking there will be an even fluorescence due to the stain in the tear film. As this breaks up areas lose their fluorescence. The time taken for this to happen is compared with the normal. In keratoconjunctivitis sicca the break-up time is reduced.

Patency of nasolacrimal ducts

If it is suspected that the nasolacrimal duct(s) could be blocked, this may be checked with fluorescein. After the nose has been blown fluorescein 2% drops are instilled into one eye and the nose blown again into a white tissue. If the duct is open, staining or fluorescence will be seen in the tissue. The procedure is repeated for the second eye.

Fluorescein is without local or systemic toxicity and there is no irritation or instillation even when the cornea is damaged.

Rose bengal

Rose bengal differs from fluorescein in staining dead and degenerate cells. Thus it is used to determine if such cells are present in the cornea and conjunctiva. After instillation of 1% drops any dead or degenerate cells will be stained a bright pink or red which is not washed away with saline. In this way, keratoconjunctivitis sicca and other abnormalities which may affect the wearing of contact lenses may be detected. Any areas of pressure from a contact lens will also be stained and may indicate that some change in the lens is needed.

Like fluorescein, rose bengal will also stain mucus but again this may be differentiated by shape and movement. False positives may also result if the stain is applied after the use of a local anaesthetic.

Rose bengal can cause considerable discomfort on instillation. Overspill onto the lids and skin must be avoided as a long-lasting stain is produced.

Drugs used in first aid and emergency procedures

Almost any of the drugs already discussed may be used in such procedures, the actual choice depending on the situation encountered.

Foreign body removal

Here a local anaesthetic may be necessary to overcome blepharospasm and to allow the eye to be examined. Any of the four available is suitable. Fluorescein may be required in order to locate the foreign body as well as to detect whether or not corneal damage has occurred. If this latter is the case then a prophylactic, such as sulphacetamide or one of the other antimicrobials, should be instilled to reduce the risk of bacterial infection.

Closed angle glaucoma

A miotic, most probably pilocarpine, may be required to cause the pupil to contract, to open the angle and the meshwork and to increase the outflow of aqueous humour to reduce the pressure. The decision whether or not to use a miotic, and the number of instillations to make, will depend on a number of factors including the possible delay before medical assistance can be received and the attitude of the local ophthalmologists. Some prefer to see patients without miotic instillation. If pilocarpine is to be instilled, 1% is used and 2 drops instilled into each eye at 10-minute intervals for 30 minutes.

Iritis

To reduce the danger of posterior synechiae and resultant block in the outflow of aqueous humour, the pupil may be dilated. The most powerful and longest lasting mydriatic available in the practice is the best choice. This is likely to be cyclopentolate (although others may be used if available). The immobilization of the sphincter and ciliary muscles will also reduce the pain. Care must be taken to distinguish the iritis from an attack of closed angle glaucoma.

Allergic responses

The best means to counteract the pain, swelling and redness associated with an allergic response is the use of an antihistamine. This is a specific antagonist to the main cause of the signs and symptoms, i.e. histamine. The only antihistamine available for use in the eye is antazoline. This is available (at 0.5%) in a preparation which also contains a vasoconstrictor, xylometazoline (0.05%). The antazoline will compete with the histamine for receptors in the blood vessels and at other sites involved in the allergic response. This will reduce the blood flow, fluid leakage and pain. Xylometazoline is an α-adrenoceptor agonist (like phenylephrine) and will interact directly with these receptors in the blood vessels to cause constriction. This will provide symptomatic relief by reducing the blood flow and capillary leakage. Weak solutions (0.12%) of the mydriatic phenylephrine may also be used as a decongestant both in allergic responses and in other situations such as contact lens moulding where vasodilatation would be a drawback. The natural hormone of the adrenal medulla, adrenaline, may also be used in both these situations as a 0.1% solution. Neither the adrenaline nor the phenylephrine will cause mydriasis at these low concentrations. As both phenylephrine and the antihistamine preparation are pharmacy medicines, they may be purchased by the patient if desired.

Patients should be warned against the regular use of decongestants to improve the appearance of a red eye (or eyes). The dilatation of the vessels may be an indication of some pathology that should be investigated. Even in the absence of any pathological problem, the overzealous use of decongestants can lead to difficulties as reactive hyperaemia often follows the vasoconstriction. This greater dilatation of the vessels may cause the patient to instil greater quantities of the decongestant with greater frequency causing the hyperaemia to increase. Excessive constriction followed by excessive dilatation may at worst lead to damage of the vessels and at best serves no useful purpose.

Whenever drugs are used in first aid or emergency treatment, it must be remembered that the first aid is rendered to alleviate discomfort on the part of the patient and to minimize any harmful processes. If further or repeated treatment is required the patient must be referred to a doctor or hospital for medical attention.

Further reading

See end of Chapter 31.

30

Side-effects of drugs

Janet Vale

In its broadest sense, a side-effect may be defined as any effect produced by a drug other than that for which the drug is being used in therapy, investigation etc. The term does not, of necessity, indicate an effect which is harmful to the patient, although of course many side-effects are indeed detrimental.

Side-effects may arise from use of ophthalmic drugs (these effects may be of either a local or systemic nature), or from the systemic use of drugs by the physician or self-administration by a patient. There must also be an awareness by the optometric practitioner of the possibility of interactions between the drugs to be used and any drugs already being taken by the patient.

Ocular side-effects of ophthalmic drugs

These drug effects are in two general categories: those which result directly from the pharmacological activity of the drug and those which are fundamentally allergic in nature.

In the first category, the problem of most significance is the possibility of inducing an attack of closed-angle glaucoma by the use of cycloplegic mydriatics, such as atropine and other muscarinic antagonists or mydriatics, such as phenylephrine.

With atropine and the other muscarinic antagonists, the problem arises because of the relaxation of the sphincter muscle, allowing the iris to fold back into the angle, and because of relaxation of the ciliary muscle. Normally, the alternate relaxations and contractions of this muscle pull on the scleral spur and encourage the flow of aqueous humour into the canal of Schlemm by altering both its diameter and the pressure within. Relaxation of the ciliary muscle may also encourage intraocular congestion through facilitated inflow and impeded

outflow of blood in the uveal tract. The possibility of a rise in intraocular pressure is more likely in the elderly patient and with the drugs producing prolonged effects, particularly atropine. Thus, the likelihood of such a problem occurring may be reduced by careful selection of the cycloplegic or mydriatic to be used, and by some prior investigation of elderly patients to determine whether or not they are predisposed to angle closure. In elderly patients, it is most likely that mydriasis is required without cycloplegia (for fundus examination), so that the practitioner should select the drug with the minimum effect on the ciliary muscle and the shortest but adequate duration of action on the sphincter muscle, which may be reliably reversed if it is felt necessary to do so once the examination is completed. In these circumstances, tropicamide 0.5% would normally be considered to be adequate or, alternatively, phenylephrine may be used. This is without effect on the ciliary muscle, has a tendency to reduce intraocular pressure, may be reliably reversed with thymoxamine and, it is claimed, causes the iris to fold in a way that is less likely to block the angle. Should an attack occur in response to the use of a mydriatic or cycloplegic mydriatic, the patient should be referred to hospital immediately. If it is likely that there will be some delay before the patient can receive attention, it is possible to instil pilocarpine (2 drops of 1% into each eye every 10 minutes for 30 minutes) in an attempt to alleviate the situation. Some ophthalmologists, however, prefer to see such patients untreated and known preferences of the local ophthalmologist should be taken into account, together with the likelihood of a delay in receiving attention, before a decision is made regarding treatment.

The problem of a rise in intraocular pressure also exists when miotics are used to reverse drug-induced mydriasis. If the reversal is incomplete and the iris remains at the midpoint between dilatation and constriction, there may be apposition between the iris and the lens. The passage of the aqueous from the posterior chamber is hindered, the pressure rises and the iris may be caused to move forward, thus blocking the angle in predisposed eyes. This is more likely to occur with those miotics which cause the ciliary muscle to contract with a resultant increase in thickness and forward movement of the lens. There is perhaps more chance of this if a muscarinic agonist or anticholinesterase is used to reverse a mydriasis unaccompanied by cycloplegia, because the miotic will be acting unopposed at the ciliary muscle, whereas the action at the iris involves either competition at the muscarinic receptors in the sphincter muscle (if a muscarinic antagonist such as tropicamide has been used) or physiological antagonism between the opposing muscles (if phenylephrine has been used). In this latter case, reversal would be best achieved with the antagonist thymoxamine, which is without activity at the ciliary muscle.

If physostigmine is used as a miotic for reversal of mydriasis, the patient may experience, not only the discomfort of a spasm of the ciliary muscle, but also an annoying twitching of the lids because of the potentiation of acetylcholine released by the nerves innervating the skeletal muscle fibres in these structures.

A further side-effect from the use of the sympathetic mydriatics (or from the use of adrenaline in the treatment of glaucoma) is the liberation of pigment from neuroepithelium of the dilator muscle. The contraction of the muscle induced by these drugs apparently results in the rupture of the pigment-containing cells. This is more often seen in older patients, is regarded as an ageing change and appears to be without detriment to the patient.

Local anaesthesia can cause desquamation of the corneal epithelial cells with resultant pitting of the cornea. This effect is most marked if the local anaesthesia is obtained with cocaine (unavailable to the optometric practitioner) and usually occurs only after prolonged or repeated anaesthesia, which is not common in optometric practice. It would appear that normal functioning of the sensory nerves is necessary for the survival of the epithelial cells. The prolonged loss of the blink reflex and associated drying of the cornea will worsen the situation. Because of the action of local anaesthetics on mitosis and cellular movement, the repair of minor corneal abrasions may be delayed by the use, even for short periods, of local anaesthetics. If possible, their use should therefore be avoided if abrasions exist or are suspected of existing.

The other category of ocular or local side-effects that may be encountered from the use of drugs in the eye is that of allergy. Allergic responses can theoretically occur to any drug that is used; however, among those used in optometry, allergy has most often been reported as occurring following the use of atropine, pilocarpine and local anaesthetics of the ester type, and even then it is not a common occurrence. The response is never shown on the first exposure to the drug and may only occur after prolonged use as, for example, with the use of pilocarpine in the treatment of glaucoma. Allergy can occur in contact lens wearers and may be due to the preservatives, particularly chlorhexidine and thiomersal, used in solutions, but care must be taken to distinguish between allergy to the preservative, allergy to protein build-up on the lenses and damage to the ocular tissues due to the attainment of high concentrations of the preservative following binding and absorption by the lens material. The true allergic response is due to an antigen–antibody reaction. In this, the immune system of the body recognizes the drug as an antigen, i.e. 'foreign', and responds with the production from plasma cells of specific antibodies. Interaction of the antigen and antibodies at the surface of mast cells results in the explosive release of the contents of these cells, namely histamine and other pharmacologically active substances such as prostaglandins and leukotrienes. The result of the release of those various substances include vasodilatation, increased permeability of capillaries allowing leakage of proteins, and stimulation or sensitization of sensory nerve endings. Thus an allergic reaction to an ophthalmic drug would be manifested as reddened, swollen conjunctiva and lids following the vasodilatation and leakage from capillaries, and discomfort or pain from the actions on the sensory nerve endings. Since the response is ultimately mediated by histamine, prostaglandins and related substances, the signs and symptoms will be essentially similar regardless of the pharmacological activities of the drug initiating the reaction. Allergic responses are not manifested on the first exposure, possibly because the production of antibodies is not rapid enough to achieve the optimum antigen–antibody concentration for interaction at the mast cell.

Should a patient show an allergic response, for example to atropine eye ointment prescribed for use at home, the first step is to discontinue use of the drug while reassuring the patient that the response is a temporary one and that there will be no lasting damage. Relief from the discomfort may be provided by a vasoconstrictor such as 0.1% adrenaline solution, which will directly constrict the blood vessels and reduce the capillary permeability, or a combined preparation of a vasoconstrictor and an antihistamine—the antihistamine will act as a competitive antagonist to histamine at its receptors. It must be remembered that should the same drug, or one closely related in chemical structure, be used again in the same patient, the allergic response is likely to recur.

The remaining side-effects which may occur from the local use of drugs in the eye are generally in response to drugs used by the ophthalmologist or general practitioner and are therefore not so likely to come to the attention of the optometric practitioner. These include the formation of cataracts from the prolonged use of the irreversible anticholinesterase ecothiopate in glaucoma and ptosis from the use of the adrenergic neurone-blocking compound guanethidine, also in glaucoma. The ptosis is due to the loss of sympathetic tone in the smooth muscle of the upper lid. The use of adrenaline in the treatment of glaucoma can result in the deposition of pigment in the ocular tissues; this may be adrenochrome, a minor metabolite of adrenaline produced by oxidation. A number of patients treated with topical adrenal steroids, for non-infective inflammatory conditions of the eye, respond with a rise in intraocular pressure due to a decreased facility of outflow. This may be the result of changes in the glycoprotein of the trabecular meshwork. The response is more frequent in patients with a family history of open angle glaucoma and is genetically determined. When treated with betamethasone 0.1% drops (4 times daily for 3 or 4 weeks), subjects may be divided into high responders (a rise of more than 15 mmHg), intermediate responders (a rise of between 6 and 15 mmHg) and nonresponders. This suggests control by a pair of allelomorphic genes (for high and low sensitivity), intermediate responders being heterozygous for this trait.

Systemic effects from locally applied drugs

Although ophthalmic drugs are applied topically to concentrate the effects in the eye, the possibility of systemic side-effects cannot be disregarded. Topically applied drugs may enter the systemic circulation by absorption through the conjunctiva (normally only a small fraction of that applied) or by absorption from the nasal mucous membranes, or the gastrointestinal tract after passage through the canaliculi. The use of ointment, as with atropine, reduces the chances of such absorption taking place, as does pressure applied over the canaliculi for some 30 seconds after instillation of drops.

The systemic side-effects from the topical use of atropine are usually limited to dry mouth and, possibly, tachycardia, the more serious problems, including central effects, occurring only from the accidental ingestion, especially by children, of ointment or drops supplied for use at home. The use of cyclopentolate drops has been associated with instances of central disturbances (hallucinations, incoherent speech etc.) particularly in children and where several drops of the higher concentration have been used (as may be necessary when the iris is heavily pigmented). Although there were no lasting effects in these cases, it would seem wise to use the lowest concentration and minimum number of drops possible and to take steps to reduce systemic absorption. Systemic absorption of pilocarpine produces signs of excess activity in the parasympathetic system, namely increased salivation, sweating and a decrease in heart rate. This is unlikely to occur from the single instillation of pilocarpine used to reverse mydriasis, but the risk is considerably higher when the drug is instilled intensively in an attempt to reduce the raised pressure of a closed angle glaucoma attack.

When considering the effects of drugs absorbed after topical administration, the possibility of interaction with drugs already being taken systemically by the patient must not be forgotten. One of the most notorious groups of drugs for causing interactions with other systemic medication is the monoamine oxidase inhibitors and this possibility must also be considered when using drops topically. In the normal situation, the amount of adrenaline or phenylephrine entering the systemic circulation after topical application is unlikely to provoke any great response (except perhaps in patients with hyperthyroidism who are extra sensitive to the catecholamines and related compounds) but, in patients being treated with monoamine oxidase inhibitors, the breakdown of such compounds may be reduced such that higher levels are achieved for a more prolonged period which may be sufficient to provoke a hypertensive response. With ephedrine, which displaces noradrenaline from storage sites in the neurones, there may be a three-fold effect: inhibition of monoamine oxidase results in a higher concentration of noradrenaline available in the stores, the noradrenaline displaced may persist longer because of enzyme inhibition and the ephedrine, normally metabolized by monoamine oxidase in the liver (also inhibited), will not be metabolized as rapidly. All these factors will contribute to the possibility of a hypertensive response. Fortunately, the monoamine oxidase inhibitors are less commonly used nowadays but the practitioner should be alerted to the possibility of interaction and sympathetic drugs should be avoided in any patient who is using, or has used in the previous 10–14 days, these compounds.

The other major group of antidepressants is the tricyclics, such as amitriptyline, which, among other actions, prevent the uptake of noradrenaline into the neurones. Adrenaline is partly inactivated by uptake (although metabolism is more important) and, therefore, any entering the systemic circulation may be potentiated by such compounds, again resulting in a hypertensive response. Phenylephrine is not a substrate for uptake and thus there should be no interaction between it and the tricyclic antidepressants; since ephedrine depends on uptake to exert its effects, there are unlikely to be any systemic problems from its use.

In patients suffering from hypertension who are being treated with β-antagonists (e.g. propranolol), drugs such as phenylephrine and ephedrine could theoretically act at the blood vessels and disturb the control of the hypertension.

It is difficult to assess how much of a real problem these theoretical interactions are in practice, because it will depend on the amount of drug absorbed systemically, the cardiovascular status of the patient etc., but it would seem sensible to err on the side of caution and avoid using drugs interacting with the sympathetic system in patients already using any of the categories of drugs discussed and to achieve mydriasis by the use of a low concentration of tropicamide.

Another possible interaction resulting from enzyme inhibition is that between certain local anaesthetics and anticholinesterases. These latter may be used by a patient in the treatment of myasthenia gravis and other situations where increased levels of acetylcholine are required. Anticholinesterases, such as neostigmine and pyridostigmine, inhibit not only acetylcholinesterase (allowing the build-up of acetylcholine at the skeletal muscle and elsewhere), but also serum cholinesterase which is responsible for the metabolism of a number of drugs including those local anaesthetics such as amethocaine, oxybuprocaine and proxymetacaine which contain an ester link in their structures. Any local anaesthetic absorbed systemically would not be destroyed as rapidly as usual. Again, it is difficult to estimate whether or not such an interaction would cause any real problem, but perhaps it would be prudent to use lignocaine (which has an amide link and is not dependent on cholinesterase) in any patient using anticholinesterase drugs.

Ocular effects from systemically administered drugs

There has been an increasing awareness during recent years that drugs administered for their effects on one structure or tissue will result in unwanted effects on other structures. This applies to drugs administered systemically for effects on non-ocular structures. A small proportion of the administered drug will find its way into the eye and may result in changes of a temporary or permanent nature which interfere with visual performance. The optometric practitioner may detect such drug-induced changes as many patients are examined on a regular basis and because patients experiencing any such problems are likely to seek advice on the visual changes, rather than connecting the change with their systemic medication (prescribed or self-administered). It is important to be aware that drug-induced changes can occur because their early recognition may be instrumental in preventing serious damage

resulting. If there is suspicion from the examination of a patient that there are changes which could be the result of systemic drugs, that patient should be referred to the general practitioner giving details of the findings. The decisions as to whether the drug is indeed responsible for the abnormality and whether to withdraw or maintain the treatment, remain the province of the doctor who must weigh the benefit of the drug against the risk to the patient. This will obviously vary with the seriousness of the disease being treated, the seriousness of the possible side-effect and the availability of alternative problem-free therapy. The referral of the patient must be done without causing undue alarm; the abrupt cessation of medication could prove more damaging to the patient than the suspected ocular side-effect. It would probably seem unnecessary to refer patients with changes in accommodation and/or pupil size from muscarinic antagonists (unless there was concern about possible angle block and raised intra-ocular pressure in predisposed patients) but an awareness of this potential problem may help in avoiding unnecessary prescription changes for what may prove to be a temporary situation.

The side-effects occurring can be divided into two main types. The side-effects which affect the pupil size, light response and accommodation are generally due to drugs possessing muscarinic blocking activity as either their major or subsidiary property. With the exception of possible angle block these side-effects result in only minor problems for the patient, often diminish during continued therapy and are reversible once the drug is withdrawn. The other side-effects which can occur are of great variety, may or may not be expected or explicable from the pharmacology of the drug and may or may not regress or reverse on withdrawal of the drug.

As with any side-effects, it is generally difficult to say how likely they are to occur and how likely the optometric practitioner is to encounter patients with such responses. In very broad terms, it can be said that side-effects are more likely to be seen with high dosage and prolonged treatment and are perhaps more likely in elderly patients because of either a predisposition to the particular problem (e.g. angle block) or because of reduced metabolism allowing higher than usual levels of the drug to persist in the body for prolonged periods. However, as responses may have a genetic basis, again giving either a predisposition (e.g. steroid-induced rise in intra-ocular pressure) or altered metabolism, this may not always be true and adverse responses may appear following only short-term or low dose administration.

Very many drugs have been implicated in causing very many ocular side-effects and it would be unreasonable to expect an optometric practitioner to remember every one of these. The more common, well proven and documented ones should be known together with the sources of information, either textual or from other professionals involved in health care, regarding the remainder.

As so many drugs have been shown, or at least suggested, to produce ocular side-effects, it is not possible to discuss them all, nor is it necessary since many of the side-effects are attributed to drugs which are used in specialized circumstances such that patients receiving such medication are unlikely to be encountered.

Because an eye examination proceeds structure by structure, it would seem reasonable to discuss possible side-effects and drugs causing them in the same way, starting however with the problem which may cause the patient to seek advice, namely blurred vision.

Blurred vision

This may of course be attributable to changes in the functions of the ciliary muscle (*see below*), but in many cases no such ready explanation exists. Such blurring has been reported for the sulphonamides, for oral hypoglycaemic drugs, such as chlorpropamide, for a number of diuretics including the thiazides, and for the anxiolytics such as the benzodiazepines (diazepam, nitrazepam etc.). In the case of the oral hypoglycaemics, the effect may be due to fluctuating carbohydrate levels, while effects on ion and fluid movement between the lens and the aqueous may be responsible for the problem in the case of diuretics. The benzodiazepines are able to produce skeletal muscle relaxation by a central action and may thus interfere with the extraocular muscles, such that precise movement of the eyes is not maintained correctly, resulting in blurring. Many other drugs have been reported as causing blurring but the problem appears to be transient, often disappearing on continued use of the drug and certainly ceasing on its withdrawal.

Conjunctiva

Among the many drugs implicated in causing conjunctivitis of one type or another are the barbiturates, for example phenobarbitone used in the treatment of epilepsy, the benzodiazepines, such as diazepam, used in anxiety and as sedatives and the non-steroidal anti-inflammatory drugs such as ketoprofen. Phenylbutazone, which belongs to this last group, has been virtually withdrawn from use because of its side-effects (including ocular problems). Rifampicin, used for prolonged periods in the treatment of tuberculosis, may produce a conjunctivitis of varying severity and also colour the tears red which can result in the staining of soft contact lenses. The sulphonamides can produce allergic responses in the conjunctiva. The most serious of these is the exudative conjunctivitis associated with the Stevens–Johnson syndrome. This syndrome affects other mucous membranes and can be fatal, but fortunately is rare. Such a response has also been reported to occur following the use of allopurinol, in the prophylaxis of gout, and carbamazepine for epilepsy. The oculomucocutaneous syndrome associated with the use of practolol, which is now restricted to hospital use, does not appear to occur in response to other β-adrenoceptor antagonists.

The phenothiazines, such as chlorpromazine, are used in schizophrenia and other behavioural disturbances. Prolonged use or high dosage has led to pigmentation of the conjunctiva which in some patients may be associated with similar problems in the cornea, retina and skin.

Cornea

As mentioned above, the use of phenothiazines can lead to deposits in the cornea as well as the conjunctiva. Indomethacin, a non-steroidal anti-inflammatory drug used in the treatment of rheumatoid conditions, can lead to punctate deposits in the cornea (and irreversible retinal damage) and patients receiving longer-term therapy with this drug should undergo regular ophthalmological checks. It is not yet clear whether this problem is characteristic of the group of drugs or unique to indomethacin. Also used in rheumatoid arthritis, sodium aurothiomalate, can lead to corneal deposition of gold at higher doses. Chloroquine use may result in subepithelial corneal deposits with a whorl-like pattern. This deposition, thought to be due to the formation of complexes with cellular phospholipids, does not normally affect vision and slowly regresses when the drug is withdrawn. It is more likely to occur when chloroquine is used in the treatment of rheumatoid arthritis than when it is used to prevent or treat malaria, because of the prolonged high dosage used in the former situation. Like the retinal changes which it usually precedes, the deposition appears to be related to the total amount of drug administered. Virtually all patients treated with amiodarone for certain types of cardiac arrhythmias show yellow-brown deposits in the cornea. Again vision appears to be unaffected and the deposits decrease when the drug is withdrawn.

A problem seen only with overdosage arises from vitamin D. Taken in excess this results in the deposition of calcium within superficial layers of the cornea. Unless this is removed by chelation (with EDTA) or surgery, vision is decreased.

The second type of drug-related corneal problem is that of oedema and, therefore, possible difficulties with wearing of contact lenses. The drugs responsible are the adrenal steroids (most often used for their anti-inflammatory effects) and the oestrogens/progestogens used for contraception. Both these groups of drugs influence water and electrolyte behaviour physiologically and it may be that such changes within the cornea are responsible for the difficulty. With the contraceptive steroids, the problems associated with contact lens wear may be compounded by a possible reduction in tear formation.

Iris and ciliary muscle

Drug effects on these structures are perhaps the most likely to be encountered in optometric practice. Changes normally result from the use of drugs which interact with the autonomic nervous system and are most likely to be associated with the systemic use of muscarinic antagonists, i.e. atropine-like drugs. As can be expected, drugs of this category have the potential to relax the ciliary muscle resulting in cycloplegia and the sphincter muscle of the iris causing mydriasis and a reduction in the light reflex. The patient may thus complain of blurred vision and/or problems with bright lights. In susceptible patients, the relaxation of the two muscles may precipitate an attack of closed angle glaucoma. The blocking activity at the lacrimal gland may reduce tear production and result in difficulties with contact lens wear. Some drugs are used first and foremost because they are muscarinic antagonists, for example hyoscine and propantheline used in the treatment of gastrointestinal problems, ipratropium used as a bronchodilator and benzhexol and orphenadrine used to treat Parkinson's disease. It should be remembered that some travel sickness antidotes and cold remedies available without prescription contain muscarinic antagonist compounds. Some drugs are less obviously muscarinic antagonists, for example the phenothiazines and tricyclic antidepressants, such as imipramine and amitriptyline. With these drugs, their primary action is exerted on receptors other than muscarinic but they have secondary or minor actions as muscarinic antagonists and may cause difficulties in some patients. Some antihistamines, mostly available without a prescription, possess muscarinic receptor blocking activity in varying degrees.

Sympathetic α-agonists, by acting at the dilator muscle, may produce mydriasis, problems with bright lights and closed angle glaucoma. Such compounds are perhaps most likely to occur in various cough and cold remedies including those available without prescription.

Muscarinic agonists, for example bethanecol, and anticholinesterases, such as distigmine, used in cases of urinary retention or atonic gut muscle, can produce spasm of accommodation for near vision and miosis which may be troublesome to a patient, especially if there are central opacities.

The problems obviously cease when the drug is withdrawn and, with the exception of closed angle glaucoma, normally cause the patient no great difficulty.

Lens

The phenothiazines may deposit in the lens, as well as the conjunctiva and cornea. The deposits begin as dot-like opacities which, with continued drug administration, may progress to form a stellate or anterior polar cataract. Long-term, high dosage treatment with the anti-inflammatory steroids, for example hydrocortisone, prednisolone, dexamethasone and triamcinolone, in rheumatoid conditions, is likely to lead to the formation of posterior subcapsular cataracts. As the steroids physiologically influence all aspects of metabolism, fat, protein, carbohydrate, electrolyte and water, this may be a consequence of abnormalities of metabolism induced by the supraphysiological doses employed in inflammatory diseases.

Retina

Probably the best known drug effect on the retina is that arising from chloroquine. Like the effects on the cornea, this is most likely to occur from the prolonged high dosage associated with treatment of rheumatoid arthritis, and the total amount of drug administered appears to be important. Problems normally only arise after a total of 100 g has been given. Because the chloroquine becomes bound to retinal pigment epithelium, the damage may progress even though administration of the drug ceases. The drug causes changes in pigmentation, particularly in the region of the macula, 'bull's eye' macula, and narrowing of retinal vessels. These changes result in defects in both peripheral and central vision. If the central retina is involved colour vision may be affected. Because medical practitioners are aware of the problems associated with the use of chloroquine, patients are normally referred for regular ophthalmological checks.

The phenothiazines may cause a purplish pigmentation of the retina and associated disturbances in vision (reduced visual acuity, problems with night vision). As with other pigmentation produced by the phenothiazines, this is normally associated with prolonged use of high dosage. It is most likely to occur with thioridazine and occasionally may result from lower dosage. Among other drugs implicated in causing retinal changes and decreased visual function are clonidine, used to treat hypertension, indomethacin and ibuprofen. With these and many other drugs the evidence for a causal relationship is not always clear.

Digoxin and other cardiac glycosides are used to treat heart failure and arrhythmias. They may result in visual problems including disturbed colour vision (a blue–yellow defect), glare phenomena and scotomata. It is not clear whether the effects are exerted directly on the retina or through a central mechanism. They are usually reversible and their importance lies in the fact that they are early indications of toxic plasma levels of the drug. Digoxin has only a very narrow therapeutic range; these visual disturbances normally precede the more serious, possible fatal cardiac disturbances which may arise.

Retinal oedema is a possible problem which has been reported for adrenal steroids, oestrogens/progestogens and certain diuretics such as chlorothiazide. This could be associated with their actions on electrolyte and fluid metabolism. Sudden cessation of adrenal steroid therapy may precipitate papilloedema.

Optic nerve

Rifampicin has already been mentioned in connection with conjunctivitis. It, and the other drugs used in the treatment of tuberculosis, have all been implicated, with varying degrees of certainty, in causing damage to the optic nerve. Isoniazid causes a general peripheral neuropathy and optic neuritis which can be prevented or reduced by administration of pyridoxine. The optic neuritis caused by ethambutol may be one of two types. If the damage is periaxial only peripheral visual field defects occur. Central vision and colour vision are unaffected. However, changes in these do occur if the damage is axial. The disturbance in colour vision is usually manifested as a red–green defect. The effects may be permanent or slowly reversible after withdrawal of the drug. By restricting the daily dose to below 15 mg/kg it is usually possible for the ocular effects to be avoided.

Colour vision

Disturbances of colour vision have already been mentioned with the antitubercular drugs and the cardiac glycosides (in association with other visual problems). Nalidixic acid, used for urinary tract infections, commonly causes objects to appear green, yellow, blue or violet. Glare phenomena may also occur. The diuretics of chlorothiazide and frusemide may also cause disturbances in colour vision.

Further reading

See end of Chapter 31.

31

Legal aspects

Janet Vale

Medicines (or drugs) comprise a large number of compounds which have beneficial effects in the treatment and prevention of disease. However, the same compounds may cause considerable harm, both immediate and long term, to either the individual or the community if used (or abused) injudiciously. For this reason, the sale and supply of medicines is controlled by a number of laws. The general aim of these laws is to apply restrictions to the sale and supply of medicines such that they are not freely available, but at the same time make it possible for individuals with a genuine requirement for the medicine to obtain a supply without undue difficulty. The Acts of Parliament thus regulating the sale and supply of medicines are the Medicines Act 1968 (introduced 1978) and the Misuse of Drugs Act 1971. (Non-medicinal poisons are covered by the Poisons Act 1972.)

Misuse of Drugs Act 1971

This act is concerned with controlling the supply of those drugs which are regarded as having abuse potential. The use of such drugs may result in both psychic and physical dependence and the appearance of withdrawal symptoms if intake is abruptly terminated. The drugs covered by the act, known collectively as controlled drugs, include the narcotic analgesics (morphine, heroin etc.), stimulants of the central nervous system (cocaine, amphetamine), hallucinogenic compounds (e.g. LSD) and cannabis. Recently the barbiturates, with the exception of those used for general anaesthesia, have been brought under varying degrees of control within the Misuse of Drugs Act.

All aspects of the controlled drugs, their manufacture, import and export, and sale and supply are covered by the act, as are matters such as the safe custody of the drugs and the registration of addicts.

In general, the possession of controlled drugs is illegal unless they have been obtained on a prescription or are being held and used by a member of one of the professions listed in the Act as entitled to possess certain controlled drugs necessary for the practice of that profession. Optometic practitioners are not listed amongst the professional groups allowed to possess controlled drugs and so may not use any such drugs in their practice. The only controlled drug which might have been of interest is cocaine which produces local anaesthesia, mydriasis and vasoconstriction when applied topically. However, there are a number of satisfactory alternatives to produce these effects and the non-availability of this drug poses no problems.

Medicines Act 1968

The Act, of eight parts in total, deals with all aspects of those compounds classed as medicines, including manufacturing licences, labelling and containers, pharmacies and much more, but the main points of relevance to optometry are contained in Part III which deals with the sale and supply of medicines.

The main principle of the Act, with regard to the sale and supply of medicines to the public, is that this should be restricted such that it is under the control of a pharmacist. It was realized, however, that in some circumstances this could prove too restrictive and the principle has been relaxed so that some medicines are more widely available. These medicines, known as general sales list medicines are not, however, completely free of restrictions on their sale and supply.

The remaining medicines are subject to increasing degrees of control and are classed as pharmacy medicines or prescription only medicines.

General Sales List

The medicines on the General Sales List comprise a group for which it was felt that the risk to health, the potential for abuse or the need for special handling was small, and that it would be to the benefit and convenience of intending users for the sale not to be restricted to a pharmacy. These medicines may thus be supplied from both registered pharmacy premises or from other permanent retail premises (but not market stalls etc.) and in some cases from vending machines. However, because some of the medicines concerned, for example aspirin, are not entirely without risk, there are restrictions concerning maximum pack size, strength of certain preparations and so on.

There are no eye drops or eye ointments on the General Sales List even though the constituents, for example sodium chloride, may be completely free of restriction (and in this case not even classed as a medicine) when not included in such formulations. All drops or ointments intended for ocular application are pharmacy or prescription only medicines. This ensures that a patient seeking preparations for use in the eye should not be able to obtain them from an outlet where no professional advice is available. Optrex eye lotion, however, is available from retail sources other than a pharmacy.

The General Sales List contains no preparations of professional interest to the optometric practitioner.

Pharmacy medicines

No list of pharmacy medicines exists as such; pharmacy medicines are those medicines which are not included in the General Sales List or the Prescription Only Medicines Order.

The requirement for pharmacy medicines is that they should be supplied from registered pharmacy premises by, or under the supervision of, a registered pharmacist. Thus, the patient wishing to obtain these medicines is able to seek, or be offered, professional advice as to their suitability, potential dangers and correct use. The pharmacist is also in a position to detect any excessive use of preparations suggestive of abuse.

All eye drops and eye ointments other than those categorized as prescription only medicines are pharmacy medicines, and include the antibacterial preparations propamidine, dibromopropamidine (Brolene) and mafenide, phenylephrine (any concentration), naphazoline drops (below a concentration of 0.015%, above which the preparation becomes a prescription only medicine), a preparation con-

taining antazoline and xylometazoline (Otrivine–Antistin) for use in ocular allergic conditions, fluorescein drops and papers, rose bengal drops, sodium chloride drops and various preparations of hypromellose, polyvinylpyrrolidine and liquid paraffin used for ocular lubrication.

The optometric practitioner may purchase any of these preparations for use in the practice with no formalities whatsoever.

Although the general requirement is that medicines in this category be supplied from a registered pharmacy by or under the supervision of a pharmacist, an exemption from these requirements is granted to optometric practitioners in that they may, in some circumstances, make a supply direct to a patient. The conditions to be satisfied are that the drug or preparation concerned would normally be used in the course of optometric practice and that an emergency exists requiring such a supply. There is no definition of an emergency, but the exemption does not constitute a permit to undertake the routine supply of pharmacy medicines to patients.

Prescription only medicines

These are listed in the prescription only medicines order and comprise those drugs where there is known abuse liability (the controlled drugs), a known or potential hazard to the individual or a danger to the health of the community from the unrestricted, unsupervised use (antibiotics and related preparations). All parenteral preparations, except insulin for human use, are also included.

The supply of prescription only medicines must be made from registered pharmacy premises, by or under the supervision of a registered pharmacist and may normally only be made in response to a prescription from a registered doctor, dentist or veterinary practitioner. In addition, doctors, dentists and veterinary practitioners may supply directly to their patients or the owners of animals under their care.

The majority of drugs employed by optometric practitioners in their practice are prescription only medicines and it might seem that problems would be experienced in obtaining supplies. This, however, is not the case for two reasons: either the drug in question is exempted from prescription only medicine control in the particular preparation required or the pharmacist is granted an exemption from the normal requirements for the supply of certain named preparations to an optometric practitioner for use in the practice, i.e. a prescription as detailed above is not required.

Examples of the first type include adrenaline and ephedrine (and their salts) which are normally prescription only medicines, but in preparations for external use, including eye drops, are classed as pharmacy medicines. Naphazoline hydrochloride is exempt from prescription only medicine requirements in concentrations below 0.015% and becomes a pharmacy medicine. The optometric practitioner may thus obtain such preparations with no formalities.

The majority of the preparations required, however, come into the second category. A supply of the drugs listed in the exemption to the prescription only medicine order may be made to an optometric practitioner, or directly to the patient of such a practitioner, on the presentation of a signed order. The details to be included in the signed order are:

Name, address and qualifications of the optometric practitioner
Date
Name and address of patient (if applicable) and age (if under 12)
Name, form (ointment or drops) and strength of medicine
Purpose for which it is required (e.g. 'for use in the practice' or more precise if the supply is to a patient for home use)
Any labelling directions
The signature of the optometric practitioner

The signed order is retained by the pharmacist. The drugs which may be supplied in this way are:

Sulphacetamine sodium, not more than 30%
Sulphafurazole diethanolamine equivalent to not more than 4% sulphafurazole
Atropine sulphate
Bethanecol chloride
Carbachol
Cyclopentolate hydrochloride
Homatropine hydrobromide
Hyoscine hydrobromide
Naphazoline hydrochloride or nitrate
Neostigmine methylsulphate
Physostigmine salicylate or sulphate
Pilocarpine hydrochloride or nitrate
Tropicamide

In addition to the exemption granted to the pharmacist, allowing the supply of these medicines, an exemption is also granted to the optometric practitioner allowing the medicines to be not only used in the practice but also supplied directly to a patient provided that this is in the course of optometric practice and in an emergency. Again an emergency is not defined. This is left to the discretion of the practitioner, who must be prepared to defend the decision if required to do so. This exemption should be seen as a privilege accorded in special circumstances, not as an indication that the routine supply of prescription only medicines may be undertaken. If such drugs are required at home by patients, the normal source of supply should be through the pharmacist.

In addition to the medicines listed above, the pharmacist is also allowed to supply to the optometric practitioner the following drugs in ophthalmic preparations:

Amethocaine hydrochloride
Lignocaine hydrochloride
Oxybuprocaine hydrochloride
Proxymetacaine hydrochloride
Oxyphenbutazone
Framycetin sulphate
Thymoxamine hydrochloride

These drugs are to be used only in the practice, the pharmacist may not supply them directly to the optometric practitioner's patient, nor in any circumstances may the practitioner supply them to a patient for use at home. As far as framycetin and oxyphenbutazone, and the local anaesthetics are concerned any need for repeated use would suggest the presence of some abnormal condition (damage, infection or inflammation) meriting medical attention.

These prescription only medicines (both groups) may also be obtained from a wholesaler when a signed order is not essential (but perhaps desirable).

The lists contain drugs which are not presently available in the UK in preparations for the eye, e.g. sulphafurazole (an antibacterial which was previously available) and bethanecol (a muscarinic agonist miotic, available in some other countries). However their inclusion in the list ensures that should preparations become available in the UK, then the optometric practitioner would be legally able to obtain supplies without any change in legislation being required.

Further reading

BARTLETT, J.D. and JAANUS, S.D. (1984) *Clinical Ocular Pharmacology*. Boston: Butterworths

BOWMAN, W.C. and RAND, H.J.(1980) *Textbook of Pharmacology*, 2nd edn. Oxford: Blackwell

BRITISH MEDICAL ASSOCIATION and THE PHARMACEUTICAL ASSOCIATION OF GREAT BRITAIN *British National Formulary* (Twice yearly publication)

DAVIES, D.M. (1981) *Textbook of Adverse Drug Reactions*, 2nd edn. Oxford: Oxford University Press

ELLIS, P. (1981) *Ocular Therapeutics and Pharmacology*, 6th edn. St Louis: C.V. Mosby

FOSTER, R.W. and COX, BARRY (1986) *Basic Pharmacology*, 2nd edn. London: Butterworths

FRAUNFELDER, F.T. (1982) *Drug Induced Ocular Side Effects and Drug Interactions*, 2nd edn. Philadelphia: Lea and Febiger

GOODMAN, L.S. and GILMAN, A. (1985) *The Pharmacological Basis of Therapeutics*, 7th edn. London: Macmillan

GRUNDY, H.F. (1985) *Lecture Notes on Pharmacology* Oxford: Blackwell

KATZUNG, B. (1987) *Basic and Clinical Pharmacology*, 3rd edn. Los Altos: Lange

KRUK, Z. and PYCOCK, C. (1983) *Neurotransmitters and Drugs*, 2nd edn. London: Croom Helm

O'CONNOR DAVIES, P.H. (1981) *The Actions and Uses of Ophthalmic Drugs*, 2nd edn. London: Butterworths

PEARCE, M. (1984) *Medicines and Poisons Guide*, 4th edn. London: The Pharmaceutical Press

VALE, J. and COX, B. (1985) *Drugs and the Eye*, 2nd edn. London: Butterworths

Part 8

Prescribing and patient management

32

General considerations in prescribing

Henri Obstfeld

When the monocular and binocular investigation techniques have been applied, the practitioner should have the following clinical details available relating to distance vision:

(1) Monocular 'vision', i.e. a measure of the ability of the brain to interpret the retinal image formed by each uncorrected eye of a distance letterchart.
(2) The monocular distance correction of each eye.
(3) The monocular 'visual acuities', i.e. the measure of the ability of the brain to interpret the retinal image formed by each corrected eye of the distance letterchart.
(4) Any anomalies of binocular distance vision.

For intermediate/near/occupational vision the details are:

(1) Monocular addition(s).
(2) Near acuities, i.e. a measure of the brain's ability to interpret the monocular retinal image formed by the correction for the appropriate object distance, of an appropriately scaled-down letterchart or paragraph of print.
(3) Any anomalies of binocular near vision.

Following this, the object is to arrive at a prescription which will provide:

(1) The best possible binocular visual acuity for distance vision, intermediate, near and/or occupational use.
(2) The most comfortable vision at all times.

Generally, the correction determined by means of a binocular balancing technique will provide such a prescription. Although it will be necessary to depart from such a prescription from time to time, it is a prerequisite to determine the full corrections first (Diepes, 1975).

If no binocular vision is possible, as in the case of the monocular patient, the correction of that eye will suffice. In other cases, binocular effects will have to be considered.

In the case of suppression of the brain's perception of one of the two foveal images, the practitioner must determine which eye is thus affected. Binocular balancing techniques may provide this information because, where there are different monocular acuities in each eye, the dominant eye is frequently associated with the higher visual acuity and the foveal image of the other eye is subject to some degree of suppression. However, in cases where alterations in the optical system of one eye have occurred relatively recently, such as a rapidly developed cataract, dominance may not yet have changed. This is a factor to be considered when prescribing; the cataractous, dominant eye should be provided with a correction which will give the best possible foveal image; any attempt to defocus the image may lead to asthenopia.

Asthenopia

According to Giles (1960), the largest percentage of patients consulting the practitioner will complain of 'eyestrain' or headaches, although it is probably more correct to say that these complaints represent the largest percentage among patients who do not come for a routine eye examination. If the practitioner cannot discover a possible optometric cause for the complaint, the patient should be referred to the general practitioner (GP). If there is an indication of marginal significance relating to the cause, the practitioner should discuss this with the patient and prescribe on the understanding that the patient will report back in due course to indicate whether the symptoms have been relieved. If there is no relief, the patient should then be referred to the GP with a letter indicating the symptoms, prescription, alteration and effect, if any, on the symptoms.

It is worth noting that presbyopes who do not yet have a near vision correction do not normally report asthenopia (Morgan, 1960), but complain about the smallness of print, bad lighting etc.

Whether to prescribe

When new patients present themselves without spectacles but with significant ametropia which, when corrected, provides a visual acuity within normal physiological limits, there is seldom reason for doubt whether to prescribe or not. Problem cases are those where the patient reports symptoms but the ametropia is small. For example, there are cases where right and left +0.25 DS or +0.50 DS with or without a very light, neutral tint can bring relief. While these cases may be psychological in origin, the relief can be real as far as the patient is concerned and can, in appropriate cases, be prescribed. This applies primarily to hyperopes, and placebos in the form of afocal lenses have sometimes been shown to provide relief (Cholerton, 1955; Nathan, 1957). The patient's mental attitude plays an important role as does the practitioner's ability to communicate with the patient (Ball, 1982).

Nixon (1984) observed a pattern of symptoms including headaches, sore, watery eyes, glare and focusing problems where a small vertical phoria could be measured after the binocular lock had been removed. Fixation disparity tests did not usually reveal a vertical slip. It was claimed that prescribing a 0.5 Δ vertical prism brought relief in many cases.

The first prescription
The very young patient

Very young patients are not able to cooperate and, in general practice, the correction will be determined by means of retinoscopy (Gruber, 1984), although other techniques are available (Obstfeld, 1971; Heilman, 1980 and Chapter 12). Where the outcome of such an examination indicates emmetropia, unless there is a significant muscle imbalance, no action is required. Cycloplegic examination is indicated in the presence of muscle imbalance and, where there is significant latent hypermetropia, a full correction may prevent any heterotropia from becoming permanent. It is necessary to monitor the patient at regular intervals. If the examination shows significant hyperopia or myopia, with or without astigmatism, the full correction is usually prescribed. In higher degrees of hypermetropia, no

reasonably sharp retinal image is formed without a correction and this will hamper the normal development of the neural system responsible for binocular vision. In the case of myopia this is less serious. The classification of ametropia is related to distant objects and, since babies are mainly occupied with vision within arms' reach, most myopic eyes will have reasonably sharp foveal images at some distance and will not develop amblyopia. Binocular problems involving convergence arise less frequently.

The need to prescribe the full astigmatic correction (reviewed at regular intervals of approximately 6 months) is similar to that in hypermetropia. In uncorrected astigmatism, the foveal image will vary in sharpness (Obstfeld, 1982) so that a certain degree of amblyopia may develop (except with normal 'against-the-rule' astigmatism in the first year of life—*see* Chapter 12). To avoid this amblyopia, the astigmatism needs to be corrected in full until such time that the patient can assist with the subjective examination. This is usually possible by 6 years of age.

Young patients, once used to a correction, tend to accept it without complaint and this equally applies to changes in the correction, especially if the examination is repeated at reasonably short intervals (e.g. 6 months) when any changes tend to be small (Weale, 1963; Sorsby, 1967).

The school child

Many first prescriptions arise at this stage in life. The first objective should be the provision of a correction which enables the child to interpret correctly writing on the chalkboard and in exercise books. A full correction may not be required since a visual acuity of 6/9 or less may well fulfil this objective. Frequently 6/9 is achieved without the correction and the practitioner must decide whether or not to prescribe. Where a correction is not prescribed, the child should be seen regularly (6-month intervals) and the parents should be advised of reasons for this. In general, children will accept a full correction as the first prescription. However, there is an inclination to reduce a high correction in both spherical and cylindrical components (which is often warranted) and then review the situation, initially at short intervals. Amblyopia arising from astigmatic anisometropia is often readily reversible once the full correction has been worn. It is not necessary to examine schoolchildren routinely under cycloplegia.

'School myopia' is considered to be the result of a number of factors, such as the personality, autonomic nervous system stimulation of the ciliary muscle and stress (Van Alphen, 1961). Irrespective of possible causes, there are a number of children with distance vision problems who are moderately myopic and respond best to a full correction. While small increases in correction may be required, it does not appear to continue much after 15 years of age and seldom exceeds 4 D.

However, the majority of school children show a remarkably small change in correction (about 0.50 DS; Hirsch, 1960) and there appear to be two distinct groups, one with almost stable corrections and a smaller group whose corrections increase steadily. This aspect has been documented by Sorsby and Leary (1970).

The adolescent

Optometrically, few changes occur during this period of life excluding those in myopia indicated above and, if any complaints do arise, they are usually associated with intensive close work (studying). A small degree of (so far) latent hyperopia may now need to be corrected or a convergence problem may be manifest. Intensive prolonged critical vision may equally have adverse effects on the compensation of heterophoria. In these cases, short-term relief is best provided by an appropriate refractive correction incorporating near additions and/or prism as indicated, but an adequate explanation must be given to the patient to ensure compliance with wearing instructions. Once the immediate need has passed, any remedial orthoptic or other therapy can be commenced as required and if appropriate.

The adult

Adults may continue with basically the same prescription with small and often insignificant changes occurring between examination until presbyopia becomes manifest. On enquiry it is often evident that prescriptions given during adolescence (usually for small degrees of hyperopia) have been abandoned and this may be related to changed visual requirements. In particular, mothers with young children often tend to do less prolonged near vision work. Pregnancy does not normally cause significant changes in visual status (Manges *et al.*, 1987).

After the age of 35 years, near vision may become more difficult. Examination of these patients often reveals a small degree of hypermetropia which, when fully corrected, relieves the symptoms. However, after a year or two, further reduction in the amplitude of accommodation causes a recurrence of symptoms and a need for an increased correction.

The presbyope

When the near point exceeds the working distance, presbyopia exists and may occur at any time after the age of 30 years depending on climatic and geographical conditions (Weale, 1982). This would agree with the general observation that the onset of presbyopia is earlier in populations nearer the Equator.

The primary requirement for presbyopia is an accurate distance correction followed by the determination of the near vision addition. The smallest addition usually prescribed is +0.50 DS and the highest does not normally exceed +3.25 DS (Obstfeld, 1967; Darras, 1968a). Unless the patient is of small stature and/or has short arms or can demonstrate to the practitioner (ideally at the patient's place of work) that a shorter than usual working distance is employed (e.g. as with a jeweller), additions over +2.75 DS are unlikely to be prescribed for patients with normal acuities. With increasing age the pupil becomes smaller which increases depth of field explaining the observation that patients over the age of 70 can 'accommodate' by 1 D or more (Ayrshire Study Circle, 1964; Charman and Whitefoot, 1977).

Prescribing too high an addition appears to cause more problems than an underestimation due to the reduced range of clear near vision as well as the shortened working distance. When the first presbyopic correction is given, it is wise to prepare the patient for what is to follow, explaining the reduction in the amplitude of accommodation, its significance and likely course. Presbyopes are advised to return at 2-yearly intervals and then may require an increase of 0.50 or 0.75 D in their addition up to the upper limit of 3.00 DS. The maximum addition may be expected to be prescribed within 10 years of the first presbyopic prescription.

It is unusual to find unequal additions between eyes with the exception of cases of significant anisometropia. If unequal additions are found, it is advisable to recheck the distance binocular balance, rebalancing of the distance correction often results in equal additions for near vision. The notion that unequal additions may be indicative of glaucoma has not been substantiated (Obstfeld, 1965).

Prescribing multifocals

Apart from functional/occupational prescribing for distances other than for 'near', the need for an intermediate prescription once an addition of +1.75 D has been reached should be considered. Because of the historical limiting influence of the British National Health Service on the prescribing of other than bifocal lenses, it is necessary to turn to a foreign source for information. Rünz (1975) estimated that almost 33% of the German population between the ages of 40 and 50 wore a bifocal, and 5% a progressive lens prescription. Over the age of 55 this changed to 33% for bifocals, 3% for trifocals and 4% for progressive lenses. Maitenaz (1985) noted that the share of progressive lenses among multifocal lenses was 12% worldwide, 6% in the USA and 60% in France.

The print you are reading now measures 9 point. Many books use print of five point size (on modern British near vision lettercharts indicated by N.5). The capital letters are about 1.75 mm high, and the small letters half that size. The visual angle of the latter subtended at the unaided eye will be 9′ of arc at 0.3 m (equivalent to a distance vision of almost 6/11), or 12′ of arc at 0.25 m (equivalent to about 6/14). This demonstrates that, although older patients may have a reduced visual acuity for distance vision, they may be able to read books with normal print without undue difficulty provided a reading correction (which may produce a slightly enlarged retinal image due to spectacle magnification, *see* Obstfeld, 1982) is used.

Apart from the presbyopic changes, there is a general tendency towards hyperopia. Between the ages of 45 and 70 years the average refraction increases by +0.75 or +1.00 D ('acquired hyperopia'). A small, but significant, number of patients show a shift towards myopia, but this occurs beyond the age of 65 ('acquired myopia') (Hirsch, 1960).

Prescribing spherical corrections

This is usually a routine matter. After binocular balancing the practitioner should be satisfied that the objective has been fulfilled (*see* beginning of chapter).

An analysis of prescription lenses has demonstrated an apparent tendency for prescribers unwittingly to round-off prescriptions. Aves (1926) was probably the first to note that the distribution characteristics of spectacle lenses occur at two levels. The upper level comprises the half and unit dioptre powers and the lower the quarter and three-quarter dioptre powers (*see Figure 32.1*). This phenomenon has been encountered by large lens manufacturers in Britain (Fletcher, 1967), France (Darras, 1968b) and Germany (Ritterman, 1969), while the same pattern can be found in American publications (Obstfeld, 1969). To date no satisfactory explanation has been proposed.

The phenomenon raises the question of whether it is necessary to determine and prescribe to 0.25 D accuracy, a doubtful proposition in view of the papers cited. However an American investigator (Appleton, 1971) stated that few practitioners would consider a trial set to be complete without lenses of 0.12 D power. Conversely the level of dissatisfaction caused by rounding-off to the nearest numerically smaller 0.50 D power (both sphere and cylinder) determined in his investigation was so low that it would be acceptable to work in 0.50 D steps. This confirms the negative view.

In practice most patients are able to make subjective judgments on ± 0.25 DS except where acuity is reduced. In these latter cases, quite large changes in refraction will not be appreciated if the acuity change is marginal and any alteration should be limited by the presenting symptoms.

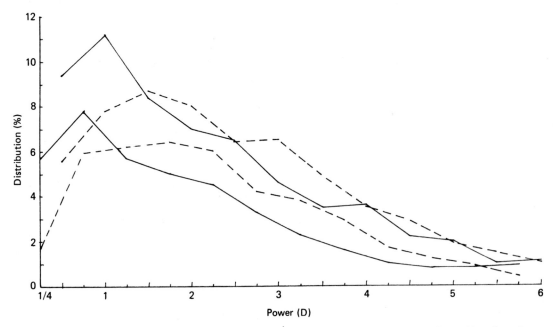

Figure 32.1 Distribution of 1109 negative and 5430 positive spherical lenses prescribed under the Supplementary Ophthalmic Service. —Negative spheres; – – – positive spheres. (Based on Bennett, 1965)

Prescribing cylindrical corrections

A large percentage of spectacle lenses (>60 %) will have a cylindrical component. The most frequently prescribed single cylindrical power is 0.50 D (30%) while few corrections (5%) will incorporate a cylinder over 1.50 D (Bennett, 1965; Obstfeld, 1967). The two-level distribution of powers described earlier has also been demonstrated for eyes with an astigmatic correction (Obstfeld, 1980).

Prescribing cylindrical corrections cannot be discussed without inclusion of the axis direction of the cylinder.

Axis direction

Since the main origin of ocular astigmatism is the anterior corneal surface (Stone, 1972) and since it can only have a positive cylindrical power, it should be corrected by negative cylindrical power. For this reason, and because negative cylinders are usually employed in subjective refraction techniques, only the negative axis directions of the correcting lenses will be discussed.

With-the-rule astigmatism (i.e. negative cylinder axis direction around the horizontal meridian) accounts for about 40%, against-the-rule and oblique astigmatism for about 30% each (Bennett, 1965; Obstfeld, 1967). A change in axis direction may occur as the patient ages. Young patients but not babies usually exhibit with-the-rule astigmatism. Sometimes this reduces or changes in middle age, and occasionally a patient will show in old age against-the-rule astigmatism, i.e. a change of some 90°. It is only possible to follow these changes in patients who remain with a particular practitioner for many years.

Prescribing spherocylindrical corrections

Quarter dioptre cylinders need only be prescribed if the patient appreciates a deterioration of the visual acuity without that component. Half-dioptre cylinders are usually prescribed. If a presbyopic patient is not corrected for distance the 0.50 DC may be omitted if the patient does not appreciate a deterioration in near vision.

Observers may notice (for instance on the fan and block chart) that in uncorrected astigmatism one of two mutually perpendicular lines will appear sharp. It is the blurred line which (normally) indicates the position of the correcting cylinder's axis position. If the blurred lines of the right and left eye of a patient are both horizontal or vertical, few if any problems are likely to arise, and the full correction may be prescribed. It is unusual for the axis of one eye to lie horizontal and that of the other eye to lie vertical, while oblique axes often lie at right angles to each other.

If the right and left axes are neither vertical nor horizontal, problems with binocular vision may occur caused by differential meridional spectacle magnification (Obstfeld, 1982), resulting in the patient's space perception being altered. This will be experienced as if the walls, ceiling and floor of a room were not meeting at right-angles, as if the floor and ceiling were sloping, and the walls were tilted towards or away from the patient. Certain groups of people (such as draughtsmen, carpenters, model makers) who have an eye for right-angles and circles, should be warned about this phenomenon as well as about the monocular distortion (a circle will look like an oval; a rectangle will appear to be obtuse or acute) which forms the basis of the problem. With the first prescription for a significant degree of astigmatism, the full prescription can be tried first accompanied by an explanation of the phenomenon that may (or may not!) present itself to the patient. As a demonstration, the patient could walk around the practice with the full correction in a trial frame. If the phenomenon is not apparent, correction is prescribed. If problems occur once the spectacles have been dispensed, a temporary correction can be prescribed incorporating a reduced cylindrical component. Meanwhile, the fully correcting lenses can be retained so that this pair of lenses may be reinserted into the same frame in a short while, after the patient has become accustomed to the reduced prescription.

Other ways to reduce distortion include: ordering back surface toric lenses, using the minimum vertex distance possible, and rotating the cylinder axes towards the horizontal or vertical meridians (in the case of an altered prescription, towards the previous axis position) and determining the cylinder powers required at these axis positions with the cross cylinder; the spherical component should be modified to give the best possible visual acuity.

If all this fails, the use of contact lenses, isogonal (Halass, 1959) or iseikonic spectacle lenses can be considered. In an exceptional case a spectacle lens/contact lens telescopic system could be considered (Douthwaite, 1987).

If the patient does not experience difficulties with distance vision, but has problems with near vision, near vision astigmatism may be the cause (Fletcher, 1952; Obstfeld, 1964). This will require a slightly different spherical and/or cylindrical component, and/or an altered axis direction due to cyclorotation, for near vision. Gross changes can be discovered using dynamic retinoscopy (Beau-Seigneur, 1946). A subjective affirmation can be obtained using the cross-cylinder technique and a near vision chart. As a result, separate reading spectacles may be found necessary or special multifocal lenses may be required (Jalie, 1984).

Guyton (1977) gave a detailed explanation of the problems and solutions. Diepes (1975) suggested that for an uncorrected patient of 50 years or over, the use of oblique cylinders should be avoided, suggesting the use of a spherical correction unless the improved visual acuity outweighed the disadvantages. It remains a problem: the patient's responses cannot be predicted. Experience and insight in the 'art of prescribing' based on educated trial and error, cannot be circumvented.

Aphakia

The only refracting component of the aphakic eye is its cornea. The consequences of removing the (approximately) +20 D crystalline lens, have been described in detail elsewhere (Obstfeld, 1982). The result is that an originally emmetropic eye will have become considerably hyperopic. The spectacle correction is usually of the order of +11 D, in addition to which an intermediate amount of astigmatism practically unrelated to any previously existing astigmatism, is created. As a result of surgical intervention, scar tissue formation often affects the corneal curvature and, although the principal meridians of the post-operative corneal curves are not always at right angles, the meridians of the astigmatism will be because of the optical properties of obliquely crossed cylinders. In his sample, Darras (1968b) found that surgery eventually resulted in a median cylinder power of +1.75 D, that 55% of the axes lay around the horizontal (against-the-rule) astigmatism and only 6% around the vertical meridian. This may measure >3 D at first, but will start to reduce and may become stable after 3 or 4 weeks. However, as a rule the cicatrization process lasts 6–8 weeks, and the astigmatism will be greater with larger incisions and increasing distance from the limbus. Further factors increasing the astigmatism are disturbance of the healing process, old age, high myopia and the presence of glaucoma (Von Gunten, 1970).

In view of the above, the following schedule may be operated, but must be adapted appropriately:

(1) On removal of bandages, the preliminary refraction is estimated and temporary spectacles provided. These are commercially available in 0.5 D steps with 2.50 and 3.00 D additions, and with a tint. The plastics, lenticular lenses can be fitted in a wrap-around dark frame, which minimizes the immediate increase in retinal illumination resulting from removal of a relatively opaque crystalline lens.

(2) At 6–8 weeks after surgery, the first accurate refraction is carried out and the temporary spectacles replaced if necessary. Reading glasses can be considered.

(3) Three months after surgery, a second accurate refraction is performed and a frame selected for definitive correction. Appropriate base curves for lenses should be selected and ultraviolet absorbing lenses considered as well as aspheric or multifocal types.

(4) Six months after surgery, a further refraction is performed. Visual problems and their possible solution should be discussed. Attention should be paid to (reduced) fields of view ('Jack-in-the-box' phenomenon; Welsh, 1961) and vertex distances.

By now, the patient will have become familiar with some other problems: the absence of any accommodation as such, the very large retinal image size(s) and, in cases of unilateral aphakia, severe anisometropia (*see below*) and aniseikonia which affects perspective. Theoretical (Obstfeld, 1982) and clinical aspects (Godio and Keating, 1984) of the retinal image sizes in unilateral and bilateral aphakia have been discussed. The patient may have discovered that reading without a special reading addition is possible. This is due to the large retinal image size(s) which may be 20–30% larger than in the phakic eye of the pair which, although being blurred, will not necessarily deter patients from reading. Some patients simply do without a reading addition (or reading spectacles), others will move distance spectacles down their nose, thus increasing the positive vergence incident on the eye (an artificial type of 'accommodation') while others will not be impressed by the sharpness of the retinal image that a near vision addition can produce.

In unilateral aphakia the phakic eye may, or may not (when a cataract is present), function in conjunction with the aphakic eye. There are patients who do not complain about problems with binocular single vision in unilateral aphakia, and it would appear that there simply is no binocular vision present (Chaston, J.M., 1975, personal communication). If, however, problems are experienced, several options are open: different vertex distances with different shape factors, one contact lens and one spectacle lens, and the fitting of an intraocular lens (Obstfeld, 1982).

One point which has not received attention is the change in prescribed prism required when a phakic (pair of) eye(s) becomes aphakic. Under favourable conditions, the patient may be able to cooperate in the determination of any prismatic component of the (temporary) prescription. However, it is possible to calculate the prismatic power component of an aphakic correction on the basis of the component of the previous phakic prescription (Obstfeld, 1986, 1987). Such a calculation shows that only about three-quarters of the phakic prescription's prismatic power will be required in the aphakic correction.

Anisometropia

Small differences in refraction in a pair of eyes are the rule rather than the exception—they do not cause problems. Trotter, quoted by Diepes (1975), found that more than 90% of a sample of 690 patients showed less than 1 D difference, and less than 4% showed a difference of 2 D or more. The main problem in these cases is the prismatic difference in the vertical meridian on looking down (for reading), or away from the optical centres of the lenses. However, occasionally problems with distance vision arise due to differences in visual acuity and/or retinal image size. Although there is elaborate (and costly) instrumentation available to detect and determine the degree of aniseikonia (retinal image size difference in a pair of eyes—*see* Chapter 27), in daily practice a simple device can be used. The patient's attention is directed to the largest optotype on the letterchart and, using vertical prisms, the right and left images are separated so that the one diplopic image lies close to and above the other. If the patient is a sufficiently good observer, a difference in image size will be noticed. Methods to equalize these are similar to those in aphakia.

If there is a difference in visual acuity, a full correction of each eye is usually acceptable. The eye with the better visual acuity will be the dominant eye, and the other will fulfil a secondary role. This appears to be less concerned with foveal rather than with peripheral vision, thus creating foveal suppression and a 'peripheral lock' in binocular vision.

If the visual acuity of the two eyes is equal, the effect of full corrections on binocular visual acuity must be considered. If there is no improvement, it may be appropriate to prescribe a lens, of a power similar to that for the dominant eye, for the non-dominant eye.

If the binocular visual acuity is improved, but the patient cannot accept the full correction for the more ametropic eye, the full correction of the eye with the 'better' visual acuity is placed in the trial frame and a similar lens power is placed in front of the other eye. While both eyes are free to look at the smallest letters on the letter chart discernible to the eye with the better acuity, and without using any device such as a septum to interfere with normal binocular vision, the spherical power in front of the other eye is gradually increased until the patient indicates that this interferes with the vision of the 'better' eye. The spherical power is reduced until the patient reports that comfortable vision has been restored. In the same way, the effect of cylindrical power (at the axis determined during monocular refraction) may be determined. It is sometimes necessary to modify (reduce) the spherical power while the cylindrical is increased. On a next visit, the whole procedure can be repeated so that in due course the undercorrected eye may be given the highest acceptable prescription compatible with comfortable binocular vision. Calder Gillie (1961) described a similar technique and questioned the need to give a full anisometropic correction.

Giles (1960) described a method developed by Turville. Using the Turville Infinity Balance and the L and F chart with the full corrections, he instructed the patient to note the position of the letters while the chin is lifted and depressed relative to the habitual position. Then, with the chin in the habitual position, the higher correction was reduced until the letters could be kept level while the chin was lifted and depressed again. The lens power thus determined was prescribed and the procedure repeated at 3–6 monthly intervals. Turville claimed that a nearly full correction could be tolerated in about one year. Recent work on prism adaptation (Henson, North and Dharamshi, 1983) might help to explain the rationale of this approach.

If there is no simultaneous vision, but alternating vision, as might be the case with a correction such as right plano and left −3.00 DS, the prescription is unnecessary. Here, the right eye will be used for distance vision and the left for near vision. A similar situation may exist in hyperopia, e.g. R +1.00 D and L + 4.00 D, the patient not being presbyopic. If such a non-presbyopic, alternating anisometropic patient needs a correction, it is sometimes useful to provide two pairs of spectacles: one pair glazed R and L with the right eye's prescription, the other similarly with that of the left eye. The one will be used for distance vision, and the other for near, the latter with the optical centres at the near visual points.

The patient presenting for the first time with anisometropia and resultant amblyopia of long standing should be prescribed a balance lens for the more ambylopic eye. Note that Winn *et al.* (1986) concluded that all anisometropes are best corrected with contact lenses.

Presbyopic anisometropes often need different reading additions, the more hyperopic eye requiring more plus. For the prescribing of bifocal corrections, *see* for instance Jalie (1984).

Prisms *(see also* Chapter 15)

Fixation disparity tests, such as the Mallett units, provide the practitioner with the prismatic power to be incorporated for decompensated heterophoria. Other devices may cause severe interference with binocular vision and be less acceptable for this purpose. However, the presence of fixation disparity should not always lead to a prismatic correction. The need for such correction should be linked to the binocular status, symptoms and objective tests (such as a cover test). An improvement in the acuity or comfort with the prism could be an indication to prescribe in itself.

When a prismatic correction is indicated for either distance or near vision, the effect of this correction should be assessed at the other viewing distance. As a consequence, a different prismatic correction may be needed for distance and for near vision. Special lenses (single vision bicentric or prism controlled bifocal lenses) may be indicated. On subsequent visits, the investigation should be repeated since changes in the amount of prismatic power required may occur.

If a spectacle-wearing patient presents with problems which could be due to incorrectly centred lenses or an alteration in a prismatic correction, a fixation disparity device can be used with the existing spectacles to check whether this is the cause for discomfort. For single vision reading spectacles, the vertical decentration of both lenses so that the optical centres lie at the near visual points should be determined taking into consideration the patient's normal head posture. It is virtually impossible to do this with a patient seated behind a refractor head.

Non-tolerance cases

These may be described as cases where the patient cannot tolerate the originally supplied lenses and/or frames, after a reasonable trial period. A British Minister of Health described (for the purposes of the National Health Service) a non-tolerance case as one 'where an ophthalmologist is satisfied that a patient is genuinely unable to use lenses which have been prescribed and supplied and that lenses to a new prescription are necessary'. It was further explained that a 'technical' non-tolerance case usually refers to the changing conditions of a patient's eyes, for example after a cataract operation (Hunter, 1985).

Priest (1979) divided the non-tolerance cases into two groups: those due to dispensing could be caused by weight intolerance, intolerance to chromatic aberration, centration, bifocal or trifocal lenses, lens form (or change thereof), to prism control of bifocals, change in vertex distance, tint or to frame materials; the other group was due to prescribing.

Priest suggested first looking at the dispensing non-tolerance aspects and eliminating these factors before the non-tolerance due to prescribing be contemplated. This should start with ascertaining that no errors occurred in the writing of the prescription, such as prism base direction or transposition errors.

Ball (1982) drew attention to the fact that a prescription may correct one eye defect and create another that the patient had not anticipated and the prescriber had overlooked or not mentioned to the patient. These include:

(1) Apparent magnification and 'drawing' of the eyes after correction of presbyopia. This may be alleviated by reducing the addition, by adding prism base-in or, if a temporary effect, it may disappear without intervention.
(2) Micropsia may occur as a result of prescribing a full myopic correction. It may be accompanied by increased contrast and unwanted clarity. These complaints are usually of a temporary nature, or can be relieved by a minimal reduction of the prescription.
(3) An increase in existing heterophoria as a result of the correction of an ametropia suggests that the heterophoria may have been the major cause of the symptom.
(4) Symptoms where none existed previously, such as the distortion caused by the correction of astigmatism, can be baffling and might be the expression of a neurotic disposition which could call for the involvement of another health practitioner. Ball collected the more common causes of intolerance succintly (*Table 32.1*).

Since anything can have happened, including the development of pathology, in the interval between final dispensing of the prescription and the patient presenting again as a non-tolerance case, a second, full eye examination should be carried out. Any findings at variance with the original examination results may point to the cause of the problem. As a result an alteration of any one, or a combination of the components of the prescription, may be found necessary. The most frequently encountered problems are probably caused by intolerance to a cylinder power or axis change, a base curve change or the prescribing of too high an addition for near vision. If non-tolerance is to be minimized, it is best to make only minimal changes to the prescription or lens type, irrespective of the examination finding and commensurate with the best possible and/or most comfortable binocular vision. However, the prescription should still fulfil the patient's visual needs in all respects and the potential benefit of any alteration will not be realized unless it is tried.

Table 32.1 Prescription-induced symptoms, transient or persistent

Symptom-type	Presenting symptoms	Examples of possible cause (non-pathological)
Referred or sympathetic	Headaches	High presbyopic additions
	Dizziness, giddiness, nausea, disorientation, unreality	Unintended prismatic effects (for example, faulty centration), prismatic corrections (*see also* spatial distortion, *below*)
Ocular	Discomfort and irritation described variously as 'drawing', 'pulling', 'straining' or 'staring' for 'clear' vision	Recent presbyopic additions
Visual		
Micropsia		Recent myopic prescriptions
		Base-out prisms
Macropsia		Recent presbyopic additions
		Base-in prisms
General spatial distortions		Unaccustomed cylinders
		Corrected anisometropia
		Change of lens form
Peripheral spatial distortion		Some multifocals
Blurred vision		Inappropriate use of prescription
		Uncorrected residual errors
		Positioning of bifocal segments
		Incorrect effective power of prescription
		Marginally over-corrected positive power resulting from maximum + routine and finite test chart distance
Diplopia		Faulty lens centration
		Improperly corrected astigmatism
		Interference from bifocal segment edge
Chromatopsia		High addition in some fused bifocals
Visual unease		Marginal blur in dominant eye
		Altered muscle balance from previous prescription
Photophobia		Recent contact lenses
		Omission of previously worn tints
Increased contrast ⎫ Unwanted clarity ⎬ 'Ghost' images ⎭		Recently and fully corrected myopia Reflections from lens surfaces
Other effects		
Lenses feel 'too strong'		Fully corrected myopia and presbyopia
Cosmetic and allied problems		For example, centre or edge thickness of lenses, visibility of bifocal segments, weight of spectacles
Stumbling, tripping		Distorting elements of prescriptions, unaccustomed bifocals

From Ball, 1982, by courtesy of the author.

References

APPLETON, B. (1971) Ophthalmic prescriptions in half-diopter intervals. *Arch. Ophthalmol.*, **86**, 263–267

AVES, O. (1926) Some notes and statistical tables on the relative distribution of refractive defects, and their correction. *Proceedings of Optical Convention 1926*, part 1, 424–450. London: Optical Convention

AYRSHIRE STUDY CIRCLE (1964) An investigation into accommodation *Br. J. Physiol. Opt.*, **21**, 31–35

BALL, G.V. (1982) *Symptoms in Eye Examinations*. London: Butterworths

BEAU–SEIGNEUR, W. (1946) Changes in power and axis of cylindrical errors after convergence. *Am. J. Optom.*, **23**, 111–121

BENNETT, A.G. (1965) Lens usage in the Supplementary Ophthalmic Service. *Optician*, 131–137, Feb. 12

CALDER GILLIE, J. (1961) The anisometropic presbyope. *Br. J. Physiol. Opt.*, **18**, 174–180

CHARMAN, W.N. and WHITEFOOT, H. (1977) Pupil diameter and the depth-of-field of the human eye as measured by laser speckle. *Opt. Acta*, **24**, 1211–1216

CHOLERTON, M. (1955). Low refractive errors. *Br. J. Physiol. Opt.*, **12**, 82–86

DARRAS, C. (1968a) Correction de la presbytie: l'addition. *Optn Lunetier*, no. 184 (May), 9–14

DARRAS, C. (1986b) Statistiques sur une clientèle d'aphaques. *Optn Lunetier*, May, 26–29

DIEPES, H. (1975) *Refraktionsbestimmung*, 2nd edn. Pforzheim: Verlag H. Postenrieder

DOUTHWAITE, W.A. (1987) *Contact Lens Optics*, p. 20 London: Butterworths

FLETCHER, R.J. (1952) Astigmatic accommodation. *Br. J. Physiol. Opt.*, **9**, 8–32

FLETCHER, T. (1967) Stock-keeping and the usage of various sights. *FMO Technical Conference Proceedings*. London: Federation of Manufacturing Opticians

GILES, G.H. (1960) *The Principles and Practice of Refraction*. London: Hammond, Hammond & Co. Ltd.

GODIO, L.B. and KEATING, M.P. (1984) Clinical determination of the corrected retinal image size in spectacle-corrected aphakes. *Am. J. Optom. Physiol. Opt.*, **61**, 160–165

GRUBER, J. (1984) Assessment of refractive status. *Optician*, 18–20, Aug. 24

GUYTON, D.L. (1977) Prescribing cylinders: the problem of distortion. *Surv. Ophthalmol.*, **22**, 177–188

HALASS, S. (1959) Aniseikonic lenses of improved design and their application. *Austr. J. Optom.*, **42**, 387–393

HEILMANN, K.(1980) *Ophthalmoscopy: Principles, Examination Technique, Application, Findings*. Stuttgart: Enke

HENSON, D.B., NORTH, R. and DHARAMSHI, B. (1983) Prism adaptation. *Optician*, 20–22, Jan. 28

HIRSCH, M.J. (1960) Refractive changes with age. In *Vision of the Ageing Patient* edited by M.J. Hirsch and R.E. Wick, pp. 63–82. Philadelphia: Chilton

HUNTER, I. (1985) Commentary. *Optom. Today*, 307, May 11

JALIE, M. (1984) *The Principles of Ophthalmic Lenses*, 4th edn. London: Association of Dispensing Opticians.

MAITENAZ .B. (1985) Discours inaugural. In *Troisième Symposium International de la Presbytie*, vol. 1, pp. 1–5. Haiti

MANGE, T.D., BANAITIS, D.A., ROTH, N. and YOLTON, R.L. (1987) Changes in optometric findings during pregnancy. *Am. J. Optom. Physiol. Opt.*, **64**, 159–166

MORGAN, M.W. (1960) Accommodative changes in presbyopia and their correction. In *Vision of the Ageing Patient*, edited by M.J. Hirsch and R.E. Wick, pp. 83–112. Philadelphia: Chilton

NATHAN, J. (1957) Small errors of refraction. *Br. J. Physiol. Opt.*, **14**, 204–209

NIXON, A.S. (1984) A clinical consideration of symptoms, measurement and correction of small vertical phorias. *Soc. Exp. Optom.*, Birmingham

OBSTFELD, H. (1964) Notes on near vision astigmatism. *Optica Int.*, **1**, 43–46

OBSTFELD, H. (1965) Change of accommodation during glaucoma. *Optica Int.*, **2**, 50–56

OBSTFELD, H. (1967) Spectacle lens prescriptions. *Opthal. Opt.*, **7**, 914–932

OBSTFELD, H. (1969) Distribution characteristics of spectacle lens powers. *Am. J. Optom.*, **46**, 882–885

OBSTFELD, H. (1971) Retinoscopy with the ophthalmoscope. *Ophthal. Opt.*, **11**, 59–72

OBSTFELD, H. (1980) A prescribing habit. *Optician*, **179**, 12–16

OBSTFELD, H. (1982) *Optics in Vision*, 2nd edn. London: Butterworths

OBSTFELD, H. (1986) The effect of prismatic spectacle and contact lens corrections on ocular rotation. *Ophthal. Physiol. Opt.*, **6**, 233–237

OBSTFELD, H. (1987) Matters arising: the effect of prismatic spectacle and contact lens corrections on ocular rotation. *Ophthal. Physiol. Opt.*, **7**, 89

PRIEST, M.J. (1979) Non-tolerance and the NHS. *Ophthal. Opt.*, 221–223, March 31

RITTERMANN, K. (1969) Das Gläserlager mit ungleichen Vorzeichen-oder- das Ende eines Mythos. *Neues Optikerj*, **11**, 103–104

RÜNZ, E. (1975) Die Versorgung der Presbyopen mit arbeidsspezifischen Augengläsern. *Optometrie, Mainz*, **23**, 127–136

SORSBY, A. (1967) The nature of spherical refractive errors. In *Refractive Anomalies of the Eye*, NINDB monograph No. 5

SORSBY, A. and LEARY, G.A. (1970) A longitudinal study of refraction and its components during growth. *Medical Research Council, Special Report Series no. 309*. London: HMSO

STONE, J. (1972) Practical optics of contact lenses. In *Contact Lenses*, edited by J. Stone and A.J. Phillips, Chap. 3, p. 89. London: Barrie & Jenkins

VAN ALPHEN, G.W.H.M. (1961) *On Emmetropia and Ametropia*. Basel: Karger

VON GUNTEN, J. (1970) Die optische Besonderheiten des aphaken Auges. *Schweiz Optiker*, **46**, 13–24

WEALE, R.A. (1963) *The Ageing Eye*. London: Lewis

WEALE, R.A. (1982) *A Biography of the Eye*. London: Lewis

WELSH, R.C. (1961) The roving ring scotoma with its Jack-in-the-box phenomenon of strong-plus (aphakic) spectacle lenses. *Am. J. Ophthalmol*, **51**, 1277–1281

WINN, B., ACKERLEY, R.G., BROWN, C.A., MURRAY, F.K., PRAIS, J and ST JOHN, M.F. (1986) The superiority of contact lenses in the correction of anisometropia. *Transactions of the British Contact Lens Association Clinical Conference*, pp. 95–100

33

Prescribing and patient management: occupational and recreational considerations

John Grundy

Visual factors have a vital influence on human activities, yet, far too often, insufficient attention is given to determining the visual abilities of patients and ensuring that they are capable of seeing adequately in relation to the demands of particular tasks.

Anything which affects visual efficiency, such as a refractive error or muscle imbalance, or the nature of the task itself, such as fine detail or poor contrast, or by the conditions under which the eyes must be used, such as poor lighting, must affect the efficiency of the individual.

In assessing occupational and recreational visual requirements, it is not sufficient to concentrate on any particular factor in isolation. The safest approach is to consider seeing as a whole, taking into account all of the relevant requirements which contribute to visual efficiency. This also requires an understanding and knowledge of the visual capability of each patient, which will differ according to the visual demands of various tasks and between individuals performing the same task. For example, a myope may be able to carry out inspection work at close range without spectacles but would be severely handicapped if asked to drive a fork lift truck. The housewife with a small degree of hypermetropia may experience no visual problems in the home, but the same person would often need a correction for clerical work if symptoms were to be avoided.

The distinction between occupational and recreational tasks may be one of degree, since what are occupations for some will be hobbies for others, for example, gardening, painting or carpentry. The visual requirements may, therefore, be similar since the size of detail, working distances etc. will often be the same, although the degree of concentration and length of time spent on the task may be very different.

Assessing recreational visual requirements usually present few problems. Most practitioners give ad-

vice on suitable hand magnifiers for the stamp collector and explain the problems of glazing a high cylindrical lens to a camera eye-piece. An appropriate remedy is given to the bifocal-wearing golfing patient who complains of difficulty. Cases of eye injuries as a result of accidents while playing squash, tennis or cricket are not infrequent, and advice is required on the most suitable frame and lenses for patients who play various sports. The visual requirements for recreational activities are known either because of participating or from spectating, but the assessment of occupational visual requirements is often a different matter.

In modern industry the various processes are becoming more and more complex and the types of work so varied that, without visiting the places of work, it is often difficult to know precisely what visual demands are likely to be made on individuals by the nature of their jobs.

As a result, a need arises to develop a logical system to determine the visual attributes required to carry out a particular visual task in order to understand the problems which exist and to give the best advice and prescribe most effectively for the work situation. Task analysis will always assist in the prescription of optimal aids for the particular activities of prime interest to the individual concerned.

Main working positions

Whether the worker is sitting, standing or moving about at work will, in presbyopes particularly, influence the type of correction to be prescribed. Careful consideration should be given to the power of the reading addition and, if multifocals are worn, to the size, height and type of segment. An example comparing groups of presbyopic workers whose visual demands differ by virtue of their working positions should make this clear.

For working at a desk, critical measurements of focal distance are usually of less importance and, provided the layout of the work is such that frequent changes in direction of gaze over a wide area can be avoided, a straightforward reading correction or relatively small segment bifocal is often satisfactory.

The machine operator, however, spends most of the day standing at work, which is often situated further from the eyes than a usual reading distance, and intermediate corrections may be necessary for the older worker when clear vision is required along the length of the machine.

When the job involves moving around the factory or office, working distances are usually variable and the objects to be viewed at different eye levels, so much more care must be taken in analysing the patient's visual requirements before deciding on the most appropriate correction.

It should also be remembered that, if the worker is moving about on elevated structures, conventional bifocals could well be dangerous (*see also* Direction of gaze and Working distances).

Direction of gaze

Those tasks which involve frequent changes in the direction of gaze, particularly at the extreme ranges of available eye movement, can be a source of visual discomfort and fatigue following the continual refocusing for different working distances and the increased amount of extraocular muscle action needed for viewing objects at very different positions in the field of view. The likelihood of symptoms also increases if the eyes are persistently turned to a position close to the limit of the binocular field of fixation.

The maximum horizontal rotation of the eyes, without moving the head, is about 90°, i.e. each eye can be turned through an angle of about 45° to the right or left of its primary position. A very similar amplitude of movement is possible vertically and obliquely, although the possible rotation downwards is greater than upwards. Usually, however, the total angle within which objects in different parts of the visual field are fixated does not exceed 35–40°, as shown in *Figure 33.1*, since it is more comfortable to turn the head when looking at objects which lie outside the field enclosed within this angle.

Also significant is the effect on those workers who are either new to the job or have changed jobs and have developed certain 'viewing habits'. They now find that they must look in different directions and at different working distances than those to which they have previously become accustomed and often complain of tiredness and visual discomfort at the start of the new work.

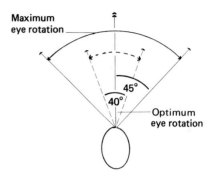

Figure 33.1 Maximum and optimum eye movements, without moving the head

Symptoms are likely to arise in those individuals with inadequate convergence and fusion, particularly when viewing very close objects. Convergence is usually held with greater difficulty in close work positions at and above the horizontal, causing problems especially for those with binocular instability.

Another common cause of complaint and discomfort occurs with bifocal wearers adopting unnatural head postures when viewing work at and above eye level.

It is necessary, therefore, to pay particular attention to muscle balances, amplitude of accommodation, convergence and fusion and, if multifocals are prescribed, to the type, height and size of segment. Recommendations can also often be made on changing the layout of the work to improve the comfort and efficiency of the individual.

Working distances

The distance between the objects being inspected and the eye affects the size of the retinal image and hence the visual acuity required to distinguish the objects. It affects the degree of accommodation and convergence demanded by the work, and the degree of uncorrected refractive error or phoria that may be tolerated.

Working distances can be classified as: far, intermediate, near and very near.

Far

Far includes those distances in which the most important objects of vision are not less than about 2 m from the eyes, for example, steel mills; transport, including cars; cranes; heavy engineering etc.

In general, jobs in this classification, because of the distance from the eyes, will have little effect on accommodation and convergence. Those people with small errors of refraction will have few problems. Usually the objects of inspection are not very small and can be discriminated fairly easily by

Age	40	42	45	48	50	52	55	60	65
Amplitude of Accommodation (D)	4.50	4.00	3.50	3.00	2.50	2.00	1.50	1.00	0.50
Usable Accommodation (D)	2.25 (3.00)	2.00 (2.67)	1.75 (2.33)	1.50 (2.00)	1.25 (1.67)	1.00 (1.33)	0.75 (1.00)	0.50 (0.67)	0.25 (0.33)
Plano	44.4 (33.3) Infinity	50.0 (37.5) Infinity	57.1 (42.9) Infinity	66.6 (50.0) Infinity	80.0 (60.0) Infinity	100.0 (75.0) Infinity	133.3 (100.0) Infinity	200.0 (150.0) Infinity	400.0 (300.0) Infinity
+0.50	36.4 (28.6) 200.0	40.0 (31.6) 200.0	44.4 (35.3) 200.0	50.0 (40.0) 200.0	57.1 (46.1) 200.0	66.7 (54.7) 200.0	80.0 (66.7) 200.0	100.0 (85.5) 200.0	133.3 (120.5) 200.0
+0.75	33.3 (26.7) 133.3	36.4 (29.2) 133.3	40.0 (32.5) 133.3	44.4 (36.4) 133.3	50.0 (41.3) 133.3	57.1 (48.1) 133.3	66.7 (57.1) 133.3	80.0 (70.4) 133.3	100.0 (92.6) 133.3
+1.00	30.8 (25.0) 100.0	33.3 (27.3) 100.0	36.4 (30.0) 100.0	40.0 (33.3) 100.0	44.4 (37.5) 100.0	50.0 (42.9) 100.0	57.1 (50.0) 100.0	66.7 (59.9) 100.0	80.0 (75.2) 100.0
+1.25	28.6 (23.5) 80.0	30.8 (25.5) 80.0	33.3 (27.9) 80.0	36.4 (30.8) 80.0	40.0 (34.3) 80.0	44.4 (38.8) 80.0	50.0 (44.4) 80.0	57.1 (52.1) 80.0	66.7 (63.3) 80.0
+1.50	26.7 (22.2) 66.7	28.6 (24.0) 66.7	30.8 (26.1) 66.7	33.3 (28.6) 66.7	36.4 (31.6) 66.7	40.0 (35.3) 66.7	44.4 (40.0) 66.7	50.0 (46.1) 66.7	57.1 (54.7) 66.7
+1.75	25.0 (21.1) 57.1	26.7 (22.6) 57.1	28.6 (24.5) 57.1	30.8 (26.7) 57.1	33.3 (29.2) 57.1	36.4 (32.5) 57.1	40.0 (36.4) 57.1	44.4 (41.3) 57.1	50.0 (48.1) 57.1
+2.00	23.5 (20.0) 50.0	25.0 (21.4) 50.0	26.7 (23.1) 50.0	28.6 (25.0) 50.0	30.8 (27.3) 50.0	33.3 (30.0) 50.0	36.4 (33.3) 50.0	40.0 (37.5) 50.0	44.4 (42.9) 50.0
+2.25	22.2 (19.1) 44.4	23.5 (20.3) 44.4	25.0 (21.8) 44.4	26.7 (23.5) 44.4	28.6 (25.5) 44.4	30.8 (27.9) 44.4	33.3 (30.8) 44.4	36.4 (34.3) 44.4	40.0 (38.8) 44.4
+2.50	21.1 (18.2) 40.0	22.2 (19.3) 40.0	23.5 (20.7) 40.0	25.0 (22.2) 40.0	26.7 (24.0) 40.0	28.6 (26.1) 40.0	30.8 (28.6) 40.0	33.3 (31.6) 40.0	36.4 (35.3) 40.0
+2.75	20.0 (17.4) 36.4	21.1 (18.5) 36.4	22.2 (19.7) 36.4	23.5 (21.1) 36.4	25.0 (22.6) 36.4	26.7 (24.5) 36.4	28.6 (26.7) 36.4	30.8 (29.2) 36.4	33.3 (32.5) 36.4
+3.00	19.1 (16.7) 33.3	20.0 (17.6) 33.3	21.1 (18.8) 33.3	22.2 (20.0) 33.3	23.5 (21.4) 33.3	25.0 (23.1) 33.3	26.7 (25.0) 33.3	28.6 (27.3) 33.3	30.8 (30.0) 33.3
+3.25	18.2 (16.0) 30.8	19.1 (16.9) 30.8	20.0 (17.9) 30./8	21.1 (19.1) 30.8	22.2 (20.3) 30.8	23.5 (21.8) 30.8	25.0 (23.5) 30.8	26.7 (25.5) 30.8	28.6 (27.9) 30.8
+3.50	17.4 (15.4) 28.6	18.2 (16.2) 28.6	19.1 (17.2) 28.6	20.0 (18.2) 28.6	21.1 (19.3) 28.6	22.2 (20.7) 28.6	23.5 (22.2) 28.6	25.0 (24.0) 28.6	26.7 (26.1) 28.6

Row labels "Plano" through "+3.50" are grouped under **Power of add**.

Figure 33.2 Ranges of clear vision with reading additions

people of less than average acuity. The objects may be moving but, because the apparent rate of movement is less with increasing distance of the objects, this may not cause difficulties. Monocular vision may be adequate, although binocular vision with highly developed stereopsis is sometimes necessary for others, e.g. crane operators.

Intermediate to near

Intermediate to near are those tasks in which the principal objects of vision are situated less than 2 m, but more than 30 cm from the eyes, i.e. the majority of indoor occupations.

Emmetropes will use more than 0.5 D but less than 4 D of accommodation with corresponding degrees of convergence. Small degrees of hypermetropia may now need to be corrected and more attention must be paid to muscle balances. The degree of visual acuity required for different jobs in this classification varies between wide limits, as does the need for binocular vision and stereopsis. Greater care must be taken in prescribing for the presbyope since a reading correction which may be suitable for typing at the shorter distance of the range may be unsuitable for occupations such as weaving at the longest distance of the range.

Very near

Very near includes all objects whose details cannot be distinguished clearly unless they are viewed at a distance of less than 30 cm. For example, sewing, many tasks in the printing industry, inspection of electrical printed circuits and in the microelectronics industry.

The greatest demands on accommodation and convergence, the need for good visual acuity, near muscle balance and stereoscopic vision occur when the details of the objects cannot be distinguished clearly unless they are viewed at these short working distances.

When the detail is very small and very close working distances are adopted, accommodation of 5–6 D is often necessary for prolonged periods and a reading prescription may become necessary at an earlier age than usual. The presbyopic patient often needs a greater near vision addition and possibly base-in prism to relieve convergence. This can be determined from the amplitude of accommodation, near point of convergence and near muscle balance. Even this may not be enough for minute work and consideration should then be given to magnifying aids to vision (*see* Size of detail of the task).

Obviously these classifications will often overlap since there are many occupations which involve the discrimination of objects and their detail at several different working distances. The visual needs of presbyopes will not always be met with a single vision prescription which may be suitable for home use. The range table (*Figure 33.2*) should make this clear.

The range table

The range table (*see Figure 33.2*) shows the range of clear vision obtainable by the emmetrope (or ametrope with distance correction), or through various additions according to the patient's usable accommodation. By careful measurement of the patient's working distances, the extent of focal ranges produced by different prescriptions can be demonstrated and compared with the needs of the job. This is particulary significant because the patient's usable accommodation becomes less and less with age, and the range of clear vision through various additions becomes constantly smaller. It then becomes much more important accurately to prescribe intermediate and near powers in accordance with the range table in order to provide clear and comfortable vision at all of the required working distances.

The average amount of accommodation which is available to individuals of various ages is shown as the 'amplitude of accommodation'. This varies widely, of course, from person to person, as does the amount of accommodation necessary for the task. General health, drugs and many other factors have a considerable effect on the amount of accommodation which can be exerted, particularly for prolonged or intricate near vision tasks. It is generally accepted that the maximum amount of accommodation which can be exerted for sustained close work is between one half and two-thirds of the total accommodation available. If the occupation is particularly visually demanding then a greater accommodative effort is required. For this reason two figures have been given for the patient's 'usable accommodation'. The figure on the left indicates the accommodation which is available when only half of the total amplitude can be exerted for prolonged periods. The figure on the right shows the amount of accommodation which can be used if two-thirds of the total amplitude can be used.

On looking down the 'age' columns, therefore, the top left figure, for various powers of addition, indicates the closest point, in centimetres, to which near objects can be viewed for prolonged periods with comfort, assuming only half the total amplitude of accommodation can be exerted. The figure on the right (in brackets) assumes that two-thirds of the total amplitude can be exerted.

'Plano' in the 'power of add ' column assumes that the eyes are emmetropic or that they have been corrected for distance. This gives a guide to the range of clear vision which can be obtained by the emmetrope or through the distance correction. There are many occupations which involve the discrimination of objects and their detail at several different working distances. The purpose of the range table is:

(1) To show that it is not always possible to satisfy the occupational visual needs of presbyopes with the same prescription which may be satisfactory for a general purpose use.
(2) To indicate what would be the most effective combination of powers of prescriptions to achieve clear vision at all of the required distances.

The following examples should make the use of the range table clear: the visual requirements at work of a patient aged 48 years are clear vision at 35 cm and 60 cm. The amplitude of accommodation will be about 3.00 D, but the usable accommodation will be 1.50 or 2.00 D, depending on whether the patient can exert either one-half or two-thirds of his total amplitude. On looking down the 'age' column it will be seen that, if the patient has only 1.50 D of usable accommodation, a +1.50 D addition will allow clear vision from 66.7 cm (focal length of the addition beyond which vision will be blurred) to 33.3 cm (closest point to which near objects can be viewed for prolonged periods with comfort). If the patient has 2.00 D of usable accommodation, a +1.00 D addition allows clear vision from 33.3–100.0 cm. In either case, the patient's visual requirements at working distances of 35 and 60 cm would be satisfied.

If, however, the patient is older (60 years), he will have an amplitude of accommodation of about 1.00 D, but only 0.50 (or 0.67) D of usable accommodation. From the 'Age' column it can be seen that no single addition will give clear vision at both 35 and 60 cm. Additions of +2.50 D include the 35-cm distance, and additions of +1.25 D include the 60-cm distance. A lens must, therefore, be selected which incorporates these powers in either bifocal, trifocal or progressive power form according to the patient's occupational needs.

Size of detail of the task

In considering working distances, the size of the detail of the task must also be taken into account in order to calculate the angle subtended at the eye and, hence, the visual acuity required to perform the task rapidly, accurately and with comfort.

The size of the retinal image of any object is inversely proportional to its distance from the eye. The smaller the object, therefore, the closer it must be if the details of its image are to be large enough to be resolved. Many of the objects which have to be viewed in different occupations are so small that only by bringing them close to the eyes and making use of amost the full powers of accommodation and

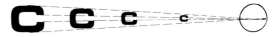

Figure 33 Diagram illustrating the concept of angular subtense

convergence, can they be seen. Obviously this cannot be sustained for long periods without giving rise to symptoms, particularly in older workers whose minimum distance for distinct vision increases with age.

At the same time, it should be remembered that objects seen in different occupations may differ considerably in physical dimensions and yet form images of similar size on the retina owing to their respective distances from the eyes (*Figure 33.3*). Therefore, on account of their same apparent size they require the same degree of acuity, even though the demands they make on the visual system may be very dissimilar.

The angle subtended at the eye, and hence the visual acuity required for the task, can be calculated in the usual way from mathematical tables (tan visual angle = size of detail of object/working distance), or a simple graphical method can be used (*Figure 33.4*).

For example, in assessing whether the visual acuity of a visual display unit (VDU) operator would be adequate for working with comfort when reading letters on the screen which are 3 mm high, the size of detail of the letters being 0.6 mm at a viewing distance of 70 cm (*Figure 33.5*), a straight line is drawn through the values of size and distance. Where the line cuts the right-hand scale indicates the corresponding visual angle (3′) and minimum visual acuity required (6/18). It is important to emphasize, however, that this value gives a measure of the resolving power of the eye and, in order for a visual task to be performed for prolonged periods with comfort, the visual acuity should certainly be higher than this minimum value. From experience, it has been demonstrated that the visual acuity necessary for any demanding visual task should be approximately twice that of the minimum value. In this example, therefore, the VDU operator should have a minimum visual acuity of 6/9 which is equivalent to N6 at 40 cm.

Most people are able to perform visual tasks requiring the perception of detail subtending an angle at the eye of 10′ of arc efficiently under ordinary conditions of lighting, provided the detail to be observed is of good contrast with its immediate background. However, the difficulty of visual tasks, even of very simple kinds, becomes progressively greater as the angular size of critical detail falls below about 3′ (*Table 33.1*), and magnifying aids to vision should be considered when very small tasks are encountered.

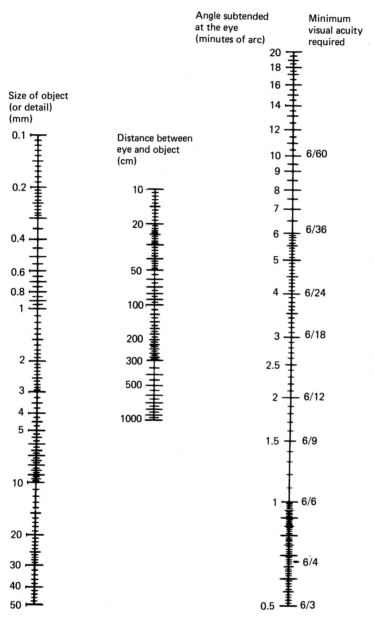

Figure 33.4 Nomogram for finding the visual angle subtended by objects of which the size and distance are known. (After Weston, 1962)

The purpose of magnification is to effectively increase the angular subtense of the task detail at the eye. Typical devices are:

(1) Hand and stand magnifiers—these differ little from those used in low vision aid work. Built-in illumination can often be helpful.

(2) Monocular and binocular loupes—incorporate positive power and, in the case of binocular loupes, prisms, they allow the task to be brought closer to the eyes.

(3) Monocular and binocular microscopes—allow a wide range of magnifications to be achieved and are particularly useful in fine assembly or inspection work.

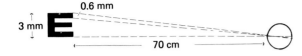

Figure 33.5 Snellen acuity in task analysis

Table 33.1 Visual acuity (VA) and angular size of critical detail

	Angular size of critical detail (minutes)	Minimum VA required	Optimum VA required	
Large	10	6/60	6/30	N20
Medium	6	6/36	6/18	N12
Small	3	6/18	6/9	N6
Very small	1.5	6/9	6/4.5	N3
Minute	0.75	6/4.5	Magnification aid + good VA required	

(4) Telescopes and binoculars—applicable to distant objects.
(5) Projection devices—although their application to all processes may be limited, they may be less tiring to use for long periods than conventional microscopes and similar instruments.

Visual acuity of the kind so far considered is related to the ability of the eye to discriminate small objects or the distance between two small parts of an object, i.e. form acuity. In many occupations, however, line detail must be appreciated, for example in detecting cracks in a casting or flaws in a ceramic tile. It may be necessary to distinguish a break of contour or alignment—vernier acuity, when reading micrometer scales, slide rules and precision gauges. The sensitivity of the visual system for these types of detail is very high, and for practical purposes it can be assumed to be of the order of one-twentieth of the corresponding angle for the details resolved in form acuity.

If, therefore, the form acuity for a given working distance is known, it is easy to calculate the equivalent visual angle for line or vernier acuity and the actual size of the detail which it should be possible to resolve, and vice versa.

Movement of the work

Unless the movement of objects in the field of view is very slow it is usually detected easily under ordinary conditions of lighting. In fact, one of the problems in many jobs is the movement of objects which are not relevant to the specific task and only act as a distraction, the eyes being attracted to the movement and away from the task. In some processes which may involve working with moving machinery, this could be dangerous. Where possible, the background to any critical viewing task should be kept free of movement and screens to cut out distractions may be necessary.

There are, however, many jobs which require the observation of moving objects and perception of detail which may be seen for only a brief time. If the direction of movement is not constant and particularly if it varies irregularly, very complicated movements of pursuit become necessary and the visual task is made very exacting.

Detection of moving detail is facilitated by:

(1) Good ocular muscle coordination and stereopsis.
(2) Perfection of the retinal image, i.e. correction of refractive errors, where necessary, and absence of ocular pathology.
(3) An adequate quantity of good quality illumination.

Stereoscopic vision

Stereoscopic vision is obviously an advantage for the performance of practically every kind of work, from threading a needle or assembling a delicate mechanism, to operating a crane.

Although individuals with monocular vision or suppression can achieve depth discrimination from other clues, it is by no means as fine or rapid as it is with stereoscopic vision. While good stereopsis is always an asset to the worker, whatever the occupation, it is essential for tasks in which persons would otherwise especially be liable to injury or where materials or objects might easily be spoilt or individual efficiency would be unduly low.

Depth perception can be affected by uncorrected refractive errors, anisometropia, uncompensated muscle balances, squints and amblyopia, but other factors may not be quite so obvious. Presbyopes wearing spectacles prescribed for a usual reading distance will find difficulty with depth perception if the working distance is situated outside the depth of field of the correction. In the dark, depth perception is of a very low order and this can be significant for certain groups of workers, such as photographers, who are often required to cut photographic papers or pour toxic chemicals in a dark-room and must, therefore, exercise greater care if accidents are to be avoided. Depth perception is better for vertical lines than horizontal lines and the job of filing, where horizontal wires are used for hanging files, is made easier if a tab is attached to the wire.

Colour vision

Whereas most employees formerly had little or no need for good colour vision, there are an increasingly large number of occupations which require good colour sensitivity and appreciation.

Reasonable colour discrimination is obviously required in the recognition of traffic and signal lights, or of electric cable colours, while excellent discrimination is required in the accurate matching of the colours of paints, dyes, fabrics and threads, both in industrial and domestic situations.

For such tasks, not only will the observer require good colour vision, but lighting giving adequate illuminance and colour rendering properties will also need to be provided. (For example, artificial daylight fluorescent sources providing an illuminance of at least 1000 lux.)

Colour may also aid in the discrimination of detail of various tasks (*see also* Visibility), as well as being important in environmental decoration. In general, lighter colours make more efficient use of light output from any lighting installation because they reflect a higher proportion of incident light, although care should be taken with gloss finishes because of the possibility of reflected glare.

Colour is often deliberately applied to components and signs as a coding system to identify hazards or to facilitate the rapid acquisition of relevant information, for example, the colour-coding of electrical resistors or pipes carrying gas, water and other services.

For any colour-coding system to be effective, adequate colour subtense and illumination is necessary, and colours should be chosen to take account of the relatively high incidence of colour deficiency in the general population. Where safety is of importance, colour combinations which can be distinguished by brightness cues (for example, the green/yellow of the mains earth lead) or shape cues should be provided (*see* Chapter 26).

Visual fields

The effects of reduced visual fields in different occupations are variable. Some jobs, such as typing, make only modest demands on visual field. In others, like driving, full fields are required. There is little doubt, however, that field loss may have a significant effect on safety in many tasks.

The monocular fields overlap to a large degree and field loss in one eye may be compensated almost entirely by the other eye. Equally important is the length of time which the field defect has been present and the degree of adaptation to it. Those engaged in operating mobile equipment and those working in environments where such equipment is in operation are greatly dependent on peripheral vision (*see* Chapter 22).

In determining the effects of reduced visual fields, the total environmental situation must be evaluated in terms of the individual's field limitations, along with experience and adjustment to the field loss. If wide peripheral vision is an occupational requirement, this should be considered in selection of frame and lens type and size. A heavy library frame, in itself, may have field restricting effects as would goggles and some side shields on protective spectacles (*see* Chapter 36).

Visibility

Consideration has been given to assessing the relationship between the individual's visual capabilities and the job requirements, but it is equally important to appreciate the effect of certain characteristics of the visual task and the environment in which it is seen.

When assessing the visual requirements for a specific task, it may be possible to suggest changes to the working conditions that will improve visibility. There are a number of important fundamental influences on visibility:

(1) The size of the working detail and its distance from the eye affects the angle subtended at the eye and hence the visual acuity required to resolve the detail. It is impossible to see an object or its detail if it subtends too small a visual angle.

(2) The ability to recognize detail in a task depends, not merely upon its subtense, but also upon the contrast, either of luminance (brightness) or colour, between the essential parts of the task and its immediate background. If the size of the detail is kept constant and the contrast is reduced, the detail becomes more difficult to see. For example, a black object on a white background provides a high contrast and is much easier to see than a black object on a grey background, even under deficient lighting conditions. Large objects are relatively easy to detect at quite low contrasts, whereas high contrast is always needed for the detection of small detail. Even in the absence of luminance

contrast, colour contrast, arising from differences in the spectral content of the light reflected or emitted by the detail and its surround, may render object detail visible. However, this may pose problems for those individuals with defective colour vision if colour contrast alone is relied upon. Increase in illumination can, to some extent, improve the visibility of low contrast detail (*see* Lighting).

(3) While the contrast and subtense of particular tasks may appear adequate, such tasks may be rendered more difficult by some form of blur (loss of high spatial frequency information), for example in carbon copies of typewritten material or photocopies.

(4) The time available for viewing the object or detail—for example, inspection personnel are often expected to examine large numbers of articles in a fixed time. If the number of articles to be inspected was reduced or the time taken for inspection increased, then the likelihood of detecting defects would be improved. However, it can be appreciated that there is often a delicate balance between productivity, efficiency and cost effectiveness.

If any one of these factors is totally insufficient, in any given case, visibility is likely to be nil. However, one factor may be considerably reduced and, by increasing one or more of the other factors, a certain level of visibility can be maintained. Similarly, increasing any or all of the factors will generally improve visibility.

Clearly the lighting of the task and the environment plays an important role.

Lighting

The amount of light necessary for accurate, strain-free work depends on the nature of the work, i.e. the complexity and visual difficulty of the task, the individual's visual acuity and age, the environment in which the work is performed and the level of performance expected, i.e. speed and accuracy of perception.

A working knowledge of the various aspects of illumination is, therefore, of considerable value to any optometric practitioner when advising patients on ways of achieving optimum vision.

Typical relationships between visual performance and illuminance for tasks of different size and contrast are shown in *Figure 33.6*. The size or contrast or both, of some tasks may be great enough to ensure the required level of visual performance at a relatively low level of illuminance, but as the difficulty of the task becomes greater, i.e. smaller size

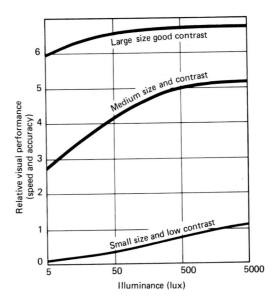

Figure 33.6 Visual performance and illuminance. (Reproduced by courtesy of the Electricity Council)

and/or lower contrast, a much higher level of illuminance becomes necessary if the task is to be performed efficiently.

Senile miosis, lowered transmittance of the ocular structures (particularly for the lens at the blue end of the spectrum), and possible macular degeneration, all contribute to the need of the elderly for more light, while the steadily increasing scattering in the eye, principally from the lens, above the age of 40 means that glare constitutes a much greater problem than for the young. The eyes of older people are slower to adapt to changes in lighting levels and the risk of accidents is increased when walking, for example, from a brightly lit room to a semi-darkened staircase.

When a group of older workers is compared with a group of young ones (*Figure 33.7*), the difference in performance between the two groups diminishes as the illuminance is increased. Where older workers are employed, it is recommended that the illumination provided for them should be some 50–100% greater than would be needed by younger workers performing the same task.

What the eye actually sees is the amount of light reflected from a surface, i.e. its brightness (luminance measured in candelas per square metre, cd/m^2). It is more convenient, however, both to measure and calculate the amount of light falling on to a surface (illuminance measured in lumens per square metre or lux), and lighting codes generally recommend illuminance levels for specific occupational or other tasks.

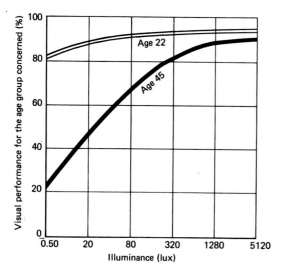

Figure 33.7 Visual efficiency with age and illuminance. (Reproduced by courtesy of the Electricity Council)

In the UK, the Lighting Division of the Chartered Institution of Building Services publishes a comprehensive code (The CIBS Code, 1984) which gives reliable recommendations on appropriate lighting arrangements and illuminances for a wide variety of interiors and tasks. These recommendations apply to tasks of normal contrast and reflectance. Where contrasts or reflectances are very low or mistakes due to wrong perception may be costly or dangerous or where eye protection is worn, the recommended illuminance should be increased.

It is possible to measure the existing level of illumination in any work place or home, easily and cheaply, by using a light meter and then to compare this value with the CIBS standard recommended in the Code. This should always be assessed in the working plane which may not be horizontal.

If specific visual tasks are to be carried out efficiently, however, consideration should be given not only to the illuminance of the task but also to its uniformity over the working area. A minimum to maximum illuminance ratio of not less than 0.7 is usually recommended. Additionally, the illuminance of the general surrounding area of the task should not be less than one-third of the task illuminance. The spectral characteristics of the task lighting are particularly important if the task involves colour discrimination. For example, light from the traditional filament lamp is rich in red and weak in blue and, therefore, unsuitable for colour matching applications. The directional effects of light can be usefully exploited to emphasize surface texture and relief and, in some cases, make it easier to recognize the details of the task. In many tasks, particular attention must be given to the adequate control of glare.

The levels of illumination used in industry are only a tiny fraction of those commonly met in nature (*Figure 33.8*). Complaints of too much light are rare outdoors on an overcast day, even though the level of illumination is generally much higher than that recommended for most industrial processes. The person who complains of too much light at work, therefore, is indicating that there is too much glare, which occurs when luminaires (light fittings), windows or other sources, seen either directly or by reflection, are too bright (relative to the eye's adaptation level) compared with the general bright-

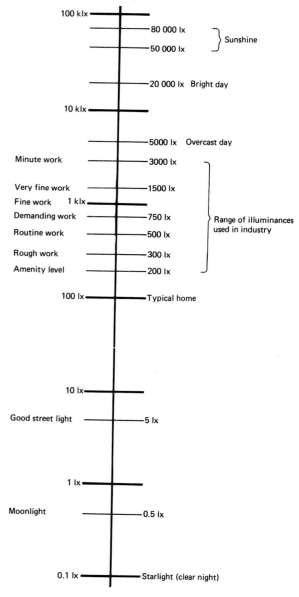

Figure 33.8 Range of naturally occurring illuminances compared with those used in industry

ness of the surroundings. Glare can impair vision (disability glare) and cause visual discomfort (discomfort glare). The two effects can be experienced separately or simultaneously. Discomfort glare has been found to be much the greater problem in interiors. Tolerance to discomfort glare varies widely among individuals and also in the same individual at different times and in varied environments. It is dependent not only upon the individual's personality, age and state of health but also upon the occupation. Glare is more likely to cause discomfort to the elderly and sick and to those carrying out visually demanding tasks; the greater the visual demand, the more important is the need to control glare. Glare can be reduced by the following:

(1) Moving the glare source away from the line of sight, although in many cases it is often easier to move the task or work position.
(2) Reducing the luminance (brightness) of the glare source and reducing the solid angle which it subtends at the eye may be helpful. Diffusers or screens could be useful.
(3) Increasing the background luminance decreases glare since glare effects from a source are worse when they are seen against a dark rather than a light background. A change in decoration of the room can be helpful.
(4) Unwanted reflections should be suppressed either by repositioning the reflecting object or by using matt surfaces—light-coloured blotting paper on highly polished desks can minimize glare effects.

Conclusion

Without accurate information concerning focal distances, size of task detail, direction of gaze etc., attempts to prescribe for the patient's complete visual needs could well prove futile. In determining the visual attributes required to carry out any parti-

cular activity, the needs and capabilities of the individual, as well as the specific demands of the task, must be carefully analysed.

If the prescribing of optical aids is to be most effective, consideration should be given to the effects of modest changes in the visual task or the environment in which the work is done. Lighting, task contrast and positioning of the work can all help to reduce the visual load and improve comfort, efficiency and safety.

Further reading

BAKER, J. (1980) Lighting for industry. *Lighting Equipment News Supplement*, October

CHARMAN, W.N. (1983) Occupational ophthalmic optics and illumination. *Course documentation*, UMIST

THE CIBS CODE FOR INTERIOR LIGHTING (1984) Chartered Institution of Building Services, London

CROSS. R.C. (1967) The optician in industry. Paper read to 1967 Annual Convention of the Association of Ophthalmic Opticians, Ireland

EYES AT WORK SYMPOSIUM (1970) *Ophthal. Opt.*, **10**, 21

FLETCHER, R.J. (1961) *Ophthalmics in Industry*. London: Hatton Press

FOX. S.L. (1973) *Industrial and Occupational Ophthalmology*. Springfield, Illinois: C.C. Thomas

GRUNDY. J.W. (1979) A professional approach to the visual problems of patients at work. *Ophthal. Opt.*, **19**, 4

GRUNDY. J.W. (1981) Visual efficiency in industry. *Ophthal. Opt.*, **21**, 17

GRUNDY. J.W. and ROSENTHAL. S.G. (1982) *VDU's on Site*. London: Association of Optical Practitioners

HOLMES. C. (1958) *Guide to Occupational and Other Visual Needs*, Vols. 1 and 2. St Cloud, Minnesota: The Vision Ease Corporation

HOPKINSON. R.G. and KAY. J.D. (1972) *The Lighting of Buildings*. London: Faber

LYONS. S.(1972) *Management Guide to Modern Industrial Lighting*. Essex: Applied Science Publishers Ltd

WESTON. H.C. (1962) *Sight, Light and Work*, 2nd edn. London: Lewis

34

Clinical applications of contact lenses

Geoffrey Woodward

The repeated or continuous application of a manufactured appliance to some of the most delicate and unusual tissues of the body is not an action to be undertaken lightly. Yet the rationale for such an action has often been far from clear and the risk–benefit ratio not appreciated by either practitioner or recipient. The evaluation of specific benefits and risks must therefore be part of the practitioner's role in contact lens practice. Furthermore, the criteria applied in such decision making must be those used by other health professionals and not those of the cosmetician or beautician. Additionally, the practitioner has an obligation to explain to the patient, in a manner consistent with their intellectual capacity, potential benefits and risks in such a way that the patient is able to give their 'informed consent' to contact lens fitting and management procedures.

This rigorous approach is in no way meant to decry many people's desire to see clearly without wearing spectacles or to suggest that there are excessively high risks in wearing contact lenses. Indeed, for many patients they offer a standard of visual correction that could not be achieved by any other method. However, in an era when new alternative methods of correction of refractive anomalies such as radial keratotomy for myopia and intra-ocular lens implantation for aphakia are becoming highly developed and subjected to close scrutiny and analysis of results, the results of contact lens fitting must inevitably be scrutinized in a similar way.

The development of contact lenses as they are currently known has been, until comparatively recently, a peculiarly haphazard affair. New materials and lens designs have appeared which, in the short term, would seem to answer many problems but they in turn have engendered new difficulties requiring the development of further procedures to resolve them. Such a sequence of events is not unexpected in any rapidly expanding technology but the practitioner must be in a position to evaluate the scientific basis of claims for new materials and lenses, discounting the wilder exaggerations of some promotional literature.

This chapter will endeavour to place the application of contact lenses within the total context of visual correction and also discuss other uses of contact lenses such as cosmesis and therapy. It is not in any way a comprehensive text dealing with techniques of contact lens fitting or properties of contact lens materials. For such information, the appropriate textbooks and journals must be consulted. By considering the indications for contact lenses in various refractive and ocular conditions, it should place the practitioner in the position of being able to prescribe the best and safest form of visual correction for the patient. It must not be forgotten for example that, in prescribing contact lenses instead of spectacles, a new area of hygiene considerations is encountered in which the evaluation of patient compliance becomes of relevance and the personality of the patient may assume major importance. Such matters are discussed in the section dealing with contraindications.

Indications for contact lens wear
Improvement in vision

Coupled with the desire to see clearly without wearing spectacles, this is undoubtedly the major motivation of most patients seeking contact lens fitting. In all cases the patient will see more clearly than without any form of optical correction, but not inevitably better than with a spectacle correction.

In considering potential improvements in vision over spectacle correction, it is helpful to consider separately the quality of peripheral vision and central visual acuity. In some situations the patient will gain in one respect and lose in the other, but generally contact lens correction affords an improvement both peripherally and centrally.

Peripheral vision

Improvement in peripheral vision compared with spectacle correction is due to the larger field of view and the relative absence of peripheral aberrations in contact lenses. The contact lens wearer has virtually the same field of view on eye movements as the emmetrope—only on extreme eye movements may degradation of vision be seen, due to the lens not remaining completely centred on the visual axis. By contrast, the field of view in the spectacle wearers is limited by both the prismatic effects at the lens periphery and the spectacle frame. The effect can be especially distressing to the aphakic patient, the so-called 'Jack-in-the-box' phenomenon.

Despite modern aspheric surfaces, high power spectacle lenses still suffer from oblique aberrations and, together with the prismatic limitations of field, these form the major reasons for intolerance to aphakic spectacle correction. Because in most directions of gaze a contact lens will remain well centred on the cornea, oblique aberrations of the lens are generally insignificant. Spherical aberration of a contact lens is not normally significant except with lenses incorporating exceptionally steep central curves—5.50 mm or less (Westheimer, 1969).
However, it has been shown at low levels of illumination that the contrast sensitivity function is reduced with contact lenses as compared with the equivalent spectacle correction, even though there is usually an absence of visual symptoms (Guillon, Lydon and Wilson, 1983). Contact lenses do suffer from chromatic aberration but fortunately the eye is very tolerant to longitudinal chromatic aberration and most contact lens materials have a dispersive power of the same order as spectacle crown glass.

It is well documented that the flexure of soft lenses when they are placed in the eye usually produces an aspheric surface, and this adventitious asphericity may often reduce aberrations.

Central vision

Improvement in central vision may be brought about in two ways:

(1) Complete or partial neutralization of corneal irregularity.
(2) Variation in the size of the retinal image.

Corneal neutralization

The concept of corneal neutralization is very old indeed, dating back to Leonardo da Vinci more than 500 years ago. In 1801, Thomas Young published his paper 'In the mechanism of the eye' in which he described an apparatus by which 'he hoped to neutralize a faulty corneal surface by substituting an artificial and accurate one; the device to abolish the action of the cornea as a refracting medium by placing in front of it a lens of known power separated from it by a layer of water of known thickness'. Thus the earlier contact lens workers who took up this notion were attempting to adjust the refractive status of the whole eye by varying the power of the cornea with the liquid lens, using afocal rather than powered contact lenses.

In contemporary contact lens practice, the main visual gain over spectacles by corneal neutralization is on irregular and scarred corneas. A distorted and semitranslucent cornea will scatter refracted and reflected light in such a haphazard manner as to drastically degrade the retinal image. The classic treatment for this was tatooing of the cornea—an extremely old procedure first described by Galen (AD 131–120).

The power of a refractive surface is equal to $(n'-n)/R_1$. In air the factor $n'-n$ is $1.376-1.00 = 0.376$, but when a liquid lens of tears is trapped against the eye by a contact lens $n'-n$ becomes $1.376-1.336 = 0.04$, so that the power of an irregularly refracting surface is considerably reduced.

For a transparent surface, the amount of light reflected for any angle of incidence depends, not only on the angle of incidence, but also on the difference between the refractive indices of the two media (Fresnel's law). Using the values of $n' = 1.376$ (cornea) and $n = 1.336$ (tears) and Fresnel's equation, it can be shown that for light incident within $15°$ of the normal the amount of light reflected from the corneal surface is reduced by more than a factor of 100 when a contact lens is placed upon it.

Variation in retinal image size

Any form of optical correction except an intraocular lens placed at the first principal plane of the eye will alter the size of the retinal image.

As can be seen from *Figure 34.1*, a myope will acquire a larger retinal image by changing from spectacles to contact lenses and a patient wearing a positive spectacle prescription, whether it be hyperopic or aphakic, a smaller retinal image. In the case of an astigmatic error there will be meridional differences in magnification.

Before considering visual improvement in specific conditions, it must not be forgotten that contact lenses will give an improvement over uncorrected ametropia, where for some reason a spectacle correction cannot be worn. This may be due to regulations specifically prohibiting the wearing of spectacles in occupations such as the police and

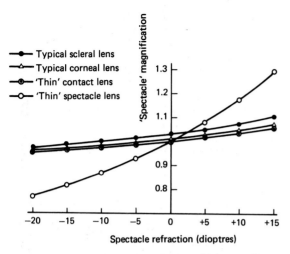

Figure 34.1 Variation of magnification with type and form of correcting lens.

certain branches of the armed services. Occasionally, but fortunately rarely, a spectacle frame cannot be tolerated or fitted owing to abnormalities of the nose, ears or underlying tissues.

Myopia

Currently, the majority of contact lenses prescribed are for the correction of myopia. The incidence and distribution of refractive errors is a racial characteristic, but in every country myopia is still the most common reason for contact lens wear.

As already shown (*Figure 34.1*), a myopic patient changing from spectacles to contact lenses will gain a larger retinal image, a wider field of view and less peripheral aberrations. In addition this patient will also have to accommodate and converge more than with spectacles. For patients with a degree of myopia of 10 D or more, a visual improvement of 2 or 3 lines of Snellen acuity is quite usual and a young myope is nearly always more satisfactorily corrected with contact lenses.

The question of the effect of wearing contact lenses on the progression of myopia is a much more contentious issue. It has been suggested that wearing specific designs of rigid lenses can arrest some cases of myopia (Black-Kelly and Butler, 1971). Stone (1973, 1976) in an extensive review of the literature and her own results concluded that unless children wear contact lenses for at least 2 years there is unlikely to be any stabilization of the progress of their myopia and that any apparent stabilization is due to change in the cornea and that axial elongation continues to occur. At the present time it would be tendentious to suggest to parents of a myopic child that the wearing of contact lenses would definitely retard the progression of the condition.

Aphakia

Over the last 20 years there has been a steady increase in the amount of cataract surgery performed worldwide. For example, in the USA Medicare estimates that the number of surgical procedures to treat cataract rose by 177% between 1965 and 1977. In England and Wales there was an increase of 71% between 1974 and 1981 (Hospital In-patient Enquiry). And in both countries removal of cataract is the most frequent surgical procedure undergone by patients over 65.

However, the method of correcting the resultant aphakia has been changing steadily over the last 10 years (*Table 34.1*).

Table 34.1 Method of aphakia correction (USA)

Method of aphakia correction (USA)	Percentage of total	
	1973	1983
Spectacles	80	20
Daily wear contact lenses	15	15
Extended wear contact lenses	0	25
Intraocular implant	5	40
	100	100

Adapted from *Vision Research*, 1983, Vol. 2, Part 3, page 100, US Department of Health and Human Sciences.

All the optical advantages of contact lenses, when compared with spectacle correction, apply equally to intraocular lenses and the predicted costs over a 10-year period for the intraocular lens is probably less (Davies *et al.*, 1986). The intraocular lens is a permanent and often irreversible form of treatment which in theory requires little or no after care. The only subsequent procedure that may really be necessary is a capsulotomy and, with the advent of lasers, this procedure has become simple and cheaper. Thus, if there is a choice between an extended wear contact lens or an intraocular lens, the main reason for choosing a contact lens would be reservations concerning the long-term effects of an intraocular lens on the eye, particularly the corneal endothelium.

As can be seen, a very fluid situation currently exists in the field of aphakia correction with a declining use of spectacle correction, a static use of daily wear contact lenses, an increasing use of extended wear contact lenses and an even greater increase in the use of intraocular lenses. At the present time, however, most ophthalmic surgeons are cautious about implanting intraocular lenses in patients under the age of 60 and most would accept that the use of daily wear contact lenses in patients capable of handling them is a relatively safe procedure. The current debate is about the complication rates and costs of intraocular lenses and extended wear lenses and this will be discussed. However, there are certain clearly defined groups of patients, where the contact lens is or is not the correction of choice.

Elderly aphakics

This group of patients with a markedly reduced visual acuity often suffer from senile macular degeneration, and therefore benefit from the enlarged retinal image produced by spectacles, particularly for near vision. This elderly group is not commonly physically active so restrictions of mobility produced by the limitations of the visual field are more than compensated for by the increased visual acuity obtained due to higher magnification with spectacles. It must not be forgotten that, in terms of central visual acuity, an accurate aphakic spectacle correction will always give the best results even though in active patients the optical disadvantages of aphakic spectacles usually outweigh this.

The aphakic of more than 60 years of age who for some reason, such as intraocular ophthalmic disease, cannot have a lens implant and is unable to handle a daily wear lens, will still be a candidate for an extended wear contact lens. Possibly some of the problems of early lens disposition, partial dehydration and early spoilage which have been encountered with hydrogel extended wear lenses may be reduced by the advent of rigid extended wear lenses fitted to aphakic patients (Benjamin and Gordon, 1984).

The aphakic infant

There is no doubt that the availability of extended wear contact lenses in high positive powers combined with new surgical techniques has had a revolutionary effect on the management of infants with cataract. It is now appreciated that most of the visual defect following congenital cataract is due to a functional amblyopia and is therefore largely preventable. In this group of patients, early cataract surgery combined with optical correction by 4 months of age is essential to mitigate the effects of visual deprivation from cataract and aphakic blur (Taylor *et al.*, 1979; *see* Chapter 11). Extended wear contact lenses are the only practical form of optical correction in such young children— particularly as the baby needs to be optically corrected for no greater distance than 30 cm as their visual and sensory world is within arms' length (Morris *et al.*, 1979; Woodward and Morris, 1982).

The younger unilateral aphakic patient has often had surgery for a traumatic cataract and here the aphakia may be complicated in terms of contact lens fitting by high or irregular corneal astigmatism and distorted or absent irides. In most cases this entails a rigid lens and at present suitable materials in terms of oxygen permeability are rarely dimensionally stable enough to allow toric lenses to be manufactured for extended wear. Although theoretically the younger unilateral aphakic patient should be a good candidate for contact lenses, in terms of retaining the advantages of binocular vision, in practice the long-term results are disappointing, many patients ceasing to wear the lens after some months. This is particularly so if the other eye is emmetropic and some time has elapsed since the original trauma. In this situation the patient can be difficult to motivate in terms of lens handling, hygiene and an adaptive schedule. Conversely, patients with bilateral traumatic cataracts usually do extremely well with contact lenses.

The speed with which contact lens fitting is carried out following cataract surgery is of great import to the patient and has cost effectiveness implications (Woodward and Drummond, 1984). The most appropriate time interval between cataract surgery and contact lens fitting is the subject of much current interest (Astin, 1984; Reading, 1984). The insertion of an extended wear hydrogel aphakic lens immediately following surgery has been suggested (Kersley, 1977), but this procedure has not been widely adopted. Currently, a period of 12 weeks following cataract extraction is recommended before definitive contact lens fitting is attempted, but new surgical procedures may change this.

The practitioner evaluating the advisability of fitting aphakic patients with contact lenses must be fully aware of the variations from the normal of the aphakic cornea. It is less prone to corneal oedema following contact lens wear even though its oxygen uptake is similar (Holden, Mertz and Guillon, 1980). Sensitivity is lower than the normal cornea as is endothelial cell density (Guillon and Morris, 1981). The implications of these findings are highly relevant to the fitting of contact lenses but outside the range of this chapter.

Astigmatism

Although contact lenses afford some optical advantages to the higher degrees of regular astigmatism, the most beneficial improvements to vision are found where the astigmatism is irregular.

In regular astigmatism, the meridional differences in retinal image size produced by spectacle correction can reduce visual acuity especially when the astigmatic axes are oblique. The reduction of these meridional differences may give an improvement in vision if contact lenses are fitted, but clinically this seems limited to astigmatism of more than 3 D. The use of diagnostic contact lenses to predict potential improvement in vision has value, but is not completely reliable as it must be appreciated that the patient has previously made a perceptual allowance for the distorted retinal image. Furthermore, high oblique astigmatism is often associated with albinism, partial albinism (Ruben, 1967) and congenital idiopathic nystagmus, such patients rarely showing any improvement in visual acuity with contact lenses. Despite this, many of these patients claim they can see better with contact lenses and this is supported to a certain extent by the finding that the contrast sensitivity function may have improved (Abadi, 1979). In Marfan's syndrome, although astigmatism may be minimal if the aphakic portion of the pupil is being used, vision through the periphery of the crystalline lens induces a high myopic astigmatism. Although this astigmatism is neutralized by the liquid lens, not being due to corneal toroidicity, most patients with Marfan's syndrome are happier in contact lenses and feel they can see better. Alternatively, if vision through the aphakic zone is better, a scleral lens with a partially occluded pupil area may be used to occlude the phakic zone (Ruben, 1975a).

It is in cases of irregular astigmatism produced by corneal distortion where the greatest visual gains may be found. The conditions where this situation occurs most commonly are: keratoconus, following keratoplasty and following trauma.

Keratoconus

The first report of a powered contact lens being used in keratoconus was by Fick (1888). Since that time use of rigid corneal and scleral contact lenses has become the standard management of the condition. By the wear of rigid lenses, nearly 80% of patients retain a visual acuity of 6/9 or better, only around 10% proceeding to keratoplasty (Cox, 1984). Several writers have suggested that contact lenses can have a direct therapeutic effect on the keratoconic eye in that the progressive deterioration may be halted; these include Hall (1963) using scleral lenses and Kemmetmuller (1983) advocating corneal lenses. However, Ruben (1976) reported no recession in the rate of progress of keratoconus with contact lens wear irrespective of the fitting and this finding was supported by Woodward (1980) who monitored the progression of the condition using serial topographic pachometry. It has also been suggested that hard contact lens wear could actually precipitate keratoconus in patients with low ocular rigidity (Hartstein and Becker, 1970; Gasset, Haude and Garcia Bengochea, 1978), but the suggestion based on retrospective studies was rejected by Foster and Yamamoto (1978).

Irrespective of these considerations, the wearing of contact lenses enables the majority of patients with keratoconus to enjoy relatively good vision and lead normal lives. Even among the group who proceed to keratoplasty, around 65% still need to wear contact lenses to reach a reasonable level of acuity (Davies, Woodward and Ruben, 1977).

Keratoplasty

If grafts are examined with the photo-electronic keratoscope, it can be shown that there are no regular corneal grafts. Ruben and Colebrook (1979) have shown that even the clearest graft giving 6/6 unaided vision has only a small area (2–3 mm) of sphericity. Astigmatism may be as high as 12 D and may be due to nipple-like protusion, tilting or eccentricity of the graft (Woodward, 1981). Although the irregular topography of a grafted cornea may make contact lens fitting technically difficult, a contact lens may be the only way to restore normal vision to an eye with an otherwise clear graft. A grafted cornea is intrinsically very vulnerable to disruption by a contact lens owing to its reduced sensitivity and lowered endothelial cell count and it may be necessary to monitor corneal swelling and deswelling with a contact lens before a final decision for contact lens wear is made. Sometimes relieving incisions may reduce the astigmatism and close cooperation between the ophthalmic surgeon and contact lens practitioner is most important in the evaluation of treatment options. Patients are naturally eager to proceed with contact lens wear as soon as possible if it improves their vision substantially, but it is unusual to fit patients before all corneal sutures have been removed. The topography of the grafted cornea may continue to vary for up to 2 years after the final removal of sutures and the necessity to refit is frequent.

Post-traumatic irregular astigmatism

This is often associated with aphakia following traumatic cataract surgery, and the same associated problems of distorted or missing irides are often present. Unless at the extreme periphery, puncture or laceration of the cornea invariably produces irregular astigmatism, especially so if suturing has been necessary. Over 90% of the irregular astigmatism can be neutralized by a liquid lens trapped between the spherical back surface of a contact lens and a traumatized cornea. Where a patient has a reduced visual acuity following corneal trauma, it is always worthwhile inserting a diagnostic contact lens to establish whether a visual improvement could be obtained by fitting.

Anisometropia

Anisometropia may be primarily due to varying degrees of ametropia between the two eyes or secondary following cataract surgery, keratoplasty or degenerative disease.

In primary anisometropia the precise difference in image size is determined by the proportion of refractive and axial ametropia contributing to the total difference in refractive error. In spite of the fact that most primary anisometropia is mainly axial, contact lenses have been found to be more acceptable than spectacles to many anisometropes. This may well be due to differences in retinal receptor spacing in the two eyes (Stone, 1981).

In unilateral aphakia, the anisometropic increase in retinal image size with spectacles may vary between 15% and 55%, but for an eye of average dimensions the figure would be in the region of 30%. Thus with spectacle correction there is an insurmountable obstacle to binocular vision, which is not usually considered possible with a difference much greater than 10%.

Calculation shows that for a previously emmetropic eye, the difference in retinal image size with unilateral contact lens correction is of the order of 10%. Despite this apparent discrepancy, most unilateral aphakic patients corrected with a contact lens are symptom free (Guillon and Warland, 1980). Furthermore aniseikonia measured subjectively is considerably lower than that calculated theoretically in this group of patients.

The successful re-establishment of binocular vision following unilateral cataract surgery varies inversely with the age of the patient (Ruben, 1975a) and as stated earlier the success rate with young unilateral aphakics of traumatic origin is not high. Despite the theoretical objections young aphakics are best corrected with contact lenses for an intermediate distance, as they are extremely loathe to wear a supplementary spectacle addition in plano bifocal form.

Corneal scarring

Scarring of the anterior surface of the cornea will produce irregular refraction and reflection of incident light and may significantly degrade the quality of vision. This degradation of vision can often be significantly reduced by the use of a contact lens. It is thus always worth evaluating any possible improvement in vision with a diagnostic contact lens before procedures, such as keratoplasty either lamellar or penetrating, are undertaken for visual reasons. Surprising improvements in vision are often obtained. If, however, the scarring is more posterior in the cornea, no improvement in vision may be anticipated.

Telescopic systems

Descriptions of a galilean telescope for the low vision patient using a minus contact lens as the eyepiece and a plus spectacle lens as the objective have appeared in many textbooks. The first edition of Mandell's *Contact Lens Practice* (1965) makes 25 references to telescopic systems and, in the text, Fildeman's Telecon system is described as 'very practical'. Bier (1970) considers them a sound prac-

tical position where a magnification of × 1.6 or less suffices. Despite these endorsements very few cases of such systems being well tolerated and worn regularly are on record.

The disadvantage of the system is that the relatively low magnification (less than 2) is insufficient to motivate the patient to tolerate the multiple disadvantages of using a high minus contact lens, a heavy spectacle which has to be kept exactly in the correct position, a limited field of vision, an effective reduction in accommodation and spatial disorientation when the eye and not the head is moved.

Silver and Woodward (1978) have suggested that factors favouring success with such a system are:

(1) A highly motivated patient.
(2) A patient with deep set eyes.
(3) A patient already wearing contact lenses with good tolerance.

Contact lenses fitted as part of such a telescopic system must be a very stable fit and this may be difficult to achieve without embarrassing corneal metabolism.

Occlusion: partial and total

Although partial occlusion produced by a contact lens may, in addition to the amelioration of symptoms such as photophobia or monocular diplopia, improve vision, it is convenient to consider this as a separate indication.

The occlusion may be partial in that light is restricted to passing along certain zones between the lens and the retina, selective in that only certain wavelengths of light are passed through the lens or disruptive in that only degraded optical images can be seen through the lens. In any of these modes of use, a contact lens is ideally suited in terms of the eye's principal phases and rotations. There is very little chance of peeping around the edge of a contact lens and within excursions of most gaze, whenever the eye moves a contact lens moves with it. If only certain wavelengths of light were to be admitted to the eye, a contact lens would be more efficient than the closest fitting spectacles. All that is lacking in the contact lens armoury at the present time is a photochromic contact lens.

Indications for partial occlusion by contact lenses include: albinism, pupil anomalies, Marfan's syndrome, pigmentary retinal degeneration, colour vision anomaly.

Albinism

Patients suffering from oculocutaneous albinism usually exhibit subnormal visual acuity (6/24–6/60), a high incidence of nystagmus and significant myopic and hyperopic astigmatism. For many years, it was suggested that the reduced visual acuity was due to light scattering within the eye and that a contact lens which occluded light from entering the eye except through the pupil could substantially improve visual acuity. It is now accepted that the most significant factor contributing to the reduction of visual acuity in albinism is macular hypoplasia with the absence of macular luteal pigment, and that there is no evidence that contact lenses with an artificial iris can significantly improve vision (Fonda, 1962; Ruben, 1967). Notwithstanding these findings, most albinos are happier when wearing contact lenses tinted or with an artificial iris; this is also true in albinoidism where the fovea is normal or nearly so, visual acuity reduced only slightly and nystagmus absent. This is probably because contact lenses are more effective in alleviating the photophobia than tinted spectacles. In addition, there is a psychological element in that patients are happier with the appearance of their eyes and other people's reaction to them when they are wearing tinted contact lenses. Theoretically, the high incidence of astigmatism would indicate the use of rigid lenses but as there is usually only minimal improvement in visual acuity most patients are happy with the various forms of tinted hydrogel lenses. Despite the visual relationship between pigmentation and corneal sensitivity it has been shown that albinos have much less sensitive corneas than normally pigmented eyes (Millodot, 1984). Providing it is not suggested to the patient that their vision will be significantly improved, contact lenses can be a highly satisfactory form of correction for this condition.

Pupil anomalies

In cases of aniridia, iris coloboma and polycoria, both an improvement in appearance and in some cases an improvement in vision may be found. The greatest improvement in vision is usually in cases of traumatic aniridia following perforating injury. An enhancement of vision to a surprising degree is not infrequently found by fitting contact lenses incorporating an iris. If, as is often the case, the traumatic aniridia is associated with corneal scarring, a visual improvement from 6/60 to 6/9 may be gained. Similar improvements in acuity may also be found in traumatic mydriasis following blunt injury or where the pupil remains permanently dilated following penetrating keratoplasty. In all of these cases, the patient's photophobia may also be alleviated by the use of an iris lens.

Marfan's syndrome

The use of contact lenses with a partially occluded pupil zone may be appropriate. As the occluding zone has to be precisely located over the phakic or aphakic zone, it is necessary to fit a scleral lens by the impression technique to achieve complete stability of the lens and avoid lens rotation.

Pigmentary degeneration of the retina

It has been suggested by some authors that in pigmentary degeneration of the retina the use of tinted lenses may decelerate the rate of progression of the condition (Adrian, Everson and Schmidt, 1977). Although this is not a commonly accepted view, clinically it does seem that patients suffering from this disease often feel more comfortable when wearing lenses with a brown tint. This is particularly so if they have also been rendered aphakic.

Colour vision anomaly

If a patient with a colour vision anomaly wears a contact lens in one eye only and this lens absorbs strongly in an appropriate waveband, it may help them to 'pass' certain occupational colour vision screening tests. It cannot be said to have improved the patient's colour vision deficiency.

Indications for the use of contact lenses where total occlusion is required are: intractable diplopia or amblyopia treatment.

Intractable diplopia

Where a paretic eye has normal vision and the patient is suffering from intractable diplopia, a contact lens may prove a more acceptable method of occlusion to the patient than an eye patch. There are technical difficulties in completely occluding an eye with normal vision with a lens of normal thickness, but successful results have been obtained in many cases.

Amblyopia treatment

Any degree of blurring to the point of total occlusion can be produced by fitting a contact lens as part of amblyopia treatment. The advantages of the method are chiefly cosmetic. There is no need to wear spectacles while the treatment is being carried out, the child's appearance is normal and it is not obvious to anyone that occlusion is being effected (Ruben and Walker, 1967). Apart from this consideration, there is little evidence that this method is any more satisfactory than more conventional methods. However, it has been suggested that extended wear contact lenses may be more satisfactory than spectacles in the treatment of accommodative esotropia (Calcutt, Mathalone and Holland, 1983).

Therapeutic indications for contact lenses

The term 'therapeutic' is often used as if it applied to a specific type of lens. This is not the case, nearly every type of lens including scleral, hydrogel and silicone rubber being able to function as a therapeutic device. Therapeutic lenses can be defined as those which are fitted with a therapeutic intent; incidentally, they may improve vision, perhaps simply by allowing the patient to keep the eye open but this was not the prime motive for lens fitting.

There are three main therapeutic actions which may be produced with contact lenses including the relief of pain, promotion of healing and protection of the eye. The relief of pain is usually effected by protecting, from trauma, areas of the cornea where epithelial breakdown and exposure of the nerve endings has occurred. The promotion of healing is assisted in two ways. Where a chronic keratitis has failed to respond to conventional treatments, a vicious circle may develop where, as part of the response to the corneal disease, the conjunctiva becomes chronically oedematous and the conjunctival vessels permanently dilated causing swelling and stiffening of the lids. These thickened lids, in turn, easily traumatize the newly forming epithelial layer retarding the normal healing of the cornea and increasing the lid response. Healing of the cornea can sometimes be promoted by protecting the delicate newly forming epithelium from the lids by the interposition of a suitable membrane in the form of a contact lens. Healing may also be promoted in a perforated cornea by helping the anterior chamber to reform by a sealing action and thus increasing apposition of the edges of the wound. Contact lenses may be used to protect the eye from trauma caused by:

(1) The environment, e.g. drying of the cornea.
(2) Aberrant lashes, e.g. trichiasis.
(3) Keratinized or cicatrized lids.
(4) Hyperkeratinized palpebral conjunctival epithelium.

Some of the conditions where therapeutic lenses have proved of value are described below.

Recurrent corneal erosions

Therapeutic contact lenses are not the first line of treatment in this painful and distressing condition which is usually associated with a primary epithelial dystrophy (Williams and Buckley, 1985). However, if other forms of treatment have not been successful, pain can be relieved with a hydrogel therapeutic lens and this may help resolution of the condition. If after 3 months of lens wear the patient is symptom free, the lens should be removed as there is always risk of complications with any form of extended wear.

Failure to re-epithelialize

This can be due to many causes. It may occur following penetration keratoplasty or be due to the non-adherence of epithelium following surgery in diabetics. A hydrogel therapeutic lens will protect the reforming epithelium, but again the lens should be removed when the epithelium is re-established.

Postkeratoplasty

In addition to cases where the donor cornea has not re-epithelialized, therapeutic lenses are useful where sutures are prominent. As well as causing severe discomfort to the patient, such sutures tend to accumulate mucus around them which can increase the risk of infection or rejection. When therapeutic lenses are fitted in such cases they should be removed for cleaning if mucus accumulates beneath them.

Bullous keratopathy

This is one of the most common indications for hydrogel therapeutic lenses particularly in elderly aphakic patients. It can be an extremely painful condition and there is no successful treatment apart from penetrating keratoplasty. Although a therapeutic lens worn on an extended wear basis inevitably produces some corneal neovascularization, in these cases the relief of pain and occasionally some improvement in vision often makes it the preferable option to further surgery. In buphthalmos the size of the cornea poses severe technical problems if keratoplasty is considered and specifically designed large flat hydrogel lenses can make the eyes more comfortable.

Abnormal tear states

Where there is a reduction in the aqueous content of the tears (keratoconjunctivitis sicca), the use of hydrogel therapeutic lenses is not indicated—in fact they may well exacerbate the condition. Some success has been reported, however, by the use of scleral lenses (Ruben, 1975b) or silicone rubber lenses (Davies and Woodward, 1978).

Where the aqueous content is normal, but the mucus and lipids are reducing rendering the corneal surface less hydrophilic and increasing the evaporation rates, hydrogel lenses are of value in relieving pain. This is especially so in Stevens–Johnson syndrome where tear abnormalities are often associated with distortion of the lid margins and conjunctival cicatrization.

Symblepharon

This may occur as a result of chemical or thermal burns or loss of the fornices due to ocular pemphigoid. Scleral lenses or rings have been used to help maintain the fornices both as an emergency treatment and following surgical procedures.

Fifth and seventh nerve lesions

Anaesthetic eyes and eyes with abnormal lid closure are very prone to exhibit an exposure keratitis. Fitting of these eyes with therapeutic lenses must be undertaken only with extreme caution. Hydrogel lenses tend to lose water rapidly, the resultant dehydration either producing a very tight lens or one that herniates forward and is blinked from the eye. Some success using therapeutic silicone rubber lenses has been reported in these cases (Woodward, 1984) and scleral lenses have also been used.

Corneal perforations and melting

In some patients, the anterior chamber has been reformed with a silicone rubber therapeutic lens following a spontaneous perforation of the cornea. There is also some evidence that a therapeutic lens will cause stromal thickening where corneal melting has occurred in rheumatoid diseases. Many of the cases will eventually need keratoplasty, but the therapeutic lens can be a useful device for temporizing until suitable donor material is available. Low water content hydrogel lenses have been used to treat small puncture wounds of the cornea, especially when in the periphery. If this does seal the wound less astigmatism is produced than by suturing.

Exposure keratitis

This condition may be produced by a wide variety of causes such as thyrotoxic exophthalmos, trauma to the lids, blow-out fracture of the orbit or surgical reconstruction of the lids following excision of a tumour. A therapeutic hydrogel lens tends to dehydrate and become unsuitable, so scleral or silicone rubber lenses are mainly used to protect the cornea, reducing discomfort and the rate of corneal vascularization.

In all of the uses of therapeutic lenses, it cannot be over emphasized that the patients need very careful monitoring in conjunction with the ophthalmologist who is responsible for the medical care, the decision when to discontinue wear being of crucial importance in the successful management of the condition. These eyes are compromised initially and the risks of secondary infection plus all the usual complications of contact lens wear are high.

Other less common uses of therapeutic contact lenses include those shown below.

Ptosis and myopathy

In carefully selected cases, a specially designed impression scleral lens may be used to produce lid elevation in ptosis (Trodd, 1971). The best chance of success is when eye movements are limited by myopathy; in other eyes normal excursion movements are problematical.

Regulation of intraocular pressure

In glaucomatous eyes where excision of a filtration bleb has produced too low an intraocular pressure, hydrogel lenses have been used to apply pressure to the leaking area to reform the anterior chamber. The effect will be produced within 2 or 3 hours or not at all.

Dispensation of drugs

Hydrophilic contact lenses presoaked in 2% or 4% pilocarpine have been used in the treatment of glaucoma (Ruben and Watkins, 1975). This method does produce intensive miotic therapy and has value in the emergency department. Because of cost and management implications, it is not widely used in the routine management of glaucoma. This technique would be applicable to many other water-soluble drugs but is not widely used at the present time.

Cosmesis

A dictionary definition of cosmetic is 'having no other function than to beautify'. This is a useful working definition of a cosmetic contact lens when used to disguise or cover an ugly and sometimes blind eye. Cosmetic lenses may also perform an incidental visual corrective function if the eye is sighted, but this is not their prime function.

The degree of personal distress produced by a scarred or disfigured eye is a very individual one and because of this it is impossible to quantify clinical indications for cosmetic contact lenses. Some patients are blithely unaware of an extremely disfigured eye while others are intensely concerned about a variation from the normal appearance which can only be detected by the closest inspection. Hence in assessing an individual patient's suitability for a cosmetic contact lens, the personality is equally, if not more, important than the technical difficulties of fitting the lens. If the patient has an obsessive personality, the worst possible case must be put to them initially otherwise they will have quite unreasonable expectations for the final appearance of the eye. The majority of cosmetic lenses are fitted to one eye only and the patient has then always the other eye with which to compare the appearance. In the case of children who have a disfigured eye through trauma, the parents not infrequently have residual guilt concerning the circumstances of the original accident. Their efforts to expunge this emotion by concealment of the damaged eye can make them extremely demanding. In this situation the child himself may not be particularly concerned about the appearance of the eye at that particular time.

The ideal patient for a cosmetic contact lens is motivated, but not obsessional, about their appearance, accepts that it is not possible to obtain a perfect match with the contralateral eye and that pupils on cosmetic lenses will not dilate or constrict.

Cosmetic lenses are available in the following forms:

(1) Hard corneal homogeneous tint.
(2) Hard corneal iris pattern.
(3) Hydrogel homogeneous tint.
(4) Hydrogel printed iris pattern.
(5) Hydrogel hand painted iris pattern.
(6) Scleral lens.

All types are available with clear or tinted powered pupil area or black pupil.

Techniques of fitting cosmetic lenses are outside the range of this chapter but the basic principle involves attempting to satisfy the patient with the simplest option first. Cosmetic contact lenses are costly and take a long time to manufacture, so patients must be given a realistic appraisal of the various options at the commencement of fitting and their hopes not unduly raised. Furthermore, with hydrogel lenses, the problems of reproducing the lens may occur when a lens ages and needs replacing. It must also be remembered that all cosmetic lenses except those with homogeneous tints are thicker than the equivalent clear lens. Thus good tolerance with a clear fitting lens does not necessarily mean that the final cosmetic lens will be well tolerated.

In spite of all these comments, fitting cosmetic contact lenses can be an interesting and rewarding field. Before embarking on this sphere of work, the practitioner must consider whether his/her own temperament is suitable for dealing with this difficult group of patients.

Contraindications

These may be considered under three headings:

Optical	*Patient specific*	*Medical*
Low refractive errors	Poor motivation	Atopy
Presbyopic and near presbyopic myopes	Poor compliance	Diabetes
	Dubious hygiene standards	Oral contraceptives
	Poor lens handling	
Presbyopia	Unavailability of after care	
	Environmental	
	Previous failure with lenses	
	Costs	

It must be emphasized that these are relative and not absolute contraindications and must be weighed against indications. For example, a high percentage of keratoconus patients are also atopic but nevertheless contact lenses are indicated in most cases. Furthermore, obvious cases of eye pathology where contact lenses would be obviously inappropriate have not been listed. Where patients are undergoing long-term topical therapy certain types of lenses may be contraindicated. Patients wearing hydrogel lenses who are using drops on a long-term basis for the control of glaucoma may develop a sensitivity to the preservative used in the drops. This may be absorbed into the matrix of the lens, its subsequent elution over a long period possibly causing toxicity problems. Such patients are better served with lenses which have little or no capacity for such absorption.

Optical

Low refractive errors

Patients who only wear spectacles on an irregular basis are in general unsuccessful contact lens wearers. The amount of time spectacles are worn is a better predictor than the dioptric value of the prescription as some patients are much less visually aware than others.

High myopes, presbyopic and near presbyopic

Although this group of patients will obtain a larger retinal image with contact lenses and enhanced distance vision, this is usually insufficient to compensate for the increased accommodation and convergence required. Only if these patients do little close work or have specific motivation to replace spectacles will they be successful.

Presbyopia

Despite claimed success rates of 50% with bifocal hard lenses (Hodd, 1983) and 40% with bifocal soft lenses (Molinari, 1984), it can be stated confidently that at the present time very few people are wearing bifocal contact lenses. In 1983, it was reported that soft lens bifocal sales represented less than 1% of the soft contact lens market (Lloyd, 1984). This is because, worldwide, the vast majority of patients fitted with contact lenses are low myopes between 20 and 30 years of age (Hamano *et al.*, 1982) and there is currently no completely satisfactory form of contact lens correction for presbyopia.

Thus it can be said that the onset of presbyopia is not in general an indication for the prescribing of contact lenses. However, this does not mean that patients already wearing contact lenses will not wish to carry on doing so when they become presbyopic. The options are:

(1) The monovision principle may be used where one eye is corrected for near and the other for distance. In spite of the theoretical objections to this, high success rates have been claimed using this technique—85% (Bayshore, 1977) and 90% (Scarborough and Loparik, 1976).
(2) Supplementary reading spectacles are, however, probably the most widely used option.
(3) Contact lens bifocals: although contemporary contact lens bifocals tend to be classified by their supposed method of operation, i.e. alternating or simultaneous vision, it is quite certain that if they function successfully it is by a combination of these two methods. Generally the most amenable patients to bifocal contact lens wear are those who have become used to unrestricted or peripheral vision and have never had completely clear stable vision with contact lenses or spectacles. High myopes and aphakics fall into this category. The arrival of bifocal contact lenses which rely on diffractive rather than refractive power for the reading addition may remove presbyopia from this section sometime in the future.

Patient specific

Poor motivation

The degree of motivation of a patient seeking contact lenses is not readily quantifiable. Paradoxically, a patient can be too highly motivated if this is based on an unrealistic expectation of the differences that contact lenses will make to his/her life. Patients are occasionally fitted through the National Health Service at the request of a consultant psychiatrist. These patients have become obsessional about wearing spectacles, feeling that the necessity to

do so has spoilt their whole life and if that necessity were removed everything would be different. Although these patients are usually successful lens wearers, their obsessional neurosis rarely disappears but is merely directed to different obsessions while their lifestyle does not undergo radical improvement. Presumably many of this group are now seeking radial keratotomy. However, many contact lens practitioners are familiar with patients who, initially withdrawn, have 'blossomed' after successfully wearing contact lenses. This is not an area amenable to controlled studies and authoritative statements can not be made.

In private practice where the patient has to pay the whole cost of the appliance case, solutions etc., plus professional fees, the willingness to pay is an indication of motivation. This is why the payment of a substantial part of the fee at the onset of fitting is highly desirable. In hospital practice careful evaluation of the precise nature of the patient's visual problems will help to avoid fitting patients with poor motivation.

Poor patient compliance

A patient who does not comply with the practitioner's instructions can be a danger to himself in terms of infection and contact lens induced disease. Yet as has been shown in all medical and paramedical fields, patient compliance is impossible to guarantee. There are only two points at which the practitioner has any influence on the situation. At the initial examination, all the implications of contact lens wear in relation to procedures and routines required of the patient must be fully explained. The importance of this first explanation cannot be over emphasized. Then, if the patient does not comply by failing to keep follow-up appointmets, the practitioner must write to the patient again pointing out all the possible risks and disclaiming all future responsibility if the patient does not attend. Furthermore, if the patient subsequently reappears when a lost or damaged lens needs replacing supply should be refused.

Dubious hygiene standards

Hygiene standards are difficult to evaluate, but patients who attend for fitting or instruction with dirty hands and nails do give the practitioner an indication that all is not well. Patients requesting refitting who present their previous unsuccessful lenses in a grubby condition and in a filthy case also indicate a lot about themselves.

Poor lens handling

Even though extended wear lenses are appropriate in some cases, patients should always be able to remove their own lenses. Only when there are overwhelming indications and the patient has 24-hour access to an emergency service should patients who are not able to remove them be fitted with contact lenses. Where only daily wear lenses are possible, patient dexterity is of obvious importance when a decision whether or not to fit is made.

Unavailability of after care

Patients who after fitting will not be able to obtain appropriate skilled after care should not be given contact lenses. Cooper and Constable (1977) reporting on two extended wear patients who lost vision to the point of blindness wrote 'a significant factor in their bad outcome was the fact that both lived in areas remote from adequate ophthalmic services'.

Environment

Polluted atmospheres of any description are undesirable for contact lens wear, more so with some types of lenses than others. Patients who are regularly exposed to them either occupationally or recreationally should be discouraged from wearing contact lenses.

Previous failure with lenses

That the patient wishes to try contact lens wear again can be construed as indicating high motivation. Nevertheless, before proceeding the specific reason for the previous failure should again be established. If the type of lens was unsuitable or the fitting satisfactory there is no reason not to try and fit the patient with a satisfactory lens. If, however, there appears to be nothing significantly wrong with the previous lenses and the patient was correctly instructed in lens wear, this must be considered a contraindiction for refitting.

Cost

In addition to the initial fees, there will always be ongoing costs for accessory solutions, care systems, maintenance and replacement of lenses. This must be explained to the patient at the initial examination. Patients unwilling or unable to bear these costs should not be fitted with contact lenses for obvious reasons.

Medical

Atopy

Patients presenting with manifestation of atopic disease such as hay fever, asthma, vernal conjunctivitis and atopic eczema are on the whole less tolerant to contact lenses than the general population.

Furthermore, they are most likely to develop giant papillary conjunctivitis (Allansmith *et al.*, 1977) or contact lens induced keratopathies (Blomfield, Jakcberc and Theodore, 1984). Also their corneal thickness and topography is different from the general population (Kerr-Muir, Woodward and Leonard, 1987). Thus the indications for fitting contact lenses must be strong before such patients are considered.

Diabetes

The use of therapeutic lenses in diabetic patients with non-adhesions of the corneal epithelium has already been described. This lower rate of epithelial healing in diabetes must be considered in the light of the possibility of minor abrasions when removing and inserting contact lenses. The necessity for caution when fitting diabetic aphakic patients with extended wear lenses has been suggested by Eichenbaum, Feldstein and Podos (1982) and Lemp *et al.* (1984).

Oral contraception

Some years ago it was suggested that women taking the contraceptive pill could become intolerant to contact lenses (Koetting, 1966). This was thought to be comparatively rare by Sabell (1970) and no relationship between the use of oral contraceptives and contact lens intolerance was found by Barry and Ruben (1980). This pattern of reporting may represent the continuing lowering of the dosage of hormones in oral contraceptives.

Risks and benefits

The concept of a contact lens as another optical appliance which may be donned or discarded at will, like a pair of spectacles, belongs to an era long passed. It may have been acceptable 30 years ago when the majority of lenses fitted were scleral, wearing times were short and corneal lenses were just becoming available. Even that is doubtful, as the long-term wear of scleral lenses may produce a low grade chronic anoxia which can initiate serious corneal changes. Nowadays, it is usual for lenses to be worn all the patient's working hours or on extended bases. This means that patients are exposed to a much higher dosage of contact lenses and the consequential ocular changes occur much sooner and become much more significant. All contact lenses cause some form of ocular change usually including both the lids and cornea. The evaluation of these contact lens induced changes is an important part of the 'fitting' of contact lenses and is a continuing process. The analogy is not with a pair of spectacles, but is more akin to the fitting of an intrauterine contraceptive device where monitoring of the effects of an appliance on tissue must be on a regular basis.

The changes produced by contact lenses vary considerably in their degree, but the practitioner must always be aware of them and in a position to evaluate their magnitude. The major changes to the environment of the outer eye produced by contact lens wear are shown below.

Occlusion of atmospheric oxygen

In spite of the power of the cornea to adapt to a lower availability of oxygen, some changes are always produced. These vary from a mild transient oedema, through localized peripheral advancement of limbal arcades to neovascularization of central corneal areas. Furthermore these changes can occur to a very great extent with an unobservant patient being quite unaware of them.

Loss of sensation

The reduction in corneal sensitivity produced by contact lens wear is well documented (Millodot, 1984). It occurs with all types of contact lenses, markedly so with hard lenses and is closely dose related.

Disruption of precorneal tear film

Contact lenses of all types disrupt the precorneal tear film and increase the rate of evaporation of tears (Tomlinson and Cederstaff, 1982). Most younger patients will have sufficient tears for this not to be as deleterious but where patients have marginally abnormal tears they may be adversely affected by the wearing of contact lenses.

Sensitization

The mild but continuous trauma produced by a contact lens combined with adhesion of the patient's own tear proteins may produce an autoimmune response as in giant papillary conjunctivitis. The degree of this response is variable, but more than 50% of eyes wearing extended wear lenses show tarsal conjunctival changes within 6 months (Prince *et al.*, 1982). A sensitivity may also develop to the preservative used in contact lens care systems producing a toxic epitheliopathy.

Infection

The cornea is surprisingly resistant to infection considering the often substantial bacterial flora in the conjunctival sac. The resistance of a healthy cornea to direct bacterial invasion is due to the impervious nature of outer epithelial layer, lid function and to tear film function. All of these can be disrupted by the wearing of contact lenses, so an increased risk of corneal infection in contact lens wearers is unsurprising. Galentine *et al.* (1984) reviewed ulcerative keratitis associated with contact lens wear at Wills Hospital, Philadelphia from 1978 to 1983; 17% of corneal ulcers were associated with the use of contact lenses and the authors concluded that contact lens use is an increasingly important risk factor for the development of corneal ulcers.

This enhanced risk of corneal infection is related to the type of lens worn, being greater with hydrogel lenses than hard lenses and greater still with hydrogel lenses worn in the extended wear mode. The severity of the infection also follows a similar pattern (Barry and Ruben, 1980). Precise figures for the incidence of corneal infection amongst contact lens wearers leading to visual loss and blindness are difficult to establish as accurate figures for the number of people actually wearing lenses are not available. Reports of such instances are, however, becoming increasingly common in the ophthalmic and optometric literature at a time when more people are wearing contact lenses and for longer periods of time.

It is thus incumbent on the practitioner to explain to the patient seeking contact lenses both the benefits and risks of their wear, particularly emphasizing the obligations the patient will have to himself in relation to lens hygiene. The standard of this can be appallingly low. Matthews, Dart and Sherwood (1983) who examined 138 patients with contact lens related disease, suggested that ocular health amongst contact lens wearers is maintained despite the use of contact lenses rather than because of it. The prescribing of a contact lens has short- and long-term implications much wider than any other optical appliance and all must be evaluated before a final decision is made.

References

ABADI. R.V. (1979) Visual performance with contact lenses and congenital idiopathic nystagmus. *Br. J. Physiol. Opt.*, **33**, 32–37

ADRIAN. W.. EVERSON. R.W. and SCHMIDT. I. (1977) Protection against photic damage in retinitis pigmentosa. In *Retinitis Pigmentosa: Clinical Implications of Current Research*, edited by M.B. Labders, pp. 233–249. New York: Plenum Press

ALLANSMITH. M.R.. KORB. D.K.. GREINER. J.V.. HENRIQUEZ. A.Z.. SIMMS. M.A. and FINENCE. V.M. (1977) Giant papillary conjunctivitis in contact lens wearers. *Am. J. Ophthalmol.*, **83**, 697–698

ASTIN. C. (1984) Aphakic contact lens fitting in a hospital department. *J. Br. Contact Lens Assoc.*, **7**(3), 164–169

BARRY. P.J. and RUBEN. M. (1980). Contact lens injuries—an analysis of 217 consecutive patients presenting to Moorfields casualty department. *Contact Lens J.* **9**, 6–10

BAYSHORE, C.A. (1977) You can fit that presbyope. *Contact Lens Forum*, December edn

BENJAMIN, W.J. and GORDON, J.M. (1984) Rigid extended wear: aphakia. *Contact Lens J.*, **12**(8), 5–16

BIER, N. (1970) *Correction of Subnormal Vision*, 2nd edn. p. 102, London: Butterworths

BLACK-KELLY, T.S. and BUTLER, D. (1971) The present position of contact lenses in relation to myopia. *Br. J. Physiol. Opt.*, **26**, 33–48

BLOMFIELD, S.E., JAKCBERC, F.E. and THEODORE, F.H. (1984) Contact lens induced keratopathy. *Ophthalmology (Rochester)*, **91**, 290–294

CALCUTT, C, MATHALONE, B. and HOLLAND, B. (1983) Contact lenses as an alternative to spectacles in accommodative esotropia, *J. Br. Contact Lens Assoc.*, **6**(4), 137–141

COOPER, R.L. and CONSTABLE, I.J. (1977) Infective keratitis in soft contact lens wearers. *Br. J. Ophthalmol.*, **61**, 250–254

COX, S.N. (1984) Management of keratoconus. *J. Br. Contact Lens Assoc.*, **7**(2), 56–64

DAVIES, P.D. and WOODWARD, E.G. (1978) The therapeutic use of silicone rubber lenses in dry eye states. *Transactions of the VIIIth European Contact Lens Society of Ophthalmologist*, Strasbourg, pp. 23–25

DAVIES, P.D., WOODWARD, E.G. and RUBEN, M. (1977) Keratoconus: an analysis of the factors which influence the optical results of keratoplasty. *Transactions of the VIIth European Contact Lens Society of Ophthalmologists*, Ghent, pp. 97–99

DAVIES, L.M., DRUMMOND, M.F., WOODWARD, E.G. and BUCKLEY, R.J. (1986) A cost-effective comparison of the intraocular lens and the contact lens in aphakia. *Trans. Ophthalmol. Soc. UK*, **105**, 304–313

EICHENBAUM, J.W., FELDSTEIN, M. and PODOS, S.M. (1982) Extended-wear aphakic soft contact lenses and corneal ulcers. *Br. J. Ophthalmol.*, **66**, 663–666

FICK, A.E. (1888) Eine Contactbrille *Arch. Augenheilk*, **18**, 279

FONDA, G. (1962) Characteristics and low vision correction in albinism. *Arch. Ophthalmol.*, **68**, 754–760

FOSTER, C.S. and YAMAMOTO, G.H. (1978) Ocular rigidity in keratoconus. *Am. J. Ophthalmol.*, **86**, 802–806

GALENTINE, P.G., COHEN, E.J., LABSON, P.R., ADAMS, C.P., MICHAUD, R. and ARENTSEN, J.J. (1984) Corneal ulcers associated with contact lens wear. *Arch. Ophthalmol.*, **102**, 891–894

GASSETT, A.R., HAUDE, W.L. and GARCIA BENGOCHEA (1978) Hard contact lens wear, an environmental risk in keratoconus. *Am. J. Ophthalmol.*, **85**, 339–341

GUILLON, M. and MORRIS, J.A. (1981) Corneal response to a provocative test in aphakic patients, *J. Br. Contact Lens Assoc.*, **4**(4), 162–167

GUILLON, M. and WARLAND, J. (1980) Aniseikonia and binocular function in unilateral aphakia. *J. Br. Contact Lens Assoc.*, **3**(1), 36–39

GUILLON, M., LYDON, D.P.M. and WILSON, C. (1983) Variations in contact sensitivity function with spectacles and contact lenses. *J. Br. Contact Lens Assoc.*, **6**(3), 120–128

HALL, C.J. (1963) Keratoconus. *Br. J. Physiol. Opt.*, **20**, 125–135

HAMANO, H., HAWABE, H. MASHIMA, J. and KOJIMA, S. (1982). Statistical trends of wearers of contact lenses. *Contact Intraoc. Lens Med. J.*, **8**, 29–38

HARSTEIN, J. and BECKER, B. (1970) Research into the pathogenesis of keratoconus: A new syndrome low ocular rigidity, contact lenses and keratoconus. *Arch. Ophthalmol.*, **84**, 728–729

HODD, N.F.B. (1983) The economics of contact lens practice. *Ophthal. Opt.*, May 21st

HOLDEN, B.A., MERTZ, G.W. and GUILLON, M. (1980) Corneal swelling response of the aphakic eye. *Invest. Ophthalmol. Vis. Sci.*, **19**, 1394–1397

KEMMETMULLER, H. (1983) Critical thoughts about the transformation of the corneal curvature by wearing contact lenses. *Contact Lens J.*, **11**(2), 3–11

KERR-MUIR, M.K.M., WOODWARD, E.G. and LEONARD, T. (1987) Atopy, corneal thickness and astigmatism. *Br. J. Ophthalmol.*, **71**, 207–211

KERSLEY, H.J. (1977) Soft contact lenses in aphakia. *Contact Lens J.*, **5**(8), 29–31

KOETTING, R.A. (1966) The influence of oral contraceptives on contact lens wearers. *Am. J. Optom.*, **43**, 268–274

LEMP, M.A., BLACKMAN, H.J., WILSON, L.A. and LEVEILLE, A.S. (1984) Gram negative corneal ulcers in elderly aphakic eyes with extended wear lenses. *Ophthalmology (Rochester)*, **91**(1), 60–63

LLOYD, M.J. (1984) Presbyopic contact lens correction. *J. Br. Contact Lens Assoc.*, **7**(3), 131–158

MANDELL, R.B. (1965) *Contact Lens Practice: Basic and Advanced*, pp. 370–378. Springfield, Illinois: Charles C. Thomas

MATTHEWS, A.M., DART, J.K.G., and SHERWOOD, M. (1983) Contact lens hygiene and related disease. *J. Br. Contact Lens Assoc.*, **6**(1), 36–50

MILLODOT, M. (1984) A review of research on the sensitivity of the cornea. *Ophthal. Physiol. Opt.*, **4**, 305–319

MOLINARI, J. (1984) New soft contact lens annular bifocal. *J. Br. Contact Lens. Assoc.*, **7**(1), 8–13

MORRIS, J.A., TAYLOR, D. ROGERS, J.E., VAEGEN and WARLAND, J. (1979) Contact lens treatment of aphakic infants and children. *J. Br. Contact Lens Assoc.*, **2**(3) 22–30

PRINCE, M.J., MORGAN, M.F., WILLIS, W.E. and WATSON, S. (1982) Tarsal conjunctival appearance in contact lens wearers. *Contact Intraoc. Lens Med. J.*, **8**(1), 16–23

READING, V.M. (1984) Astigmatism following cataract surgery. *Br. J. Ophthalmol.*, **68**, 97–104

RUBEN, M. (1967) Albinism and contact lenses. *Contact Lens J.*, **1**(2), 5–8

RUBEN, M. (1975a) *Contact Lens Practice, Visual, Therapeutic and Prosthetic*, p.240. London: Baillère and Tindall

RUBEN, M. (1975b) The medical uses of contact lenses. *Austr. J. Optom.*, **58**, 239–246

RUBEN, M. (1976) Treatment of keratoconus. *Contact Lens Intraoc. Lens. Med. J.*, **2**(1), 18–20

RUBEN, M. and COLEBROOK, E. (1979) keratoconus, keratoplasty curvature and lens wear. *Br. J. Ophthalmol.*, **63**, 268–273

RUBEN, M. and WALKER, J. (1967) Contact lenses used as occluders. *Br. J. Orthop.*, **24**, 120–125

RUBEN, M. and WATKINS, R. (1975) Pilocarpine dispensation from the soft hydrophilic contact lens. *Br. J. Ophthalmol.*, **59**, 455–458

SABELL, A.G. (1970) Oral contraceptives and the contact lens wearer. *Br. J. Physiol. Opt.*, **25**(2), 127–137

SCARBOROUGH, S.T. and LOPANIK, R.W. (1976) A two eyed look at the presbyopic patient. *Contact Lens Forum*, Sept.

SILVER, J.H. and WOODWARD, E.G. (1978) Driving with a visual disability. *Ophthal. Opt.*, **18**(21), 794–796

STONE, J. (1973) Contact lens wear in the young myope. *Br. J. Physiol. Opt.*, **28**(2), 90–134

STONE, J. (1976) The possible influences of contact lenses on myopia. *Br. J. Physiol. Opt.*, **31**(3), 89–114

STONE, J. (1981) Practical optics of contact lenses and aspects of contact lens design. *Contact Lenses*, 2nd edn, edited by J. Stone and A.J. Phillips, Chap. 4, p. 103. London: Butterworths

TAYLOR, D. VAEGAN, MORRIS, J.A., ROGERS, J.E. and WARLAND, J. (1979) amblyopia in bilateral infantile and juvenile cataract. *Trans. Ophthalmol. Soc. UK*, **99**(1), 170–176

TOMLINSON, S. and CEDERSTAFF (1982) Tear evaporation from the human eye. *J. Br. Contact Lens Assoc.*, **5**(4), 141–152

TRODD, T.C. (1971) Ptosis props in ocular myopathy. *Contact Lens J.*, **3**(4), 3–6

WESTHMEIMER, G. (1969) Abberations of contact lenses. *Am. J. Optom.*, **38**(8), 445–448

WILLIAMS, R. and BUCKLEY, R.J. (1985) Pathogenesis and treatment of recurrent corneal erosions. *Br. J. Ophthalmol.* (in press)

WOODWARD, E.G. (1980) Progression of keratoconus in eyes fitted with contact lenses. *The Cornea in Health and Disease*, Transactions of 16th European Society of Ophthalmology, Brighton 40.1, 531–536

WOODWARD, E.G. (1981) Contact lens fitting after keratoplasty. *J. Br. Contact Lens Assoc.*, **5**(2), 42–49

WOODWARD, E.G. (1984) Therapeutic silicone rubber lenses. *J. Br. Contact Lens. Assoc.*, **7**(1), 39–41

WOODWARD, E.G. and DRUMMOND, M.F. (1984) Cost effectiveness in a hospital contact lens department. *Ophthal. Physiol. Opt.*, **4**(2), 161–167

WOODWARD, E.G. and MORRIS, J.A. (1982) Contact lenses in aphakic infants. *Nursing Times*, **78**(17), 725–727

YOUNG, T. (1801) On the mechanism of the eye. *Philos. Trans. R. Soc. Lond.*, **16**, 23–88

Part 9

Dispensing the correction

35

The choice of lens form and type

Colin Fowler

The choice of a suitable form and type of spectacle lens with which to dispense a correction is becoming more complex with the ever increasing number of lenses and lens materials becoming available. This chapter can only offer a brief outline of the concepts involved in lens selection and perusal of the references and specialist textbooks will be required for a comprehensive view of this subject.

General considerations

Prescription

The prescription is an all important concept in lens selection: not only whether a given lens is suitable for a given prescription, but whether it is *available* in that prescription. For this, it is essential for every dispensing professional to be equipped with suitable reference works on lens availability. Most lens manufacturers and the larger prescription laboratories publish catalogues of lens availability, but there are independent publications, for example, *Lens Forms*, published in London by the Optical Information Council. Such publications are invaluable in giving not only the prescription ranges in which each lens type is manufactured, but also the uncut lens diameter for determining if the lens is large enough to glaze the required frame.

Existing lenses

The type of lens (if any) worn previously is naturally an invaluable starting point in deciding on the type of lens to be dispensed. The difficulty comes when deciding to give a new type of lens or lens material, rather than simply deciding to repeat a similar lens type for the patient. In many cases, a change in lens type is unavoidable due to requirements of the frame, change of occupation, requirement for a tint

etc. Certainly, it is not always good practice to change a lens type just for the sake of it.

Functional requirements

Occupational requirements can often be difficult to analyse in the consulting room, particularly if the task is unknown to the dispenser. With presbyopes, occupational dispensing is not just a question of choosing the correct lens, but also involves the correct reading addition, determined at a suitable working distance. Where the occupation is hazardous, the process itself should be screened, and protective eye-wear may have to be provided by the employer.

Patient requirements

Dealing with the wishes of the patient can be one of the most difficult dispensing tasks. This can often be a case of steering a patient away from using an unsuitable type of frame rather than difficulties over a choice of lens. But there can be other instances, for example, where an individual wants a very dark tint to be incorporated into spectacles which are going to be used for constant wear, including use at night.

Industrial protection

The problems of industrial protective equipment are dealt with elsewhere (Chapter 37), but there is an increasing demand for spectacle lenses of the protective type. With the advent of plastic lenses, such lenses no longer have an inherent weight penalty as found with the conventional type of heat toughened glass. Recent years have seen many developments in the field of eye protection, often in response to legislation for protective lenses.

Cost

The cost of a finished pair of spectacles is undoubt-edly one of the major considerations for many selecting a lens. In this discussion, however, it will not be a prime point, as lens costs can be very variable from individual practitioners, depending on their fee structure.

Frame type

Without doubt, the fashion for large aperture spec-tacle frames has been the major influence in the design of many spectacle lenses and the dispenser must constantly consider whether a particular lens size and shape can be edged from a particular lens uncut.

Lens manufacturers are constantly seeking ways of glazing lenses of ever increasing power into large frames without weight or thickness penalties.

Lens material

Irrespective of lens type or form, the first decision on lens selection is the type of material. For many years, all lenses were glass, but optical plastics became available in the 1930s (Twyman, 1952). Since then, development of lens materials has been along two main routes, that of plastics with different and improved properties, and glass with high refractive index. *Table 35.1* illustrates some of the commonly available types of glass material. The parameters of refractive index, constringence and density are commonly used to describe a lens material and give an indication of the thickness variation, dispersive effect on white light and lens weight, respectively. White ophthalmic crown has been the standard material for many years, and is the comparative material by which all others are judged.

Traditional methods of increasing the refractive index involved the incorporation of lead or barium compounds, with an ensuing weight penalty.

However, in the early 1970s, Schott perfected a lens material (SF64) using titanium oxide for raising the index (Fowler, 1976). The effect of this on the weight of the finished lens is shown in *Figure 35.1*, where lenses of three materials are compared. It is interesting to note that although SF64 is denser than crown glass, the finished lens is lighter above a certain power due to a reduction in lens volume from the increased refractive index of the glass. The exact trade-off point will depend on the precise conditions. However, it would be inadvisable to promote such materials as having a noticeable saving in weight at high powers, as the effect is subjectively slight.

Figure 35.1 also shows that CR39 plastic lenses are appreciably lighter than the equivalents in glass, as would be expected from their low densities. However, they will be thicker than the equivalent glass lens, as is shown in *Figure 35.2*. In fact, the finished thickness of plastic lenses is often greater than that expected purely from the change in

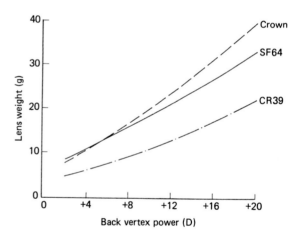

Figure 35.1 Relationship of lens weight to back vertex power for a series of circular plus power lenses, 50 mm in diameter, all with an edge thickness of 1 mm. Material parameters are as shown in Table 35.1

Table 35.1 Some examples of ophthalmic lens materials

Name	Manufacturer	Refractive index	Constringence*	Density (g/ml)
Crown	Various	1.523	58	2.54
CR39	P.P.G.	1.498	58	1.32
Polycarbonate	G.E., Bayer	1.586	30	1.20
SF64	Schott	1.701	31	2.99
BaSF 64	Schott	1.706	39	3.20
LHI	Hoya	1.702	40	2.99
OC 70	Pilkington	1.700	51	3.38

* The value of constringence (reciprocal dispersive power) gives an indication of the chromatic aberration properties of finished lenses; a large value is ideal, indicating low dispersive power.

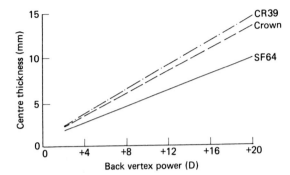

Figure 35.2 Relationship of lens centre thickness to back vertex power for a series of circular plus power lenses, 50 mm in diameter, all with an edge thickness of 1mm. Material parameters are as shown in *Table 35.1*

refractive index since plastic lenses are often made thicker, particularly in minus powers, for reasons of mechanical stability.

Durability

There are some important properties relevant to lens materials which are not covered in *Table 35.1*, namely impact resistance, surface hardness and ease of manufacture. Plastic materials are inherently much stronger than glass, although glass can be toughened by heat and chemical means. Increasingly, hybrid glass and plastic laminations are being used (*see Figure 35.3*) which enable the impact resistance qualities of plastic to be combined with the low thickness and tint qualities of glass— particularly in relation to photochromic tints (Merigold, 1984).

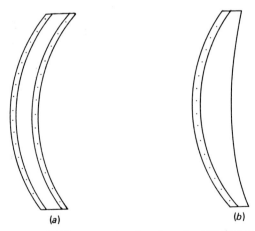

Figure 35.3 Two examples of modern glass/plastic composite lens designs. (*a*) Essilor 'CS' with a plastic layer bonded between thin glass shells, which can be photochromic; (*b*) Chance-Pilkington 'RR PL' with photochromic glass front surface bonded to CR39. (After Merigold, 1984)

All plastic materials are more easily scratched than glass, but quantifying the degree of 'scratchability' of a material is difficult, due to the lack of a standard test procedure. All manufacturers tend to use different tests, which give somewhat variable results. It is now possible to obtain a wide range of different coatings for plastic lenses, designed to reduce the surface scratches. These are principally for CR39 lenses, but polycarbonate lenses are also supplied with a scratch-resistant coating as a matter of routine.

Tint

There is, unfortunately, no known way of scientifically prescribing tinting lenses. Glass-tinted lenses with the tint incorporated into the lens material (generally known as 'solid' tints) can have their transmission characteristics very accurately specified and duplicated. Plastic lenses (and vacuum-coated glass lenses) are not so reproducible in their tint characteristics, and are normally used for general purpose glare protection. It is a present trend to incorporate an ultraviolet-inhibiting agent into CR39 plastic lenses, in order to cut out near visible ultraviolet light. This does not colour the lens, although lenses with total absorption up to 400 nm have been produced which are slightly tinted (for example the UV400 from the Orcolite Corporation).

For general purpose spectacles, the most common glass lens tint is one of the many photochromic varieties now available. It is unfortunate that most of the sales literature on these materials tends to concentrate on the performance of plano samples and ignores the effects of increased thickness from high prescription values changing the photochromic properties. However, figures are available (*Table 35.2*) which give the effects of lens thickness on the properties of Reactolite Rapide.

Table 35.2 Effect of thickness on transmission of Reactolite Rapide

| Thickness (mm) | Transmission | | |
	Unexposed (%)	Fully exposed (%)	Faded overnight (%)
1.0	90.5	28.0	90.0
2.0	90.0	16.0	88.0
3.0	89.5	10.5	86.0
4.0	89.0	8.0	84.0
5.0	88.5	6.0	83.5

Data of Chance-Pilkington.

For high powered prescription lenses, therefore, it would be advisable either to use a material which darkens to a medium density in a plano sample, rather than one of the very wide acting types, or alternatively to use a hybrid lens, composed of plano photochromic in conjunction with white glass or plastic for the powered portion (*Figure 35.3*).

Virtually all types of lens material can now be given an anti-reflection coating. Originally these were only available for glass lenses, but now plastic lenses as well can be coated. Single and multilayer coatings can be applied (Fincham and Freeman, 1980), multiple layers increasing the efficiency of the coating. Although a coated lens of this type transmits more light, it is unlikely that this will be noticed by the wearer. The main advantages are the improved cosmetic appearance of the lens, and also the reduction in surface reflections visible to the wearer.

Lens form

Single vision lenses

It is important to distinguish between two major classifications of lens form, namely curved lenses having 'one surface convex in all meridians and one surface concave' and flat lenses, being 'any other type of lens' (B5 3521, 1962). Originally, all lenses were of flat form but now curved forms predominate, with flat lenses only being used for special purposes.

The reason for the change to curved lenses was to try to reduce the off-axis aberrations of spectacle lenses. The well-known graph of Tscherning's ellipse (*Figure 35.4*) shows the required thin lens form necessary for the reduction of oblique astigmatism (Bennett, 1974). The graphs given here also illustrate the change in *radius* of the front surface required when changing from crown glass to high index glass for a given power. Over a wide range of powers, there are two forms of lens giving zero oblique astigmatism, but it is only the shallower lens forms that are practical for the production of actual lenses, particularly in large diameters. The illustrated graphs are for distance vision, the near vision forms being flatter for a given power, and hence, any form is a compromise, particularly when other aberrations are considered as well. The correction of distortion, for example, requires very steep lens forms which, for reasons mentioned above, are not practical.

Lens ordering

When dispensing prescriptions, many practitioners do not specify the precise lens form required, simply stating that the lens should be meniscus or toric (the spherical and astigmatic forms of curved, respectively) or flat. In many instances this is quite adequate, as the mass-produced single vision lenses of major manufacturers are supplied in a reasonable range of base curves to provide reasonable control

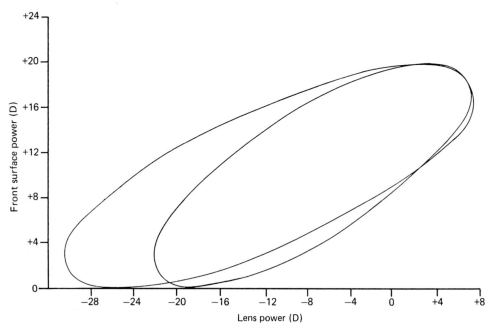

Figure 35.4 Tscherning ellipses, illustrating the distance vision 'third order' forms for thin lenses to give zero oblique astigmatism. The small ellipse is for 1.523 index material, the larger being for 1.701 index, but expressed in terms of 1.523 surfacing tool power

of aberrations across the 'normal' prescription range (less than ±8.00 D). It may also prove quite difficult to decide what would be the best base curve in any particular set of circumstances.

Problems can arise when ordering new lenses for a patient of high prescription if the base curve is changed dramatically, for example, from curved to flat form or vice versa. Despite the theoretical considerations on lens design, which indicate that over the vast majority of lens powers curved forms are superior, there are some individuals who prefer flat form lenses. In addition, judicious lens design can improve the cosmetic appearance of a finished lens in a frame. For example, prescriptions involving a large oblique cylinder will often look better made up in minus cylinder toric form, rather than plus cylinder toric. This is because the cylinder will cause a large variation in edge thickness on the lens, which is unsightly. If this is made on the rear surface of the lens, then this edge thickness varation will occur behind the rim, with the spherical curve on the front surface.

Dispensing high power single vision lenses

It is the dispensing of prescriptions over 8.00 D that calls for the greatest amount of care and skill. The decision on type of lens is very much related to the frame aperture and decentration required. In very large frames, full aperture spherical curve lenses will become physically impossible to manufacture, thus the choice has to be made between a full aperture lens in high refractive index glass, using a lenticular, or reduction of the frame aperture. With high plus lenses there is another option, that of using a lens incorporating an aspheric surface.

Lenticulars

Although lenticular lenses do not always have a pleasing cosmetic appearance, they are very light in weight, and can sometimes be appreciated for this reason, particularly if made in plastic material. For the high myope, even quite small lenticular apertures do not affect the field of view unduly, as a result of the prismatic effect of the lens. But this is certainly not the case with the high hypermetrope, where the peripheral prismatic effect acts in a way that reduces the field of view. This is one of the reasons why so many aspheric designs have been developed for high plus prescriptions, and not for high myopia. The other main reason can be gleaned from inspecting Tscherning's ellipse where it can be noted that it is not possible to have a lens free from oblique astigmatism over +7 D or so, whereas the negative range of astigmatism-free lenses covers the vast majority of myopic prescriptions. Some of the main types of lenticular are illustrated in *Figure 35.5*. It should be noted that most negative designs

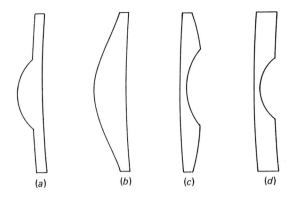

Figure 35.5 Some examples of single vision lenticular lenses for high power prescriptions. (*a*) Solid lenticular, round or oval aperture; (*b*) blended aspheric lenticular; (*c*) flattened lenticular; (*d*) plano margin lenticular. (In each case the front surface is on the left)

are produced as individual special lenses by prescription laboratories, rather than being mass produced by major lens manufacturers. Plus lenticulars, however, are not essentially modified full aperture lenses and require specialist manufacture if supplied as a one-piece solid lens.

A feature of recent years has been the development of lenses that combine a high power control zone and low power flange of a lenticular with the near full aperture lens appearance. This was suggested by Davis (1959) for plus prescriptions and has since been applied to minus prescriptions as well (Fowler, 1983a). These 'blended lenticulars' have much larger effective apertures in plus prescriptions than in the 'Super-Lenti' (*Figure 35.6*) for reasons of field of view as mentioned earlier.

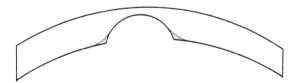

Figure 35.6 Wrobel 'Super Lenti' blended lenticular for high minus lenses. The shaded zones represent the parts of the rear surface that are removed to improve the cosmetic appearance of the lens compared with a conventional lenticular. (Reproduced from Fowler, 1983a, with permission)

Asperics

With the advances that have now taken place in plastic lens moulding techniques, it is now possible to mould quite complex aspheric curves. Aspheric lenses for high hypermetropia have developed along a number of different lines, depending on the philosophy of the design. These can be summarized (Fowler, 1983b) as:

(1) *Conic section lenses*—lenses made with one surface a conic of revolution, usually an ellipsoid.
(2) *Polynomial surface lenses*—lenses made with one surface described by a polynomial curve, in order to try to improve on the properties of the first group.
(3) *'Drop' type lenses*—lenses based on the 'Welsh Four Drop' concept (Welsh, 1978) where the power drop towards the edge of the lens is greater than that necessary for the correction of oblique astigmatism and curvature, but does provide a low distortion value and a good field of view. This group includes such lenses as the Armorlite 'Multi-Drop', Sola 'Hi-Drop' and Signet 'Hyperaspheric'.
(4) *Blended lenticulars*—these are lenses designed to overcome the limitations in uncut size found in all the previous designs. Thus the uncut diameter is in the order of 66/67 mm, compared with a maximum of approximately 60 mm in the previous designs, if made in full aperture form. Effectively, they are lenticulars with a large central aperture and a narrow peripheral flange, but without a conspicious dividing line between these zones. The original lens in this group was the American Optical 'Ful-Vue' (Whitney, Reilly and Young, 1980), although other designs have now appeared, such as the Essilor 'Omega' and the Rodenstock 'Perfastar'.

Table 35.3 gives some guidance on the use of these various types of lens.

Irrespective of whether a high powered lens is positive or negative, there are some rules that should be followed:

(1) The decentration of full aperture lenses should be limited to as small an amount as possible, in order to avoid excessive variations in edge thickness. For similar reasons, frames with an exaggerated shape should be avoided.
(2) The lens should be fitted as close to the eye as possible, to optimize the field of view.
(3) The lens should be centred accurately, both vertically and horizontally. This is not only to reduce any unwanted relative prismatic effect between the two eyes, but also in aspheric lenses in particular to give the best visual acuity.

Multifocal lenses

Bifocals

Many of the considerations of single vision lenses also naturally apply to bifocal lenses. The basic concepts of aberration control, choice of material and form are similar, but the extra power zone further complicates the choice.

Bifocals can be considered under a number of classifications, such as whether or not the lens is prism controlled in the segment, shape of segment, type of construction etc., all of which have some relevance to the choice.

Table 35.3 Comparison of the properties of various types of aspheric lens for aphakia

Desirable lens properties	Full aperture conic	Aspheric lenticular	'Drop' type lens	Blended lenticular
Wide field of good acuity	1	2	3	2
Low centre thickness	3	1	3	2 (1*)
Low peripheral distortion				
Large eyesize	2	+	1	1
Small eyesize	2	2	1	2
Good cosmetic appearance				
Large eyesize	2	3	2	1
Small eyesize	2	1	2	2
Low weight	3	1	2	2 (3*)

1 = good.
2 = reasonable.
3 = poor.
* = high index glass version, all others CR39.
+, note prismatic jump at edge of lenticular aperture.
Reproduced from Fowler, 1983b, with permission.

Size and shape of segment

In general, the larger the segment, the greater will be the field of view at near, and the more the segment will interfere with distance vision. Hence, any occupational requirements will have an influence here depending on the ratio of distance/ near tasks, and the width of field, required at near. Thus draughtsman require a large near field, as do copy typists. A large segment, however, can be a disadvantage when driving, particularly when looking backwards on reversing.

The shape of the segment will control the change in prism that occurs when looking from distance to near or vice versa, sometimes known as 'jump' because of the apparent effect of the prism on objects. This depends on the distance of the optical centre of the addition (not the near optical centre) below the top of the segment. If this is placed at the top of the segment, then there will be no 'jump' as occurs in semicircular straight top bifocals, sometimes known as 'C' segment bifocals. Many bifocals are 'D' shaped, which reduces the jump compared with the equivalent round segment. These latter round lenses exhibit the most 'jump'—the larger the segment the worse the effect. Thus, for a round segment downcurve bifocal of the 'invisible' type:

$$\text{Jump } (\Delta) = \text{Segment radius (cm)} \times \text{Addition (D)}$$

An 'invisible' lens always has the optical centre of the addition at the centre of the segment in order to reduce the visibility of the addition. A 'visible' bifocal, or prism-controlled bifocal, has the optical centre of the addition positioned at a point designated by the prescriber, which renders the segment more visible. Some prism-controlled bifocals are supplied with a fixed optical centre position for a specific purpose. Thus an 'Executive' bifocal (American Optical) is manufactured with the optical centres for distance and near coincident and placed on the segment top, unless vertical prism is incorporated on the non-segment side.

Prism-controlled multifocals

As a result of the method of construction used in conventional bifocals, it is not possible to control the prism independently at distance and near. Thus, any prism worked on the lens, at the stage of second side working in the prescription house, will affect both distance and near prescriptions.

It is occasionally necessary to supply a lens, however, where the distance and near prism are independently controlled. This is usually for one of two reasons: first to incorporate a prescribed prism at distance and not at near, or vice versa, and second for the control of near prismatic imbalance in the case of anisometropia with binocular vision. An example of the first type might be where base-in prism is prescribed at near only in each eye to assist

convergence. Also, cases occur where distance vision prism only is required; on these occasions, prism-controlled bifocals are required with a prism in the segment, which neutralizes the distance prism to give zero prism at near.

Anisometropia

Much consideration has been given to the problem of bifocals for anisometropia (for example, see Emsley and Moore, 1954). This type of dispensing problem can be illustrated by the prescription: R plano; L −5.00 DS; add +2.00.

If it is assumed that the myopic lens is centred for distance, then, if the wearer looks down the lens at a distance of 10 mm for near vision, the left eye will experience a prismatic effect (from Prentice's rule) of 5 Δ base-down, with zero prism in the other eye. This relative prismatic effect of 5 Δ in the vertical direction would be uncomfortable and disruptive to binocular vision. This prism is due solely to the effects of the distance prescription, but since near additions are usually fitted symmetrically, the near segment will have no effect on the relative prism in such a case. In order to reduce this prism, without inducing any prism in the distance portion, several choices are available:

(1) If unequal size 'invisible' segments are used, then the larger segment will exert more base-down prism than the smaller, for the same power of reading addition. Unfortunately, the differential in segment sizes is large if any effective prism control is to be achieved, making the resultant cosmetic appearance poor. The amount of prism overcome can be calculated from: Difference in segment radius (in cm) × Addition (D).
(2) Prism can be incorporated into the segment using a prism-controlled bifocal. In the UK, this generally takes the form of a 22 mm round segment glass bifocal, although specials can be made up as cement or Franklin split forms.
(3) A conventional bifocal can be rendered prism controlled in the vertical direction by working a bi-prism on the front surface. This is usually carried out on a 'D' segment, or an 'Executive' bifocal, and gives, in combination with a rear surface prism, very effective prism control with little cosmetic disadvantage (*Figure 35.7*).

This discussion assumes that the wearer has binocular vision. Many individuals with large degrees of anisometropia are amblyopic in one eye and do not have binocular vision. Similarly, long-term wearers of anisometropic prescriptions will have adapted to the relative prismatic effect at the near visual point and will be in no different position with bifocals than with single vision lenses. It is therefore a question of

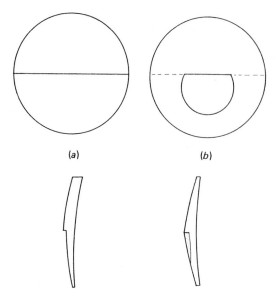

Figure 35.7 Two examples of bi-prism bifocals, shown in plan view (upper diagrams) and sectional view (lower diagrams). (*a*) Executive bifocal bi-prism; (*b*) fused 'D' segment bi-prism

clinical judgement when deciding on the appropriate type of bifocal.

Effectivity of near addition

It is natural to believe that, if two lenses give the same reading of back vertex power (BVP) on a focimeter, then they will have the same optical effect under all conditions. This is not true for near vision, and can be illustrated by an example. If a reading prescription is determined using a plano/convex trial case lens, with a prescription of +7.00 DS, and then dispensed in meniscus form, the difference in effective power can be as follows:

	Trial lens	*Spectacle lens*
Form	Plano/convex	Meniscus
BVP	+7.00 DS	+7.00 DS
F_1	Plano	+ 10.00 D
t	3.0 mm	6.0 mm
n_d	1.523	1.523
Object distance	250 mm	250 mm
Exit vergence	+3.03 D	+2.74 D

where F_1 = power of the front lens; t = axial thickness of the lens; n_d = mean refractive index of lens material.

This effect is due to the difference in form and thickness of the two lenses, and considers the paraxial power effects only. In a bifocal or multifocal, the effect of a near object is more complex, and consists of three components: the form and thickness of the lens, oblique vision through the lens and the change in vertex distance as the eye looks away from the optical centre of the lens towards the segment.

These three effects will all mean that the effectivity of a near addition may well be different to the value determined on the focimeter (Jalie, 1981). Some lens manufacturers have recognized this problem and give calculated or measured near vision powers taking the above effects into consideration. For example, Carl Zeiss (Oberkochen) give a measured power on the lens packet, as well as the 'nominal' power determined on a focimeter by conventional means.

The concept of near addition of a bifocal or multifocal is somewhat confused by the standard methods for determining the addition on a focimeter. British Standard 2738 (1985) 'Spectacle Lenses' states that the major portion of a multifocal is always specified in terms of back vertex power. However, the near addition is given in terms of the difference in vertex power measured on the segment side. This means that the correct near addition is given by the difference between the distance and near front vertex powers for most lenses, where the segment is manufactured on the front surface. It is only where the segment is on the rear surface that a back vertex power difference is correct. The reason for this procedure is because, when a bifocal manufacturer makes a semi-finished lens, the finished centre thickness is unknown. This method of measurement makes the addition power independent of the lens thickness, but it still only gives a 'nominal' addition; the effectivity still has to be taken into account.

Occupational bifocals and trifocals

The limitation with the majority of bifocal designs is that it is assumed that the wearer is always going to look downwards for near vision. Coupled with the fact that, by definition, there are only two focal lengths on the lens, this means that a significant number of wearers are going to have problems either due to the positioning of the segment, or because intermediate vision is required between the far and near limits of a bifocal.

Examples of occupations where near vision at the top of the field is required include librarians, shopkeepers and airline pilots. Two examples of occupational bifocals are given in *Figure 35.8*, the up-curve bifocal having the major portion for near vision, with a negative addition for distance, and the double bifocal having distance vision in the centre of the lens, with two near vision segments situated above and below.

Bifocal lenses are only really satisfactory where the depth of field of the two portions of the lens overlaps. However, as accommodation drops with age, the depth of field of each zone becomes

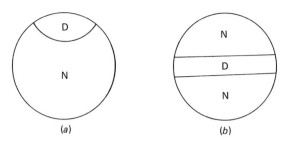

Figure 35.8 Two examples of occupational bifocals, showing distance (D) and near (N) zones of the lens. (*a*) 38-mm segment up-curve solid bifocal; (*b*) Sola double bifocal, with 10-mm deep distance zone

progressively reduced as the addition increases. This, therefore, gives poor intermediate vision, which can be a considerable handicap. Trifocals are available in a wide variety of designs for such cases, the intermediate addition bearing a fixed relationship to the power of the reading addition, usually having 50% or 60% of the power of the latter. Such lenses can be extremely satisfactory in use if fitted correctly. It is important to place the top of the intermediate segment as high as possible without interfering with distance vision, otherwise there will not be enough reading segment within the frame aperture. In recent years, progressive power lenses have increasingly been used instead of trifocals, although the trifocal will still give a better field of intermediate vision.

Progressive power lenses

The pre-presbyope is accustomed to having completely variable focus between infinity and the near point. Bifocal and trifocals restore near and intermediate focusing ability to presbyopes, but only in discreet intervals of power. It was, therefore, predictable that lenses would be designed to give

presbyopes a smooth range of near focusing distances, with no sudden jumps between power zones. There have been many approaches to this problem (Bennett, 1972), but the current commercially available designs have all followed the same basic approach (*Table 35.4*) including a large distance area with stable (or near stable) power, stable reading area and a progressive power zone in between.

This has been the pattern for progressive power lenses since the French optical manufacturer Essilor produced the Varilux lens in the late 1950s.

Because there are no sudden changes in power on the lens, a progressive power surface gives a completely 'invisible' multifocal, and indeed many are used purely for this cosmetic advantage. Unfortunately, however, the progressive power zone cannot be made as short as would be liked (6–8 mm) without causing blurring intermediate vision. It is therefore spread over 12–14 mm, which means that a progressive lens wearer will have to look a greater distance down the lens to find the stable reading zone than would be the case in an equivalent power bifocal or trifocal.

As shown in *Figure 35.9* when the power increases on the lens, so does lateral magnification, if spherical curves are used. This change in magnification can cause visual discomfort, particularly if head movements are made when viewing vertical lines. Hence with Varilux 2, Essilor used horizontal sections of conic form, prolate ellipsoids in the progressive area to reduce the peripheral power and magnification, and oblate ellipsoids in the distance to increase peripheral magnification and balance the effect at near. This spreading of the distortion control across virtually the whole lens gives a very good low distortion effect when the lens is photographed against a grid pattern target, but this does mean that the stabilized power for both distance and near occupies a narrow zone. An alternative approach is found in the American Optical A040

Table 35.4 Classification of progressive power lenses

Grid pattern appearance	Characteristics	Varifocal lenses
A = good	Lenses with low peripheral distortion, but narrow central reading area	Varilux 2, Truvision M3, Progressive R
B = medium	Lenses with moderate peripheral distortion and medium size stabilized near power zone	NZ, AO 7, Unison
C = poor	Lenses having a large stabilized near zone, but surrounded by areas of marked distortion	Youngers 10/30, AO 40

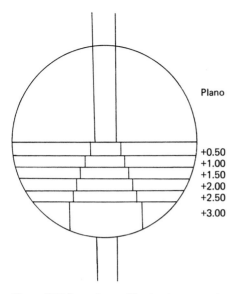

Plano
+0.50
+1.00
+1.50
+2.00
+2.50
+3.00

Figure 35.9 Lateral magnification in progressive power lenses illustrated by a mythical lens with discreet power steps in the intermediate. This is being used as a spectacle magnifier to view an object consisting of two vertical lines. (Reproduced from *The Optician*, Vol. 184, no. 4750, p. 21 (1982) with permission)

lens, where the distance power is completely stabilized, and there is a large effective stabilized near zone. But this means that the change from distance to near power is compressed into a much smaller area than in the Varilux 2, giving a more distorted grid photograph.

It is certainly very difficult to predict which type of progressive lens, if any, will suit a given presbyope, because often the feature of a successful wearer is not the prescription or occupation, but personal motivation to succeed with this type of lens. However, there does seem to be one type of individual that persistently has difficulty with progressive lenses—someone who is accustomed to making large lateral eye movements at near, without any head movement.

Because progressive lenses have relatively small areas of useful progressive power, it is imperative that they are fitted accurately. This usually means specifying monocular centration distances to allow for facial asymmetry, as well as specifying separate left and right fitting heights.

Acknowledgements

Parts of this chapter are based on a lecture entitled 'Matters to be taken into consideration when deter-

mining lenses to order', given at a series of spectacle lens symposia organized by the Worshipful Company of Spectacle Makers.

References

BENNETT, A.G. (1972) Variable and progressive power lenses. *Mfg. Opt. Int.*, Part 1, **25**(12), 759–762

BENNETT, A.G. (1973) Variable and progressive power lenses. *Mfg. Opt. Int.*, Part 2, **26**(1), 42–45; Part 3, **26**(2), 88–91; Part 4, **26**(3), 137–141; Part 5, **25**(4), 199–204

BENNETT, A.G. (1974) A guide to ophthalmic lens design. *Optician*, **167**, Part 1 (4312), 4–9; Part 2 (4313), 4–12; Part 3 (4314), 4–9

BS 2738 (1985) *Tolerances on Optical Properties of Mounted Spectacle Lenses*. London: British Standards Institution

BS 3521 (1962) *Glossary of Terms Relating to Ophthalmic Lenses and Spectacle Frames*. London: British Standards Institution

DAVIS, J.K. (1959) Problems and compromises in the design of aspheric cataract lenses. *Am. J. Optom. Arch. Am. Acad. Optom*, **36**, 279–288

EMSLEY, H.H. and MOORE, A.A.S. (1954) Solid bifocals, available types and methods of ordering them. *Optician*, Part 1, **128** (3318), 393–398; Part 2, **128**(3319), 426–428

FINCHAM, W.H.A. and FREEMAN, M.H. (1980) *Optics*, 9th edn. London: Butterworths

FOWLER, C.W. (1976) A comparison of high index glasses for single vision lenses. *Mfg. Opt. Int.*, **29**, (11) 479–485

FOWLER, C.W. (1983a) The Wrobel Super Lenti. *Optician*, **185** (4796), 26

FOWLER, C.W. (1983b) Choosing and using aspheric spectacle lenses. *Optician*, **185** (4780), 13–15

JALIE, M. (1981) *The Reading Addition of Bifocal Lenses*. Work reports of the Second International Symposium on Presbyopia. Paris: Essilor

MERIGOLD, P.A.(1984) Ophthalmic photochromic materials. *Trans. Br. Coll. Ophthal. Opt. Int. Cong.*, **1**, 158–164

TWYMAN, F. (1952) *Prism and Lens Making: A Textbook for Optical Glassworkers*, 2nd edn. London: Adam Hilger Ltd

WELSH, R.C. (1978) Spectacle lenses for aphakia patients. US Patent No. 4, 073, 578

WHITNEY, D.B., REILLY, J.A. and YOUNG, J.M. (1980) Aspheric Lens Series, US Patent No. 4, 181, 409

Further reading

BENNETT, A.G. and BLUMLEIN, S.J.L. (1983) *Ophthalmic Prescription Work*, 2nd edn. London: Butterworths

JALIE, M. (1984) *The Principles of Ophthalmic Lenses*, 4th edn. London: Association of Dispensing Opticians

36

Non-aesthetic criteria for frame selection

Richard Earlam and Rachel North

Materials

Throughout the history of spectacles, many different materials have been used. There are examples of frames in many collections made of wood, leather, bone, horn, tortoiseshell, together with the precious metals, gold and silver, and some of the interesting alloys such as pinchbeck. As the spectacle manufacturers could, in the past, have been likened to a cottage industry, the variation found in antique spectacles is endless. Indeed, it is particularly interesting to note that sides (temples) as we now know them, which fit snugly behind the ear, were only a recent innovation. The Chinese, who are well known for their inventiveness, used to support a front on the nose by attaching strings. These were positioned where the sides are now attached, and passed backwards over the ears to counterweights which applied the force necessary to support the front firmly. It may be that the wig delayed the development of the side, in its present form, as they would have been difficult to use.

Today many of the materials used for antique spectacles would be extremely expensive to obtain. Real shell, obtained from the Hawkesbill turtle, is now banned in the UK. As plastics materials were developed, they replaced the natural ones which were becoming more difficult to obtain. The working properties of these newer synthetic substances are much more predictable and they are ideal for the mass production techniques used today. Goldfilled is the only material to survive the changes in frame manufacture. It is now found in good quality metal frames. In the past, spectacles and quizzers were articles of fashion, but probably only for the rich. These days spectacles are still fashion items but the mass production techniques make it possible to obtain good quality at a reasonable price.

Properties required of frame materials

The properties required can be listed as:

(1) They must not injure—cause dermatitis etc.
(2) They must be rigid—hold the shape and measurements.
(3) They must take and hold a good polish.
(4) They must resist attack from skin acids.
(5) They must be durable.
(6) They must be light.
(7) They must hold colour, which won't fade in use.

Must not injure

To fit a face both comfortably and firmly, a frame must rest on the nose preferably bearing over a large area, and the sides must lie against the head behind the ears and grip slightly. It is surprising that there are not more problems of dermatitis among the spectacle-wearing population. The skin does occasionally object to the presence of many substances, and these can cause discomfort by irritation or dermatitis.

The materials used for spectacle frames generally do not cause skin problems. Of the many thousands of people who wear spectacles, very few will have any symptoms. Those who do are often wearing metal frames that have a poor quality nickel alloy base metal. When nickel salts come into contact with the skin, they invariably set up a site of dermatitis. As this is just one of the many skin irritants, it should be remembered that the plasticizers and colouring agents can also cause problems. Even gold can cause dermatitis. It should be remembered that nickel is frequently plated to enhance its appearance and occasionally this plating cracks and the nickel salts can be leeched out. It has been observed that sweat, blood or saliva can leech the nickel from stainless steel. The problem of nickel dermatitis is much enhanced if there is marked perspiration because this contains sodium chloride.

A chapter about frame fitting would not normally contain any biochemistry but it is most useful to understand the mechanism of dermatitis as it relates directly to the problems a patient may experience.

Contact dermatitis

This is of two types—irritant contact dermatitis (ICD) and allergic contact dermatitis (ACD). Both are caused by an agent coming into contact with the skin: an irritant and allergen.

Irritants

An irritant directly damages the tissues of the skin if applied for sufficient time and in sufficient concentration. The time and concentration required may vary from person to person, depending on intrinsic differences in the barrier properties of the skin. Susceptibility is increased when the skin is very dry or fair and when there is a tendency to atopic eczema. Most irritants seem to work by gradually overwhelming the barrier and repair functions of the skin.

Allergens

An allergen (or sensitizer) is a substance that can induce a specific immunological reaction. However, most substances causing ACD have to initially combine with a tissue protein before they become an active allergen—these are known as haptens. In order to penetrate the skin barrier, this reactive substance must have a low molecular weight. The reaction with the tissue protein or proteins (the exact identity of which is not known) usually occurs at the junction between the dermis and epidermis.

Sensitization then proceeds by what is known as a type IV allergic mechanism, in which the hapten–protein complex is first processed by special cells lying within the epidermal layer. Information from this processing is then passed along an immune cell chain to lymphocytes which are the effector cells. These 'triggered' lymphocytes pass into the dermal lymphatic vessels and arrive in the local lymph nodes, where they develop into two populations of sensitized lymphocytes: memory T cells and effector T cells. The memory T cells, which circulate throughout the lymphatic and blood systems, remain active for a long time. On any subsequent contact with the identical hapten–protein complex, these cells multiply and transform into effector cells. Effector T cells circulate in the blood and, at the site of penetration of the hapten, release substances that initiate and maintain the inflammatory process—which is dermatitis. These substances, known

as lymphokines, cause increased vascular permeability and attract more lymphocytes and damage the surrounding tissues. This damage is due to increased cell membrane permeability with resultant osmostic lysis, allowing the cell contents to escape.

Sensitization may occur on the first contact with a substance, or not for weeks or even years. Once triggered, there is a latent period of 14–21 days during which time the hapten–protein complex is processed, and competent lymphocytes produced. After this period, any persisting or subsequent contact with the allergen will initiate the allergic inflammatory response, which will begin within 12 hours, peak at 48–72 hours, then subside.

An allergy may well be life-long, and can be initiated on any area of skin subsequently contacted. It will be specific to the one substance or sometimes to a closely related one.

Factors which influence the development of the allergy relate to:

(1) The allergen itself, dose–concentration, vehicle, and the presence of occlusion, i.e. covering of the skin, which through increased humidity increases permeability.
(2) The host—the presence of a persisting ICD which compromises the skin barrier, age/sex, genetic predisposition.
(3) The environment—temperature, humidity and, therefore, the season.

The solution to dermatitis is sometimes difficult to find. If the frame concerned is made of metal, it is wise to first swap the lenses to a plastics frame. As the patient may also be allergic to a component of the plastic, it is essential to be prepared to keep changing materials until one is found which does not produce any response.

Looking at this problem from the practitioner's point of view, it must be accepted that many of the sore nose problems result, not from dermatitis, but from ill fitting spectacles. With age there are pronounced physiological changes to the elasticity and fat content of the skin and, therefore, frames do not always sit well on old skin.

Rigidity and maintenance of shape

The materials for spectacle frames can not be described in engineering terms as rigid. However, they certainly can resist the bending forces sufficiently well and maintain the pressures applied across the bridge and joints. It is important that the dimensions and shape of a spectacle frame be maintained after manufacture. If the material will not allow this, the lenses will become loose and the fit will spontaneously change. An unstable material is not of any use for spectacle frames. Of the two groups of frame materials, plastics and metal, the metal frames are probably the most rigid.

Polishing properties

Polishing any material imparts the appearance of a totally flawless surface. This is enhanced further when a very 'high' shine is present. If a well polished surface is viewed with progressively increasing magnification, there will come a time when the surface texture can again be seen. The art of applying a good 'shine' is to reduce the surface abrasions until they become so fine that they cannot be seen. As this technique advances, the surface reflections become more obvious. If a material is very soft it will probably be deformed by local heating. If the material is hard it will require considerable effort to polish it to the required quality but it will maintain the finish for a long time. This is demonstrated when comparing the plastic and metal frames.

Acid resistance

This is probably not a problem as patients generally tend to change their frames well before the material is seriously attacked. It is well known that cellulose-nitrate becomes yellow and crazed with time. When looking at a very old cellulose acetate frame, there is most often evidence of attack by sweat. Many of the more recent materials are reported to perform better in this respect.

Durability

This property should not be confused with rigidity, as a rigid object is one which can resist bending forces and is often referred to as stiff. As a force is applied to an object, it will bend and return to its original shape, if not bent beyond the elastic limit. Once this limit has been exceeded it stays bent or breaks. A durable material is usually quite elastic and will bend readily but return again to the original shape when the force is removed. An 'ideal' frame material is one where rigidity and durability are in harmony.

Light weight

Spectacle frame materials are fairly light and if the style of frame is not so exaggerated that it substantially increases the bulk, the weight of the frame alone is not very important when compared with some lenses (Humphrey, 1980).

Colour retention

In this respect spectacle frame materials behave just like other substances which contain pigments—they fade with time. This is not regarded by patients as a problem and illustrates the success of the dye manufacturers.

Materials frequently used in frame manufacture

Cellulose nitrate

Nitrate material was patented in the late 1800s, and manufactured by steeping cotton linters in a sulphuric/nitric acid bath. The nitrated material was then made plastic by the addition of camphor. This now quite old and infrequently used material is an ideal spectacle frame material, in that it is both rigid and takes a good finish. Unfortunately, it is also inflammable. This is not too surprising when it is remembered that Gun Cotton, an explosive still used most successfully by the military forces today, is also a cellulose nitrate. The nitrating process is of course carried much further to produce a lively explosive. This frame material has been banned in some parts of the world, and in others it simply went out of fashion. When considering how easily the eyebrows and hair burn in comparison to a nitrate frame, it would appear that this excellent material has been unfairly maligned. Although not now popular, the material can still be obtained.

Cellulose acetate

Many frames are made of this material. Cellulose acetate is made by hydrolysing cellulose triacetate to remove some of the acetyl groups. The manufacturing process involves steeping the cellulose polymer in acids, and converting it into a solid. This is then ground into a powder which is mixed with the required pigments and a plasticizer. It is then stirred, filtered and rolled into sheets which are finally pressed.

To form extruded cellulose acetate sheet, the powder and plasticizer are squeezed through nozzles. This makes a more suitable material for spectacle frames, as it can be coloured in a more imaginative way. The British Standards specification of cellulose acetate frames can be found in BS 3352 (1962).

Cellulose propionate

This material is closely related to cellulose acetate. It is produced by a similar process in which propionic acid is substituted for the cellulose triacetate. This material is springy, quite light and strong. It is reported to resist attack from skin acids.

Frames of this material are manufactured by moulding. The plastic at this stage is colourless and the required colours are added later by a dyeing process. As this colour can be leeched out with methylated spirit, care is needed when cleaning the lenses.

Nylon

This is a very durable plastic which has been used in engineering for a long time. Like cellulose propionate, the frames are moulded. The moulds are very expensive so the styles are not changed too often. The grooves in these frames are very deep so it is usual to glaze the lenses about 2 mm oversize to ensure a tight fit. The very flexible nature of this material makes it more difficult to obtain an ideal fit, as adjustment is very difficult. It must be acknowledged that there is a place for this material, particularly where a frame is likely to be abused, but as it is so difficult to adjust it is not the material of choice.

Carbon X

Carbon fibre is a very rigid inflexible material and is now used in aircraft and racing car construction and to make sports equipment. Carbon X is a fairly new material which contains 60% nylon and 40% carbon fibre. This is very strong and is again moulded to form a range of spectacle frames. As these frames often have rather thin rims, the suitability of this material will be proved with time.

Perspex

This material (acrylic-polymethylmethacrylate, produced by ICI as Perspex) is widely used today in the engineering field. However, it has been very popular as a frame material. Perspex works well by hand and on a grindstone as the cuttings clear well. This, together with the large range of bright colours available, would still make this a useful material bearing in mind the frame styles of today. Unfortunately, while this material works well and facilitates such techniques as hidden pinning, it is quite awkward to adjust, as a large amount of heat is required to make it flexible. Practitioners with delicate skin on their fingers disliked being burnt and consequently spent less time than that needed to correctly adjust the frame. When heated to an extremely high temperature, this material exhibits a thermo-memory and will return to the original shape fashioned by the frame maker. This aspect is quite useful as it is easy to remove an adjustment if required. If, however, insufficient heat was applied while carrying out the adjustment, the material usually broke. When it was popular, the making of Perspex sides formed a major part of a frame repairer's job. As many of the Perspex frames of yesterday were of an exaggerated style, some being individually made to patient's requirements, most of the work was done by hand.

Before this material is written off as one only used in the past, it must be mentioned that it has a low water absorption and it resists many solvents. Very few, if any, people develop dermatitis from a Perspex frame.

Optyl (epoxy resin)

This material is made from thermoplastic epoxy resin, mixed with selected hardeners. Optyl is a thermosetting material that can only be formed into frames by moulding techniques (Anon, 1980). Moulding is an expensive method of frame production which does not lend itself towards frequent changes in frame styles. The frames are made in a colourless form and coloured later to comply with the orders received from the frame stockists. These frames are quite fashionable.

It would be ungenerous to mention that this material is not liked by some practitioners. It, like Perspex, needs a lot of heat to soften it so that it can be manipulated easily. Breakages are frequent if the material is not handled correctly. Workshops have a tendency to stretch frames when glazing them, which is a serious problem as experience has shown that stretched rims have a predisposition to breaking. The resulting characteristic crack either runs along the groove, or starts at the front, runs along the groove and passes through the back half of the rim. In many cases this crack occurs after some months have elapsed.

SPx

This transparent thermoplastic material is in the co-polyamide group. These days there are many frames made of SPx, a material used by Silhouette to produce a range of fashion frames which are injection moulded. This material is very stable and is slightly lighter than cellulose acetate. It has a hard surface like Perspex and is resistant to many solvents. It can be shrunk and stretched, but when doing this great care is needed. It resists attack by skin acids and would appear to be unlikely to cause dermatitis. Further technical information can be obtained from Silhouette Fashion Frames Ltd.

Plastics frames

Most plastics frames are made of a thermoplastic material. This means that heat will soften it, so that it can be manipulated to adjust the fitting or insert the lenses.

In the past, frames were heated with a naked flame. Nowadays, the heat is supplied with a bead bath or, more frequently, with an electric 'blow heater'. With the 'blow heater', air is forced through an element by a small fan—rather like a very hot hair dryer. This instrument is found in most optical practices and can easily supply the required temperature to carry out all the manipulations. Blow heaters have now been used for a long time and were very popular during the cellulose nitrate era.

Metal frames

Gold

This expensive metal is no longer generally used on its own for spectacle frames. 'Solid gold' frames are still available, but they are extremely expensive. Pure gold is represented as 24 carat and in this form is extremely soft and pliable and totally unsuitable for a spectacle frame. A 'solid gold' frame is usually made from 14 or 18 carat gold which contains, together with the gold, metals such as copper and silver. It is alloyed to make it more rigid.

GF (goldfilled or rolled gold)

Practitioners know this material as 'goldfilled', which is abbreviated to GF. It is formed by covering a base metal with a layer of protective gold. This is an ideal material for a metal frame. The base metal can be made of monel, manganese, nickel, tin, bronze, and other alloys, but most often nickel silver. A nickel silver base is fairly robust, and the gold coating is quite inert, not generally causing dermatitis. (Cases of gold dermatitis have been recorded.) A good quality nickel silver contains no silver but is made of up to 61% copper, 18% nickel and zinc. A poor quality alloy contains much less nickel.

High quality frames may not use nickel silver as the base metal. Instead an alloy called monel may be used, which, according to DIN specifications, should contain 63–70% nickel, 1–2.5% iron, 1.25% manganese together with copper (Hardy, 1983).

GF material should be clearly marked using notations such as 1/10th 12 carat or 1/20th 10 carat, or as a fraction, i.e. 500/1000 (*see* British Standard BS 3462 (1962)). A material that is now becoming popular for the top quality metal frames is copper beryllium. This is an age-hardening springy material which has been used for some years in the electrotechnical industry, for example for the springs of switches. As it is springy, hard and durable, it can be used in the manufacture of thin metal frames (Kremmler, 1980).

Production of GF

The coating of gold, on goldfilled, is applied by first melting the gold with an induction furnace. The gold sheet produced is then rolled into thinner sheets and forged into a tube which exactly fits a core of base metal, to which it is welded. After this union has taken place, the cylinder of base metal with its gold coat is drawn continuously to form a thin wire. This is then forged into the sections required. This lovely material is, as can be imagined, rather expensive. These days other alternatives are often used and the market is declining.

Plated frames

An alternative to GF is produced by gold plating. In this, the base metal is first plated with platinum to produce a non-corrosive layer, which is subsequently covered with a very thin gold coat. It is estimated that, at the moment, about 30% of all metal frames used are plated.

The quality of gold plating used on spectacle frames is not well defined. It can vary from as little as a gold flash applied by the manufacturers of very cheap sunglasses, to a gold layer which can be 5, 10 or even 15 μm thick. With this large variation of the gold layer, the quality of a plated frame is not immediately obvious. It is regrettable that there is no approved marking to identify the quality of a plated frame as there is for hallmarked silver items. It should be noted that some of the poorer quality metal frames, which are covered with a coloured lacquer, are likely to suffer chipped/cracked colouring layers. Soldering processes frequently burn a coloured coating, leaving a discoloured area where the heat has 'run'. This means that painted frames do not repair well.

Aluminium

Alloys of aluminium are formulated so that they do not tarnish, are durable, and light. Frames made of aluminium are usually anodized to provide an attractive colour range. As the surface colour provided is not particularly scratch resistant, the frames lose their surface quality rather quickly. This metal is not particularly hard wearing and it is difficult to weld, braze, or solder, so the components are frequently assembled with a nut and bolt. This method of construction is, in some ways, unsatisfactory as the metal is easy to forge and the nuts are apt to 'pull through' the frame. This renders the frame useless.

Aluminium is a 'cold' metal to wear as it is a good conductor of heat which is emphasized by its use for cooling heat sinks in the electronics industry. These frames are usually made with rather thick rims and sides which do not hold the adjustments well. The material does not flex and can be uncomfortable to wear. Aluminium is therefore not an ideal frame material.

Titanium

This is a fairly recently introduced metal, which has proved most useful in industries that manufacture components for ships and aeroplanes. It is particularly light and flexible, with a good surface hardness. It is also very resistant to corrosion. However, with all these attributes this metal is difficult to machine. The problems are well illustrated by the titanium dust, which is produced while the metal is being ground. This dust is highly explosive and is usually removed from the working environment by passing the extracted air through water. Titanium makes very expensive, good quality frames.

Summary

The materials used for spectacle frames are being constantly modified by the manufacturers and new materials are often introduced. From a practice point of view there is no doubt that there are many patients who would benefit from having a plastics frame made to fit their noses correctly. In these cases the material chosen would probably be cellulose acetate. There are many colours available in this material, but sometimes they are quite difficult to match. Hand-made frames, while infrequently used, are available and can be ordered and supplied to meet a patient's specific needs.

Bridge fitting

Having chosen the material, the variety of bridge fitting must now be considered. This decision will depend on the shape of the nose and its relation to the cheeks, brow and eyes. In most cases it is desirable to fit a frame so that there is a back vertex distance of between 8 and 12 mm. The lenses will be tipped inwards slightly towards the cheeks.

There are two basic bridge types: pad and regular. These are defined later. There are, of course, those that can be described as a mixture of both varieties, where the individual qualities of each are selected and combined.

Fitting criteria

Pad

The pad bridge, as the name suggests, supports the weight of the frame and lenses on the pads, which project backwards behind the frame. As the weight is only rested on these pads, it is not necessary for any other part of the bridge to touch the nose. This approach is strictly applied to rocking/toggle pads.

The rims of a frame perform a dual function of holding the lenses and the pads. In the plastics pad type of frame, where the front is made in a plastics material, the rims should conform to the shape of

the nose and rest gently against the skin. The lower edge of the bridge should not rest on to the crest of the nose but leave a measurable clearance. It is unnecessary for there to be any sculpting of this lower edge to accommodate the slope of the nose (crest angle) as it should not touch. With this type of bridge there is a free passage of air around the nose, except where the pads bear. When the bridge measurements are well conceived a plastics pad bridge can be extremely comfortable. A pad bridge is frequently adapted for the mass-produced frames. When the parameters of this bridge are wisely chosen, the frame looks cosmetically well balanced and will fit many different noses.

There are three varieties of this bridge which are all commonly used:

(1) Plastics pad—this variety previously described, is very frequently found on stock frames.
(2) Toggle/rocking pad—a variety usually associated with the metal frames where the pad is attached to an arm allowing the pad enough movement to conform to the shape of the nose.
(3) Keyhole—as the name suggests, this is a bridge that looks like a keyhole. It allows large clearance at the top of the nose. This is probably the most satisfactory bridge and it is discussed further under the heading Bridge design.

The regular bridge

This bridge is usually tailored to fit an individual nose. It can be inserted/attached to a metal frame, but is more usually constructed as part of a plastics frame made of cellulose acetate.

The regular bridge is built so that it presents a large bearing surface to the nose. This should extend from one side of the nose over the crest and down the other, encompassing a strip which should be wider than 4 mm if possible. In this way the weight per unit area is decreased, producing a most comfortable fit. With this method of fitting, air is not free to circulate around the nose and may cause problems in hot, humid weather.

There are three different varieties of a regular bridge which are referred to as: regular, flush and inset. These names indicate if the bridge profile projects: forwards, backwards, or has no projection either forwards or backwards. By selecting the appropriate bridge type, the back vertex distance can be changed allowing adequate clearance for the eyelashes.

Facial measurements

Facial measurements are often totally ignored in favour of the 'suck it and see technique' usually applied in practice. Indeed, this practical method of fitting, which involves the viewing of the total fit with an experienced eye, is very satisfactory. The mass-produced frames usually have pad bridges which are kept in several different measurements so that the various fixed contours and sizes can be assessed.

Facial measurements are useful when a patient has a nose that does not conform to the standard bridge profiles of the stock, mass-produced frames or where the eye or eyelashes protrude forwards so that they would touch the rear surface of the lenses.

The essential measurements can be subdivided into two groups: those that relate to the bridge, and those that relate to the sides and their adjustment. More attention is usually devoted to the bridge, as a competent practitioner will be well able to both measure and adjust a side.

Facial measurements

These include:

(1) Interpupillary distance (PD).
(2) Bridge height.
(3) Apical radius.
(4) Distance between rims (DBR) on datum.
(5) DBR at 10 mm below crest.
(6) DBR at 15 mm below crest.
(7) Angle of crest.
(8) Splay.

The temporal width and the lens size have not been listed for the following reasons. The lens size depends to some degree on the lens shape used and the prescription of the lens to be fitted, and as such is not a facial measurement. The temporal width is a measurement which related to the frames of the past in which the lenses were very small by today's standards. This measurement relates to the distance between the sides at points located 25 mm from the front. It is many years since the sides have been made to graze the temples. It is more usual these days to have about 10–15 mm clearance. With modern methods of frame fitting, this measurement is now obsolete.

Interpupillary distance
The interpupillary distance is measured between the pupils when the eyes are in the primary position. This measurement is needed so that the lenses may be accurately centred. If it is ignored, an unwanted prismatic effect results. It is not necessary or desirable to measure a near centration distance as it is fraught with inaccuracies and can easily be calculated. The list below gives the approximations to the calculated values for use at one-third of a metre which are of use in practice:

Pupillary distance	Inset in each eye
60 mm	2 mm
64–66 mm	2.5 mm
70 mm	3 mm

It must be remembered that the inset will increase substantially as the near vision distance is decreased.

Before any facial measurements can be taken, it is important to establish the position of a reference line, known as the 'datum line'. This is used to locate the vertical position of the bridge measurements in their relation to the lens shape. It is usually made to coincide with the lower lid margin so that a patient will ultimately look above the centres of the lenses when they are placed on datum. This allows the patient to look perpendicularly through the optical centres when reached. There is also a cosmetic advantage to this approach, as spectacle frames usually look better when the brow cannot be seen directly through the lenses. Otherwise the patient acquires a surprised look.

Bridge height
This is a measurement of the height of the crest of the nose above the datum line. It is important to locate this position very carefully as it has a profound effect on the final fit of the frame and its cosmetic appearance. As a general rule, any error in this measurement should serve to lift the frame, as frames frequently slip slightly when adjusted to comfortable tension. Great care should be exercised to ensure that this measurement is taken at the same level as the patient. Discrepancies caused by this fundamental error of measurement are usually rather large.

Apical radius
The apical radius allows the curve at the crest of the nose to be duplicated. It is needed to make the bridge of the frame and usually has a value between 5 and 12 mm, or more typically about 8 or 9 mm.

Distance between rims on datum
This is the distance across the nose at the same height as the imaginary datum line.

DBR at 10 mm and 15 mm below crest
In the past, these measurements were referred to as base measurements. In this way they were easily distinguished from the other measurements which are taken in relation to the datum line. Both of these measurements give the width of the nose at the defined points below the crest. It is possible, when the patient has a very high bridge, that the DBR at 10 mm below crest is the same measurement as the DBR on datum.

Having taken a measurement for the bridge height, apical radius, DBR on datum and the DBRs at 10 and 15 mm below the crest, it is advisable, even when very experienced, to plot these locations onto a piece of card. This can be cut out and fitted to the patient's nose to ensure a good fit. Even a small error of about 1 mm in a DBR will usually ruin an otherwise perfect contour. With the profile drawn on to the card, it is easy to isolate any inaccuracies, and speculate what a correct measurement might be. This is illustrated in *Figure 36.1*

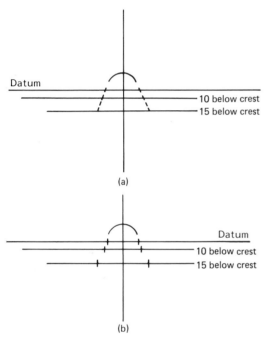

Figure 36.1 (*a*) The measurements forming a satisfactory bridge profile: bridge height = 7 mm; apical radius = 6 mm; DBR at 10 mm below crest = 16; DBR at 15 mm below crest = 21 mm; DBR on datum = 14 mm. (*b*) The appearance of a bridge profile where the measurement of the DBR datum is too small (DBR on datum = 12 mm)

Angle of crest and splay

Having established the overall profile of a nose, the way in which the nose splays and thickens as it joins the face is stated by the splay angle and the angle of crest. Using these measurements the inside of the bridge is opened up so that the bearing surfaces lie comfortably against the skin.

These measurements can easily be taken with the City Rule which was designed and developed by the late Paul Fairbanks. Other rulers are available. The method of taking the measurements is well described in the books accompanying the rule.

Bridge design

This aspect can be better described as the art of choosing a suitable bridge type for the facial contours presented. At first sight it might be felt that a regular bridge would suit all noses. Indeed this type of bridge will always produce a comfortable fit, but it is not always sensible to use a regular bridge as it can be cosmetically very poor.

The controlling factor governing the use of a regular bridge is primarily the bridge height. When the facial measurements indicate a low bridge, i.e. lower than 4 mm above datum, the shape of the bridge distorts the symmetry of the front. *Figure 36.2* shows the top rims plunging downwards towards the bridge. This is not the usual contour adopted for a stock bridge and as such a low regular bridge looks unusual. When the bridge is low and the bridge projection is inset, it is difficult to make the frame cosmetically appealing. When a regular bridge is chosen, care must be taken to sculpt the profile of the crest angle so that the front edge of the bridge neither clears the crest of the nose so well as to leave a large gap, or fit so tightly that the front edge digs in. It is an advantage here if the practitioner concerned has some practical skill so that minor profile adjustments can be made.

If this practical approach is ignored, it is well to remember the potential suffering a dentist could cause if he did not adjust the height of crowns and fillings!

When the bridge required is low and a large amount of inset is needed, it is often prudent to use a keyhole bridge. It is useful to remember that a large frontal angle can also be accommodated if needed. A bridge of this type is tailored so that there is a large clearance at the top of the nose and in doing this it is possible to construct a frame where the underside of the bridge is about 7 mm above the datum line. The characteristic of this bridge is that the top part is relieved in the shape of a keyhole. The rims which form the bearing surface and touch the nose may or may not be fitted with pads. When the splay angle is large it is impossible to include pads as the bearing surfaces may splay outwards at an angle as extreme as 45°.

With a keyhole bridge, the projection of the patient's nose can often be ignored and the frame manufactured with the more usual 2 mm bump found on the stock frames. In this way a frame that will fit an awkward nose can be made to appear like a fashionable stock frame and the patient can continue to ardently follow the fashion.

Lens shape

The lens shape is an important factor these days as large frames are fashionable. Where the prescriptions are low, the lenses are fairly thin, even when

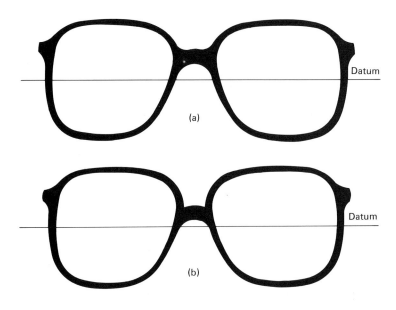

Datum

(a)

Datum

(b)

Figure 36.2 The cosmetic effect of changing the bridge height. Bridge height (*a*) 6 mm above datum; (*b*) 2 mm above datum. (The bridge measurements are the same for each design)

made in a plastics material where the lens is thickened for mechanical stability. As the lens power increases, the lens size and shape becomes progressively more important. When the lens power is very high, not only would it be cosmetically unacceptable to use a large lens but it might be technically impossible to fulfil the order.

The usual method of choosing a lens shape is to try on the various frames that have the desired characteristics. Before the chosen shape is ordered together with the special bridge and side measurements, consideration must be given to the proportion of the end product. If the bridge being ordered is somewhat low, it may be prudent to modify the top nasal corner of the shape to make the bridge and rim contours compatible. It must be borne in mind that the aesthetic qualities of a well designed mass-produced frame depend on carefully worked out dimensions. A practitioner who upsets the symmetry with an ill-conceived modification is likely to be disappointed with the final result.

When the lens power is large, it becomes much more difficult to make a pair of spectacles that are cosmetically pleasing. In these cases a very fine balance must be achieved between the lens size and the lens thickness. In these instances the decentration of the lens, both horizontally and vertically, must be considered. It is sometimes helpful to draw out the lens shape showing the position of the optical centre so that the edge substance can be calculated at various important positions, such as the lower and top temporal corners. In this way the practitioner will appreciate the effectiveness of small modifications to the lens size and shape. With care it is sometimes possible to substantially improve the cosmetic appearance of a pair of spectacles without

compromising the practical considerations of frame making.

Designing frames for individual patients can be quite difficult. As with other skills, competence improves with practice. Having ordered many special frames, it will become easier to achieve the desired effect. In this respect, it is important to appreciate the undoubted skills of the frame maker who has to interpret the written specifications. There are many small characteristics of a spectacle frame which are not given on an order. These are left to the discretion of the frame maker, who also imparts an artistic touch.

Special frames

These days, there are many leisure pursuits which are visually demanding and require special frames. In the past little attention was given to this aspect as most of the specialized appliances are related to helping people who have received hospital treatment.

The mass-production market, particularly the sports companies, have embraced the need for special frames, as they are constantly seeking new lines. They realized that there are many sporting activities which require eye protection. It is now possible to obtain specialized safety products from sporting outlets. The role of the qualified practitioner is rather ill defined in this respect as many practices are not interested in providing special frames, but it is within the scope of an optical practice to supply, service and adjust these appliances for their patients. When becoming involved in this work the practitioners must fully understand how the appliance will be used as they will then be able to choose the best fitting technique and materials.

Acknowledgment

The authors wish to thank Dr P. Groom, General Practitioner, Cyncoed, Cardiff, for his contribution on dermatitis.

References

ANON (1980) Frame materials and manufacture. Part 3. *Mfg Opt. Int.*, **33** (6), 52–55

BRITISH STANDARDS INSTITUTE, BS 3352 (1962) Specification for spectacle frames made of cellulose acetate

BRITISH STANDARDS INSTITUTE, BS 3462 (1962) Specification for metal spectacle frames

HARDY, S. (1983) Frame materials: metal. *Mfg Opt. Int.*, **36**(2), 13

HUMPHREY, B. (1980) Plastics frame material. *Mfg Opt. Int.*, **33**(5), 44–47

KREMMLER, J. (1980) Copper-beryllium for modern spectacle frames. *Mfg Opt. Int.*, **33**(5), 49

Further reading

ADAMS, R.M. (1983) *Occupational Skin Disease*. New York: Grune & Stratton

CRONIN, E. (1980) Spectacle frame allergy. In *Contact Dermatitis*, pp. 643–646. Edinburgh: Churchill Livingston

FISHER, A.A. (Ed.) (1986) *Contact Dermatitis*. Philadelphia: Lea & Febiger

MAIBACH, H. I. and GELLIN (Eds) (1982) *Occupational and Industrial Dermatology*. Chicago: Year Book Medical Publishers Ltd

POLAK, L. (1977) Immunological aspects of contact sensitivity. In *Dermatotoxicology and Pharmacology*, edited by F.N. Marzulli and H.I. Maibach, pp. 225–288. New York: John Wiley & Sons

37

Eye protection

Rachel North and Richard Earlam

Potential ocular hazards, such as flying particles, chemical splashes etc. should be eliminated or controlled at source. If this is not possible, eye protection must be provided, and worn. Screens or fixed shields can be used to protect against potential hazards in some industrial situations, but in sports such as squash, where a ball can easily cause serious damage on impact, eye protection must be worn. Eye protectors should not only be provided to fulfil legal obligations but also for many leisure activities such as do-it-yourself (DIY), skiing, squash and ice hockey. The ideal requirements of an eye protector are:

(1) It must provide adequate protection against the hazard for which it is designed, e.g. flying particles or radiation.
(2) It should be comfortable during wear and not steam up.
(3) It should be light in weight and not interfere with movements.
(4) It needs to be easily cleaned.
(5) It must be readily replaced at a reasonable cost.
(6) It must be durable, non-flammable and non-irritant to the skin.
(7) It must be of suitable optical quality and not impair visual function.
(8) It must be cosmetically acceptable.
(9) It must be compatible with other protective devices, such as ear and respiratory protective equipment.

Eye protectors may be made in the form of spectacles, goggles (cup or box type), screens or visors supported by a headband, or in the form of a helmet.
The lenses for these eye protectors may be made of the following materials:

(1) Glass:
      heat and special heat toughened
      chemically toughened
      laminated.
(2) Plastics:
      polymethylmethacrylate (PMMA)
      allyl diglycol carbonate (CR39)
      polycarbonate cellulose acetate.
(3) Wire gauze.

The frames or lens housing may be made of:

(1) Metal, e.g. nickel.
(2) Plastics:
      cellulose acetate butyrate (CAB)
      cellulose acetate
      polycarbonate
      nylon

Lens materials

Glass

Heat toughened (= heat tempered or thermo-tempered)

Glass is fragile, brittle and breaks into very sharp slivers or splinters. It is therefore unsuitable for an impact resistant eye protector, unless it is heat or chemically toughened.
Heat-toughened lenses are usually made from spectacle crown glass. After the lenses have been manufactured, they are glazed so that they fit the frame/housing. The toughening process begins when the shaped lens is placed into a furnace and heated to 637 °C for 50–300 s. The time spent in the oven depends on the weight, size and average thickness. After heating, it is withdrawn and rapidly cooled, usually by a jet of cold air. The sudden cooling of the lens creates a state of compression at the lens

surface and a state of tension in the lens mass. This produces a compression–tension coat, often referred to as the compression envelope. As glass is stronger in compression than in tension, it improves the impact resistance.

Advantages

It is a comparatively quick, cheap process, not needing skilled labour, the equipment requires little bench space, and is inexpensive.

Disadvantages

(1) Prescription lenses over +5.00 D are not ideal for toughening as the bulk of glass requires prolonged heating. This can cause warping which degrades the optical qualities. Warping can be seen easily when viewing the focimeter image of the reading portion in fused bifocals. Lenses of over −5.00 D have poor impact resistance due to the relatively small centre substance.
(2) A heat-toughened lens will always be thicker than an untoughened lens of equivalent power. The minimum substance for conventional heat-toughened lenses is around 3.3 mm for reasonable robustness. However, in the UK, Birch Stigmat have managed to produce protective prescription lenses with a good performance that have a smaller centre thickness. It is pleasing to note that the impact resistance of this lens is well above the general robustness requirements of the British Standard governing eye protectors (BS 2092) and, because they are thinner than the conventionally heat-toughened lenses, they are lighter.
(3) Impact resistance is markedly reduced by scratches and other surface abrasions. Therefore, the lenses which conformed to BS 2092 when first received from the factory, would not retain the same level of impact resistance throughout life. As the lens surface will naturally become scratched with use, lenses should be inspected regularly, and replaced when distinct scratches are present. It has been estimated that scratches reduce the effectiveness of a heat-toughened lens by about 20%.
(4) The heat-toughening process has an adverse effect on the photochromic salts present in photochromic lenses. It reduces the range of activity and the lens does not lighten to the original transmission. To restore most of this activity, it is necessary to apply a secondary annealing process.

Chemically toughened

This is a more recent method of toughening glass which is very popular in Europe. As with heat toughening, the impact resistance is created by the formation of a compression–tension coat. In this instance, however, it is produced by a chemical process. The lenses are first pre-heated and then lowered into a potassium nitrate solution at 440 °C for 16 hours. The compression coat is produced by exchanging the larger potassium ions present in the solution for the smaller sodium ions present in the glass. As this treatment occurs on the surface of the glass only, it produces a very thin but tough compression coat (100 μm thick). For photochromic lens toughening, the solution is changed to 40% potassium nitrate and 60% sodium nitrate at a reduced temperature of 400 °C. This process does not significantly affect the photochromic activity of lenses.

Advantages

(1) As this lens generally performs well it need not be as thick as its heat-toughened counterpart.
(2) It has greater impact resistance to large missiles than the conventionally toughened lens.
(3) Chemical toughening is suitable for many lenses of stock thickness. Therefore specially surfaced lenses are required less often.
(4) The toughening process takes the same time for all lenses.
(5) The chemical toughening process requires lower temperatures; therefore warping is not a problem.

Disadvantages

(1) Chemical toughening requires expensive equipment as it must withstand the chemicals and the high temperatures involved.
(2) It is not ideally suited for crown glass. For the best results a special type of glass is needed, which is far more expensive.
(3) The impact resistance of the lens is markedly affected by scratches to the lens surface as the compression coat is very thin. It has been estimated that the safety factor is reduced by about 30%.
(4) It is difficult to identify if the lens has been toughened as no stress pattern can be seen.

A comparison of heat and chemically toughened lenses is given in *Table 37.1*.

When heat-toughened glass lenses are viewed through a polariscope or strain tester, a shadow or stress pattern can be seen. The Maltese cross shape is typical. This is induced during the heat-toughening process when the lens is cooled. New methods of thin lens toughening do not give the characteristic Maltese cross stress pattern. A visual inspection of the stress pattern cannot be relied upon to determine if a lens has been correctly toughened.

Table 37.1 Comparison of properties of heat and chemically toughened lenses

	Heat toughened	Chemically toughened
Material	Crown glass	Preferably not crown glass
Lens thickness and weight compared to untoughened	Increased*	Similar
Compression coat	Thick	Thin
Effect of surface scratches on impact resistance	Reduced	Further reduced
Prescription available	Limited	Less limited
Impact resistance to large particles	Less	Greater
Photochromic activity	Reduced	—

*Thin lens toughening—2.1 mm thick instead of 3 mm.

If these toughened glass lenses (chemical or heat) are fractured, they generally give a radial fracture pattern; concentric cracks can also occur. Therefore, only a few splinters of glass are produced and the fragments tend to stay in the frame

Laminated glass

These lenses are made by adhering two layers of crown glass to an inner layer of plastics material. This type of lens has an impact resistance only slightly higher than crown glass, but when it shatters the components are supposed to stick to the plastics interlayer. However, it can be particularly dangerous when a large, low velocity missile hits the lens as slivers emanating from the back surface can injure the eye. This material is becoming increasingly popular for car windscreens.

Plastics

Plastics lenses have many advantages over glass and hence they are widely used for eye protectors, especially where impact resistance is required.

Advantages

(1) They offer greater impact resistance, particularly against high velocity particles.
(2) If the lens is fractured it tends to break into relatively less sharp, larger fragments.
(3) Surface scratches do not obviously affect the impact resistance.
(4) The weight is about 50% that of a glass lens of equivalent power (*Figure 37.1*).

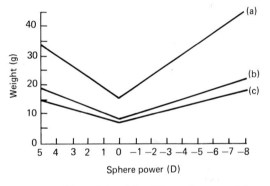

Figure 37.1 The weight of the different lens materials. (*a*) Glass; (*b*) hard resin; (*c*) polycarbonate. (After Herbert, 1984)

(5) A plastics lens can be thinner than a glass lens of equivalent power as it may not be necessary to thicken the lens as much to maintain the impact resistance.
(6) Plastics generally withstand hot sparks and molten metal splashes better than glass as the metal does not fuse to the lens surface.
(7) They have greater resistance to steaming up due to the lower thermal conductivity.
(8) They offer greater protection against ultraviolet radiation.

Disadvantages

(1) The lens surface is soft and scratches easily. It needs a scratch-resistant coating which has been

shown to reduce the impact resistance of some lenses.

(2) For plastics lenses, the range of refractive index extends between 1.49 and 1.60. The higher index is usually accompanied by a lower *v*-value (Abbé number) which can seriously degrade the marginal performance of a lens due to the chromatic aberration.

Polymethyl methacrylate and Columbia Resin 39

Polymethyl methacrylate (PMMA, ICI Perspex) was the first plastics material used for prescription lenses (Igard/Igard Z). These lenses are not so popular at the moment and to a large extent have been replaced by the thermosetting plastic Columbia Resin 39 or (CR39; allyldiglycol carbonate) which offers a greater impact resistance. However, when a CR39 lens breaks it gives slightly sharper fragments than one made of PMMA, although both are suitable for eye protectors. Lenses can be made up as a combination of PMMA and CR39. Prescription lenses for eye protectors are commonly made from CR39, which can also be tinted easily if required using a dyeing technique. This method of tinting can not be applied to PMMA lenses as they become deformed.

Polycarbonate

This has the highest impact resistance of all the lens materials, but unfortunately it has a very soft surface which is easily scratched. To avoid these surface scratches, a quartz coating is often used. As it is suitable for injection moulding, it is commonly used for plano eye protectors where the lenses and front are moulded in one piece. Polycarbonate is becoming increasingly more popular for prescription lenses in eye protectors, particularly as it is now accepted for BS 2092.2.

Advantages

(1) Excellent impact resistance; much greater than heat-toughened glass. If the lens does fracture upon impact it cracks but does not break into particles.
(2) No warpage, chipping or discolouration of the lenses with age.
(3) Silica-coated lenses are much more scratch resistant than uncoated lenses.
(4) Polycarbonate is the lightest lens material (specific gravity, 1.2).
(5) Polycarbonate has a fairly high refractive index (1.586).
(6) The material absorbs ultraviolet radiation readily.

Disadvantages

(1) The surface quality is poor when it is compared with glass or CR39.
(2) Lenses can not be tinted by a dyeing process. They must be vacuum coated.
(3) The *v*-value is poor (30) and causes colour fringes. This is most marked when viewing through the periphery of the lens, especially with high power prescriptions.
(4) Anti-scratch coatings can reduce the impact resistance from 800 feet/s (240 m/s) to 500 feet/s (150 m/s).This is a considerable reduction.

Cellulose acetate

This has a relatively poor impact resistance when compared to polycarbonate and is commonly used for general purpose eye protectors. It does, however, have good resistance to chemicals and is more often used for chemical visors and box goggles.

Wire gauze

Gauze goggles have a very good impact resistance but are generally not accepted as they degrade the visual function and give no protection against splashes of molten metal etc.

Testing procedures of protective lenses

The lenses used in eye protectors have to be tested. This establishes whether they are suitable for the specific hazard for which they were designed. The following functions are assessed:

(1) Impact resistance.
(2) Surface hardness.
(3) Chemical resistance.
(4) Thermostability.
(5) Flammability.
(6) Resistance to hot particles.
(7) Radiosensitivity.

Impact resistance

The impact resistance of a lens can be influenced by:

(1) Abrasions/scratches of the lens surface.
(2) Size and speed of missile/particle.
(3) Lens thickness.
(4) Type of material.

Abrasions/scratches of the lens surface

The impact resistance of all types of lenses is reduced if the surface is abraded. Abrasions have the greatest influence upon the impact resistance of heat or chemically toughened glass lenses which have a thin tension coat. There are two modes of failure of a lens, which depend partly upon the size of the missile. Large particles (22 mm) hitting a lens cause it to bend and hence the fracture is initiated on the back surface. Therefore, any scratches to the front surface will not affect the impact resistance significantly. Smaller particles (3.2 mm) do not cause the lens to bend upon impact so the fracture is generally initiated on the front surface. This means that any front surface scratches will reduce the impact resistance to smaller particles (Welsh *et al.*, 1974).

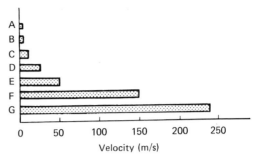

Figure 37.2 Fracture velocity of a 3 mm thick sample of the different lens materials when impacted by a 6.5 mm diameter steel ball.
(A) Laminated glass; (B) untoughened glass; (C) Toughened glass; (D) PMMA; (E) CR39; (F) coated polycarbonate; (G) uncoated polycarbonate

Size of missile

In general, as the missile size decreases, the lens impact resistance (measured as the fracture velocity) increases (Wigglesworth, 1971a). When a 3 mm heat-toughened glass lens is hit by a large missile (19.1–28.6 mm), it demonstrates more impact resistance than a CR39 lens of similar thickness. However, when the missile is small (3.2–6.3 mm) the CR39 lens performs best.

Thickness of lens

As the lens thickness increases, the impact resistance also increases. Lenses with a 3 mm centre thickness or more meet the drop ball test for Australia, and the USA standards for heat-toughened or CR39 lenses. It is not advisable to use a 2.00 mm thick lens, particularly if it is to be heat toughened (Wigglesworth, 1971b).

Impact resistance increases slightly as the lens is bent but only small differences were noted when the curves were adjusted between 6.00 and 10.00 D, with both heat-toughened and CR39 lenses (Wigglesworth, 1971b).

Type of materials

The type of material used for an eye protector gives an indication of the mean fracture velocity which can be resisted. *Figure 37.2* shows the fracture velocity for some of the materials available. The samples were all the same thickness and were struck by a 6.5 mm steel ball (standard test for the UK). In comparison to the other materials, polycarbonate offers the greatest fracture resistance (*see Table 37.2*).

Surface hardness

Glass has a hard surface, unlike plastics, which are soft and can be easily abraded. There have been many efforts to study the problems associated with surface abrasion, not all of which fully represent the natural wear and tear. A measure of the haze produced by an abrasion test is one that has been used. (The Taber abrasion test—500 cycles with CS 10F abrasive wheels under a 430 g load; Galic, 1980.) There are distinct advantages in coating plastics lenses particularly polycarbonate, a soft thermoplastic. The coated polycarbonate lens with a thin coat (5 μm) is superior to the uncoated CR39 lens. Other tests for surface hardness include: diamond point scratch resistance, recoil, indentation under load and residual indentation. Other than the diamond point test these do not indicate how well these lenses will wear.

Chemical resistance

Glass lenses are resistant to most chemicals. Plastics may, however, show surface clouding and crazing with some strong chemical solutions. CR39 has quite good chemical resistance and is frequently used for chemical visors and box goggle windows.

Thermostability

Polycarbonate and polymethyl methacrylate are materials which distort more readily than glass. PMMA softens at 80°C, CR39 at 100°C and polycarbonate at 120°C.

Flammability

All the plastics materials are flammable but they have high ignition temperature and therefore it is

Table 37.2 Mean fracture velocities of spectacle lens materials (metres per second)

Lens material	Thickness (mm)	Mean fracture velocities (m/s) of diameter missiles		
		1 inch (25.4 mm)	$\frac{1}{4}$ inch (6.5 mm)	$\frac{1}{8}$ inch (3.2 mm)
Allyl resin	3	6.6	49	88
Allyl resin	2	5.0	39	63
Polymethyl methacrylate	3	4.5	34	58
Toughened glass	3	7.6	18	29
Toughened glass	2	3.7	12	23
Untoughened glass	3	3.1	12	23
Laminated glass	3	2.2	12	25
Polycarbonate				
Coated	3		152	
Uncoated	3		244	

Modified from Wigglesworth, 1972.

not considered a significant contraindiction for their use.

Resistance to hot particles

Eye protectors must be able to withstand hot particles impinging upon them, as can occur in such processes as grinding or welding. A glass surface is very easily pitted by such particles as they fuse to the surface. Plastics on the other hand do not pit easily. This is possibly due to the elasticity of the surface when heated by the particle.

Radiosensitivity

This should be considered when a lens is broken and particles penetrate the eye. In this situation, a series of X-ray pictures may be taken from different angles to locate the particle. If the material is nearly invisible to X-rays it will be most difficult to find. Glass fragments can be observed by X-ray techniques if they are not too small (>0.5 mm) but plastics particles are very difficult to detect.

A summary of the properties of the various materials used for lenses in eye protectors is given in *Table 37.3*.

Materials for lens housing

The lens housing may be made of: metal, such as a nickel alloy, or plastics like polycarbonate, nylon and cellulose acetate/butyrate. These materials may be used in the manufacture of: spectacle frames;

goggles, both cup or box type; face shields and helmets.

Spectacle frames

Protective spectacle frames may be manufactured by three methods:

(1) Front cut from a flat sheet of plastics material —frames manufactured by this process are generally used for prescription eye protectors and made from cellulose acetate.
(2) Frame formed by injection moulding from plastics granules—this technique again uses cellulose acetate for frames, which are generally glazed with prescription lenses. In plano eye protectors, nylon or polycarbonate is often used.
(3) Frames made from wire, e.g. nickel type —these frames have been shown to cause more damage upon impact than a plastics frame, when the blow forces it against the upper brow and cheek (Fatt, 1979). Frames with the adjustable toggle pads can cause more injury to the nose than a plastics bridge.

Particular concern has been expressed about the use of metal frames for prescription eye protectors. The reasons are:

(1) The screws quickly work loose, notably the rim securing screws.
(2) Accurate glazing of the lens is critical, since if the lens is too small it may fall out, or if too

Table 37.3 A comparison of the major properties of glazing materials for eye protectors

Material	Impact* resistance (m/s)	Hardness	Chemical resistance	Thermo-stability	Fracture pattern	Resistance to hot particles	Weight
Glass							
Heat toughened	18	V. good	V. good	V. good	Fair	Poor	Heaviest
Chemically toughened	>18	V. good	V. good	V. good	Fair	Poor	Heavy
Laminated	12	Good	Good	Fair	Poor	Poor	Heavy
Plastics							
PMMA	34	Poor	Good	Fair	V. good	V. good	Light
CR39	49	Poor	Good	Good	Good	Good	Light
Polycarbonate (uncoated)	>152	Poor	Fair?	Good	V. good	Good	Lightest

*Impact resistance: fracture velocity of a 3 mm thick lens impacted with a quarter inch (6.5 mm) steel ball. Modified from Collins, 1983.

large it may induce stresses at the edge of the lens.

(3) Metal frames have narrower rims than plastics frames, which makes the glazing of high power lenses more difficult.

Recommendations relating to the use of metal frames:

(1) Rim screws should be secured by: a lock nut, peening, or adhesives which bond the thread.
(2) Plastics lenses should be used instead of glass.

Sideshields for spectacle frames

These must not restrict the wearer's field of vision, and should therefore be composed of a transparent material which does not discolour with age. Injection moulded sideshields are the best as their shape does not alter. Those made from a flat sheet tend to warp. Any warping of the sideshield will produce gaps between the shield and the front allowing particles direct access to the eye. Many of the sideshields are made of injection-moulded polycarbonate. They may also be made from wire gauze or perforated plastics, to allow a better air flow.

The main advantage of spectacle protectors is that they fit well. There is a range of sizes available. Spectacles are not suitable for grade 1 impact protection under BS 2092.

Plano one-piece eye protection

These are usually moulded in one piece from polycarbonate. This type has the advantage that the lenses cannot be dislodged as may occur with a spectacle frame. They are suitable for emmetropes

but are usually only manufactured in one size. As the fit required is different for each individual, they do not always fit well. If eye protectors are not fitted correctly they will not provide the necessary protection. Prescription eye protectors are normally fitted by an optometric practitioner, and should be carefully adjusted on collection. It is most unfortunate that plano eye protectors are often handed out by the safety officer who does not have the training or the facilities to fit them.

Plano eye protectors are often disliked by employees who do not normally wear spectacles and are therefore worn very reluctantly. The employees, complaints may be as follows:

(1) Restricted field of view, due to the frame.
(2) Magnification effect—afocal lenses can give a small magnification, caused by the shape of the lenses (base curve effect).
(3) Reflections from the lens surfaces give rise to unwanted ghost images.
(4) Peripheral displacement effects of afocal lenses increase with centre thickness, base curve and angle of ocular rotation. The vertical displacement effect induced on ocular rotation is only normally a problem if the lenses have different base curves.

Goggles—cup type

These may be used to provide protection against molten metal, flying particles or dust etc. A good tight fit to the face is required. The housing is generally made of polyvinyl chloride (PVC).

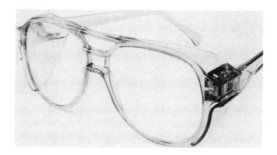

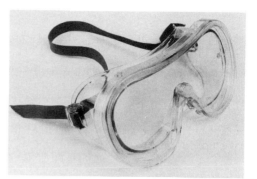

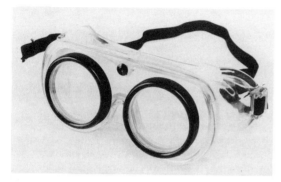

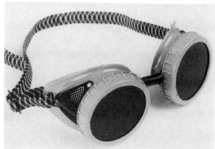

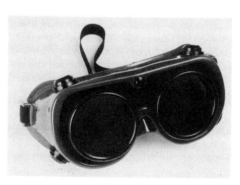

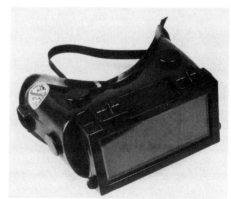

Figure 37.3 Some of the eye protection currently available (by kind permission of British American Optical Company)

Advantages

(1) Adjustable nasal fitting, i.e. distance between lenses.
(2) Screw rim types allow the lenses to be replaced or changed to another type of lens, e.g. tinted or impact resistant.

Disadvantages

(1) Cup type goggles can not normally be worn over prescription spectacles.
(2) Ventilation is usually poor, which causes the lenses to mist. If present, the ventilation holes must be adequately screened to prevent penetration by dust or chemicals etc.

(3) They are sometimes uncomfortable as the cup is hard and often the separation of lenses is too large causing obstruction of central vision.

Goggles—box types

These are normally made of PVC which gives a good fit around the brows and cheeks. The one-piece lens may be of cellulose acetate, polycarbonate or possibly toughened glass.

Advantages

(1) They can normally be worn comfortably over prescription spectacles.
(2) They usually have good ventilation.

(3) They are light weight.
(4) There is no central obstruction of vision.

Disadvantages

(1) The nasal fitting is not adjustable.
(2) The one-piece lenses are not always easy to replace and hence the whole eye protector may have to be discarded.

Face shield

These are usually headband-supported visors or full face shields. They cover the face and neck, and are used to provide protection from flying particles and chemical splashes. They can easily be worn over prescription spectacles or other types of eye protection if required. The face shield is generally made from either polycarbonate or cellulose acetate. They can also be made so that they can be hand-held like the arc welding screens, which have a tinted window. Face shields are also used to provide protection for motorcyclists, cricketers and security guards, among others.

Helmets

Helmets are generally used for welding, as they also provide protection of the face and neck from intense radiation and spatter. There is a window containing a filter to prevent the harmful radiations reaching the eyes. The filter may be designed so that it can be flipped up to expose a clear impact-resistant lens used for grinding and chipping operations. There are some superior variations of this appliance, where the window is fitted with a polarizing cell which darkens to welding density as soon as the arc is struck. These usually have their own air supply as the gases from welding rods are toxic.

Table 37.4 shows the different types of eye protectors and the range of hazards for which they may be used (according to BS 2092 and 1542). Some of the eye protectors discussed are shown in *Figure 37.3*.

British standards for eye protectors

There have been various guidelines given concerning the construction and marking of eye protectors. The British Standards relating to the various types are listed as follows:

BS 2092—specification for industrial eye protectors.
BS 679—filters for use during welding and similar operations.
BS 1542—equipment for eye, face and neck protection against radiation arising during welding and similar operations.
BS 1729—green protective spectacles and screens for steelworks operatives.
BS 2742—filters for protection against intense sun glare (for general and industrial use).
BS 4803—guide to protection of personnel against hazards from laser radiation.
BS 4110—eye protection for vehicle users.

The British Standard of most interest to the optometric practitioner is *BS 2092*. This covers eye protectors such as prescription safety spectacles. The 'Protection of Eyes Regulations 1974' state that the eye protectors supplied must conform to the safety standards given in the Certificates of

Table 37.4 Type of eye protector (Ref. BS 2092 and BS 1542)

		Spectacle	Cup goggles	Box goggles	Face screen
General purpose	(GP)	x	x	x	x
Impact grade 2	(I2)	x	Poss	x	x
Impact grade 1	(II)	N/A	Poss	x	x
Molten metal	(MM)	N/A	x	x	x
Chemical splash	(CS)	N/A	N/A	N/A	x
Chemical droplet	(CD)	N/A	Poss	x	N/A
Dust	(D)	N/A	x	x	N/A
Gas	(G)	N/A	N/A	x	N/A
Combination of impact					
	+ MM	N/A	Poss	x	x
	+ CS	N/A	N/A	N/A	x
	+ CD	N/A	Poss	x	N/A
	+ D	N/A	Poss	x	N/A
	+ G	N/A	Poss	Poss	N/A

N/A = not applicable; Poss = possibly obtainable; x = definitely available.
After Rousell (1979).

Approval. These certificates are issued by the Chief Inspector of Factories and refer to specific British Standards.

BS 2092: specification for industrial eye protectors*

Types of eye protection listed for use against industrial hazards are:

(1) Impact.
(2) Molten metal.
(3) Dust.
(4) Gas.
(5) Chemicals.
(6) Any combination of (1)–(5).

The eye protectors include spectacles, goggles box and cup type, eye screens (visors) and face screens (one-piece eye protectors).

Construction of eye protectors

The eye protectors should be constructed and designed to withstand the tests shown in *Table 37.5*. The various tests can be briefly summarized as shown below.

Temperature test
This tests the stability of the material used by heating it in an oven at 60 °C for half an hour and is followed immediately by the robustness test and then the optical test.

Robustness test
This test involves striking the lens and housing with a quarter inch (6.5 mm) steel ball at 40 ft/s (12.2 m/s). This test is approximated by dropping a 7/8 inch steel ball through a distance of 50 inches onto the lens.

Optical quality
This tests the accuracy and quality of the protective lens. The lenses should transmit at least 80% of

(visible) light except when they are impact resistant and double layered, when the transmission should be at least 70%. The lenses must be made of a toughened or laminated glass, or a plastics material, or of a combination of these materials.

Flame test
This tests that the materials used are self-extinguishing or do not burn at a rate greater than 3 inches/min (7.5 cm/min).

Corrosion test
This test is applied to all the metal parts of the protector to eliminate which are metals or alloys affected by perspiration.

Disinfection test
All this is to test that all eye protectors should be capable of effective cleaning and disinfection.

All the above tests allow the eye protector to be classified as a general purpose type. The following additional tests have to be carried out to allow the protector to be classified specifically for impact, molten metal etc.

Impact resistance
This test is carried out using a quarter inch (6.5 mm) steel ball impacting the protector at 390 ft/s (119 m/s) for grade 1 and at 150 ft/s (45.7 m/s) for grade 2. Grade 1 lenses must be made of a plastics material except when double lenses are used.

Molten metal and hot solids
Lenses must be resistant to the penetration of hot solids and all parts of the protector must not allow the molten metal to adhere to them. Splash, dust and gas protectors are tested for resistance to penetration of the appropriate hazard.

Lenses

Tinted lenses can be used in eye protectors. Prescription protectors can only be made to comply with

Table 37.5 Schedule of tests

Type of eye protection	Tests for all appliances	Additional tests
General purpose	Temperature	– –
Impact	Robustness	Impact
Molten metal	Optical	Molten metal and hot solids
Chemical	Flame	Splash and dust
Dust	Corrosion	Dust
Gas	Disinfection	Gas
Combination of above		As appropriate

* Note: since the completion of this chapter the British Standard 2092 has been amended BS2092: 1987, Eye-protection for industrial and non-industrial uses.

the general purpose or impact resistance grade 2. A manufacturer of prescription eye protectors must state the minimum substance of their lenses, and samples of the lenses should be tested. Prescription lenses must also comply with the requirements of BS 2738 spectacle lenses.

Sideshields

Impact resistance spectacles must provide lateral protection to the orbital cavities and therefore must be fitted with sideshields (Clause 39). Any spectacles claiming to be impact resistant grade 2 should have sideshields which must at least meet the requirement of the general robustness test. The sideshields will not be marked if they are as strong as the rest of the eye protector, but if they are only to general robustness strength they must be marked BS 2092. General purpose spectacles do not have to have sideshields, but if they do they must also withstand the robustness test.

Note that grade 1 impact resistant eye protectors can only be made in the form of a goggle or visor and not spectacles.

Marking of eye protectors

The identification marks used for eye protectors are shown in *Table 37.6*. All appliances should be accompanied by a description, in words, of the purpose for which the eye protectors have been designed.

The Kitemark is the registered mark of the British Standards Institution and, for it to be used, a manufacturer must hold a current licence granted by the BSI. To obtain and hold the licence, the quality control of the products must be under the surveillance of the BSI.

If the eye protector is Kitemarked the user has the assurance that it conforms to the relevant British Standard. It is not mandatory for eye protectors to be Kitemarked, but if there is no Kitemark the purchaser must rely solely on the manufacturer's assurance.

Supply of prescription eye protectors

Only companies which have accepted the requirements of The British Standards Institute (BSI) Quality Assessment Schedules, are allowed to provide Kitemarked prescription eye protectors. This scheme allows companies to become registered firms if they can satisfy the very high level of internal quality control. This allows other firms to buy from these BS 2092 licence holders, without having to carry out the usual tests themselves. Lists of registered firms are available.

Table 37.6 BS 2092—marking of eye protectors

Type	Lens marking	Housing marking
General purpose	(1) BS 2092 (2) Manufacturer's mark or licence number	(1) BS 2092 (2) Manufacturer's mark or licence number
Chemical	As for general purpose	As for general purpose, and letter 'C'
Dust	As for general purpose	As for general purpose, and letter 'D'
Gas	As for general purpose	As for general purpose, and letter 'G'
Impact Grade 1 Grade 2	As for general purpose and the figure 1 or 2*	As for general purpose and the figure 1 or 2*
Molten metal	As for general purpose; additionally mark with letter 'M'*	As for general purpose; additionally marked with letter 'M'
Combination impact and/or molten metal with chemical, dust or gas	As for impact and/or molten metal*	As for impact and/or molten metal and letter 'C', 'D' or 'G' as appropriate

*Glass lenses supplied for use in impact and/or molten metal eye protectors in combination with plastics lenses shall be additionally marked with the word 'outer'.
Reproduced by kind permission of BSI. (Copies of BS 2092 obtained from Linford Wood, Milton Keynes, MK14 6LE.)

Problems associated with BS 2092

The tests for impact resistance and general robustness have been criticized for the following reasons:

(1) Only one size of missile is used (6.5 mm=1/4 inch). Many perforating eye injuries are due to sharp particles of 1 mm or less (0.034 inch) travelling at high velocity. This is not taken into account when testing an eye protector. (The American Standard ANSI Z87.1 uses a 1 inch diameter steel ball dropped from 50 inches onto the whole eye protector.)

(2) The tests do not take into account the effect of scratches or abrasions to the lenses, which will normally occur during use. These will definitely change the impact resistance of an eye protector.

(3) The recognized ballistic tests are carried out with the eye protector mounted on an approved dummy head. The BSI have considered it unsatisfactory to ballistics test prescription eye protectors as the characteristics of prescription lenses are too variable. Instead they have instigated a system where a cross-section of the daily work is periodically tested. This is essential as it ensures the standard of the Kitemark is maintained. The test used by the workshops is known as the 'drop ball' test. A steel ball of 7/8th inch diameter is dropped onto the lens from a height of 50 inches. It is recognized in BS 2092 as the test which approximates the general robustness standard. The drop ball test is widely misinterpreted to mean that a lens tested with the drop ball test is eligible to be marked BS 2092. It must be remembered that, when lenses are poorly glazed into badly designed frames, the wearers will not be provided with the full protection intended.

(4) The 'general purpose' eye protector category is also often misunderstood. It is sometimes thought to mean that it is adequate for all purposes and therefore issued in error.

Future developments

The BSI has decided to reissue the BS 2092. There may well be three major changes which take into account some of the criticisms previously mentioned:

(1) The drop ball test may be omitted to avoid confusion.

(2) The 'general purpose' eye protector may be renamed the 'basic grade' eye protector.

(3) The title of the standard may be altered to include non-industrial occupations, such as dentists, school children, students etc. who require eye protectors.

There is now a European Committee for Standardisation (CEN) which has a technical committee dealing with matters concerning eye protection. If the CEN Standard is agreed and issued as a European Directive, then the present British Standards will be replaced by the CEN which may well be inferior, especially if the concept of the Kitemark system is removed (Davey, 1986).

In conclusion, an optometric practitioner must remember the legal responsibilities outlined in the Health and Safety at Work Act 1974, and the Protection of Eyes Regulations 1974. Optometric practitioners must be responsible, and ensure that the eye protectors supplied are suitable in all aspects, as well as conforming to the relevant safety standard. It would be highly desirable if the appliances supplied were Kitemarked as this would both ensure and demonstrate that they are of the highest standard. In a case of litigation, this could be a most important factor.

References

BRITISH STANDARDS INSTITUTE. BS 2092 (1967) Specification for industrial eye protectors

COLLINS, M. (1983) *Occupational Public-Health Optometry*. Department of Optometry, Queensland Institute of Technology, Brisbane, Queensland, Australia 4000

DAVEY, J.B. (1986) Standards in eye protection. *Dispensing Optics*, March 14–17

FATT, I. (1979) Is the frame safe? *Mfg. Opt. Int.*, March, 109–110

GALIC, C. (1980) Polycarbonate, the spectacle lens with a future. *Mfg. Opt. Int.*, June/July, 57–61

HERBERT. S. (1984) The polycarb story could have a happy ending. *Optical World*, April/May, 4–8

PROTECTION OF EYES REGULATIONS, 1974/161. London: HMSO

PROTECTION OF EYES REGULATIONS, 1976/303 (amendment). London: HMSO

ROUSSEL, D.F. (1979) *Eye Protection*, A ROSPA Publication

WELSH, K.W., MILLER, J.W., KISLIN, B., TREDICI, T.J. and RAHE, A.J. (1974) Ballistic impact testing of scratched and unscratched ophthalmic lenses. *Am. J. Optom. Physiol. Opt.*, **51**, 304–311

WIGGLESWORTH, E.C. (1971a) A ballistic assessment of eye protector lens material, *Invest. Ophthalmol.*, **10**, 985–991

WIGGLESWORTH, E.C. (1971b) The impact resistance of eye protector lens material. *Am. J. Optom. Arch. Am. Acad. Optom.*, **48**, 245–261

WIGGLESWORTH, E.C. (1972) A comparative assessment of eye protective devices and a proposed system of acceptance testing and grading. *Am. J. Optom. Arch. Am. Acad. Optom.*, **49**, 287–304

Part 10

Partial sight and its management

38

Visual disability

Janet Silver

More and more frequently, practitioners encounter the situation where their best efforts leave the patient unable to perform everyday tasks. The modern professional function can no longer be considered simply as supplying the best correction for ametropia, but must also include the supply of aids and advice that will enable visually handicapped people to function to the limit of their capability.

It is now well accepted by the medical, teaching and other professions concerned with rehabilitation, that the intelligent prescribing of low vision aids will enable many people with an acquired visual disability to use previous experience, skills and training. The congenitally disabled can be enabled to join in nearly all so-called 'normal' activities and, in most cases, be educated with fully sighted children (Parlett, Jamieson and Pocklington, 1976).

It is only relatively recently that the visually handicapped have been encouraged to use residual vision and to employ optical and other appliances to maximize this. Most of the principles have been well understood for centuries, but within the last 25 years aids have become significantly less expensive and far more acceptable in terms of weight and performance. This has coincided with changes in attitude both from the patients and from the health care professions, and a dramatic change from an agrarian to an industrial (or even largely clerical) society. The appearance of the ubiquitous visual display unit has created for the visually handicapped a new range of problems, although the computer technology that it so often represents has solved quite a few.

Prevalence

Definitions of visual disability are different for nearly every country that publishes a definition.

Nizetic (1975) quoting World Health Organisation data, gives prevalence rates varying between 29/100 000 for El Salvador to 4000/100 000 in the Yemen, countries where similar rates might have been expected. Clearly not only do definitions differ, but reporting rates are less than completely reliable.

In countries where some breakdown of the statistics on visual disability is available, the age distribution is remarkably similar. Less than 5% of all recognized visual disability occurs in children under 16 years of age and over 70% are over retirement age in the UK. Visual disability can reasonably be considered to be one of the penalties of old age. Less than one in 3000 people under the age of 16 will have a registered visual disability compared with one in 30 of those over 75 years (Silver and Jackson, 1982). Similar distributions are found in all the highly developed countries (Sutherland, 1982). Even in these countries, it is well established that much disability is unreported. Cullinan (1977) in community-based studies in Canterbury, using WHO definitions (i.e. less than 6/18 or equivalent), found that as much as 40% of registerable visual disability may be unrecognized by any of the professions concerned with visual welfare.

Estimates of world figures vary from 6 million (Genensky, 1973) to the same figure for the USA alone (Goldish and Marx, 1973). Cullinan (1982, personal communication) suggests 30 million as reasonable. Sorsby (1972), in an analysis of data from the register of the blind in England and Wales, found that some 15% had only perception or no perception of light. There is every reason to believe that this sort of proportion exists throughout the world. Therefore, 85% of the recognized blind, plus those recognized and unrecognized as 'partially sighted', are continuing to use vision for some things.

Use of residual vision

With most visual disability acquired in middle or late life, it is of great benefit both to the individual and the community if the person with an acquired disability is enabled to maintain independence.

Visually handicapped patients frequently believe that they can damage their remaining vision by sitting too close to a television screen or by watching it too much. There is also frequently the unspoken belief that the residual vision can in some way be used up and should, therefore, be conserved and drawn on only for essentials. Alternatively, it is believed that using already damaged eyes will further exacerbate the disease process. These superstitions are barriers to true cooperation and must be confronted and swept away.

Much benefit can be derived from very simple strategies such as using contrast intelligently. Steak will be difficult to see on a brown plate, boiled fish disappears on white; reverse them add a green vegetable and a common problem is resolved. If one or two such suggestions are made, the patient will usually adopt the principles and apply them generally.

There are many tasks which can be performed if a visually handicapped person is given some magnification. This can be achieved in many ways; the simplest is just to make the material larger. For example most banks will supply statements in large print on request, and libraries hold large stocks of books in 14 or 16 point; Prestel and Ceefax can be zoomed up. The easiest way of gaining magnification is simply to move close to the object; halving the distance from the object will double the angle it subtends at the retina. As well as being the least expensive and most comfortable method, it is also the most easily available. For specific tasks, such as perhaps viewing television where the optimum distance may be a metre, it will be necessary to ensure that the patient has an appropriate spectacle correction especially if presbyopic or aphakic.

Some problems can simply be sidestepped. A push-button telephone with enlarged digits and a memory solves several problems, a microwave oven is easier to manage than a radiant heat cooker. When such strategies are inappropriate, the person can derive great benefit from intelligently prescribed low vision aids.

The optics

Magnification is normally considered to be quarter power in dioptres (D/4) for simple hand, stand and spectacle magnifiers. There is considerable difference of opinion between authorities in the field, and indeed from one manufacturer to another, on how the actual magnification is calculated (Bennett, 1982; Weale, 1982; Bailey, 1984), with some manufacturers quoting D/4 + 1.

Even if simple dioptric power is used, this may be given as the back vertex power, the front vertex power or the equivalent power. The back vertex power is the reciprocal of the distance between the back surface of a lens and its second principal focus (in metres). The back vertex is the surface closest to the eye. Front vertex power is the reciprocal of the distance between the front surface of the lens and its first principal focus (in metres). The equivalent power is the reciprocal of the distance between the principal point and the second focal point, which is very difficult to measure in practice. In low-powered lenses, the difference between front vertex power, back vertex power and equivalent power is negligible, but in higher powered or combinations of lenses the differences may be significant. The practitioner needs to be aware of the method used if true comparisons are to be made.

Telescopic lenses used as low vision aids are frequently galilean but may also be astronomical if hand held when bulk and weight are less important. Galilean (or terrestrial) telescopes have two main components: an eyepiece lens, which is negative (F_1), and a positive objective (F_2). The magnification of the system F_1/F_2, and the distance between the components is the difference between their focal lengths. Thus an eyepiece lens of -20 D combined with an objective of $+10$ D will produce an afocal telescope with an erect image, magnification of $\times 2$, and the space between the components will be 5 cm. The system can be modified to allow for refractive errors or closer objects by altering the distance between the lenses, or by appropriate modifications to the powers of the components.

Astronomical telescopes have a positive eyepiece, and the space between the components is the sum of their focal lengths. Thus a $+20$ combined with a $+10$ will need 15 cm between the components, and produce an inverted image magnified $\times 2$. A prism can be added to provide an erect image, with the inevitable penalty of an increase in weight and bulk. Several manufacturers now produce roof prism telescopes using a Pechan Schmidt prism to present a compact system with a bright image.

For the practitioner, magnification is purely how much larger the object actually appears to the patient, and until a coherent and universally adopted describing method comes into existence it is advisable to treat both manufacturer's claims and the various formulae with scepticism and adopt a pragmatic approach. When descriptions are essential, a sensible policy is either to state the back vertex power (in D), or the manufacturer's description and name; for example $+20.00$ plastic aspheric lenticular or $\times 5$ COIL hyperocular, or Keeler $\times 5$ Full-field telescope.

The appliances

A wide variety of aids is available, each of them with disadvantages for the individual patient and each of them more suited for some functions than others. Every practitioner develops preferences for certain aids but these should never be allowed to become prejudices. Alternatives of every type of aid should be available; it is impossible to meet every contingency from one manufacturer's products.

Effective prescribing for the low vision patient is dependent upon the availability of a comprehensive range of devices. Several manufacturers, notably, 'Designs for Vision', using methods and instruments devised by Dr William Feinbloom, or the intelligent and flexible system devised by Charles Keeler and marketed under his name, have produced 'fitting sets' that cover many functions. Depending on local circumstances one of these can be used as a foundation and other ranges or individual aids can be added until the practitioner has acquired sufficient to match his needs.

Low vision aids are classified in many ways — but only function in the clinical context is considered here. Every type of aid, indeed every aid, has different characteristics — both advantages and disadvantages. Ultimately the function of the practitioner is to use his expertise to prescribe the aid with fewest disadvantages for the specific patient's requirements.

For near vision there are many alternatives.

Hand and stand magnifiers

Most readily accessible and accepted are hand and stand magnifiers which are available in enormous variety. In fact, they meet different needs and are described in different ways by different manufacturers. They can be found made of glass or plastics materials and may be described in focal length (inches or centimetres), the diameter of the lens, or most usefully in dioptres. Unfortunately no coherent method of describing them has been adopted. The simplest approach is to neutralize any lens and quote its back vertex power in dioptres. Integral illumination can be an advantage. Both types have a relatively small field unless the patient can be persuaded to use the appliance close to the eye.

If carefully placed, a stand magnifier may allow a task requiring both hands; they have particular advantages when there are additional handicaps. Stand magnifiers are often very bulky, but they have frequent applications in industry if low power is acceptable and a large field is essential (*Figure 38.1*).

The simple hand magnifier is the most widely used aid. Hand lenses are usually held well within their focal length and the resultant magnification may in practice be considerably less than might be expected. Even where other devices are used, a hand lens is a great advantage in pocket or handbag. A good low vision clinic will hold perhaps 50 alternative hand and stand magnifiers, each of which will have significantly different characteristics (*Figure 38.1*).

Theoretically, magnifiers should be used with a distance vision correction. In practice, the patient will often prefer to wear a normal reading correction, selecting the material with normal near-vision spectacles, then reading the small print with the magnifier.

Spectacle magnifiers

Sometimes called 'microscopes', high-powered convex lenses may be mounted in spectacle frames, attached to them with clips, or simply held in the orbit as watchmaker's loupes. Such lenses, which may be spherical or aspheric, are normally described in magnification powers (*Figure 38.2*). The standard formula for simple magnifiers can be applied in reverse, thus a ×4 spectacle magnifier will have the power of 16 D, a ×9, 36 D etc. However, it is generally accepted that the main function of the lens is to focus the image at the retina, most of the magnification being due to the proximity of the object.

It must be remembered that magnification and working distance will be modified by the patient's own refractive error. If a ×5 spectacle magnifier (i.e. +20.00 D) is used by an aphakic patient where 12 D is used to correct the surgical hypermetropia, only 8 D will remain for the near vision correction. This will give ×2 magnification and a working distance of 12 cm. Conversely, if a similar lens is put before a 12 D myopic eye the total positive power would be 32 D, the working distance 3 cm and the actual magnification ×8.

Spectacle magnifiers are excellent cosmetically and have a relatively good field. Several manufacturers produce them in bifocal form which is an advantage in many situations. Disadvantages are the short working distance in higher powers and the inevitable loss of binocular vision where more than about ×2 magnification is indicated. Spectacle magnifiers are usually single lenses, although sometimes two or more lenses in combination are used. Powers currently available are up to about ×20, and again integral illumination is available for some high-powered aids.

Clearly, if high reading additions are to be given binocularly, problems will arise with convergence. In practice, patients can rarely cope with more than 10 D addition and then base-in prism is needed to relieve the convergence. Lehbensohn (1949) suggests that the near interpupillary distance can be calculated by dividing the distance interpupillary distance (in mm) by the reading distance plus 1 (in

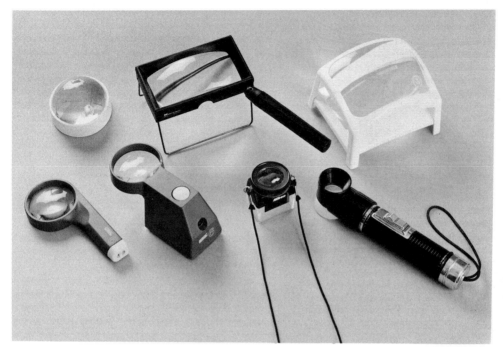

Figure 38.1 Hand and stand magnifier. *Top*: left—dome magnifier × 2, which has excellent light gathering qualities; centre—Eschenbach folding stand magnifier × 2.5; right—double lens stand magnifier × 3. (Schweizer Optics). *Bottom*: left—aspheric × 6 hand magnifier (Combined Optical Industries Ltd); centre left— × 6 stand magnifier which can be battery or mains illuminated (Combined Optical Industries Ltd); centre right— × 8 stand magnifier (Nikon). The neck cord is a useful extra; right—× 15 stand magnifier battery illuminated by Peak

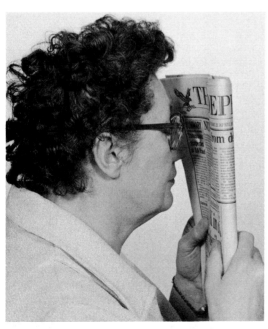

Figure 38.2 Spectacle magnifier × 5—note the short working distance and inevitable illumination problems (Combined Optical Industries Ltd). Similar ones are available from other manufacturers, some in bifocal form

inches). For practitioners used to thinking entirely metric, this is a messy calculation, and a useful rule of thumb is to incorporate 1 Δ for each dioptre of addition divided between the two eyes. It must be borne in mind that normal convergence will reduce the interpupillary distance and, therefore, small eyesizes are essential. Inevitably, chromatic aberrations are increased and a thick lens is created.

Telescopes

For distance vision (for these purposes from 25 cm to infinity) only telescopic systems are in normal use. The major disadvantages of telescopes are that they reduce field, are very heavy, have a conspicuous appearance, disrupt normal spatial relationships, and are relatively expensive (*Figures 38.3–38.5*).

Small low-powered telescopes can be mounted on spectacle frames for distance vision use. Several different types are available. Most face-mounted telescopes use a straightforward galilean principle. Simple binocular sports-spectacles are mass produced with adjustable interpupillary distances, individual focusing, and magnification up to about ×3. Several manufacturers (Zeiss, Keeler, Designs for Vision, Hamblin, Stigmat etc.) produce monocular

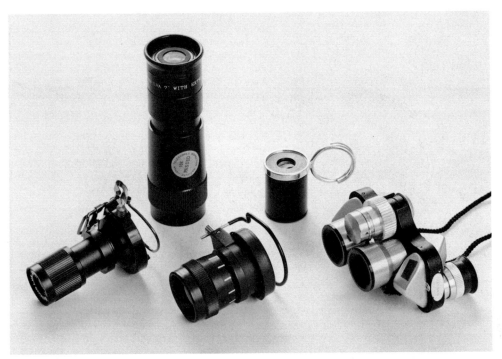

Figure 38.3 *Top*: left—× 8 roof prism monocular tele-scope—supplied through Edward Marcus Ltd, but similar ones are available, also rubber covered; right—finger ring telescope × 2.5 focusable, by Keeler. *Bottom*: left—focusable × 2.75. Here it is mounted on a clip, but it can also be normally spectacle mounted (from Mar-cus). Similar ones are available incorporating prescrip-tions from Keelers. Centre—Eschenbach × 3 distance telescope; clips over existing spectacles; also available in × 3 and × 4 for near vision use. *Right*—Tohyoh × 6 miniature binocular

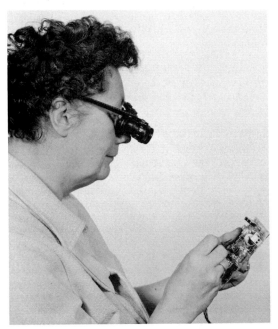

Figure 38.4 Eschenbach × 4 binocular telescopic spec-tacle—eyes can be focused individually, p.d. adjustable

or binocular telescopes which can incorporate a correction for ametropia. These can sometimes be mounted high on a lens to allow vision below; the head is dropped slightly to allow vision 'along the tubes' — these are called 'bioptic telescopes'; magnification is again no more than ×3. They have obvious applications in the classroom. Certain States in the USA license visually disabled people to drive using such appliances. It is claimed that suit-able patients can easily learn the use of such devices, the actual use being similar to glancing in a rear view mirror; the inevitable field loss is deemed unimpor-tant. Similar telescopes are placed centrally or low on the carrier lens and also have convex 'cap' lenses of varying power which can be added to reduce the focal length for near vision. Flexible working dis-tances may also be achieved if the system is designed so that the space between the components can be adjusted to allow focusing.

Telescopic spectacles incorporating any correc-tion for ametropia can be supplied at up to ×8 binocular or ×10 monocular for near. A few tele-scopes will clip onto or suspend from spectacles, apparently producing the best of both worlds, but they are monocular, only up to ×4, and unbalance the spectacles.

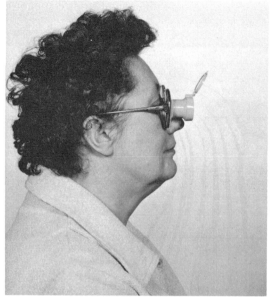

(a)

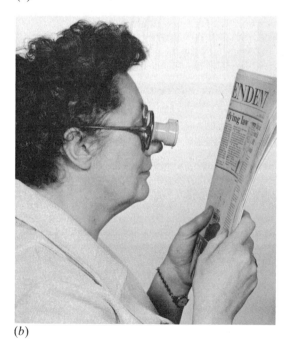

(b)

Figure 38.5 Keeler flip-up telescope shown (*a*) for distance use and (*b*) with the flap down at × 3 for near

Near vision telescopes are the only optical appliance that can allow manipulative skills such as writing, or sewing, to be sustained or acquired. The same disadvantages apply to near as distance vision telescopes and, in that they are often used for longer periods, to neglect refractive errors results in discomfort and reduced performance.

Small hand-held monocular or binocular telescopes are used for a wide range of purposes. For most patients the maximum is around ×8.

It is possible to use a contact lens as an eyepiece and a spectacle lens as an objective, with the back vertex distance replacing the normal tube. While, superficially, a very attractive idea, the magnification available is low and the system uncomfortable to wear.

For severe field loss, small reversed galilean telescopes are available. Little used in practice, they simply minify and most patients rapidly learn to scan and prefer to do so.

Electronic aids

Since the early 1970s, electronic aids utilizing closed circuit television (CCTV) techniques have become widely available (*Figure 38.6*). They permit far

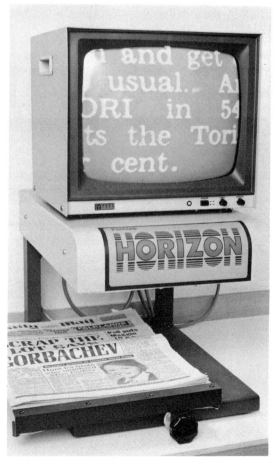

Figure 38.6 Closed circuit television reader shown here at × 15 with a white-on-black image—by Focus; many alternatives are available, each with marginally different characteristics

higher levels of magnification than have previously been available (up to ×50 on most machines), allow image reversal, i.e. white print on a black background, and a normal reading position with the distance from the screen selected by the subject who wears the appropriate spectacle correction. Such aids allow enormous flexibility, particularly when a zoom lens is incorporated, as a wide range of magnification is then available by making a simple adjustment. Disadvantages are the cost, currently at least £1000 and its bulk — CCTV is transportable rather than portable. Flat screen and liquid crystal technology should produce a truly portable CCTV of acceptable quality very soon.

In the early 1980s, a new device was introduced using a hand-held multiple photoreceptor which is slid across the line of print. The image is orange on very dark red, and the image quality limited by the number of receptors, but the machine is about briefcase size and allows up to ×64.

Electronic reading machines can be linked to computers — this development opens up new fields of activity to the visually handicapped, especially in employment and education.

Image intensifiers originally developed for military use, have been suggested as an aid for those with night-blindness. They are still relatively expensive, and not very easy to use. Under most circumstances it is easier and more effective simply to increase the light level. Several firms produce very good high power torches — a halogen bulb is often an advantage.

Illumination

Every practitioner needs to be familiar with the principles and be equipped with flexible lighting in order to be able to provide optimum conditions for individual patients and advise them accordingly. Some patients benefit from very high levels of illumination, a normal tungsten lamp producing an unacceptable level of heat at high wattage, but this can be reduced significantly by using a focused luminaire which at 60 W will give 3000 lux at 30 cm from source compared with 500 lux from a standard tungsten lamp (Gill and Silver, 1982).

Halogen luminaires are becoming widely available as an attractive alternative, and some of the new looped fluorescent tubes mounted in flexible arm stands produce little heat, but are disliked by some patients possibly because they can cause hyperfluorescence in the crystalline lens.

Any luminaire must be carefully sited to avoid veiling glare, and should not be in the sight-line where it will cause discomfort.

The low vision examination

Patients should be referred for low vision assessment when they wish to perform tasks that they cannot manage with normal spectacle correction.

At the assessment the ophthalmological findings should be available including fields, electrodiagnostic investigations etc., where appropriate, and a family and medical history along with information on present and planned treatment. These data give the low vision practitioner some insight into how the patient perceives the environment and the prognosis of preservation of vision, both long and short term.

The most important part of the procedure is the full elucidation of the patient's visual problems. This process is beset with traps for the unwary practitioner. First, patients come to the clinic in a very complex psychological state. They have usually been told that they are 'blind' and have attempted to adjust to this by abandoning all ambition to acquire information visually. Such patients will state very modest aims, 'to read my bank statement and letters' being very common, but close questioning will reveal far more. Another patient presents a wide range of diffuse problems, 'I want to see better' and it becomes evident that what is being sought is an overall improvement, i.e. a cure for the eye condition, rather than the means to cope with the disability. In both cases, the true situation must be confronted and the function of the low vision aids explained and understood. Patients should be encouraged to bring examples of 'problem materials' with them to the assessment, along with any aids prescribed, purchased or improvised. It is important to create a sympathetic environment as only without fear of disapproval or ridicule will patients disclose their own unconventional solutions. These may include wearing two or more pairs of glasses or convex lenses 'borrowed' from other devices. This provides invaluable information about the motivation and adaptability of the patient. Most patients request help with reading but for one patient it will be checking the occasional telephone number, for another reading notes at meetings and masses of letters, for a third checking printer's proofs for publication.

It is of benefit if some priority order is established and agreed, with the most important tasks taking precedence. If such an order is not established, it is common for the practitioner to prescribe against what is perceived as normal needs rather than actual ones. Patients should be encouraged to present examples of material which they wish to be able to manage. It is common to find patients with unrealistic expectations of what can be achieved with optical appliances but also, among the elderly particularly, expectations may be very low.

The patient must be refracted with care. Visual acuity of 2/60 may well improve to 6/60 which, while possibly not significant in terms of improving mobility, may well be crucial at near. Best vision should be established for each eye and near vision acuity recorded with a +4.00 addition. This makes a useful starting point as it represents not only unit magnification but also the limit to which reading material is normally held. The working distance should always be measured and recorded. In most disorders, one eye has rather better vision than the other and the appropriate magnification level should be established for each eye in turn starting with the better eye. Plus lenses can be added in 2.00 D steps; a normal trial case will give up to ×5 magnification with a working distance of 5 cm. The main magnification effect is due to the increased angle subtended at the retina by the print as the material is moved closer. The function of the lens is simply to bring this larger retinal image into focus. Steps of 2 D will allow the patient to become accustomed to holding things closer in several steps rather than one jump. If more than ×5 magnification is indicated it is necessary to move to hyperoculars or magnifiers remembering to modify both expected effective magnification and working distance by the patient's refractive error. The second eye should be assessed in the same way.

Prescribing

The choice of appropriate aids is governed by the problem tasks. For example, if the first priority task is reading newsprint but the patient merely wishes to be able to check a television programme or perhaps the value of investments, then a simple magnifier may well fill the need. If, however, large blocks of newsprint need to be read then a spectacle magnifier may be most appropriate. If the newspaper also includes a crossword puzzle then a telescope is indicated. When there is any evidence of binocular function, and the power required is within the limitations of the hardware, binocular telescopic lenses should be tried. Assuming disability of similar aetiology and distance acuity of about 6/60 (N24 with a +4.00 add) magnification of perhaps ×5 would be indicated. In the first example, a simple hand magnifier would apparently provide an adequate solution, the second suggests a spectacle magnifier, probably in bifocal form, the third demands a telescope to make the necessary editorial marks. This sort of thinking should prevent the practitioner from exhausting the patient and wasting consultation time with a long series of inappropriate aids. It is good standard practice to establish magnification requirements with high plus additions up to 20 D, which is equivalent to ×5 and, while concentrating on the type of aid indicated by the patient's originally defined problems, ensure that at least one aid of the alternative types is demonstrated. If patients have low expectations, the possibilities revealed may encourage at that stage a revision of the requests. The patient's response to each type of appliance should be noted — the correct aid is the most acceptable one, at least at the first visit. Broadly, telescopes are indicated where there is a manipulative task or a long working distance is required, spectacle magnifiers where cosmetic considerations are important and a monocular aid is acceptable, stand magnifiers where grip is impaired or the patient has difficulty sustaining the correct lens position, hand magnifiers for infrequent use or as an extra aid for shopping etc., CCTV when very high magnifications, extra contrast or the ergonomic advantage is essential or there is a great deal of reading. Whenever possible, patients prefer binocular vision.

Most patients will attend with an escort and it is of benefit to involve this person towards the end of the assessment, both to confirm that the desired level has indeed been reached and to reinforce the message of illumination and range. Very few patients can absorb too many changes into their way of life at one time, therefore it is wise to supply the aid that appears to meet the first priority need and allow that aid to be absorbed into the patient's way of life before introducing other appliances to meet other needs.

The diagnosis

While without doubt the single most important prognostic factor for success in using low vision aids is the motivation of the individual patient, some groups do appear to do better than others. Motivation tends to be better in younger people, as does the ability to acquire the skills necessary to use the aids.

The success rate is high among albinos, and in the various forms of juvenile macular degeneration. Indeed most disorders causing damage at the posterior pole, which include diabetic maculopathy, central serous retinopathy etc., can be considered relatively benign. However, when untreated, disciform macular degeneration usually results in a very large central scotoma and requires levels of magnification so high as to preclude reading except for vital information. When treated by laser, patients with disciform macular degeneration have a better visual acuity, and then frequently do quite well (Moorfields Macular Study Group, 1982).

Generally speaking, patients with disorders resulting in tunnel vision do not do well, except with electronic aids.

Conditions causing opacities of the media are, of course, a very disparate group. Patients with such opacities need a highly contrasted image, and special attention to the illumination.

Many visually handicapped people also have another disability, and attention must be paid to tremor, grip, posture as well as other sensory deficiencies such as hearing and touch.

Training

Several groups, mainly in the USA and Sweden, advocate training patients in the use of aids and eccentric fixation (Goodrich and Quillman, 1977; Backman and Inde, 1979). The ideas and methods seem reasonable, but very labour intensive. So far no properly controlled trials have been published that demonstrate the cost benefits.

Romayanda *et al.* (1982) advocate the use of a prism to shift the image off a damaged macula onto useful adjacent retina. The underlying theory is questionable.

Light sensitivity

Many patients with early opacity of the media complain about glare. The real problem is light scatter due to oblique light and a tinted lens does very little, if anything, to alleviate this and may reduce contrast below safety levels under some circumstances. A hat with a brim or peak will often provide protection from oblique light.

The group of disorders collectively known as retinitis pigmentosa severely affects light/dark adaptation. It has been suggested that such patients should wear a filter that reduces the transmission of the short wavelengths. The best known of these is the Corning 550 photochromic lens which has a red appearance. Some people do appear to like them, but for most patients a plastics lens with a brown or red tint is equally beneficial (Silver and Lyness, 1985). It is necessary to provide shielding at the sides, and order the light transmission appropriate for the individual situation; possibly 30% for most situations in Northern Europe, but 10 or 15% for the beach and even less for snow.

The only other group where there are indications for tinted lenses are where cone function is severely reduced. This group frequently derives benefit from very dark tinted lenses with perhaps 2% transmission. This can be ordered as a plastics lens or be achieved by coating a solid tint with a surface tint, a good combination being Crookes B2 coated with Astor C2.

Dispensing

A range of hand/stand magnifiers and hand-held telescopes should be available from stock. A supply of half eye and full aperture high-plus spectacles, similar to those used as a temporary post-operative correction for aphakia, can be used as spectacle magnifiers on a temporary or permanent basis.

Accurate dispensing is essential if aids are to give maximum benefit. Fitting a binocular telescopic spectacle requires a similar approach to dispensing varifocals. The frame should be sturdy and semi-library weight. A useful technique is to place a strip of transparent sticky tape over each rim and for the practitioner to mark the pupil centre by aligning the pupil with his own. It is a wise precaution to cross-check with a normal pupillary distance (p.d.) rule. Mass-produced binocular aids should be centred correctly before they are given to the patient.

Spectacle magnifiers can be fitted into any normal spectacle frame, but the choice is limited by the limited diameter of the blank. Although accurate centration is less important than with telescopes, it is nonetheless very desirable. The back vertex distance, normally an essential part of the specification for high power lenses, can be ignored, the variation in effectivity making only a tiny modification to the working distance. However, if the lens is worn close to the eye, the field is larger.

Follow-up

The importance of follow-up cannot be overstressed. Even the most experienced practitioner may not prescribe the ideal appliance at the first visit. Indeed many patients reject the 'ideal' appliance, particularly if it is conspicuous or demands major behavioural modifications. Such a rejection is probably multifactorial, but changes in attitudes and skill will have taken place by first follow-up and a sophisticated aid may then be accepted. Many patients are seen with progressive disease or active disease that will ultimately stabilize. Such patients should be given either a series of simple magnifiers until stability is reached or aids such as the Stigmat telescope which, by the addition of alternative caps, can be modified in the light of changed circumstances.

A reasonable follow-up regimen is to see the patient 3 months after any aid is supplied and, when the management is stabilized, at yearly intervals. Patients often use a number of aids for different purposes, e.g. a personnel manager might use a hand-held monocular to enable him/her to select the correct bus to get to work, a spectacle magnifier to interview staff, a hand magnifier in the supermarket on the way home, and a face-mounted telescope to watch a favourite television programme after dinner. Few patients actually use this number of aids, but it is not unknown.

Delivery of service

Different countries have alternative ways in which aids are provided. Clinics may be associated with medical and surgical units, medical or optometry schools, the rehabilitation services or the special education system for the visually handicapped. In most countries, some contribution is payable by the patient towards the cost of aids and services, though many allow a trial period. Health insurance covers many people, and war veterans are usually well served.

In the UK through the National Health Service, low vision aids are prescribed at the request of an ophthalmologist. Treatment is completely free and all aids are given to patients 'on loan'. Under the Manpower Services 'Aids to Employment' scheme, any aid or modification to the environment that can be considered essential can be supplied on loan at the work place. By this means several hundred persons have been supplied with electronic aids. These are prescribed through low vision clinics at centres able to perform a full assessment.

Interdisciplinary relationships

The practitioner needs a good working relationship with others involved in rehabilitation, social workers, mobility teachers, educationalists, technical officers etc. and close interaction with the ophthalmologist responsible overall. Patients using low vision aids will often use non-visual methods for some things and the sort of arrangement where information can be given informally (and fast) by telephone can be greatly to the advantage of all concerned.

The practitioner needs to be aware of other services available to the visually handicapped. There are an increasing number of special interest groups such as the Retinitis Pigmentosa Society, the Albino Fellowship etc. which do much to disseminate information and remove the common feeling of isolation caused by the disability.

There are, of course, methods of obtaining information that do not involve the use of sight at all. These involve braille and other tactile systems. But, more and more, the trend is towards methods that do not impose a delay, i.e. microprocessors interpreting optical information and giving an audible or tactile output.

A social worker and the rehabilitation services can provide much practical day-to-day advice on daily living skills, but it is the clinician who has the best information on how the patient perceives the world and, therefore, who is uniquely fitted to provide encouragement in the optimum use of reduced vision.

Attitudes to disability will continue to change. With appropriate low vision aids the visually disabled may be given the ability to function as effectively as most sighted people.

Acknowledgements

The author is grateful to the Consultants at Moorfields Eye Hospital for their cooperation and support, to Carole Clark for clerical assistance and to the Medical Illustration Department for the photographs in this chapter.

References

BACKMAN, O. and INDE, K. (1979) *Low Vision Training*. Malmo: LiberHermods

BAILEY, I.L. (1984) Magnification of the problem of magnification of the . . . *Optician* May 25th, 14–18.

BENNETT, A.G. (1968) *Ophthalmic Lenses*. London: Hatton Press

BENNETT A.G. (1982) Spectacle magnification and loupe magnification. *Optician*, **183**, 16–18, 36

CULLINAN, T.R. (1977) Visually disabled people in the community (Table 21). *Health Services Research Unit Report 28*. University of Kent at Canterbury

GENENSKY, S. (1973) *Binoculars: a Long-ignored Aid for the Partially Sighted*. pp. 6–7. Santa Monica: Rand

GILL, J.M. and SILVER, J.H. (1982) Illumination from domestic lamps. *Ophthal. Opt.*, **22**, 282

GOLDISH, L.H. and MARX, M.H. (1973) The visually impaired as a market for sensory aids and series for partially sighted persons. *New Outlook for the Blind*, **67**, 289–296

GOODRICH, G.L. and QUILLMAN, R.D. (1977) Training eccentric viewing. *J. Vis. Impair. Blind.*, **71**, 377–381

LEHBENSOHN, J.E. (1949) Practical problems relating to presbyopia. *Am. J. Ophthalmol.*, **32**, 22

MOORFIELDS MACULAR STUDY GROUP (1982) Treatment of senile disciform macular degeneration: a single-blind randomised trial by argon laser photocoagulation. *Br. J. Ophthalmol.*, **66**, 745–753

NIZETIC, B. (1975). Public Health Ophthalmology. In *Theory and Practice of Public Health*, edited by W. Hobson. Oxford: Oxford Medical Publications

PARLETT, M., JAMIESON, M. and POCKLINGTON, K. (1976) *Towards Integration*. National Foundation for Education Research, Slough

ROMAYANANDA, M., WONG, S.W., ELZENENY, I.H. and CHAN, G.H. (1982) Prismatic method for improving visual acuity in patients with low vision. *Ophthalmology*, **89**, 937–945

SILVER, J., GOULD, E. and THOMSITT, J. (1974) The provision of low vision aids to the visually handicapped. *Trans. Ophthalmol. Soc. UK*, **94**, 310

SILVER, J.H. (1976) The place of optimum low vision aids in the management of visual handicap. *MPhil Thesis*, City University, London

SILVER, J.H. and JACKSON, J. (1982) Visual disability series, Part 1. *Ophthal. Opt*, December 18th, 841–842

SILVER, J.H. and LYNESS, A.L. (1984) Do red lenses solve the light problem? *Ophthal. Physiol. Opt.*, **5**, 87–89

SORSBY, A. (1972) The incidence and causes of blindness in England and Wales 1963–1968. *DHSS Reports on Health and Medical Subjects*. No 128. London:DHSS

SUTHERLAND, A.T. (1982) *Disabled We Stand*. London: Souvenir Press

WEALE, R.A. (1982) The loupe and the eye. *Optician*, **183**, 29

Index